Clinical Research on Type 2 Diabetes and Its Complications

Clinical Research on Type 2 Diabetes and Its Complications

Editor

Fernando Gómez-Peralta

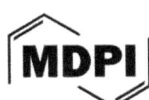

Basel • Beijing • Wuhan • Barcelona • Belgrade • Novi Sad • Cluj • Manchester

Editor
Fernando Gómez-Peralta
Segovia General Hospital
Segovia, Spain

Editorial Office
MDPI
St. Alban-Anlage 66
4052 Basel, Switzerland

This is a reprint of articles from the Special Issue published online in the open access journal *Journal of Clinical Medicine* (ISSN 2077-0383) (available at: https://www.mdpi.com/journal/jcm/special_issues/Type_2_Diabetes_Complications).

For citation purposes, cite each article independently as indicated on the article page online and as indicated below:

Lastname, A.A.; Lastname, B.B. Article Title. *Journal Name* **Year**, *Volume Number*, Page Range.

ISBN 978-3-0365-9418-7 (Hbk)
ISBN 978-3-0365-9419-4 (PDF)
doi.org/10.3390/books978-3-0365-9419-4

© 2023 by the authors. Articles in this book are Open Access and distributed under the Creative Commons Attribution (CC BY) license. The book as a whole is distributed by MDPI under the terms and conditions of the Creative Commons Attribution-NonCommercial-NoDerivs (CC BY-NC-ND) license.

Contents

Fernando Gómez-Peralta and Cristina Abreu
Clinical Research on Type 2 Diabetes: A Promising and Multifaceted Landscape
Reprinted from: *J. Clin. Med.* **2022**, *11*, 6007, doi:10.3390/jcm11206007 1

Mamunur Rashid, Mohanad Alkhodari, Abdul Mukit, Khawza Iftekhar Uddin Ahmed, Raqibul Mostafa, Sharmin Parveen and Ahsan H. Khandoker
Machine Learning for Screening Microvascular Complications in Type 2 Diabetic Patients Using Demographic, Clinical, and Laboratory Profiles
Reprinted from: *J. Clin. Med.* **2022**, *11*, 903, doi:10.3390/jcm11040903 5

Dae Youp Shin, Bora Lee, Won Sang Yoo, Joo Won Park and Jung Keun Hyun
Prediction of Diabetic Sensorimotor Polyneuropathy Using Machine Learning Techniques
Reprinted from: *J. Clin. Med.* **2021**, *10*, 4576, doi:10.3390/jcm10194576 29

Li-Ying Huang, Fang-Yu Chen, Mao-Jhen Jhou, Chun-Heng Kuo, Chung-Ze Wu, Chieh-Hua Lu, et al.
Comparing Multiple Linear Regression and Machine Learning in Predicting Diabetic Urine Albumin–Creatinine Ratio in a 4-Year Follow-Up Study
Reprinted from: *J. Clin. Med.* **2022**, *11*, 3661, doi:10.3390/jcm11133661 47

Alexandra Filipov, Heike Fuchshuber, Josephine Kraus, Anne D. Ebert, Vesile Sandikci and Angelika Alonso
Measuring of Advanced Glycation End Products in Acute Stroke Care: Skin Autofluorescence as a Predictor of Ischemic Stroke Outcome in Patients with Diabetes Mellitus
Reprinted from: *J. Clin. Med.* **2022**, *11*, 1625, doi:10.3390/jcm11061625 61

Ekaterina B. Luneva, Anastasia A. Vasileva, Elena V. Karelkina, Maria A. Boyarinova, Evgeny N. Mikhaylov, Anton V. Ryzhkov, et al.
Simple Predictors for Cardiac Fibrosis in Patients with Type 2 Diabetes Mellitus: The Role of Circulating Biomarkers and Pulse Wave Velocity
Reprinted from: *J. Clin. Med.* **2022**, *11*, 2843, doi:10.3390/jcm11102843 71

Da Young Lee, Jaeyoung Kim, Sanghyun Park, So Young Park, Ji Hee Yu, Ji A. Seo, et al.
Fasting Glucose Variability as a Risk Indicator for End-Stage Kidney Disease in Patients with Diabetes: A Nationwide Population-Based Study
Reprinted from: *J. Clin. Med.* **2021**, *10*, 5948, doi:10.3390/jcm10245948 83

José Ignacio Martínez-Montoro, Beatriz García-Fontana, Cristina García-Fontana and Manuel Muñoz-Torres
Evaluation of Quality and Bone Microstructure Alterations in Patients with Type 2 Diabetes: A Narrative Review
Reprinted from: *J. Clin. Med.* **2022**, *11*, 2206, doi:10.3390/jcm11082206 95

Alessandro Mantovani, Andrea Dalbeni, Giorgia Beatrice, Davide Cappelli and Fernando Gomez-Peralta
Non-Alcoholic Fatty Liver Disease and Risk of Macro- and Microvascular Complications in Patients with Type 2 Diabetes
Reprinted from: *J. Clin. Med.* **2022**, *11*, 968, doi:10.3390/jcm11040968 109

Laurence J. Dobbie, Mohamed Kassab, Andrew S. Davison, Pete Grace, Daniel J. Cuthbertson and Theresa J. Hydes
Low Screening Rates Despite a High Prevalence of Significant Liver Fibrosis in People with Diabetes from Primary and Secondary Care
Reprinted from: *J. Clin. Med.* **2021**, *10*, 5755, doi:10.3390/jcm10245755 125

Virginia Bellido, Cristina Abreu Padín, Andrei-Mircea Catarig, Alice Clark, Sofía Barreto Pittol and Elias Delgado
Once-Weekly Semaglutide Use in Patients with Type 2 Diabetes: Results from the SURE Spain Multicentre, Prospective, Observational Study
Reprinted from: *J. Clin. Med.* **2022**, *11*, 4938, doi:10.3390/jcm11174938 137

Joshuan J. Barboza, Mariella R. Huamán, Beatriz Melgar, Carlos Diaz-Arocutipa, German Valenzuela-Rodriguez and Adrian V. Hernandez
Efficacy of Liraglutide in Non-Diabetic Obese Adults: A Systematic Review and Meta-Analysis of Randomized Controlled Trials
Reprinted from: *J. Clin. Med.* **2022**, *11*, 2998, doi:10.3390/jcm11112998 151

Eugene Yu-Chuan Kang, Chunya Kang, Wei-Chi Wu, Chi-Chin Sun, Kuan-Jen Chen, Chi-Chun Lai, et al.
Association between Add-On Dipeptidyl Peptidase-4 Inhibitor Therapy and Diabetic Retinopathy Progression
Reprinted from: *J. Clin. Med.* **2021**, *10*, 2871, doi:10.3390/jcm10132871 165

Blake J. McKinley, Mariangela Santiago, Christi Pak, Nataly Nguyen and Qing Zhong
Pneumatosis Intestinalis Induced by Alpha-Glucosidase Inhibitors in Patients with Diabetes Mellitus
Reprinted from: *J. Clin. Med.* **2022**, *11*, 5918, doi:10.3390/jcm11195918 177

Dilvin Semo, Julius Obergassel, Marc Dorenkamp, Pia Hemling, Jasmin Strutz, Ursula Hiden, et al.
The Sodium-Glucose Co-Transporter 2 (SGLT2) Inhibitor Empagliflozin Reverses Hyperglycemia-Induced Monocyte and Endothelial Dysfunction Primarily through Glucose Transport-Independent but Redox-Dependent Mechanisms
Reprinted from: *J. Clin. Med.* **2023**, *12*, 1356, doi:10.3390/jcm12041356 191

Anna Ramírez-Morros, Josep Franch-Nadal, Jordi Real, Mònica Gratacòs and Didac Mauricio
Sex Differences in Cardiovascular Prevention in Type 2: Diabetes in a Real-World Practice Database
Reprinted from: *J. Clin. Med.* **2022**, *11*, 2196, doi:10.3390/jcm11082196 209

Tigestu Alemu Desse, Kevin Mc Namara, Helen Yifter and Elizabeth Manias
Development of a Complex Intervention for Effective Management of Type 2 Diabetes in a Developing Country
Reprinted from: *J. Clin. Med.* **2022**, *11*, 1149, doi:10.3390/jcm11051149 225

Ana Lopez-de-Andres, Rodrigo Jimenez-Garcia, Javier de Miguel-Díez, Valentin Hernández-Barrera, Jose Luis del Barrio, David Carabantes-Alarcon, et al.
Sex-Related Disparities in the Prevalence of Depression among Patients Hospitalized with Type 2 Diabetes Mellitus in Spain, 2011–2020
Reprinted from: *J. Clin. Med.* **2022**, *11*, 6260, doi:10.3390/jcm11216260 245

Daniel J. Rubin, Naveen Maliakkal, Huaqing Zhao and Eli E. Miller
Hospital Readmission Risk and Risk Factors of People with a Primary or Secondary Discharge Diagnosis of Diabetes
Reprinted from: *J. Clin. Med.* **2023**, *12*, 1274, doi:10.3390/jcm12041274 257

Virginia Bellido and Antonio Pérez
COVID-19 and Diabetes
Reprinted from: *J. Clin. Med.* **2021**, *10*, 5341, doi:10.3390/jcm10225341 271

Ricardo Gómez-Huelgas and Fernando Gómez-Peralta
Perceptions about the Management of Patients with DM2 and COVID-19 in the Hospital Care Setting
Reprinted from: *J. Clin. Med.* **2022**, *11*, 4507, doi:10.3390/jcm11154507 . . . . **287**

Domingo Orozco-Beltrán, Juan Francisco Merino-Torres, Antonio Pérez, Ana M. Cebrián-Cuenca, Ignacio Párraga-Martínez, Luis Ávila-Lachica, et al.
Diabetes Does Not Increase the Risk of Hospitalization Due to COVID-19 in Patients Aged 50 Years or Older in Primary Care—APHOSDIAB—COVID-19 Multicenter Study
Reprinted from: *J. Clin. Med.* **2022**, *11*, 2092, doi:10.3390/jcm11082092 . . . . **301**

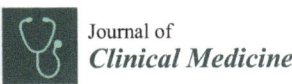

Editorial

Clinical Research on Type 2 Diabetes: A Promising and Multifaceted Landscape

Fernando Gómez-Peralta * and Cristina Abreu

Unidad de Endocrinología y Nutrición, Hospital General de Segovia, 40002 Segovia, Spain
* Correspondence: fgomezp@saludcastillayleon.es

Type 2 diabetes constitutes an imposing epidemiological, economic, and scientific global challenge. The chronic complications of type 2 diabetes are a major cause of mortality and disability worldwide [1,2]. Clinical research is the main way to gain knowledge about long-term diabetic complications and reduce the burden of diabetes. This allows for designing effective programs for screening and follow-up and fine-targeted therapeutic interventions. However, new research methodologies are needed to obtain more accurate and useful insights into the biological and clinical processes involved in diabetic complication development.

During the last few years, new approaches for clinical research have incorporated digital tools to analyze the complex physiopathological background of type 2 diabetes. In this *Special Issue*, entitled *"Clinical Research on Type 2 Diabetes and Its Complications"* and published in the *Journal of Clinical Medicine* (https://www.mdpi.com/journal/jcm/special_issues/Type_2_Diabetes_Complications), some valuable digital methodologies were used in different studies focusing on the type 2 diabetes syndrome. Novel machine learning techniques for predicting long-term complications are one of these approaches, as the studies of Huang, Rashid, and Shin et al. depict [3–5]. The data presented by these authors suggest that machine learning may be more accurate in predicting diabetic microvascular complications than traditional methods. Additionally, digital tools such as artificial intelligence and machine learning can be implemented through an automated and rapid process.

Among the frequent causes of frustration for people with diabetes and the health care providers involved in their management is the delayed detection of diabetic complications. The outlook of clinical research appears promising in the near future owing to the development and implementation of advanced methods for the detection of early alterations in the micro- and macrovascular complications associated with diabetes. Two papers in this *Special Issue* cover the use of specific biomarkers tracing the progress of diabetic cardiovascular complications [6,7]. In another contribution, Lee et al. revisit the long-term glycemic variability and its relationship with end-stage kidney disease [8].

Besides the genetic approach, the application of digital techniques, including machine learning and artificial intelligence, and novel biomarkers could be crucial for individualized type 2 diabetes management, which is the backbone of precision medicine.

Two review papers address the complications that are non-traditionally linked to type 2 diabetes, although currently under exhaustive research: bone health and non-alcoholic fatty liver disease [9,10]. The multifaceted nature of type 2 diabetes is clearly visualized owing to the holistic angle used by these approaches.

The efficacy and safety of new type 2 diabetes pharmacological treatment are covered by three original papers [11–13]. The Yu-Chuan Kang et al. study includes a large population sample and an extended follow-up to evaluate the association between dipeptidyl peptidase-4 inhibitors and diabetic retinopathy [13]. This could be the first signal for a new safety risk of a pharmacological class of drugs used by millions worldwide.

The COVID-19 pandemic was first reported in China in December 2019 and continues to be a devastating condition for global health and economy. The COVID-19 disease has

Citation: Gómez-Peralta, F.; Abreu, C. Clinical Research on Type 2 Diabetes: A Promising and Multifaceted Landscape. *J. Clin. Med.* **2022**, *11*, 6007. https://doi.org/10.3390/jcm11206007

Received: 27 September 2022
Accepted: 5 October 2022
Published: 12 October 2022

Publisher's Note: MDPI stays neutral with regard to jurisdictional claims in published maps and institutional affiliations.

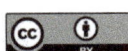

Copyright: © 2022 by the authors. Licensee MDPI, Basel, Switzerland. This article is an open access article distributed under the terms and conditions of the Creative Commons Attribution (CC BY) license (https://creativecommons.org/licenses/by/4.0/).

immediate implications for common chronic metabolic disorders such as type 2 diabetes. Both direct infection and the associated distress due to preventive measures in the general population have worsened the control of type 2 diabetes. Some factors indicate that COVID-19 or other coronavirus-caused diseases can be seasonal or persistent in the future. Type 2 diabetes has a strong negative effect on the prognosis of patients with COVID-19. Three papers in this *Special Issue* review the implications of this disease in relation to diabetes [14–16].

Finally, the aim of researchers in this field should be to make all these remarkable advances accessible to those populations experiencing more difficulties due to sociodemographic factors such as cultural deprivation, sex discrimination, or limited income [17–19].

Author Contributions: Conceptualization, writing—original draft preparation, writing—review and editing were equally done by F.G.-P. and C.A. All authors have read and agreed to the published version of the manuscript.

Funding: This research received no external funding.

Acknowledgments: The authors acknowledge the continuous editorial assistance of Nicole Quinn, Always English S.L.

Conflicts of Interest: The authors declare no conflict of interest.

References

1. Roth, G.A.; Abate, D.; Abate, K.H.; Abay, S.M.; Abbafati, C.; Abbasi, N.; Abbastabar, H.; Abd-Allah, F.; Abdela, J.; Abdelalim, A.; et al. Global, regional, and national age-sex-specific mortality for 282 causes of death in 195 countries and territories, 1980–2017: A systematic analysis for the Global Burden of Disease Study 2017. *Lancet* **2018**, *392*, 1736–1788. [CrossRef]
2. James, S.L.; Abate, D.; Abate, K.H.; Abay, S.M.; Abbafati, C.; Abbasi, N.; Abbastabar, H.; Abd-Allah, F.; Abdela, J.; Abdelalim, A.; et al. Global, regional, and national incidence, prevalence, and years lived with disability for 354 diseases and injuries for 195 countries and territories, 1990–2017: A systematic analysis for the Global Burden of Disease Study 2017. *Lancet* **2018**, *392*, 1789–1858. [CrossRef]
3. Rashid, M.; Alkhodari, M.; Mukit, A.; Ahmed, K.I.U.; Mostafa, R.; Parveen, S.; Khandoker, A.H. Machine Learning for Screening Microvascular Complications in Type 2 Diabetic Patients Using Demographic, Clinical, and Laboratory Profiles. *J. Clin. Med.* **2022**, *11*, 903. [CrossRef]
4. Shin, D.Y.; Lee, B.; Yoo, W.S.; Park, J.W.; Hyun, J.K. Prediction of Diabetic Sensorimotor Polyneuropathy Using Machine Learning Techniques. *J. Clin. Med.* **2021**, *10*, 4576. [CrossRef]
5. Huang, L.Y.; Chen, F.Y.; Jhou, M.J.; Kuo, C.H.; Wu, C.Z.; Lu, C.H.; Chen, Y.L.; Pei, D.; Cheng, Y.F.; Lu, C.J. Comparing Multiple Linear Regression and Machine Learning in Predicting Diabetic Urine Albumin–Creatinine Ratio in a 4-Year Follow-Up Study. *J. Clin. Med.* **2022**, *11*, 3661. [CrossRef]
6. Filipov, A.; Fuchshuber, H.; Kraus, J.; Ebert, A.D.; Sandikci, V.; Alonso, A. Measuring of Advanced Glycation End Products in Acute Stroke Care: Skin Autofluorescence as a Predictor of Ischemic Stroke Outcome in Patients with Diabetes Mellitus. *J. Clin. Med.* **2022**, *11*, 1625. [CrossRef] [PubMed]
7. Luneva, E.B.; Vasileva, A.A.; Karelkina, E.V.; Boyarinova, M.A.; Mikhaylov, E.N.; Ryzhkov, A.V.; Babenko, A.Y.; Konradi, A.O.; Moiseeva, O.M. Simple Predictors for Cardiac Fibrosis in Patients with Type 2 Diabetes Mellitus: The Role of Circulating Biomarkers and Pulse Wave Velocity. *J. Clin. Med.* **2022**, *11*, 2843. [CrossRef]
8. Lee, D.Y.; Kim, J.; Park, S.; Park, S.Y.; Yu, J.H.; Seo, J.A.; Kim, N.H.; Yoo, H.J.; Kim, S.G.; Choi, K.M.; et al. Fasting Glucose Variability as a Risk Indicator for End-Stage Kidney Disease in Patients with Diabetes: A Nationwide Population-Based Study. *J. Clin. Med.* **2021**, *10*, 5948. [CrossRef] [PubMed]
9. Martínez-Montoro, J.I.; García-Fontana, B.; García-Fontana, C.; Muñoz-Torres, M. Evaluation of Quality and Bone Microstructure Alterations in Patients with Type 2 Diabetes: A Narrative Review. *J. Clin. Med.* **2022**, *11*, 2206. [CrossRef] [PubMed]
10. Mantovani, A.; Dalbeni, A.; Beatrice, G.; Cappelli, D.; Gomez-Peralta, F. Non-Alcoholic Fatty Liver Disease and Risk of Macro- and Microvascular Complications in Patients with Type 2 Diabetes. *J. Clin. Med.* **2022**, *11*, 968. [CrossRef]
11. Bellido, V.; Abreu Padín, C.; Catarig, A.M.; Clark, A.; Barreto Pittol, S.; Delgado, E. Once-Weekly Semaglutide Use in Patients with Type 2 Diabetes: Results from the SURE Spain Multicentre, Prospective, Observational Study. *J. Clin. Med.* **2022**, *11*, 4938. [CrossRef] [PubMed]
12. Barboza, J.J.; Huamán, M.R.; Melgar, B.; Diaz-Arocutipa, C.; Valenzuela-Rodriguez, G.; Hernandez, A.V. Efficacy of Liraglutide in Non-Diabetic Obese Adults: A Systematic Review and Meta-Analysis of Randomized Controlled Trials. *J. Clin. Med.* **2022**, *11*, 2998. [CrossRef] [PubMed]
13. Kang, E.Y.C.; Kang, C.; Wu, W.C.; Sun, C.C.; Chen, K.J.; Lai, C.C.; Chen, T.H.; Hwang, Y.S. Association between Add-On Dipeptidyl Peptidase-4 Inhibitor Therapy and Diabetic Retinopathy Progression. *J. Clin. Med.* **2021**, *10*, 2871. [CrossRef]
14. Bellido, V.; Pérez, A. COVID-19 and Diabetes. *J. Clin. Med.* **2021**, *10*, 5341. [CrossRef] [PubMed]

15. Gómez-Huelgas, R.; Gómez-Peralta, F. Perceptions about the Management of Patients with DM2 and COVID-19 in the Hospital Care Setting. *J. Clin. Med.* **2022**, *11*, 4507. [CrossRef]
16. Orozco-Beltrán, D.; Merino-Torres, J.F.; Pérez, A.; Cebrián-Cuenca, A.M.; Párraga-Martínez, I.; Ávila-Lachica, L.; Rojo-Martínez, G.; Pomares-Gómez, F.J.; Álvarez-Guisasola, F.; Sánchez-Molla, M.; et al. Diabetes Does Not Increase the Risk of Hospitalization Due to COVID-19 in Patients Aged 50 Years or Older in Primary Care—APHOSDIAB—COVID-19 Multicenter Study. *J. Clin. Med.* **2022**, *11*, 2092. [CrossRef] [PubMed]
17. Ramírez-Morros, A.; Franch-Nadal, J.; Real, J.; Gratacòs, M.; Mauricio, D. Sex Differences in Cardiovascular Prevention in Type 2: Diabetes in a Real-World Practice Database. *J. Clin. Med.* **2022**, *11*, 2196. [CrossRef] [PubMed]
18. Desse, T.A.; Namara, K.M.; Yifter, H.; Manias, E. Development of a Complex Intervention for Effective Management of Type 2 Diabetes in a Developing Country. *J. Clin. Med.* **2022**, *11*, 1149. [CrossRef] [PubMed]
19. Dobbie, L.J.; Kassab, M.; Davison, A.S.; Grace, P.; Cuthbertson, D.J.; Hydes, T.J. Low Screening Rates Despite a High Prevalence of Significant Liver Fibrosis in People with Diabetes from Primary and Secondary Care. *J. Clin. Med.* **2021**, *10*, 5755. [CrossRef]

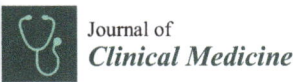

Article

Machine Learning for Screening Microvascular Complications in Type 2 Diabetic Patients Using Demographic, Clinical, and Laboratory Profiles

Mamunur Rashid [1,†], Mohanad Alkhodari [2,*,†], Abdul Mukit [1,3], Khawza Iftekhar Uddin Ahmed [1], Raqibul Mostafa [1], Sharmin Parveen [4] and Ahsan H. Khandoker [2]

1. Department of Electrical and Electronic Engineering, United International University, Dhaka 1212, Bangladesh; mrashid152005@bseee.uiu.ac.bd (M.R.); abdul.mukit64@gmail.com (A.M.); khawza@eee.uiu.ac.bd (K.I.U.A.); rmostafa@eee.uiu.ac.bd (R.M.)
2. Healthcare Engineering Innovation Center (HEIC), Department of Biomedical Engineering, Khalifa University, Abu Dhabi 127788, United Arab Emirates; ahsan.khandoker@ku.ac.ae
3. Department of Electrical and Computer Engineering, University of Oklahoma, Tulsa, OK 74135, USA
4. Department of Health Informatics, Bangladesh University of Health Sciences, Dhaka 1216, Bangladesh; sharminparveen@yahoo.com
* Correspondence: mohanad.alkhodari@ku.ac.ae
† These authors contributed equally to this work.

Abstract: Microvascular complications are one of the key causes of mortality among type 2 diabetic patients. This study was sought to investigate the use of a novel machine learning approach for predicting these complications using only the patient demographic, clinical, and laboratory profiles. A total of 96 Bangladeshi participants with type 2 diabetes were recruited during their routine hospital visits. All patient profiles were assessed by using a chi-squared (χ^2) test to statistically determine the most important markers in predicting three microvascular complications: cardiac autonomic neuropathy (CAN), diabetic peripheral neuropathy (DPN), and diabetic retinopathy (RET). A machine learning approach based on logistic regression, random forest (RF), and support vector machine (SVM) algorithms was then developed to ensure automated clinical testing for microvascular complications in diabetic patients. The highest prediction accuracies were obtained by RF using diastolic blood pressure, albumin–creatinine ratio, and gender for CAN testing (98.67%); microalbuminuria, smoking history, and hemoglobin A1C for DPN testing (67.78%); and hemoglobin A1C, microalbuminuria, and smoking history for RET testing (84.38%). This study suggests machine learning as a promising automated tool for predicting microvascular complications in diabetic patients using their profiles, which could help prevent those patients from further microvascular complications leading to early death.

Keywords: microvascular complications; cardiac autonomic neuropathy; diabetic peripheral neuropathy; diabetic nephropathy; diabetic retinopathy; patient profiles; machine learning

1. Introduction

Diabetes is called a 'silent killer' that is killing around 1.6 million people each year, making it the 5th leading cause of death worldwide [1]. There are two types of diabetes, type 1 and type 2. Type 2 is a chronic metabolic disorder and an expanding global health problem in the past decades. It results in hyperglycemia, which reduces the ability of the body's cells to respond fully to insulin. This situation is called 'insulin resistance'. In this state, insulin production increases, due to the inaction of the hormone. The global prevalence of type 2 diabetes in low- and middle-income countries was estimated to be 415 million in 2015 and is predicted to rise to 642 million by 2040 [2]. Type 2 diabetes mellitus has been rapidly rising worldwide over the past three decades, particularly in developing countries, including Bangladesh [3]. The prevalence of type 2 diabetes in Bangladesh will be more than 50% within the next 15 years, placing Bangladesh as the country with the 8th largest diabetic population in the world [4]. A study suggests that diabetic prevalence will more than double between 2020 and 2030 [5]. The IDF (International Diabetes Federation) Diabetes Atlas has estimated that if nothing is done, the number of diabetes patients may rise to 629 million in 2045 [6] and cases may double from 151 million [7] from 2000 to 2025 [8]. The prevalence of diabetes is higher in rural areas [9], but it was high for males in urban areas, whereas it was lower in rural areas compared to females in Bangladesh [10,11].

Neuropathies are a common persistent complication of both types of diabetes mellitus that confer morbidity and mortality to diabetic patients. Cardiac autonomic neuropathy (CAN) is associated with an increased risk of mortality [12,13]. A study including 1171 patients with type 1 and type 2 diabetes mellitus using a predefined HRV and spectral analysis of R-R intervals reported abnormal findings for 34.3% of type 2 patients [14]. Neuropathy is the most common microvascular complication of both type 1 and type 2 diabetes mellitus [15–17]. A study conducted in the outpatient section of BIRDEM Hospital, Dhaka, Bangladesh found that 19.7% of all registered type 2 patients have diabetic peripheral neuropathy (DPN) [18]. The prevalence of DPN among type 2 diabetic patients is much higher in Europe. A study concludes that 32.1% of the diabetic patients in the United Kingdom, 17.6% in Turkey, and 35.4% in Spain have DPN [19]. The prevalence of DPN increases with the age of the patient and also with the diabetic duration [18,20]. A multi-country study conducted in Asia shows a 58.6% prevalence of micro or macroalbuminuria, indicating an impending pandemic of diabetic renal (i.e., nephropathy) and cardiovascular diseases in Asia [21]. A cross-sectional study with 836 rural Bangladeshi patients showed a high prevalence of retinopathy in Bangladesh [22]. Results from 35 studies from 1980 to 2008 with 22,896 subjects with diabetes showed that the global prevalence for any RET was 34.6% (95% CI 34.5–34.8) [23]. Analyses of the exponential trend revealed an increase in diabetes prevalence among the urban and rural populations at a rate of 0.05% and 0.06% per year, respectively [24]. Increasing age, hypertension, and higher BMI were found to be significant risk factors in the urban and rural communities of Bangladesh [25]. However, the patients with type 2 diabetes in Bangladesh have limited knowledge of its risk factors, cause, and management [26,27]. Depressive diabetic symptoms were found in 29% of males and 30.5% of female participants with diabetes and 6.0% of males and 14.6% of female subjects without diabetes [28].

Most recently, machine learning has emerged in many biomedical applications as a promising tool to aid in decision-making regarding many diseases, including diabetes. In [29], the authors managed to implement a machine learning approach based on decision trees to identify the diabetic patients with or without treatment procedures from their lipid profiles. In addition, Koren et al. [30] developed a trained model capable of diagnosing diabetic patients with drugs that lower blood glucose levels. Moreover, in [30,31], the authors proposed a deep neural network to diagnose diabetic patients from clinical profiles. To recognize patterns among diabetic patients, Alloghani et al. [31] presented several machine learning models that were able of characterizing patients and explain the readmission procedures. Several other studies [32–35] utilized machine learning and deep neural networks in many other applications in diabetes diagnostics. However, even though the implementation of machine learning models for diabetes diagnostics showed high levels of performance, there is still a lack of knowledge about its impact on discriminating between the various microvascular complications. In addition, it is essential to be able to determine, both statistically as well as from a machine perspective, which features play a critical role in characterizing these complications in type 2 diabetic patients.

In this paper, a study is conducted to investigate the efficiency of applying a machine-learning-based approach in discriminating between diabetic patients, according to their microvascular complication status (Figure 1). The novelty of the presented approach lies in utilizing only the demographic, laboratory, and clinical information of patients within the framework of machine learning for diabetes diagnostics. Therefore, time-consuming clinical testing using advanced medical equipment can be avoided, which is essential in communities with economic hardship or a lack of clinical expertise. In addition, the proposed study allows for elaborating on the most important information within patient profiles when testing for each microvascular complication. To the best of the authors' knowledge, there have been very limited attempts towards identifying certain types of microvascular complications using machine learning. Therefore, a gap still exists in the literature about how certain patient information impacts the discrimination between diabetes complications. The present study provides a complete clinical testing approach for CAN-, DPN-, and RET-positive cases by looking into patient information from a machine-based perspective. NEP cases were not used in a separate machine-learning-based testing scenario because they can be easily identified from their patient profile information. Further, with a focus on CAN cases, the study investigates the ability of trained models to deeply discriminate between CAN-only patients and patients with additional complications alongside CAN.

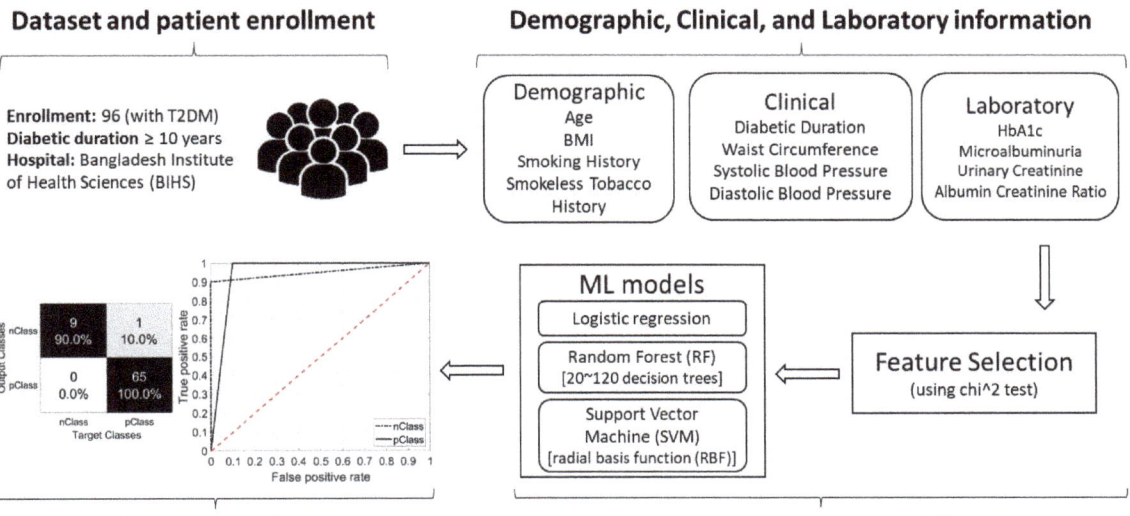

Figure 1. A graphical view of the complete research work in this study, including patient enrollment; demographic, clinical, and laboratory information acquisition; machine learning modeling; and performance evaluation of the model.

2. Materials and Methods

2.1. Study Type

This is a cross-sectional study of Bangladeshi patients from Dhaka who have had type 2 diabetes mellitus for more than 10 years. We followed the STROBE cross-sectional reporting guidelines [36]. The study was approved by the ethical review committee of the Bangladesh University of Health Sciences (BUHS/BIO/EA/17/01) and conforms to the ethical principles outlined in the declaration of Helsinki and the Ministry of Health and Family Welfare of Bangladesh.

2.2. Inclusion and Exclusion Criteria

The parameters that were included in the inclusion criteria: Bangladeshi national, diagnosis of type 2 diabetes mellitus, above 40 years of age, able to give written consent, and the diabetes duration was 10 years or more. The exclusion criteria included: stroke history, having any heart disease, not being able to give consent, diabetes duration of less than 10 years, and the presence of any other pathophysiology that may lead to one or more similar complications, such as cancer.

2.3. Participants and Complications

One hundred and three (47 males and 56 females) unrelated patients of more than 40 years of age that had type 2 diabetes for 10 years or more were randomly selected and enrolled in the study during routine visits to the BIHS [37] Hospital between 18 December 2017 and 26 April 1018. This hospital is one of the most visited hospitals for diabetic patients in Bangladesh.

In this study, the recruited patients were diagnosed with complications, such as CAN, DPN, NEP, and RET (Table 1). The presence of these complications was confirmed by a qualified physician, based on the criteria outlined by the report of the WHO consultation group [38]. A diagnosis of cardiac autonomic neuropathy (CAN) was obtained from the Ewing test, which included five tests: deep breathing, lying to standing, the Valsalva maneuver, lying to standing BP, and sustained handgrip BP [39]. A diagnosis of diabetic peripheral neuropathy (NCV) was obtained using a nerve conduction velocity (NCV) test. There were several tests for recognizing polyneuropathy, CTS (carpal tunnel syndrome), peroneal neuropathy, and other types of neuropathies. A diagnosis of nephropathy (NEP) was determined by the ACR (albumin–creatinine ratio) level >30 mg/mmol for microalbuminuria, and >300 mg/mmol for macroalbuminuria [40]. A diagnosis of retinopathy (RET) was obtained from the fundus image test and classified according to the WHO criteria [41]. Fundus imaging is a process where 3-D retinal semi-transparent tissues are projected onto the imaging plane using reflected light and represented in 2-D [42].

Table 1. Types of complications of patients included in this study.

Name of the Complication	Type	Number of Patients, N (%)	Total, N
CAN	pCAN (with CAN)	65 (67.708)	96
	nCAN (without CAN)	10 (10.417)	
	Test result unavailable	21 (21.875)	
DPN	pDPN (with DPN)	44 (45.833)	96
	nDPN (without DPN)	46 (47.917)	
	Test result unavailable	6 (6.250)	
RET	pRET (with RET)	7 (7.292)	96
	nRET (without RET)	89 (92.708)	

Among these subjects, 70 were able to complete the diagnostic tests for all three complications (CAN, DPN, and RET). There were several combined complications found in some patients. The frequency of complications is shown in Table 2. To observe the importance of demographic, clinical, and laboratory profiles, a multiclass analysis (3-class analysis) was conducted using the classes marked in bold in Table 2 (CAN vs. CAN + DPN vs. CAN + DPN + Others). CAN + DPN + Others are the combinations of CAN + DPN + NEP, CAN + DPN + RET, and CAN + DPN + NEP + RET. These three classes were selected from Table 2 with higher numerals.

Table 2. Types and frequency of complications of diabetes patients.

Types of Complications		Numerals, N (%)	Total, N
nComp (no complication)		4 (4.16)	
Single Complications	CAN	21 (21.875)	
	DPN	3 (3.125)	
	NEP	0 (0.00)	
	RET	0 (0.00)	
Combined Complications	CAN and DPN	16 (16.67)	96
	CAN and NEP	6 (6.25)	
	DPN and NEP	2 (2.083)	
	CAN, DPN, and NEP	12 (12.5)	
	CAN, DPN, and RET	2 (2.083)	
	CAN, DPN, NEP, and RET	4 (4.16)	
Not sure (due to unavailable test results)		26 (27.08)	

2.4. Types of Variables

2.4.1. Demographic and Clinical Variables

The demographic data were collected from the patients at the time of enrollment. We measured the waist circumference, height, and weight at the time of enrollment and listed the value for the diabetic duration, age, gender, smoking history, and smokeless tobacco history. All of these data were verified from the necessary and relevant documents. The clinical data were measured at the time of enrollment. The blood pressure was measured on the first day before starting their Ewing test. If the systolic blood pressure was >130 mm Hg and diastolic blood pressure was >80 mm Hg or they were taking antihypertensive medications, it was called hypertension. Dyslipidemia was diagnosed from the medications of the patient or by checking the history of dyslipidemia of that patient. The data and its basic analysis are shown in Table 3.

Table 3. Demographic and clinical variables of patients.

Variables and their subdivisions	Demographic Variables					
	Male		Female		All	
	Mean ± SD	N (%of M)	Mean ± SD	N (% of F)	Mean ± SD	N (% of total)
Patients		47 (45.63)		56 (54.37)		103 (100)
Age (years)	57.70 ± 9.78	47 (100)	54.60 ± 7.93	56 (100)	56.01 ± 8.91	103 (100)
≥40 and <50	44.8 ± 3.22	10 (21.28)	45.6 ± 2.95	15 (26.79)	45.28 ± 3.02	25 (24.27)
≥50 and <60	53.2 ± 2.7	15 (31.91)	52.86 ± 3.17	22 (39.29)	53 ± 2.95	37 (35.92)
≥60	66.63 ± 4.78	22 (46.81)	63.73 ± 3.79	19 (33.93)	65.29 ± 4.54	41 (39.80)
CAN	58.74 ± 9.63	31 (65.95)	53.32 ± 7.40	37 (66.07)	55.79 ± 8.85	68 (66.01)
DPN	58.95 ± 10.33	21 (44.68)	52.58 ± 6.33	24 (42.85)	55.55 ± 8.93	45 (43.68)
Nep	58.5 ± 10.37	12 (25.53)	54.37 ± 8.75	16 (28.57)	56.14 ± 9.52	28 (27.18)
Ret	56.8 ± 11.64	5 (10.63)	47.5 ± 0.707	2 (3.571)	54.14 ± 10.54	7 (6.796)
BMI (kg/m^2)	25.53 ± 3.47	47 (100)	27.93 ± 5.08	56 (100)	26.84 ± 4.56	103 (100)
Underweight: <18.5	0	0 (0)	0	0 (0)	0	0 (0)
Normal: ≥18.5, <25	23.54 ± 1.45	**27 (57.45)**	22.93 ± 1.69	17 (30.36)	23.31 ± 1.56	44 (42.72)
Overweight: ≥25.0, <30	26.54 ± 1.03	15 (31.91)	27.58 ± 1.32	**24 (42.86)**	27.18 ± 1.31	39 (37.86)

Table 3. *Cont.*

	Mean ± SD	N (%)	Mean ± SD	N (%)	Mean ± SD	N (%)
Obese: ≥30	33.23 ± 4.09	5 (10.638)	34.18 ± 4.77	15 (26.79)	33.94 ± 4.52	20 (19.42)
CAN	26.26 ± 3.71	31 (65.95)	27.94 ± 5.82	37 (66.07)	27.17 ± 5.01	68 (66.01)
DPN	25.52 ± 3.56	21 (44.68)	28.75 ± 5.01	24 (42.85)	27.24 ± 4.64	45 (43.68)
Nep	26.17 ± 4.22	12 (25.53)	29.18 ± 5.60	16 (28.57)	27.89 ± 5.19	28 (27.18)
Ret	26.79 ± 5.53	5 (10.63)	26.29 ± 2.09	2 (3.571)	26.65 ± 4.60	7 (6.796)
Smoking history		9 (19.15)		0 (0)		**9 (8.74)**
Smokeless tobacco history		10 (21.28)		17 (30.357)		**27 (26.21)**

	Clinical variables					
Name of the Variables and their subdivisions	Male		Female		All	
	Mean ± SD	N (%of M)	Mean ± SD	N (% of F)	Mean ± SD	N (% of total)
Diabetes duration (years)	16.17 ± 6.07	47 (100)	15.55 ± 5.76	56 (100)	15.83 ± 5.88	103 (100)
≥10 and <20	13.54 ± 2.76	37 (78.72)	12.60 ± 2.64	41 (73.21)	13.05 ± 2.73	78 (75.73)
≥20 and <30	24 ± 3.116	8 (17.02)	22.30 ± 1.93	13 (23.21)	22.95 ± 2.52	21 (20.39)
≥30	33.5 ± 2.12	2 (4.26)	32 ± 2.828	2 (3.57)	32.75 ± 2.22	4 (3.88)
CAN	16.54 ± 6.20	31 (65.95)	16.13 ± 6.01	37 (66.07)	16.32 ± 6.05	68 (66.01)
DPN	17.33 ± 7.43	21 (44.68)	**14.16 ± 4.80**	24 (42.85)	15.64 ± 6.30	45 (43.68)
Nep	18.91 ± 8.11	12 (25.53)	16.81 ± 6.63	16 (28.57)	17.71 ± 7.24	28 (27.18)
Ret	13 ± 2.828	5 (10.63)	17.5 ± 3.535	2 (3.571)	14.28 ± 3.49	7 (6.796)
Waist Circumference (cm)	90.84 ± 8.61	47 (100)	97.38 ± 9.46	56 (100)	94.39 ± 9.61	103 (100)
Men ≥90	97.40 ± 6.7	23 (48.94)				
Women ≥80			97.72 ± 9.19	**55 (98.21)**		
CAN	92.09 ± 8.47	31 (65.95)	96.58 ± 9.30	37 (66.07)	94.54 ± 9.15	68 (66.01)
DPN	92.64 ± 8.13	21 (44.68)	**98.63 ± 9.07**	24 (42.85)	95.84 ± 9.06	45 (43.68)
Nep	91.22 ± 6.71	12 (25.53)	97.31 ± 9.80	16 (28.57)	94.70 ± 9.00	28 (27.18)
Ret	89.91 ± 5.26	5 (10.63)	93.98 ± 14.36	2 (3.571)	91.07 ± 7.53	7 (6.796)
Systolic blood pressure (mmHg)	141.2 ± 19.5	47 (100)	136.0 ± 20.14	56 (100)	138.4 ± 19.94	103 (100)
≤119	108 ± 5.29	4 (8.51)	108.3 ± 8.96	12 (21.43)	108.2 ± 8.03	16 (15.53)
≥120 and <14	129.2 ± 6.67	19 (40.43)	130.1 ± 4.98	19 (33.93)	129.7 ± 5.82	38 (36.89)
≥140 and <160	148.2 ± 7.52	15 (31.91)	148.3 ± 5.71	19 (33.93)	148.2 ± 6.47	34 (33.01)
≥160	169.6 ± 9.72	9 (19.15)	171.3 ± 6.40	6 (10.714)	170.3 ± 8.33	15 (14.56)
CAN	145.0 ± 20.16	31 (65.95)	134.0 ± 21.30	37 (66.07)	139.0 ± 21.35	68 (66.01)
DPN	148.5 ± 20.82	21 (44.68)	134.8 ± 15.96	24 (42.85)	141.2 ± 19.43	45 (43.68)
Nep	153.0 ± 15.16	12 (25.53)	136.1 ± 17.22	16 (28.57)	143.4 ± 18.19	28 (27.18)
Ret	158.6 ± 16.14	5 (10.63)	137.5 ± 17.67	2 (3.571)	152.5 ± 18.21	7 (6.796)
Diastolic blood pressure (mmHg)	78.97 ± 9.86	47 (100)	76.42 ± 11.96	56 (100)	77.59 ± 11.07	103 (100)
≤79	71.36 ± 7.45	22 (46.81)	67.96 ± 6.98	32 (57.14)	69.35 ± 7.30	54 (52.43)
≥80–89	82.73 ± 2.83	19 (40.43)	83.81 ± 3.08	16 (28.57)	83.22 ± 2.95	35 (33.98)
≥90–99	94 ± 3.39	5 (10.64)	94.14 ± 2.61	7 (12.5)	94.08 ± 2.81	12 (11.65)
≥100	100 ± 0	1 (2.13)	105 ± 0	1 (1.79)	102.5 ± 3.54	2 (1.94)
CAN	78.45 ± 11.40	31 (65.95)	75.48 ± 12.76	37 (66.07)	76.83 ± 12.16	68 (66.01)
DPN	78.19 ± 12.23	21 (44.68)	76.87 ± 10.63	24 (42.85)	77.48 ± 11.29	45 (43.68)
Nep	74.91 ± 13.48	12 (25.53)	75.93 ± 10.81	16 (28.57)	75.5 ± 11.79	28 (27.18)
Ret	84.6 ± 10.13	5 (10.63)	72.5 ± 3.54	2 (3.571)	81.14 ± 10.27	7 (6.796)

2.4.2. Laboratory Data

The laboratory data were taken from the laboratory of the hospital after the enrollment. The laboratory test parameters were hemoglobin A1c (HbA1c), microalbuminuria, urinary creatinine, and the albumin–creatinine ratio. The data and its basic analysis are shown in Table 4.

Table 4. Laboratory variables of patients.

Types and Their Variables	Male		Female		All	
	Mean ± SD	N (%of M)	Mean ± SD	N (% of F)	Mean ± SD	N (% of total)
			HbA1c (mmol/mol,%)			
Not specified	9.066 ± 1.944	47 (45.63)	8.621 ± 1.453	56 (54.37)	8.824 ± 1.701	103 (100.0)
Optimal: <7		2 (4.26)		8 (14.29)		10 (9.71)
Fair: 7–8		12 (25.53)		11 (19.64)		23 (22.33)
High: >8		33 (70.21)		37 (66.07)		70 (67.96)
CAN	9.213 ± 1.790	31 (45.59)	8.716 ± 1.491	37 (54.41)	8.943 ± 1.640	68 (66.02)
Optimal: <7		1 (3.23)		4 (10.81)		5 (7.35)
Fair: 7–8		6 (19.35)		8 (21.62)		14 (20.59)
High: >8		24 (77.42)		25 (67.57)		49 (72.06)
DPN	9.291 ± 1.988	21 (46.67)	8.930 ± 1.667	24 (53.33)	9.098 ± 1.810	45 (43.69)
Optimal: <7		2 (9.52)		3 (12.50)		5 (11.11)
Fair: 7–8		3 (14.29)		4 (16.67)		7 (15.56)
High: >8		16 (76.19)		17 (70.83)		33 (73.33)
Nephropathy	9.9750 ± 2.221	12 (42.86)	8.763 ± 1.902	16 (57.14)	9.282 ± 2.094	28 (27.18)
Optimal: <7		1 (8.33)		3 (18.75)		4 (14.29)
Fair: 7–8		1 (8.33)		4 (25.00)		5 (17.86)
High: >8		10 (83.33)		9 (56.25)		19 (67.86)
Retinopathy	10.720 ± 3.334	5 (71.43)	11.100 ± 1.980	2 (28.57)	10.829 ± 2.846	7 (6.80)
Optimal: <7		0 (0.00)		0 (0.00)		0 (0.00)
Fair: 7–8		2 (40.00)		0 (0.00)		2 (28.57)
High: >8		3 (60.00)		2 (100.00)		5 (71.43)
			Microalbuminuria (mg)			
Not specified	60.6164 ± 99.490	47 (46.08)	49.571 ± 82.123	55 (53.92)	54.661 ± 90.247	102 (99.03)
Optimal: <30		34 (72.34)		38 (69.09)		72 (70.59)
Microalbuminuria: 30–300		10 (21.28)		15 (27.27)		25 (24.51)
Macro albuminuria: >300		3 (6.38)		2 (3.64)		5 (4.90)
CAN	88.439 ± 113.172	31 (45.59)	56.981 ± 93.199	37 (54.41)	71.322 ± 103.204	68 (66.02)
Optimal: <30		18 (58.06)		25 (67.57)		43 (63.24)
Microalbuminuria: 30–300		10 (32.26)		10 (27.03)		20 (29.41)
Macro albuminuria: >300		3 (9.68)		2 (5.41)		5 (7.35)
DPN	121.925 ± 124.49	21 (47.73)	55.2565 ± 87.479	23 (52.27)	87.075 ± 110.720	44 (42.72)
Optimal: <30		10 (47.62)		15 (65.22)		25 (56.82)
Microalbuminuria: 30–300		8 (38.10)		7 (30.43)		15 (34.09)
Macro albuminuria: >300		3 (14.29)		1 (4.35)		4 (9.09)
Nephropathy	210.308 ± 91.414	12 (42.86)	144.519 ± 98.407	16 (57.14)	172.7143 ± 99.417	28 (27.18)
Optimal: <30		0 (0.00)		1 (6.25)		1 (3.57)
Microalbuminuria: 30–300		9 (75.00)		13 (81.25)		22 (78.57)

Table 4. Cont.

Types and Their Variables	Male			Female			All	
Macro albuminuria: >300		3 (25.00)			2 (12.50)			5 (17.86)
Retinopathy	158.62 ± 140.295	5 (71.43)		136.15 ± 178.691	2 (28.57)		152.20 ± 136.247	7 (6.80)
Optimal: <30		2 (40.00)			1 (50.00)			3 (42.86)
Microalbuminuria: 30–300		2 (40.00)			1 (50.00)			3 (42.86)
Macro albuminuria: >300		1 (20.00)			0 (00.00)			1 (14.28)
			Urinary Creatinine (mg/dL)					
Not specified	194.46 ± 139.83			130.87 ± 117.85			160.17 ± 131.70	102 (99.03)
Target 20–320 mg/dL		41 (87.23)			50 (90.91)			91 (89.22)
Non-Target >320 mg/dL		6 (12.77)			4 (7.27)			10 (9.80)
CAN	236.15 ± 150.39	31 (45.59)		123.28 ± 107.24	37 (54.41)		174.74 ± 139.68	68 (66.02)
Target 20–320 mg/dL		25 (80.65)			34 (91.89)			59 (86.76)
Non-Target >320 mg/dL		6 (19.35)			2 (5.41)			8 (11.76)
DPN	236.84 ± 160.20	21 (47.73)		157.52 ± 149.63	23 (52.27)		195.34 ± 158.11	44 (42.72)
Target 20–320 mg/dL		17 (80.95)			20 (86.96)			37 (84.09)
Non-Target >320 mg/dL		4 (19.05)			3 (13.04)			7 (15.91)
Nephropathy	256.43 ± 205.44	12 (42.86)		152.65 ± 77.99	16 (57.14)		197.13 ± 152.68	28 (27.18)
Target 20–320 mg/dL		9 (75.00)			16 (100.0)			25 (89.29)
Non-Target >320 mg/dL		3 (25.00)			0 (0.00)			3 (10.71)
Retinopathy	211.36 ± 55.58	5 (71.43)		159.95 ± 135.98	2 (28.57)		196.67 ± 75.96	7 (6.80)
Target 20–320 mg/dL		5 (100.0)			2 (100.0)			7 (100.0)
Non-Target >320 mg/dL		0 (0.00)			0 (0.00)			0 (0.00)
			Albumin–Creatinine Ratio (mg/mmol)					
Not Specified	32.09 ± 52.45	47 (46.08)		39.28 ± 74.58	55 (53.92)		35.97 ± 65.11	102 (99.03)
Optimal: <3		12 (25.53)			10 (18.18)			22 (21.57)
Borderline high: 3–30		23 (48.94)			29 (52.73)			52 (50.98)
High: >30		12 (25.53)			16 (29.09)			28 (27.45)
CAN	44.35 ± 60.99	31 (45.59)		45.36 ± 86.19	37 (54.41)		44.90 ± 75.22	68 (66.02)
Optimal: <3		7 (22.58)			6 (16.22)			13 (19.12)
Borderline high: 3–30		12 (38.71)			20 (54.05)			32 (47.06)
High: >30		12 (38.71)			11 (29.73)			23 (33.82)
DPN	60.73 ± 68.22	21 (47.73)		35.97 ± 51.28	23 (52.27)		47.79 ± 60.55	44 (42.72)
Optimal: <3		6 (28.57)			5 (21.74)			11 (25.00)
Borderline high: 3–30		4 (19.05)			11 (47.83)			15 (34.09)
High: >30		11 (52.38)			7 (30.43)			18 (40.91)
Nephropathy	105.960 ± 57.952	12 (42.86)		111.404 ± 109.675	16 (57.14)		109.071 ± 89.771	28 (27.18)

Table 4. Cont.

Types and Their Variables	Male		Female		All	
Optimal: <3		0 (0.00)		0 (0.00)		0 (0.00)
Borderline high: 3–30		0 (0.00)		0 (0.00)		0 (0.00)
High: >30		12 (100.0)		16 (100.0)		28 (100.0)
Retinopathy	86.567 ± 87.999	5 (71.43)	58.923 ± 61.616	2 (28.57)	78.671 ± 77.312	7 (6.80)
Optimal: <3		0 (0.00)		0 (0.00)		0 (0.00)
Borderline high: 3–30		2 (40.00)		1 (50.00)		3 (42.86)
High: >30		3 (60.00)		1 (50.00)		4 (57.14)

2.5. Machine Learning Modeling

2.5.1. Clinical Testing Approach

To provide a complete diagnosis of a type 2 diabetes patient, four tests in two steps were applied sequentially (Figure 2) on patients' demographic, clinical, and laboratory (DCL) information. This study supports type 2 diabetic patients with microvascular complications having a better screening from their DCL information. The approach combines a single-class binary classification model with three different classifiers and a multiclass classification model. The single-class classification model can run three tests in parallel to classify CAN, DPN, and RET separately. If all three tests result in a negative class, it means the patient with type 2 diabetes has no microvascular complications. If the test shows positive results, the patient goes for that specific complication treatment. However, obtaining a positive class from the CAN test leads to a multiclass classification model. This model can determine whether the patient has other microvascular complications along with CAN. Thus, this results of this model include: CAN (having only CAN), CANDPN (having DPN with CAN), CANDPN+ (having NEP or RET with CAN and DPN). The resulting class determines the treatment that should be provided to the patient.

2.5.2. Analysis of the Demographic Clinical and Laboratory Profiles

The demographic variables (such as gender, height, age, weight, smoking history, tobacco history, and diabetes duration), clinical measurements (waist circumference, BMI, systolic blood pressure, and diastolic blood pressure), and measured laboratory values (such as HbA1c, microalbuminuria, urinary creatinine, and albumin–creatinine ratio) were selected for further analysis as patient information.

A feature selection approach was then followed based on the univariate chi-squared test to choose the foremost critical factors among all the demographic, clinical, and laboratory variables. In this test, a statistical hypothesis investigation is performed for each DCL feature to test whether the observed calculations coordinate with the anticipated ones, i.e., patient's complication type. Moreover, it gives a noteworthy distinction *p*-value measure (p-value < 0.05) between categories based on the statistical calculations and desire [43]. A feature with a lower *p*-value signifies that this variable is most likely dependent on the complication label. Hence, it is vital for anticipating the complication and has discriminatory characteristics. In this way, a score of significance is returned for each DCL profile utilized within the test as score = $-\log(p)$. In this work, we call this score importance. We calculated importance using a function called fscchi2 () in MATLAB 2021a.

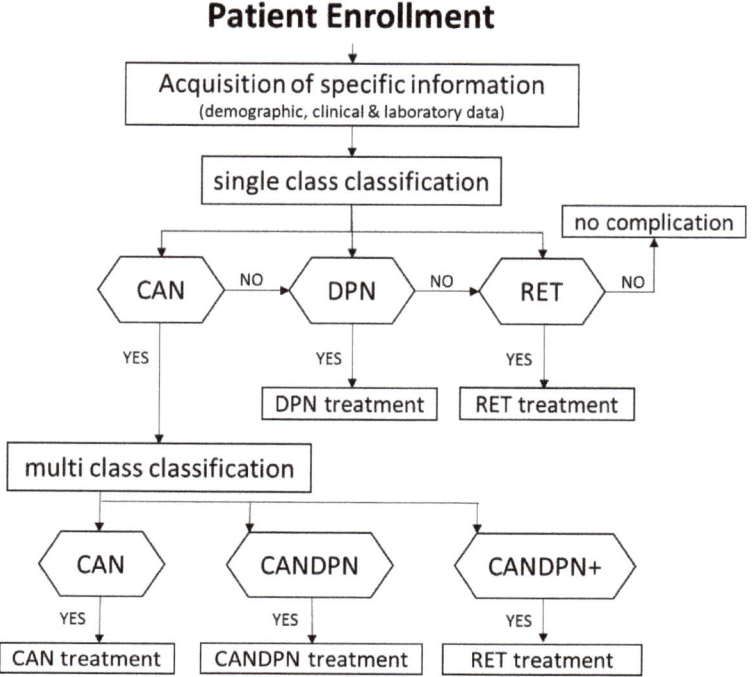

Figure 2. The proposed procedure for screening diabetic patients. Every patient initially goes through the information acquisition of this clinical diagnosis flowchart. Five tests are then applied in two stages. The second stage (multiclass class is only for the patients who go through the CAN test and have a positive CAN. A single-class classification can predict the presence of microvascular complications (CAN, DPN, or RET) and can predict whether there is any presence of complications. Multiple complications with CAN could be classified using the multiclass classifier.

2.5.3. Support Vector Machine (SVM)

SVM is an exceedingly popular machine learning algorithm used in classification and regression problems. It is one of the classic machine learning techniques that can help to solve big data classification problems. SVM allows the classification of single-class as well as multiclass classification problems. It is commonly utilized as an exception finder, where the model is prepared to recognize training data from any other irrelevant information [44]. The model tends to distinguish which unused objects are closely representing the selected class in the training phase, which is generally called a positive class [45]. A set of probabilities has been returned by the model to show the degree of matching between the testing and training samples. In this paper, a single-class SVM was used for the training model in the CAN, DPN, and RET tests. Having the complication has been considered as the positive class in the single-class classification. However, a multiclass SVM was for training in the CANDPNOthers test. To guarantee the highest performance from the model, a non-linear RBF (radial basis function) kernel was used with fine-tuned hyper-parameters.

2.5.4. Random Forest (RF)

Random forest (RF), also known as classification and regression tree (CART), is a form of decision trees, where a set of tree-like trait nodes is associated with a set of sub-trees of decision nodes [46,47]. This algorithm is considered a conglomeration strategy that employs the concepts of bagging. All the decision trees are calculated based on the corresponding resource cost, outcome chances, and utility to provide a prediction. The prediction preparation begins by doling out an occasion at each tree to its root node. At that point, for each of the subsequent sub-nodes, the results are calculated successively. Once a leaf is experienced, the tree-like nodes halt and an occasion is relegated with a prediction. All of the occasions and predictions shape the ultimate choice made by the tree model [48]. In this work, 20–120 decision trees were utilized to construct the model. The choice of the number of trees for each single-class test, as well as the multiclass test, was fine-tuned to guarantee the greatest conceivable performance from the model.

2.5.5. Logistic Regression

Logistic regression is one of the most commonly used machine learning algorithms in statistics. It is a statistical model that uses a logistic function to represent a binary dependent variable in its most basic form, though there are many more advanced variants. Logistic regression is a technique for estimating the parameters of a logistic model in regression analysis. The natural logarithm of the odds is used as a regression function of the predictors in the logistic regression model. The expression for a one predictor (X) one outcome (Y) logistic regression model is $\ln[\text{odds}(Y=1)] = \beta_0 + \beta_1 X$, where ln is the natural algorithm, $Y = 1$ or $Y = 0$ refers to the event occurrence of the event, β_0 is the intercept term, and β_1 is the regression coefficient that refers to the change in the logarithm of the event's odds with a 1-unit change in the predictor X [49].

2.5.6. Training and Testing

A leave-one-out scheme was followed in the single-class models, as well as in the multiclass model, to ensure the incorporation of the highest possible number of samples within the prepared models. Besides, it was fundamental to supply a prediction for each and every patient. An iterative process was applied in this scheme by selecting one subject as testing data, whereas the remaining subjects were used for training. The method repeated on each cycle until a prediction was given for every subject.

2.5.7. Parameter Optimization

In each test, several model parameters were fine-tuned to ensure the highest acquirable model performance. Performance was measured in the form of accuracy, sensitivity, specificity, precision, f1-score, and area under the curve (AUC). To handle data imbalance (65 positive classes vs. 10 negative classes in the CAN test and 7 positive classes vs. 89 negative classes in the RET test), a model parameter called 'prior probability' was introduced in the algorithm during the training phase. The prior probabilities were found observationally, where the initial weight was set to each class that was equal to its number of samples relative to the whole number of samples [50]. Prior probability was not used in the DPN test, as it had balanced classes. The minimum leaf size and bag fraction value were used as per the behavior of the RF model, on an iterative basis and keeping the optimum value.

3. Results

3.1. Demographic, Clinical, and Laboratory Profiles

Demographic and clinical data, along with major comorbidities with type 2 diabetes, are shown in Table 3, and laboratory profiles are shown in Table 4. There were 47 (45.63%) male patients and 56 (54.37%) female patients. The mean age of the patients was 56 years (±8.913), the mean ages of the male and female patients were 57.1 years (±9.78) and 54.6 years (±7.93), respectively. This is consistent with the finding that the diabetic population in Bangladesh, as well as south Asia, are comparatively younger than in the west [51,52]. The sub-variables under 'Age' show that 46.8% of the male subjects were greater than 60 years old, but about 40% female subjects were between 40 and 50, though, overall, the patients showed an increasing prevalence for a higher age. A study in Spain also showed that an increase in patient age increases the prevalence of diabetic complications [19]. In this study, 27 (57.45%) males, 35 (62.50%) females, and a total of 62 (60.19%) patients had a history of hypertension (mean systolic blood pressure was 138.4 mm Hg). A total of 35 (33.98%) patients had dyslipidemia, where 14 (29.79%) were male and 21 (37.5%) were female. Only nine (8.74%) patients had a history of smoking, and they were all male. In addition, the overweight condition (42.86%) was common for female diabetic patients, with more than 98% female subjects having a waist circumference higher than 80 cm, while 57.45% of the male subjects had a normal weight. Though obesity was relatively common for female patients (27%), a total of 20 (19.42%) patients were obese (mean BMI (body mass index) = 33.94 kg/m^2 and mean waist circumference = 90.84 cm for males and 97.38 cm for females). For the retinopathy patients, the waist circumference was 89.91 cm for males and 93.98 cm for females, where 15 (26.79%) were female and 5 (10.638%) were males.

More than 67% of the patients for any type of complication had a high HbA1c (mean HbA1c = 8.824, male mean HbA1c = 9.066, and female mean HbA1c = 8.621 for the patients with CAN). The retinopathy patients had very high HbA1c (mean HbA1c = 10.829, male mean HbA1c = 10.720, and female mean HbA1c = 11.100). Microalbuminuria was found in 25 (24.51%) patients, where 10 were male and 15 were female. In the case of nephropathy, a total of 22 (78.57%) patients had microalbuminuria. All the retinopathy patients had a creatinine level of 20 to 320 mg/dL. The mean ACR (albumin–creatinine ratio) for the patients was 35.967 mg/mmol, where 47 (46.08%) males had a mean ACR of 32.092 mg/mmol, and 55 (53.92%) females had a mean ACR of 39.280 mg/mmol. Neuropathy was the most common complication in Bangladeshi diabetic type 2 patients of more than 40 years' old who had diabetes for more than 10 years. Besides, there were very few retinopathy patients, so it implies that the rate of retinopathy in Bangladeshi type 2 diabetes patients is very low.

3.2. Complications of Type 2 Diabetes

Overall, more than one clinically diagnosed complication was present in 99 subjects out of the cohort of 103 diabetics included in this study. Most of the subjects had CAN (66.02%), followed by diabetic peripheral neuropathy (43.69%), nephropathy (27.18%), and retinopathy (6.8%). Those patients who had retinopathy also had CAN and DPN. The rate of retinopathy complication was very low. Only seven retinopathy patients were found, and five patients out of them had all types of complication, while the other two had CAN and DPN. This trend suggests that RET should be the final stage of the above four diabetes microvascular complications in Bangladesh. We did not find any subject with only NEP or only RET. If a patient had RET, we can say that he/she had CAN and DPN both or CAN, DPN, and NEP, i.e., all the complications. The average diabetic duration of the male patients with CAN and DPN was high (17.33 years for CAN and 18.91 years for DPN) and comparatively lower for RET (13 years). The female patients with retinopathy had a high diabetic duration of 17.5 years. They did not check for DM until they became very ill, so their reported DM duration is from the day they first found out, not from the actual moment of DM development. The overall result indicates a high prevalence of complications in Bangladeshi type 2 diabetes patients.

3.3. Classification of Cardiac-Related Microvascular Complications

To assess the association between any complication (as an outcome) and significant demographic, clinical, and laboratory variables of the patients, several machine learning models (logistic regression, RF, and SVM) were trained by changing the model parameters in an iterative way and observing the sensitivity, specificity, precision, f1-score, and accuracy of the model. The chi-squared (χ^2) test was used to choose significant variables and we use only these significant variables to determine the classification accuracy. The threshold for a significant importance level was different for each test.

3.3.1. CAN

We found diastolic BP (importance 2.1), albumin–creatinine ratio (importance 1.6), and gender (importance 1) to be the significant predictors for screening CAN, which is the most common complication among Bangladeshi patients with type 2 diabetes. We had 65 positive and 10 negative CAN patients in our study. To find the best suitable result and to maximize the model performance, we used prior probability in the classification model of CAN. We found that RF was the best model at the weight of (1.05 and 0.9). The performance (shown in Table 5) of the model was obtained as accuracy 98.68%, sensitivity 98.48%, and specificity 100%. The performance is shown in Figure 3. In Table 6, the 95% confidence intervals, including the mean values of the features, are provided for CAN patients to represent the true mean of the population.

Table 5. Comparison between two machine learning models for each test.

Tests		CAN (pCAN vs. nCAN)	DPN (pDPN vs. nDPN)	RET (pRET vs. nRET)
logistic regression	Accuracy, %	80	55.56	88.54
	Sensitivity, %	85.71	55.77	93.33
	Specificity, %	85.71	55.26	16.67
SVM	Accuracy, %	77.33	67.8	80.5
	Sensitivity, %	29.41	68.89	96.05
	Specificity, %	91.34	66.67	20
RF	Accuracy, %	98.67	67.8	84.38
	Sensitivity, %	100	68.09	97.44
	Specificity, %	98.48	67.44	27.78

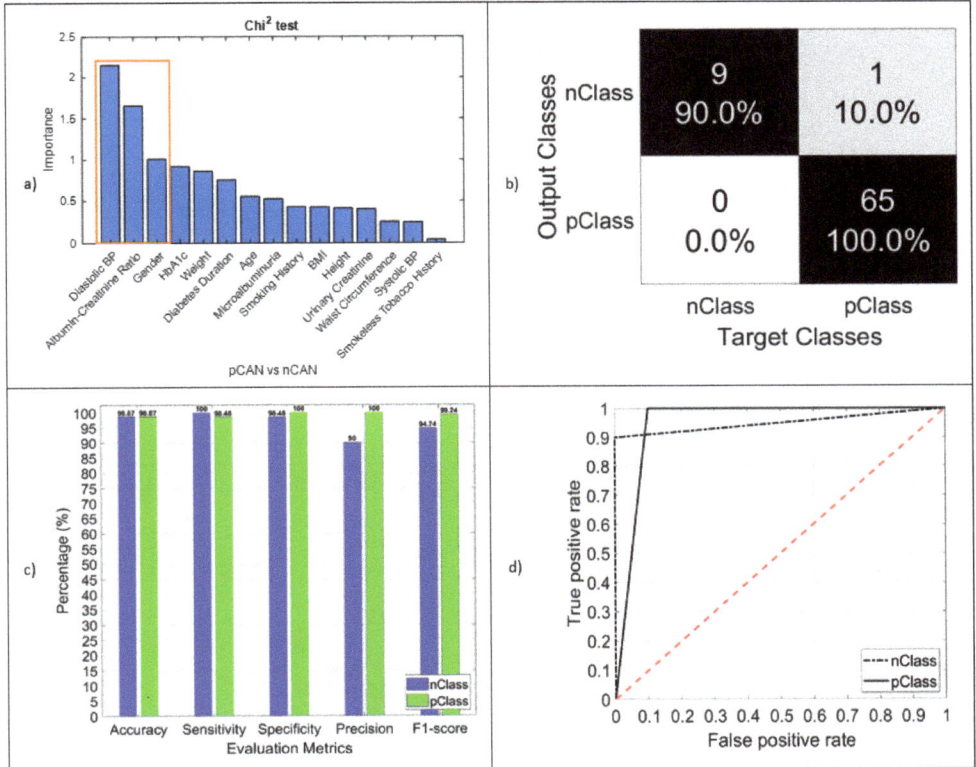

Figure 3. (a) Chi-squared test result. The importance of different marked features was used in the model as an identifier; (b) confusion matrix of the CAN test (pClass vs. nClass); (c) performance evaluation matrices; (d) TPR vs. FPR, graphical view of the CAN classifier model performance.

Table 6. 95% Confidence intervals for cardiac autonomic neuropathy patients (categorical features, such as gender, smoking history, and smokeless tobacco history, have been omitted from the table);. The subject count is 75 (65 pCAN, and 10 nCAN patients), and the features that are used in the model classifier are marked in bold text.

Features	Mean	95% CI (Lower Limit to Upper Limit)	
'Age'	56.167	54.315	58.018
'Waist Circumference'	141.382	136.503	146.262
'Diabetes Duration'	15.844	14.571	17.117
'BMI'	26.657	25.694	27.621
'Systolic BP'	138.900	134.847	142.953
'Diastolic BP'	**77.600**	**75.355**	**79.845**
'Weight'	65.517	63.634	67.400
'Height'	157.399	155.252	159.546
'HbA1c'	8.799	8.465	9.133
'Microalbuminuria'	55.741	36.539	74.943
'Urinary Creatinine'	160.656	131.724	189.588
'Albumin–Creatinine Ratio'	**37.387**	**23.178**	**51.595**

3.3.2. DPN

Similarly, microalbuminuria (importance 5.1), smoking history (importance 2.9), smokeless tobacco history (importance 2.7), HbA1c (importance 2.4), albumin–creatinine ratio (importance 1.9), systolic BP (importance 1.8), diastolic BP (importance 1.4), and urinary creatinine (importance 1.4) were found to be the most significant predictors for determining DPN from type 2 diabetes patients in Bangladesh. This is consistent with other findings that age and diabetic duration are insignificant [15,53–58] here, since all the patients were more than 40 years of age and the diabetic duration was a minimum of 10 years. Both the RF and SVM models showed the highest accuracy for classifying DPN in the patients with type 2 diabetes mellitus from Bangladesh. Figure 4 illustrates the result of classifying DPN, and the numeric values are stored in Table 5. Table 7 shows the true means and 95% confidence intervals of the populations included in the DPN test.

Table 7. 95% confidence intervals for diabetic peripheral neuropathy patients (categorical features, such as gender, smoking history, and smokeless tobacco history, have been omitted from the table). The subject count is 90 (44 pDPN, and 46 nDPN patients), and the features that are used in the model classifier are marked in bold text.

Features	Mean	95% CI (Lower Limit to Upper Limit)	
'Age'	55.844	54.017	57.671
'Waist Circumference'	140.642	135.853	145.432
'Diabetes Duration'	15.781	14.580	16.983
'BMI'	26.657	25.713	27.600
'Systolic BP'	**138.385**	**134.449**	**142.322**
'Diastolic BP'	77.615	75.473	79.756
'Weight'	65.658	63.824	67.491
'Height'	157.603	155.475	159.730
'HbA1c'	8.902	8.554	9.251
'Microalbuminuria'	**55.269**	**36.692**	**73.847**
'Urinary Creatinine'	160.770	133.508	188.032
'Albumin-Creatinine Ratio'	**36.744**	**23.202**	**50.286**

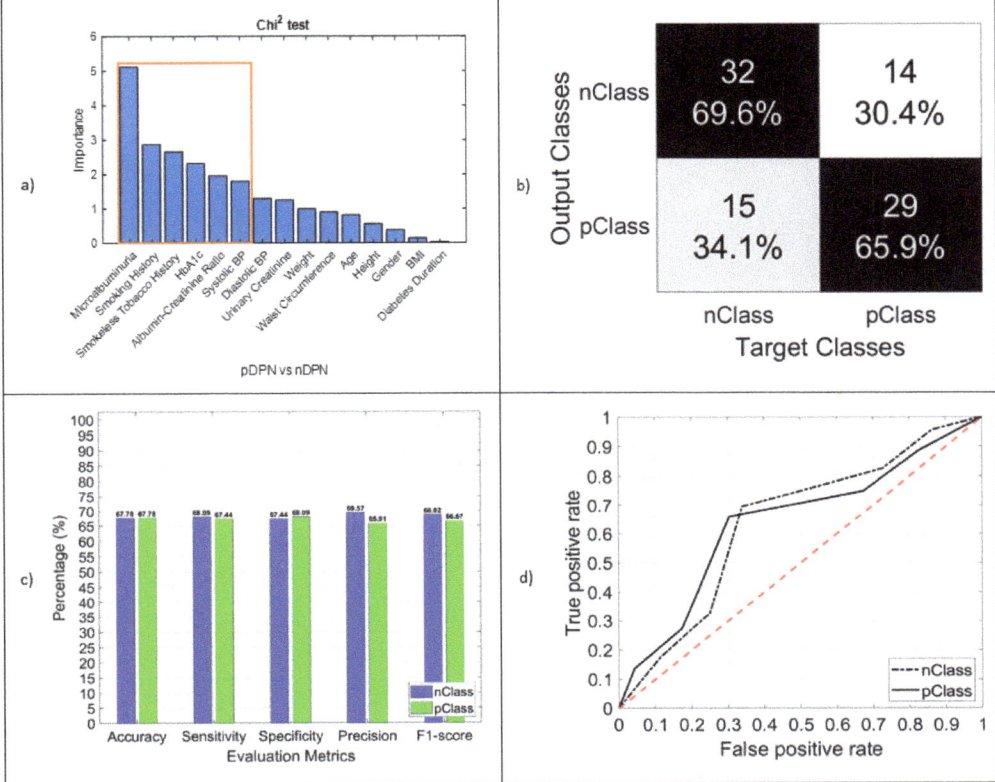

Figure 4. (**a**) Chi-squared test result. The importance of different marked features was used in the model as an identifier; (**b**) confusion matrix of the DPN test (pClass vs. nClass); (**c**) performance evaluation matrices; (**d**) TPR vs. FPR, graphical view of the DPN classifier model performance.

3.3.3. RET

In the case of diabetic retinopathy (RET), HbA1c (importance 6.1), microalbuminuria (importance 4.7), smokeless tobacco history (importance 2.8), weight (importance 1.9), gender (importance 1.8), urinary creatinine (importance 1.7), and albumin–creatinine ratio (importance 1.7) were found to be significant predictors to classify whether a type 2 diabetes mellitus patient has retinopathy (Figure 5). A previous study in Bangladesh showed a 5.4% prevalence of retinopathy patients [22], and in our study, we had 6.8% of type 2 diabetes patients with retinopathy. The accuracy (shown in Table 5) of the RF model was 84.38%. To show the true mean of the features in diabetic retinopathy test, Table 8 is added with means and 95% confidence interval information.

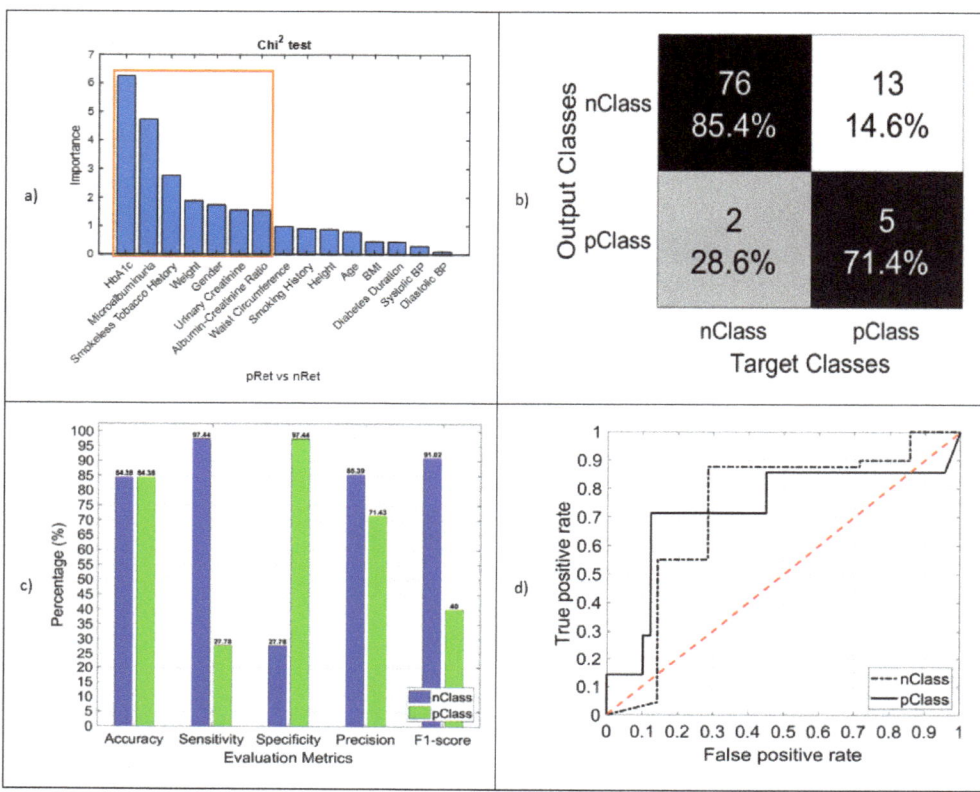

Figure 5. (**a**) Chi-squared test result. The importance of different marked features was used in the model as an identifier; (**b**) confusion matrix of the RET test (pClass vs. nClass); (**c**) performance evaluation matrices; (**d**) TPR vs. FPR, graphical view of the RET classifier model performance.

Table 8. 95% confidence interval for diabetic retinopathy patients (categorical features, such as gender, smoking history, and smokeless tobacco history, have been omitted from the table). The subject count is 96 (7 pRet and 89 nRet patients) and the features that are used in the model classifier are marked in bold text.

Features	Mean	95% CI (Lower Limit to Upper Limit)	
'Age'	55.707	53.651	57.763
'Waist Circumference'	139.958	134.525	145.391
'Diabetes Duration'	15.827	14.486	17.167
'BMI'	26.817	25.683	27.951
'Systolic BP'	138.813	134.153	143.474
'Diastolic BP'	77.347	74.802	79.891
'Weight'	**65.601**	**63.476**	**67.727**
'Height'	157.177	154.610	159.744
'HbA1c'	**8.955**	**8.553**	**9.356**
'Microalbuminuria'	**67.648**	**44.636**	**90.660**
'Urinary Creatinine'	172.120	139.197	205.044
'Albumin-Creatinine Ratio'	44.128	27.134	61.123

3.3.4. CANDPNOthers

The multiclass analysis test provides a comprehensive picture of patients who have other diabetic neuropathies in addition to CAN. A total of 55 patients were considered as training and testing inputs for machine learning models, with 16 suffering from CANDPN and 14 suffering from CANDPN+, where 'Others' included NEP and RET. In the CANDP-NOther test, three classes were assigned to the model, i.e., CAN vs. CANDPN (the patients with both CAN and DPN complications) vs. CANDPN+ (the patients with CAN, DPN, and NEP; CAN, DPN, and RET; or CAN, DPN, NEP, and RET). We only included these classes due to the insufficient number of patients in the other classes. SVM performed better in this multiclass classification rather than RF. The confusion matrix (Figure 6) illustrates that the CAN and CANDPN+ classes could be classified effectively. However, identifying CANDPN patients using this model might be inefficient. The features used in this model were the albumin–creatinine ratio and microalbuminuria. These two features are common for all the binary tests that have been performed in this study.

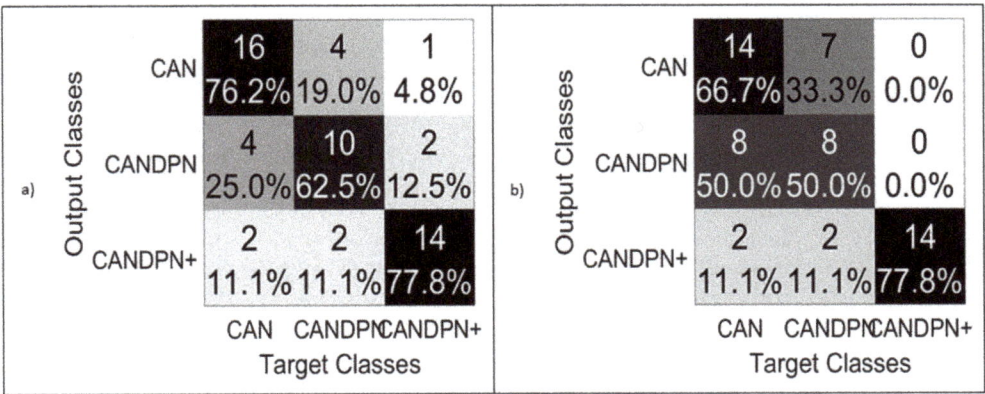

Figure 6. Performance comparison (confusion matrix) between the multiclass SVM classifier and the multiclass RF classifier. (**a**) Confusion matrix of SVM classifier; (**b**) confusion matrix of RF classifier; classes: 1. CAN, patients with CAN; 2. CANDPN, with DPN and CAN; 3. CANDPN+, patients with NEP and/or RET with CAN and DPN.

4. Discussion

This study demonstrated the importance of demographic, clinical, and laboratory profiles in the machine learning domain for the classification of diabetic microvascular complications. Moreover, this study illustrated a complete machine-learning-based clinical approach to screen diabetic patients suffering from diabetic microvascular complications. It also provides an association of other microvascular complications along with CAN. It provides a stepwise clinical approach to screen diabetes microvascular complications for the Bangladeshi type 2 diabetic cohort. The high performance achieved in each test strongly suggests that DCL profiles should be included as features in the machine learning approach to ensure a high classification accuracy. In our study, we also showed the DCL profiles that are highly associated with a kind of complication. Thus, the clinician can easily coordinate the physiological grounds.

4.1. Demographic, Clinical, and Laboratory Profiles

In this study, we demonstrated the significance of DCL profiles to screen a microvascular complication of the type 2 diabetic population in Bangladesh. The profiles that were used in this study are easily collectible by any hospital in Bangladesh. Moreover, gathering this information from a patient is not costly. Furthermore, all the DCL profiles used in this study are not required to be collected for screening using the proposed method. Only the significant features that are listed (Section 3.3) for each test will be needed to execute the test. However, to execute all the tests proposed in this study, a mathematical union of all the significant features that are used in each test would be required.

Diastolic BP, Albumin–Creatinine Ratio, and Gender were highly associated with CAN in our CAN test. Thus, we have found the highest accuracy for the CAN classifier by using these three predictors. In [59,60], the authors showed the influence of hypertension on diabetic complications, and our study we found that diastolic BP was a good predictor variable to classify CAN. However, we have found that HbA1c was not required for testing CAN. On the other hand, microalbuminuria was significantly associated with peripheral neuropathy, nephropathy, and retinopathy. This finding supports both the studies in [61,62], where the authors showed the association of microalbuminuria with nephropathy and retinopathy. Moreover, in [63], Bell et. al. observed the significant association of microalbuminuria with diabetic neuropathy. HbA1c was significantly associated with retinopathy in our study. It was also associated with peripheral neuropathy. In [64,65], the authors established the relationship between HbA1c and microvascular complications. Many authors showed the significance and association of different demographic, clinical, and laboratory parameters with diabetic microvascular complications. However, in our study, we found significant DCL profiles using a statistical model and used these significant profiles with a machine learning model to show the performance.

4.2. Machine Learning as a Screening Tool

This work describes the application of a modern machine learning model, combining the use of statistically significant features to exploit demographic, clinical, and laboratory data to extract a classifier that can classify type 2 diabetes microvascular complications. To address the class imbalance, a machine learning hyper-parameter 'prior probability' was used. Picking up the benefits of the recent advances of machine learning in the area of diabetes diagnosis is considered to be fundamental. It makes a difference within the investigation of colossal healthcare records and changes them into clinical experiences that can help healthcare experts in prompt and intelligent decision-making. Even though the involvement of a clinician within the diagnosis and treatment of diabetic patients may be necessary, machine learning models might be able to provide an early-stage screening that can avoid numerous complications from further development. Besides, when there is a tremendous request for medical specialists or unbounded data available, it is quite hard to provide a complete diagnostic for each quite effectively. In this manner, pre-trained machine learning models can make the process faster and less rigorous for healthcare suppliers and practitioners. Different sorts of machine learning algorithms, such as support vector machines (SVM), K-nearest neighbor (KNN), choice trees, etc., have been utilized broadly within the research associated with type 2 diabetes microvascular complications [66].

CAN plays a major role in myocardial ischemia and infarction, heart arrhythmias, hypertension, and heart disappointment and it increases the risk of sudden cardiac death. Jelinek and Cornforth [67] proposed a novel clustering technique using a graph-based machine learning system that enables the identification of severe diabetic neuropathies in 2016. This proposed model outperforms SVM, RF, and KNN. Cho et al. [68] showed an accuracy of 88.7% (AUC 0.969 and specificity 0.85) using SVM classifiers along with a feature selection method for the prediction of diabetic nephropathy from the data of 4321 patients. Reedy et. al. [69] proposed a multi-model ensemble-based machine learning algorithm to classify diabetic retinopathy. The authors included several machine learning classifiers in their research and concluded that the ensemble model provides better accuracy with better sensitivity and specificity. Sambyal et. al. [66] provided a review of using machine learning models to classify diabetes microvascular complications in 2020. The authors showed that most of the work for classifying RET had been conducted using fundus image as the input, and he compared the different achieved accuracies of the different classifiers by different authors. By only using the demographic, clinical, and laboratory profiles, our model outperforms all the models reviewed by the author in terms of classifying diabetic retinopathy. The authors also have reviewed several machine learning models proposed by different authors for classifying cardiac autonomic neuropathy and nephropathy. However, we only used DCL profiles as independent features to classify microvascular complications.

4.3. Clinical Relevance

The test schemes followed in this work offer physicians an important clinical diagnostic method in the evaluation and diagnosis of type 2 diabetes microvascular complications. The single-class classifiers can operate individually in parallel or sequentially. However, for finding combined complications with CAN, the model works sequentially with the CAN testing classifier. Since this model is sequential, this digs deeper by analyzing diabetics with single and combined complications. Single-class classifiers identify any microvascular complication that is present in a patient, regardless of whether the multiclass classifier predicts the presence of other complications with CAN. Such a clinical test will ensure a better diagnose of type 2 diabetes microvascular complications by distinguishing the cause of single CAN and other related complications. Furthermore, the silent nature of these complications makes it difficult to diagnosis correctly, especially when combined with other microvascular complications. The performance achieved through machine learning using only DCL profiles in this study provides a path to prevent many undiagnosed CAN-only cases. Since a CAN-only medical procedure may not provide effective treatment if additional complications are not properly identified. It is vital to know about combined complications. The multiclass classification test helps to identify multiple complications with autonomic neuropathy.

4.4. Key Message to the Health Community of Bangladesh

Globally, healthcare stakeholders are entering a new era of data-driven clinical detection and prognostication. The application of modern machine-learning-based approaches offers great promises for early diagnosis or prognosis of various health complications. The early identification of patients at risk of microvascular complications due to type 2 diabetes can mitigate the burden on the healthcare system, especially in the context of a resource-limited setup. As the present study shows that screening is feasible from the demographic, clinical, and laboratory (DCL) variables using a proper machine learning classification model, the health community can utilize this benefit for screening that can avoid numerous complications from further development. It also can help healthcare experts in prompt and intelligent decision-making and save the patients from incurring greater healthcare costs.

5. Conclusions

This study explored the present status of microvascular complications in a cohort of type 2 diabetes patients in Bangladesh. Higher comorbidities and microvascular complications were found as compared with neighboring countries, most likely due to the increased levels of hypertension in this cohort. This study also suggests that a high diastolic BP and albumin-creatinine ratio are related to CAN; high microalbuminuria, HbA1c, and blood pressure are related to DPN; high HbA1c and microalbuminuria are related to RET. These findings may be useful in finding risk factors for the development of diabetic complications. Using these risk factors as the independent features, a machine learning model could be designed to screen microvascular complications. This study shows a machine learning model could be utilized to identify diabetes complications in Bangladesh, where the majority of its population is poor. We believe this study could contribute to more effective and affordable screening techniques [70] for diabetes-related microvascular complications.

It is worth noting that the proposed study should be further validated on a wider patient cohort to strengthen the observations. Although the findings of this study were promising and correlate with the observations found in the literature, one limitation to the current work was the small sample size, which is a common situation in biomedical studies that rely on patient data. Overall, RF and SVM are known to handle small sample sizes with high performance capabilities [71–73], especially when compared to other artificial intelligence algorithms, such as deep neural networks, that require large datasets. Therefore, an essential future direction to the current study is to be tested on large clinical data and with additional machine/deep learning algorithms.

Author Contributions: Conceptualization, M.R., A.M., K.I.U.A., and A.H.K.; data curation, M.R. and A.M.; formal analysis, M.R. and M.A.; investigation, M.R. and M.A.; methodology, M.R., M.A., A.M., K.I.U.A., and A.H.K.; project administration, K.I.U.A., R.M., and A.H.K.; software, M.R. and M.A.; supervision, K.I.U.A., R.M., and A.H.K.; validation, M.R., M.A., A.M., K.I.U.A., R.M., S.P., and A.H.K.; visualization, M.R. and M.A.; writing—original draft, M.R. and M.A.; writing—review and editing, M.A., A.M., K.I.U.A., R.M., S.P., and A.H.K. All authors have read and agreed to the published version of the manuscript.

Funding: This work was funded by United International University [UIU-RG 162013] and was partially supported by another grant (award number 8474000132) from the Healthcare Engineering Innovation Center (HEIC) at Khalifa University, Abu Dhabi, UAE.

Institutional Review Board Statement: The study was approved by the ethical review committee of Bangladesh University of Health Sciences (BUHS/BIO/EA/17/01) and conforms to the ethical principles outlined in the declaration of Helsinki and the Ministry of Health and Family Welfare of Bangladesh.

Informed Consent Statement: A consent form was taken from every participant to be eligible for enrollment in the study.

Data Availability Statement: Data and models could be shared under research agreement with any other researchers working in non-profit organizations.

Acknowledgments: This work would not have been possible without the research funding from Institute of Advance Research (IAR) and United International University. Their support for this study is greatly appreciated.

Conflicts of Interest: The authors declare no conflict of interest.

Abbreviations

CAN	cardiac autonomic neuropathy
DPN	diabetic peripheral neuropathy
Nep	nephropathy
Ret	retinopathy
NCV	nerve conduction velocity
CTS	carpal tunnel syndrome
ACR	albumin–creatinine ratio

References

1. Diabetes. Available online: https://www.who.int/health-topics/diabetes#tab=tab_1. (accessed on 23 August 2021).
2. Ogurtsova, K.; da Rocha Fernandes, J.D.; Huang, Y.; Linnenkamp, U.; Guariguata, L.; Cho, N.H.; Cavan, D.; Shaw, J.E.; Makaroff, L.E. IDF Diabetes Atlas: Global estimates for the prevalence of diabetes for 2015 and 2040. *Diabetes Res. Clin. Pract.* **2017**, *128*, 40–50. [CrossRef]
3. Chen, L.; Magliano, D.J.; Zimmet, P.Z. The worldwide epidemiology of type 2 diabetes mellitus—Present and future perspectives. *Nat. Rev. Endocrinol.* **2012**, *8*, 228–236. [CrossRef]
4. Whiting, D.R.; Guariguata, L.; Weil, C.; Shaw, J. IDF diabetes atlas: Global estimates of the prevalence of diabetes for 2011 and 2030. *Diabetes Res. Clin. Pract.* **2011**, *94*, 311–321. [CrossRef]
5. Wild, S.; Roglic, G.; Green, A.; Sicree, R.; King, H. Global prevalence of diabetes: Estimates for the year 2000 and projections for 2030. *Diabetes Care* **2004**, *27*, 1047–1053. [CrossRef]
6. International Diabetes Federation, 8th ed. 2017. Available online: https://diabetesatlas.org/upload/resources/previous/files/8/IDF_DA_8e-EN-final.pdf (accessed on 15 November 2021).
7. International Diabetes Federation, Diabetes Atlas. 2000. Available online: https://suckhoenoitiet.vn/download/Atla-benh-dai-thao-duong-2-1511669800.pdf (accessed on 15 November 2021).
8. International Diabetes Federation, 7th ed. 2015. Available online: https://www.diabetesatlas.org/upload/resources/previous/files/7/IDF%20Diabetes%20Atlas%207th.pdf (accessed on 15 November 2021).
9. Hira, R.; Miah, M.A.W.; Akash, D.H. Prevalence of Type 2 Diabetes Mellitus in Rural Adults ($\geq$31years) in Bangladesh. *Faridpur Med. Coll. J.* **2018**, *13*, 20–23. [CrossRef]
10. Saquib, N.; Saquib, J.; Ahmed, T.; Khanam, M.A.; Cullen, M.R. Cardiovascular diseases and type 2 diabetes in Bangladesh: A systematic review and meta-analysis of studies between 1995 and 2010. *BMC Public Health* **2012**, *12*, 434. [CrossRef]

11. Katulanda, P.; Ranasinghe, P.; Jayawardena, R.; Constantine, G.R.; Sheriff, M.R.; Matthews, D.R. The prevalence, patterns and predictors of diabetic peripheral neuropathy in a developing country. *Diabetol. Metab. Syndr.* **2012**, *4*, 21. [CrossRef] [PubMed]
12. Maser, R.E.; Mitchell, B.D.; Vinik, A.I.; Freeman, R. The association between cardiovascular autonomic neuropathy and mortality in individuals with diabetes a meta-analysis. *Diabetes Care* **2003**, *26*, 1895–1901. [CrossRef] [PubMed]
13. Suarez, G.A.; Clark, V.M.; Norell, J.E.; Kottke, T.E.; Callahan, M.J.; O'Brien, P.C.; Low, P.A.; Dyck, P.J. Sudden cardiac death in diabetes mellitus: Risk factors in the Rochester diabetic neuropathy study. *J. Neurol. Neurosurg. Psychiatry* **2005**, *76*, 240–245. [CrossRef]
14. Ziegler, D.; Dannehl, K.; Mühlen, H.; Spüler, M.; Gries, F.A. Prevalence of Cardiovascular Autonomic Dysfunction Assessed by Spectral Analysis, Vector Analysis, and Standard Tests of Heart Rate Variation and Blood Pressure Responses at Various Stages of Diabetic Neuropathy. *Diabet. Med.* **1992**, *9*, 806–814. [CrossRef]
15. Abbott, C.A.; Carrington, A.L.; Ashe, H.; Bath, S.; Every, L.C.; Griffiths, J.; Hann, A.W.; Hussein, A.; Jackson, N.; Johnson, K.E.; et al. The North-West Diabetes Foot Care Study: Incidence of, and risk factors for, new diabetic foot ulceration in a community-based patient cohort. *Diabet. Med.* **2002**, *19*, 377–384. [CrossRef] [PubMed]
16. Daousi, C.; MacFarlane, I.A.; Woodward, A.; Nurmikko, T.J.; Bundred, P.E.; Benbow, S.J. Chronic painful peripheral neuropathy in an urban community: A controlled comparison of people with and without diabetes. *Diabet. Med.* **2004**, *21*, 976–982. [CrossRef] [PubMed]
17. Sima, A.A.F. Diabetic Neuropathy, 2nd Edition. P.J. Dyck and P.K. Thomas. Philadelphia: W.B. Saunders, 1999. No. of pages: 560. Price: £85.00. ISBN: 0721661823. *Diabetes. Metab. Res. Rev.* **1999**, *15*, 379. [CrossRef]
18. Mørkrid, K.; Ali, L.; Hussain, A. Risk factors and prevalence of diabetic peripheral neuropathy: A study of type 2 diabetic outpatients in Bangladesh. *Int. J. Diabetes Dev. Ctries.* **2010**, *30*, 11–17. [CrossRef] [PubMed]
19. Cabezas-Cerrato, J. The prevalence of clinical diabetic polyneuropathy in Spain: A study in primary care and hospital clinic groups. Neuropathy Spanish Study Group of the Spanish Diabetes Society (SDS). *Diabetologia* **1998**, *41*, 1263–1269. [CrossRef] [PubMed]
20. Hussain, A.; Vaaler, S.; Sayeed, M.A.; Mahtab, H.; Ali, S.K.; Khan, A.A. Type 2 diabetes and impaired fasting blood glucose in rural Bangladesh: A population-based study. *Eur. J. Public Health* **2007**, *17*, 291–296. [CrossRef]
21. Wu, A.Y.T.; Kong, N.C.T.; De Leon, F.A.; Pan, C.Y.; Tai, T.Y.; Yeung, V.T.F.; Yoo, S.J.; Rouillon, A.; Weir, M.R. An alarmingly high prevalence of diabetic nephropathy in Asian type 2 diabetic patients: The MicroAlbuminuria Prevalence (MAP) Study. *Diabetologia* **2005**, *48*, 17–26. [CrossRef]
22. Akhter, A.; Fatema, K.; Ahmed, S.F.; Afroz, A.; Ali, L.; Hussain, A. Prevalence and Associated Risk Indicators of Retinopathy in a Rural Bangladeshi Population with and without Diabetes. *Ophthalmic Epidemiol.* **2013**, *20*, 220–227. [CrossRef]
23. Yau, J.W.; Rogers, S.L.; Kawasaki, R.; Lamoureux, E.L.; Kowalski, J.W.; Bek, T.; Chen, S.J.; Dekker, J.M.; Fletcher, A.; Grauslund, J.; et al. Global prevalence and major risk factors of diabetic retinopathy. *Diabetes Care* **2012**, *35*, 556–564. [CrossRef]
24. Biswas, T.; Islam, A.S.M.N.; Rawal, L.B.; Islam, S.M.S. Increasing prevalence of diabetes in Bangladesh: A scoping review. *Public Health* **2016**, *138*, 4–11. [CrossRef]
25. Rahman, M.M.; Rahim, M.A.; Nahar, Q. Prevalence and risk factors of Type 2 diabetes in an urbanizing rural community of Bangladesh. *Bangladesh Med. Res. Counc. Bull.* **2007**, *33*, 48–54.
26. Islam, S.M.S.; Niessen, L.W.; Seissler, J.; Ferrari, U.; Biswas, T.; Islam, A.; Lechner, A. Diabetes knowledge and glycemic control among patients with type 2 diabetes in Bangladesh. *Springerplus* **2015**, *4*, 1–7. [CrossRef]
27. Saleh, F.; Mumu, S.J.; Ara, F.; Begum, H.A.; Ali, L. Knowledge and self-care practices regarding diabetes among newly diagnosed type 2 diabetics in Bangladesh: A cross-sectional study. *BMC Public Health* **2012**, *12*, 1–8. [CrossRef]
28. Asghar, S.; Hussain, A.; Ali, S.M.K.; Khan, A.K.A.; Magnusson, A. Prevalence of depression and diabetes: A population-based study from rural Bangladesh. *Diabet. Med.* **2007**, *24*, 872–877. [CrossRef]
29. Alcalá-Rmz, V.; Galván-Tejada, C.E.; García-Hernández, A.; Valladares-Salgado, A.; Cruz, M.; Galván-Tejada, J.I.; Celaya-Padilla, J.M.; Luna-Garcia, H.; Gamboa-Rosales, H. Identification of people with diabetes treatment through lipids profile using machine learning algorithms. *Healthcare* **2021**, *9*, 422. [CrossRef] [PubMed]
30. Alcalá-Rmz, V.; Zanella-Calzada, L.A.; Galván-Tejada, C.E.; García-Hernández, A.; Cruz, M.; Valladares-Salgado, A.; Galván-Tejada, J.I.; Gamboa-Rosales, H. Identification of Diabetic Patients through Clinical and Para-Clinical Features in Mexico: An Approach Using Deep Neural Networks. *Int. J. Environ. Res. Public Health* **2019**, *16*, 381. [CrossRef]
31. Zhou, H.; Myrzashova, R.; Zheng, R. Diabetes prediction model based on an enhanced deep neural network. *EURASIP J. Wirel. Commun. Netw.* **2020**, *2020*, 1–13. [CrossRef]
32. Bae, S.; Park, T. Risk prediction of type 2 diabetes using common and rare variants. *Int. J. Data Min. Bioinform.* **2018**, *20*, 77–90. [CrossRef]
33. Kannadasan, K.; Edla, D.R.; Kuppili, V. Type 2 diabetes data classification using stacked autoencoders in deep neural networks. *Clin. Epidemiol. Glob. Health* **2019**, *7*, 530–535. [CrossRef]
34. Alharbi, A.; Alghahtani, M. Using Genetic Algorithm and ELM Neural Networks for Feature Extraction and Classification of Type 2-Diabetes Mellitus. *Appl. Artif. Intell.* **2019**, *33*, 311–328. [CrossRef]
35. Alkhodari, M.; Rashid, M.; Mukit, M.A.; Ahmed, K.I.; Mostafa, R.; Parveen, S.; Khandoker, A.H. Screening Cardiovascular Autonomic Neuropathy in Diabetic Patients with Microvascular Complications Using Machine Learning: A 24-Hour Heart Rate Variability Study. *IEEE Access* **2021**, *9*, 119171–119187. [CrossRef]

36. Von Elm, E.; Altman, D.G.; Egger, M.; Pocock, S.J.; Gøtzsche, P.C.; Vandenbroucke, J.P. The Strengthening the Reporting of Observational Studies in Epidemiology (STROBE) statement: Guidelines for reporting observational studies. *J. Clin. Epidemiol.* **2008**, *61*, 344–349. [CrossRef] [PubMed]
37. Bangladesh Institute of Health Sciences Hospital. Available online: http://www.bihsh.org.bd/ (accessed on 12 September 2019).
38. James, P.A.; Oparil, S.; Carter, B.L.; Cushman, W.C.; Dennison-Himmelfarb, C.; Handler, J.; Ortiz, E. Guía basada en la evidencia de 2014 para el manejo de la presión arterial alta en adultos: Informe de los miembros del panel designados para el Octavo Comité Nacional Conjunto (JNC 8). *JAMA* **2014**, *311*, 507–520. [CrossRef] [PubMed]
39. Lin, K.; Wei, L.; Huang, Z.; Zeng, Q. Combination of Ewing test, heart rate variability, and heart rate turbulence analysis for early diagnosis of diabetic cardiac autonomic neuropathy. *Medicine* **2017**, *96*, e8296. [CrossRef] [PubMed]
40. Kaplow, L.; Shavell, S. *Fairness Versus Welfare*; Havard University Press: Cambridge, MA, USA, 2006; Chapter 3.
41. McCarty, C.A.; Taylor, K.I.; McKay, R.; Keeffe, J.E.; Working Group on Evaluation of NHMRC Diabetic Retinopathy Guidelines. Diabetic retinopathy: Effects of national guidelines on the referral, examination and treatment practices of ophthalmologists and optometrists. *Clin. Experiment. Ophthalmol.* **2001**, *29*, 52–58. [CrossRef] [PubMed]
42. Abràmoff, M.D.; Garvin, M.K.; Sonka, M. Retinal imaging and image analysis. *IEEE Rev. Biomed. Eng.* **2010**, *3*, 169–208. [CrossRef]
43. Antoch, J. A Guide to Chi-Squared Testing. *Comput. Stat. Data Anal.* **1997**, *23*, 565–566. [CrossRef]
44. Müller, K.R.; Mika, S.; Rätsch, G.; Tsuda, K.; Schölkopf, B. An introduction to kernel-based learning algorithms. *IEEE Trans. Neural Netw.* **2001**, *12*, 181–201. [CrossRef]
45. Moya, M.M.; Koch, M.W.; Hostetler, L.D. One-class classifier networks for target recognition applications. *STIN* **1993**, *93*, 24043.
46. Ho, T.K. Random Decision Forest. In Proceedings of the 3rd International Conference on Document Analysis and Recognition, Montreal, QC, Canada, 14–16 August 1995; pp. 278–282.
47. Wu, X.; Kumar, V.; Quinlan, J.R.; Ghosh, J.; Yang, Q.; Motoda, H.; McLachlan, G.J.; Ng, A.; Liu, B.; Philip, S.Y.; et al. Top 10 algorithms in data mining. *Knowl. Inf. Syst.* **2008**, *14*, 1–37. [CrossRef]
48. Quinlan, J.R. {C4}.5—Programs for Machine Learning. In *The Morgan Kaufmann Series in Machine Learning*; Morgan Kaufmann: Burlington, MA, USA, 1993.
49. LaValley, M.P. Logistic regression. *Circulation* **2008**, *117*, 2395–2399. [CrossRef] [PubMed]
50. Nisbet, R.; Miner, G.; Yale, K. Data Understanding and Preparation. In *Handbook of Statistical Analysis and Data Mining Applications*; Elsevier: Amsterdam, Netherlands, 2018; pp. 55–82.
51. Ramachandran, A. Specific problems of the diabetic foot in developing countries. *Diabetes. Metab. Res. Rev.* **2004**, *20*, S19–S22. [CrossRef] [PubMed]
52. Hussain, A.; Rahim, M.A.; Azad Khan, A.K.; Ali, S.M.K.; Vaaler, S. Type 2 diabetes in rural and urban population: Diverse prevalence and associated risk factors in Bangladesh. *Diabet. Med.* **2005**, *22*, 931–936. [CrossRef] [PubMed]
53. Boulton, A.J.M.; Cavanagh, P.R.; Rayman, G. *The Foot in Diabetes*, 4th ed.; Boulton, A.J., Cavanagh, P.R., Rayman, G., Eds.; Wiley: Toronto, ON, Canada, 2006.
54. BÖRü, Ü.T.; Alp, R.; Sargin, H.; Koçer, A.; Sargin, M.; Lüleci, A.; Yayla, A. Prevalence of peripheral neuropathy in type 2 diabetic patients attending a diabetes center in Turkey. *Endocr. J.* **2004**, *51*, 563–567. [CrossRef] [PubMed]
55. Mimi, O.; Teng, C.L.; Chia, Y.C. The prevalence of diabetic peripheral neuropathy in an outpatient setting. *Med. J. Malays.* **2003**, *58*, 533–538.
56. Yang, C.P.; Lin, C.C.; Li, C.I.; Liu, C.S.; Lin, W.Y.; Hwang, K.L.; Yang, S.Y.; Chen, H.J.; Li, T.C. Cardiovascular risk factors increase the risks of diabetic peripheral neuropathy in patients with type 2 diabetes mellitus. *Medicine* **2015**, *94*, e1783. [CrossRef]
57. Young, M.J.; Boulton, A.J.M.; MacLeod, A.F.; Williams, D.R.R.; Sonksen, P.H. A multicentre study of the prevalence of diabetic peripheral neuropathy in the United Kingdom hospital clinic population. *Diabetologia* **1993**, *36*, 150–154. [CrossRef]
58. Ashok, S.; Ramu, M.; Deepa, R.; Mohan, V. Prevalence of neuropathy in type 2 diabetic patients attending a diabetes centre in South India. *J. Assoc. Physicians India* **2002**, *50*, 546–550. [PubMed]
59. Hirsch, I.B.; Brownlee, M. Beyond hemoglobin A1c—Need for additional markers of risk for diabetic microvascular complications. *JAMA J. Am. Med. Assoc.* **2010**, *303*, 2291–2292. [CrossRef]
60. Ayad, F.; Belhadj, M.; Pariés, J.; Attali, J.R.; Valensi, P. Association between cardiac autonomic neuropathy and hypertension and its potential influence on diabetic complications. *Diabet. Med.* **2010**, *27*, 804–811. [CrossRef] [PubMed]
61. Karar, T.; Alniwaider, R.A.R.; Fattah, M.A.; Al Tamimi, W.; Alanazi, A.; Qureshi, S. Assessment of microalbuminuria and albumin creatinine ratio in patients with type 2 diabetes mellitus. *J. Nat. Sci. Biol. Med.* **2015**, *6*, S89. [PubMed]
62. Parving, H.H.; Hommel, E.; Mathiesen, E.; Skøtt, P.; Edsberg, B.; Bahnsen, M.; Lauritzen, M.; Hougaard, P.; Lauritzen, E. Prevalence of microalbuminuria, arterial hypertension, retinopathy, and neuropathy in patients with insulin dependent diabetes. *Br. Med. J.* **1988**, *296*, 156–160. [CrossRef]
63. Bell, D.S.; Ketchum, C.H.; Robinson, C.A.; Wagenknecht, L.E.; Williams, B.T. Microalbuminuria Associated with Diabetic Neuropathy. *Diabetes Care* **1992**, *15*, 528–531. [CrossRef] [PubMed]
64. Škrha, J.; Šoupal, J.; Prázný, M. Glucose variability, HbA1c and microvascular complications. *Rev. Endocr. Metab. Disord.* **2016**, *17*, 103–110. [CrossRef]
65. Nathan, D.M.; McGee, P.; Steffes, M.W.; Lachin, J.M.; DCCT/EDIC research group. Relationship of glycated albumin to blood glucose and HbA(1c) values and to retinopathy, nephropathy and cardiovascular outcomes in the DCCT/EDIC study. *Diabetes* **2014**, *63*, 282–290. [CrossRef] [PubMed]

66. Sambyal, N.; Saini, P.; Syal, R. Microvascular Complications in Type-2 Diabetes: A Review of Statistical Techniques and Machine Learning Models. *Wirel. Pers. Commun.* **2020**, *115*, 1–26. [CrossRef]
67. Jelinek, H.F.; Cornforth, D.J.; Kelarev, A.V. Machine Learning Methods for Automated Detection of Severe Diabetic Neuropathy. *J. Diabet. Complicat. Med.* **2016**, *1*, 1–7. [CrossRef]
68. Cho, B.H.; Yu, H.; Kim, K.W.; Kim, T.H.; Kim, I.Y.; Kim, S.I. Application of irregular and unbalanced data to predict diabetic nephropathy using visualization and feature selection methods. *Artif. Intell. Med.* **2008**, *42*, 37–53. [CrossRef]
69. Reddy, G.T.; Bhattacharya, S.; Ramakrishnan, S.S.; Chowdhary, C.L.; Hakak, S.; Kaluri, R.; Reddy, M.P.K. An Ensemble based Machine Learning model for Diabetic Retinopathy Classification. In Proceedings of the International Conference on Emerging Trends in Information Technology and Engineering, ic-ETITE 2020, Vellore, India, 24–25 February 2020.
70. Walker, B.A.; Khandoker, A.H.; Black, J. Low cost ECG Monitor for Developing Countries. In Proceedings of the 2009 International Conference on Intelligent Sensors, Sensor Networks and Information Processing (ISSNIP), Melbourne, VIC, Australia, 7–10 December 2009; pp. 195–199.
71. Khandoker, A.H.; Lai, D.T.; Begg, R.K.; Palaniswami, M. Wavelet-based feature extraction for support vector machines for screening balance impairments in the elderly. *IEEE Trans. Neural Syst. Rehabil. Eng.* **2007**, *15*, 587–597. [CrossRef]
72. Qi, Y. Random forest for bioinformatics. In *Ensemble Machine Learning*; Springer: Boston, MA, USA, 2012; pp. 307–323.
73. Alkhodari, M.; Jelinek, H.F.; Werghi, N.; Hadjileontiadis, L.J.; Khandoker, A.H. Estimating Left Ventricle Ejection Fraction Levels Using Circadian Heart Rate Variability Features and Support Vector Regression Models. *IEEE J. Biomed. Health Inform.* **2020**, *25*, 746–754. [CrossRef]

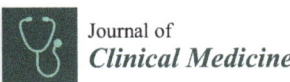 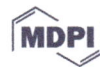

Article

Prediction of Diabetic Sensorimotor Polyneuropathy Using Machine Learning Techniques

Dae Youp Shin [1], Bora Lee [2], Won Sang Yoo [3], Joo Won Park [4] and Jung Keun Hyun [1,5,6,*]

1. Department of Rehabilitation Medicine, College of Medicine, Dankook University, Cheonan 31116, Korea; sindae90@dkuh.co.kr
2. Deargen, Co., Ltd., Daejeon 34051, Korea; 2bora@deargen.me
3. Department of Endocrinology and Metabolism, College of Medicine, Dankook University, Cheonan 31116, Korea; smff03@hanmail.net
4. Department of Laboratory Medicine, College of Medicine, Dankook University, Cheonan 31116, Korea; joowon@dankook.ac.kr
5. Department of Nanobiomedical Science & BK21 NBM Global Research Center for Regenerative Medicine, Dankook University, Cheonan 31116, Korea
6. Institute of Tissue Regeneration Engineering (ITREN), Dankook University, Cheonan 31116, Korea
* Correspondence: rhhyun@dankook.ac.kr; Tel.: +82-10-2293-3415

Abstract: Diabetic sensorimotor polyneuropathy (DSPN) is a major complication in patients with diabetes mellitus (DM), and early detection or prediction of DSPN is important for preventing or managing neuropathic pain and foot ulcer. Our aim is to delineate whether machine learning techniques are more useful than traditional statistical methods for predicting DSPN in DM patients. Four hundred seventy DM patients were classified into four groups (normal, possible, probable, and confirmed) based on clinical and electrophysiological findings of suspected DSPN. Three ML methods, XGBoost (XGB), support vector machine (SVM), and random forest (RF), and their combinations were used for analysis. RF showed the best area under the receiver operator characteristic curve (AUC, 0.8250) for differentiating between two categories—criteria by clinical findings (normal, possible, and probable groups) and those by electrophysiological findings (confirmed group)—and the result was superior to that of linear regression analysis (AUC = 0.6620). Average values of serum glucose, International Federation of Clinical Chemistry (IFCC), HbA1c, and albumin levels were identified as the four most important predictors of DSPN. In conclusion, machine learning techniques, especially RF, can predict DSPN in DM patients effectively, and electrophysiological analysis is important for identifying DSPN.

Keywords: machine learning; diabetes mellitus; diabetic sensorimotor polyneuropathy; random forest; prediction; electrophysiology

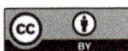

1. Introduction

Type 2 diabetes mellitus (T2DM), the most common form of diabetes, is a major disease in humans worldwide [1], and its incidence is increasing with aging and lifestyle changes [2]. There is evidence that half of T2DM patients experience neurological disorders and a progressive disability of nerve fibers in the course of diabetes, and serious neurological symptoms lead to poor quality of life [3]. Diabetic sensorimotor polyneuropathy (DSPN) is a common neurological complication resulting from neuroinflammation, mitochondrial dysfunction, and apoptosis due to hyperglycemia, dyslipidemia, and altered insulin signaling, and leads to various symptoms and signs, including neuropathic pain, decreased sensation, and foot ulceration [4,5]. The management of DSPN is not limited to controlling hyperglycemia, and multidisciplinary programs, such as patient education, lifestyle modification, and physical activity, are required to control various physical and psychological symptoms and foot complications [6]. Therefore, early detection and prediction of DSPN is very important in DM patients.

The classification of DSPN has been defined in previous studies [7–10]. Typical DSPN is the most common form in DM patients and chronic, symmetrical, and length-dependent sensorimotor polyneuropathy [11]. Tesfaye et al. defined the minimal criteria for typical DSPN to estimate severity: possible, probable, confirmed, and subclinical based on clinical symptoms and signs and electrophysiology [7]. Numerous staging and scoring systems have been developed to assess the severity of DSPN; however, choosing the optimal scoring system is confusing because the results of previous studies are different regarding which system is effective [12–14]. Electrophysiological assessments, including nerve conduction studies (NCS), are important for diagnosing DSPN objectively [15,16]; however, special equipment is needed, and these assessments cannot be performed routinely for patients without clinical symptoms or signs because of the discomfort caused by electrical stimulation or needle insertion. Because the pathophysiology of diabetic neuropathy reveals a broad spectrum of axonal involvement and segmental demyelination, electrophysiological findings also indicate both axonal degeneration and demyelination [17]. Numerous predisposing factors for the development of DSPN have been found [18–21]. DSPN is significantly correlated with poor glucose control [18,19], longer duration of diabetes, poor metabolic management, smoking and the presence of cardiovascular disease, and DSPN severity is correlated with hypertension, dyslipidemia, microalbuminuria, alcohol consumption, and body mass index [20,21]. Most previous studies on the prediction of DSPN used various statistical methods. While traditional statistical methods draw only population inferences from clinical information, recently developed machine learning (ML) methods focus on developing predictive models from general-purpose learning algorithms [22]. Therefore, ML is considered to be a better way to predict DSPN in DM patients.

ML is a computationally broad and powerful data mining technique that can accommodate a large set of proposed variables as inputs to identify factors related to the results of interest [23], and ML develops algorithms that can learn patterns and decision rules, such as early detection, prediction and diagnosis, from data that are attributable to the medical field. Recent studies have used various ML techniques to predict complications, including retinopathy, nephropathy, foot ulceration and DSPN, in T2DM patients [24–28], and ML was effective for prediction of DSPN severity [24], 3-year complication developments [25], high-risk retinopathy, and numerous complications in nonadherent T2DM [27]. Haque et al. found that machine learning algorithms, especially random forest (RF), were effective in predicting DSPN severity based on the scoring system using Michigan Neuropathy Screening Instrumentation [29], which is not used widely, and that study assessed only type 1 diabetes mellitus (T1DM) patients.

The purpose of the current study was to delineate whether machine learning techniques are more useful than traditional statistical methods for predicting DSPN in type 2 DM patients, and whether the widely used classification for DSPN, which is based on clinical and electrophysiological findings, is amenable to the use of predictive models.

2. Materials and Methods

2.1. Subjects

Medical records of patients with T2DM who visited Dankook University Hospital for the management of DM were collected, and 746 subjects were initially enrolled (Figure 1). Patients were diagnosed with T2DM by a physician at the Department of Endocrinology, based on the guideline of the American Diabetes Association [30]. Patients who did not undergo electrophysiological studies ($n = 206$) or had incomplete clinical data ($n = 53$) were excluded at first, and then patients who had other types of polyneuropathies, including heavy alcohol use ($n = 3$), hepatic failure ($n = 2$), renal failure ($n = 4$), chemotherapy for malignancy ($n = 7$), and typical musculoskeletal anomalies ($n = 1$), were subsequently excluded. As a result, 470 patients were included in the study (Figure 1). This study was approved by the Dankook University Hospital Institutional Review Board (IRB No. 2019-12-009).

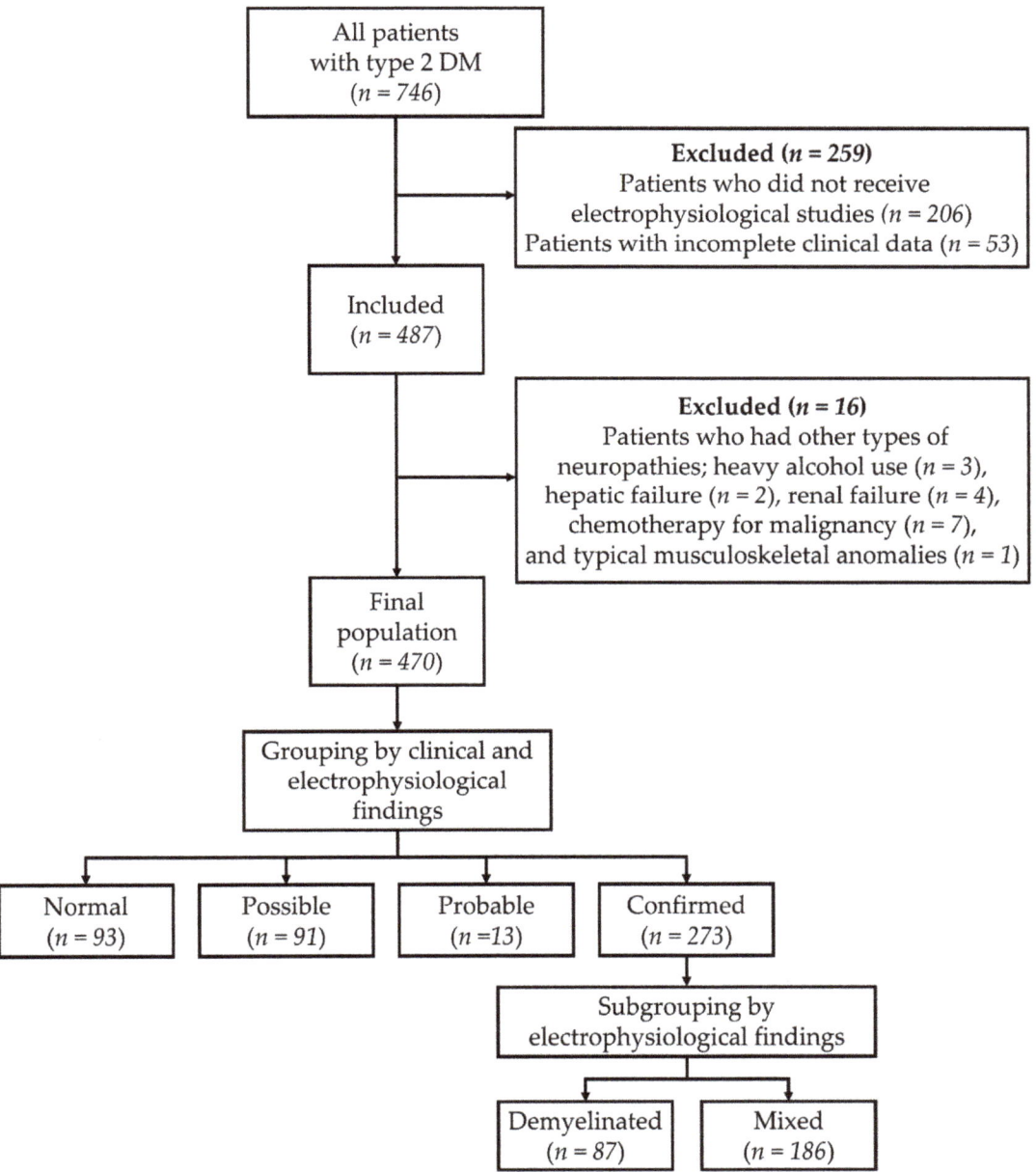

Figure 1. Flow and grouping of patients.

2.2. Classification

Subjects were classified into 4 groups according to definitions of minimal criteria for typical DSPN based on the area of clinical care by Tesfaye et al. [7]: normal, possible, probable, and confirmed. The normal group ($n = 93$) consisted of subjects without any neurological symptoms or signs as previously described [7], and the possible group ($n = 91$) comprised subjects with one of the neurological symptoms or signs. The probable group ($n = 13$) comprised subjects with two or more neurological symptoms or signs. The confirmed group ($n = 273$) consisted of subjects with abnormal electrophysiological findings and neurological symptoms or signs. Electrophysiological assessments were performed according to the guidelines of the American Academy of Neurology [16], and NCS and electromyography of the upper and lower extremities were conducted. According to electrophysiological findings, the confirmed group was divided into two subgroups: A demyelinated subgroup (n = 87) with subjects who predominantly showed demyelination and a mixed subgroup (n = 186) with subjects who showed abnormal spontaneous activities during needle electromyography and demyelination (Figure 1).

2.3. Clinical Data

All subjects' clinical information, such as baseline characteristics, past medical history, current health status, diabetic complications, and medications, was analyzed. Baseline characteristics included age, sex, weight, height, body mass index (BMI), disease duration (from initial diagnosis of T2DM to the date of the last follow-up at the hospital), smoking (current smoking, past smoking, or nonsmoking), family history of T2DM, and diabetes education. Past medical history included hypertension (HTN), dyslipidemia, and history of stroke and coronary artery disease. HTN was defined as systolic blood pressure > 140 mmHg, diastolic blood pressure > 90 mmHg or the use of antihypertensive medications. Diabetic retinopathy was included in diabetic complications. Medications for DM, HTN and dyslipidemia were included; medications for DM were metformin, sulfonylureas, thiazolidinediones (TZDs), dipeptidyl peptidase-4 inhibitors (DPP4is), sodium-glucose cotransporter-2 inhibitors (SGLT2is), and insulin; medications for HTN were calcium channel blockers (CCBs), angiotensin-converting-enzyme inhibitors (ACEis), angiotensin II receptor blockers (ARBs), beta blockers (BBs) and thiazides; and medications for dyslipidemia were statins. BMI was calculated as weight in kilograms divided by the square of height in meters.

2.4. Laboratory Data

A total of 432 laboratory codes from blood and urine tests were obtained from all subjects, and we divided subjects into a control group (n = 197) with normal electrophysiological findings and a test group (n = 273) with abnormal electrophysiological findings within the criteria of DSPN to identify the optimal number of laboratory codes (Figure 2). Forty-eight codes could be obtained for more than half of the subjects (n = 98) in the control group, and 62 codes could be obtained for more than half of the subjects (n = 135) in the test group (Figure 2a). When the results of the two groups were combined, 39 laboratory codes were ultimately selected (Figure 2b). Each laboratory code was assessed several times during the follow-up periods (range: 31–18368 days, mean value: 5202.9 days), and various changes in the values were observed within the period (Figure 2c).

Three methods were used to standardize the values of laboratory codes for ML analysis. Method 1 refers to the average value of each laboratory code during the follow-up period, method 2 is the first value of each laboratory code when T2DM was initially diagnosed while visiting the hospital, and method 3 refers to the pattern of laboratory code changes. The pattern was defined as −1, 0, and 1 as follows. If the initial value was 10% or more lower than the overall average of the values excluding the initial value, it was considered −1; if the change was less than 10%, it was regarded as 0; and if the initial value was greater than 10% of the overall average of the values excluding the initial value, it was regarded as 1.

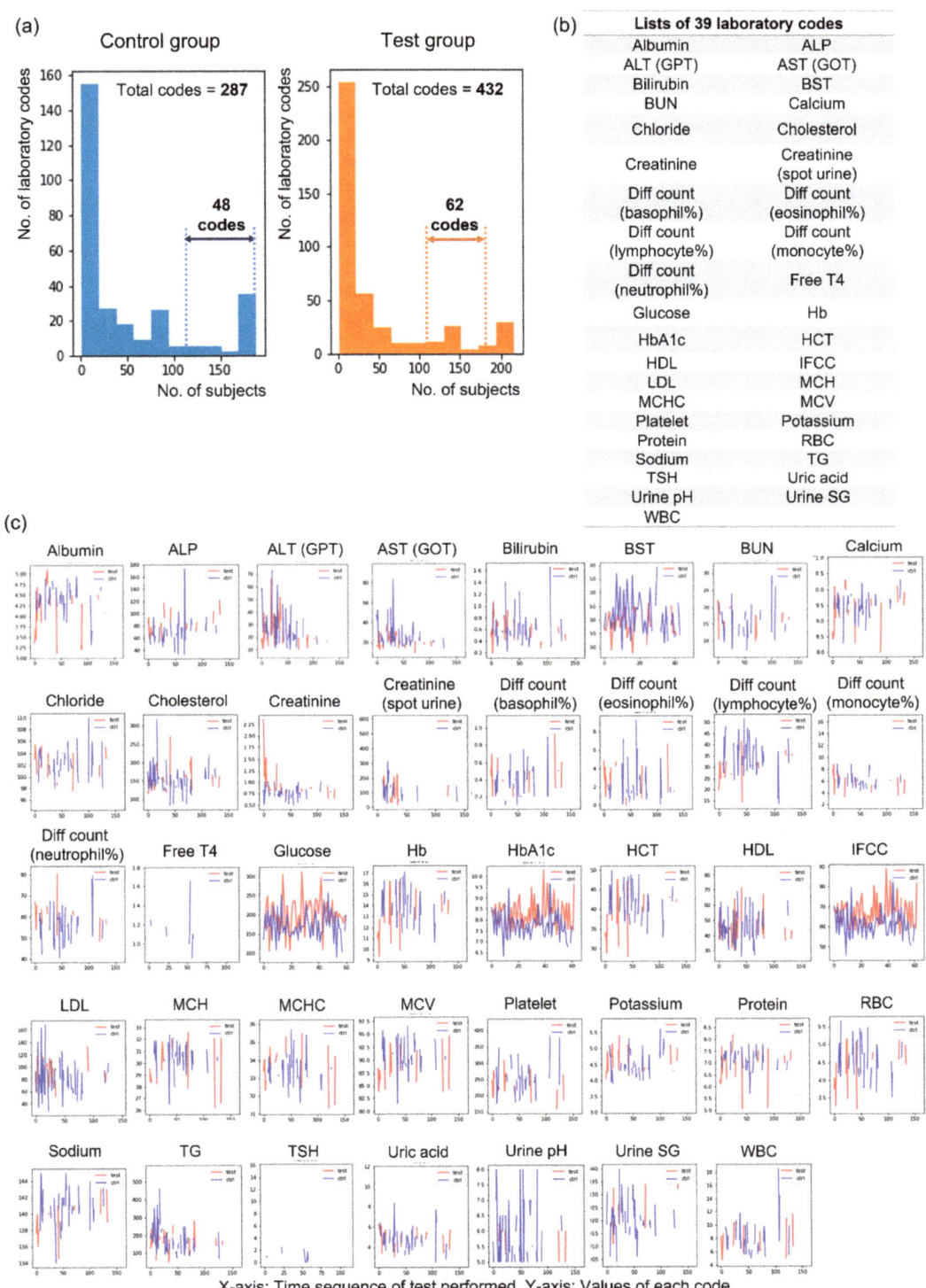

Figure 2. Selection of laboratory codes for machine learning analysis. (**a**) The distribution of laboratory codes according to tested subject numbers in the control and test groups, (**b**) lists of 39 selected laboratory codes, (**c**) graphs showing the changes

in 39 selected laboratory codes at the initial and follow-up periods. Abbreviations: ALP = alkaline phosphatase; ALT (GPT) = alanine aminotransferase (glutamic pyruvate transaminase); AST (GOT) = aspartate aminotransferase (glutamic oxaloacetic transaminase); BST = blood sugar test; BUN = blood urea nitrogen; Diff = differential; T4 = thyroxine; Hb = hemoglobin; HbA1c = hemoglobin A1c; HCT = hematocrit; HDL = high-density lipoprotein cholesterol; IFCC = International Federation of Clinical Chemistry; LDL = low-density lipoprotein cholesterol; MCH = mean corpuscular hemoglobin; MCHC = mean corpuscular hemoglobin concentration; MCV = mean cell volume; PLT = platelet; RBC = red blood cell; TG = triglyceride; TSH = thyroid-stimulating hormone; SG = specific gravity; WBC = white blood cell.

2.5. Machine Learning Analysis

First, to define which variable set will be used for the classification model, a random forest (RF) model trained by different variable combinations was tested. As described above, there are four different variable sets: clinical data and methods 1, 2, and 3 for laboratory data. RF was trained with all possible combinations of four variable sets. Because of the limitation of the sample size, the sample was divided into ten groups, and each group was used as the test set. For each test set, the remainder of the samples were divided into a training set and a validation set at a 4:1 ratio by preserving the percentage of samples for each class. Fivefold cross-validation was performed for each test set, and the final performance was defined as the average of the performance over 10 iterations [31]. The combination set of clinical data and methods 1 and 3 for laboratory data (total, 105 variables) showed the best performance in cases of classifying patients [area under the curve (AUC) = 0.8350 and accuracy = 74.85%, Table 1; therefore, the combination set was used as an input variable for model training.

Table 1. Identification of the selection of data and methods for machine learning analysis of subjects.

Feature Set Used	Lab Feature Extraction Method	Feature Counts	AUC	Accuracy (%)
Laboratory data only	Method 1	39	0.7954	73.74
	Method 2	39	0.7790	71.53
	Method 3	36	0.7226	65.32
	Method 1 + 3	75	0.8095	73.83
	Method 2 + 3	75	0.7950	72.26
	Method 1 + 2 + 3	114	0.8012	73.06
Clinical data only	-	30	0.7493	69.79
Laboratory and clinical data	Method 1	69	0.8284	76.09
	Method 2	69	0.8096	72.68
	Method 3	66	0.8100	72.98
	Method 1 + 3	105	0.8350	74.85
	Method 2 + 3	105	0.8141	73.02
	Method 1 + 2 + 3	144	0.8219	74.21

Note: method 1 = average value of each laboratory code during the follow-up period; method 2 = the first value of each laboratory code when T2DM was diagnosed initially; method 3 = the pattern of laboratory code changes (−1, 0, or 1), Abbreviations: AUC = area under the curve.

The DSPN predictor model was trained with the input variables identified above. The model performance was tested with the same method used when identifying the input variables. Three ML algorithms were used: XGBoost (XGB) [32], support vector machine (SVM) [33], and random forest (RF) [23], which were used alone or in combinations of two or more, that is, an ensemble of models for improvement of the model performance by fusion of the contents learned by different models and reduction of overfitting problems [34]. Among the various methods, the model averaging method for averaging the predicted values of several models was used in this work. AUC, accuracy, sensitivity, and specificity were used as performance metrics.

Finally, the feature importance of the best model among 7 models (XGB, SVM, RF, ensemble of XGB and SVM, ensemble of XGB & RF, ensemble of SVM and RF and ensemble of XGB and SVM and RF) was extracted from each model. If the best model was an ensemble of more than two models, the average feature importance obtained from each model was used as the feature importance of the ensemble model. Next, the models were retrained and evaluated with input features by adding features one by one, from the most to the least important. This was done to select the best set of features for DSPN prediction based on feature importance, and the performance was better when using the top 69 features for AUC and top 38 features for accuracy rather than all 105 features.

2.6. Statistics

To compare the predictability of ML results, traditional statistical methods were also carried out. All statistical analyses were performed with SPSS 26 (IBM, Armonk, NY, USA). The Shapiro-Wilk test was performed to assess the normal distribution of all quantified histological and functional data from each group. Categorical parameters were compared by likelihood ratio, and numerical parameters among groups were compared by one-way analysis of variance (ANOVA) and the Games–Howell post hoc test. Logistic regression was performed using statistically significant parameters and parameters that were identified to be important in previous studies, and the AUC, accuracy, sensitivity, and specificity were analyzed. p-values less than 0.05 were considered to indicate statistical significance.

3. Results

3.1. Baseline Characteristics among the Four Groups

When comparing baseline characteristics among the four groups, disease duration was significantly longer in the confirmed group than in the normal and possible groups (4543.18 ± 2849.75 days and 4464.03 ± 2934.87 days vs. 5686.67 ± 3648.57 days and in the normal, possible, and confirmed groups, respectively), and height was higher in the confirmed group than in the normal group (1.61 ± 0.09 m vs. 1.64 ± 0.09 m in the normal and confirmed groups, respectively). BMI and the initial values of BST and HbA1c were also different between the confirmed group and normal group and between the confirmed group and possible group (Table 2). The incidence of diabetic retinopathy was higher in the confirmed group (51.6%) than in the other groups (23.1–28.6%). Age; sex; weight; incidence of hypertension and dyslipidemia; smoking habit; past medical history of coronary artery disease, cerebrovascular disease, and stroke; and number of subjects who received diabetes education were not different among the groups (Table 2). Medications for diabetes control were different among groups; metformin (89.2–94.5%), sulfonylureas (68.1–68.8%), dipeptidyl peptidase-4 inhibitors (66.7–71.4%), and sodium-glucose cotransporter-2 inhibitors (17.2–20.9%) were used by a higher proportion of subjects in the normal and possible groups, whereas the proportion of subjects in the confirmed group who used insulin (65.6%) was higher than that in other groups (Table 2).

Table 2. Baseline characteristics of participants.

	Normal (A) (n = 93)	Possible (B) (n = 91)	Probable (C) (n = 13)	Confirmed (D) (n = 273)	p-Value	Post Hoc
Disease duration (days)	4543.18 ± 2849.75	4464.03 ± 2934.87	4933.46 ± 3463.31	5686.67 ± 3648.57	0.004	A<>D, B<>D
Age (years)	51.33 ± 12.30	49.74 ± 11.51	53.85 ± 8.92	51.32 ± 14.91	0.676	
Sex (male)	48 (51.6)	48 (52.7)	5 (38.5)	176 (64.5)	0.027	
Height (m)	1.61 ± 0.09	1.62 ± 0.09	1.59 ± 0.09	1.64 ± 0.09	0.006	A<>D
Weight (kg)	66.10 ± 11.76	66.26 ± 11.14	62.21 ± 11.41	64.29 ± 11.92	0.308	
BMI (kg/m^2)	25.33 ± 3.81	25.26 ± 3.48	24.65 ± 4.07	23.82 ± 3.66	0.001	A<>D, B<>D
Initial BST	211.78 ± 98.75	196.51 ± 87.62	178.21 ± 104.57	249.06 ± 117.68	0.000	A<>D, B<>D
Initial HbA1c	8.69 ± 2.18	8.72 ± 2.06	9.03 ± 3.09	9.59 ± 2.54	0.002	A<>D, B<>D
DM retinopathy	25 (26.9)	26 (28.6)	3 (23.1)	141 (51.6)	0.000	
Hypertension	54 (58.1)	56 (61.5)	8 (61.5)	186 (68.1)	0.304	
Dyslipidemia	76 (81.7)	70 (76.9)	10 (76.9)	197 (72.2)	0.29	
Smoking						
No	61 (65.6)	57 (62.6)	12 (92.3)	163 (59.7)		
Current	18 (19.4)	19 (20.9)	1 (7.7)	57 (20.9)	0.172	
Past smoking	14 (15.1)	15 (16.5)	0 (0.0)	53 (19.4)		
Family history of DM	28 (30.1)	51 (56.0)	4 (30.8)	106 (38.8)	0.003	
CAD Hx	25 (26.9)	24 (26.4)	6 (46.2)	93 (34.1)	0.248	
CVD Hx	43 (46.2)	33 (36.3)	6 (46.2)	134 (49.1)	0.205	

Table 2. Cont.

	Normal (A) (n = 93)	Possible (B) (n = 91)	Probable (C) (n = 13)	Confirmed (D) (n = 273)	p-Value	Post Hoc
Stroke Hx	25 (26.9)	16 (17.6)	2 (15.4)	63 (23.1)	0.427	
Diabetes education	43 (46.2)	36 (39.6)	8 (61.5)	128 (46.9)	0.412	
Medications						
Metformin	83 (89.2)	86 (94.5)	11 (84.6)	201 (73.6)	0.000	
Sulfonylureas	64 (68.8)	62 (68.1)	5 (38.5)	159 (58.2)	0.048	
TZDs	11 (11.8)	5 (5.5)	1 (7.7)	3 (13.6)	0.158	
DPP4is	62 (66.7)	65 (71.4)	8 (61.5)	147 (53.8)	0.011	
SGLT2is	16 (17.2)	19 (20.9)	1 (7.7)	21 (7.7)	0.004	
Insulin	37 (39.8)	32 (35.2)	8 (61.5)	179 (65.6)	0.000	
CCBs	32 (34.4)	26 (28.6)	7 (53.8)	104 (38.1)	0.204	
ACEis	10 (10.8)	10 (11.0)	1 (7.7)	32 (11.7)	0.965	
ARBs	51 (54.8)	54 (59.3)	7 (53.8)	156 (57.1)	0.933	
BBs	21 (22.6)	24 (26.4)	6 (46.2)	76 (27.8)	0.355	
Thiazides	15 (16.1)	20 (22.0)	2 (15.4)	47 (17.2)	0.723	
Statins	78 (83.9)	70 (76.9)	10 (76.9)	192 (70.3)	0.058	

Note: Values are presented as the mean ± standard deviation or number of subjects (%). $p < 0.05$ among the four groups by one-way ANOVA for continuous data or likelihood ratio for categorical data. Post hoc testing was performed using the Games–Howell test. Abbreviations: BMI = body mass index; BST = blood sugar test; HbA1c = hemoglobin A1c; DM = diabetes mellitus; Hx = history; CAD = coronary artery disease; CVD = cerebrovascular disease; TZDs = thiazolidinediones; DPP4is = dipeptidyl peptidase-4 inhibitors; SGLT2is = sodium-glucose cotransporter-2 inhibitors; CCBs = calcium channel blockers, ACEis = angiotensin-converting-enzyme inhibitors; ABRs = angiotensin II receptor blockers; BBs = beta blockers.

3.2. Identification of an Appropriate Classification for Prediction Using Machine Learning Analysis

Using ML algorithms, four groups of normal (A), possible (B), probable (C), and confirmed (D) samples were analyzed with various combinations. When comparing all groups separately (A vs. B vs. C vs. D) using the combined analysis of XGB and RF, the AUC was 0.8546, and the accuracy was 60.85% (Table 3). One of the classifications set to three groups (combination of A and B vs. C vs. D) showed the highest AUC value (0.8925) using the same analysis (XGB + RF); however, this classification was not appropriate because the number of group C patients was small ($n = 13$), which can result in imbalanced results [35]. When looking at the classification that combined group C with other groups, rather than alone, the classification with the combination of A, B and C vs. D showed a higher value of AUC (0.8250) than the other classifications and the highest value of accuracy (74.47%) (Table 3). Therefore, we performed all ML analyses and statistics based on this classification (A + B + C vs. D).

Table 3. Values of AUC and accuracy of machine learning analysis when comparing each group or their combinations.

Classification	ML Model Which Showed the Best Result	AUC	Accuracy (%)
A vs. B vs. C vs. D	XGB + RF	0.8546	60.85
A vs. B vs. C + D	RF	0.8105	62.34
A vs. B + C vs. D	RF	0.8075	61.32
A + B vs. C vs. D	XGB + RF	0.8925	73.40
A + B vs. C + D	RF	0.8103	72.68
A + B + C vs. D	RF	0.8250	74.47

Note: A = normal group, B = possible group, C = probable group, D = confirmed group. Abbreviations: AUC = area under the curve; XGB = XGBoost; RF = random forest; SVM = support vector machine.

3.3. Identification of an Appropriate ML Algorithm for the Prediction of DSPN and Analysis of Predictive Values

When we compared various ML techniques (XGB, SVM, RF, and their combinations), RF showed the best AUC (0.8250) and accuracy (74.47%), and the sensitivity and specificity were also higher (0.7940 and 0.6720, respectively) than those of any other single algorithm or their combination (Table 4). Logistic regression analysis was performed to compare the combination of normal, possible, and probable groups with the confirmed group using meaningful parameters of the following basic characteristics and laboratory data: disease duration, initial value of HbA1c, DM retinopathy, family history of DM, use of metformin and insulin, serum levels of glucose, HDL cholesterol, albumin, and creatinine. The results of logistic regression analysis showed lower AUC (0.6620) and specificity (0.3519) values than RF. The receiver operating characteristic (ROC) curves of each ML algorithm and logistic regression analysis are shown in Figure 3. The AUC of RF was the highest (0.8250) among the 7 ML models, as described earlier, whereas the AUC of logistic regression was the lowest AUC value (0.6620).

Table 4. Values of machine learning and logistic regression analysis using the classification of the combination of the normal, possible, and probable groups versus the confirmed group.

Model	AUC	Accuracy (%)	Sensitivity	Specificity
XGB	0.7604	69.83	0.7708	0.5899
SVM	0.7535	66.81	0.6643	0.6721
RF	0.8250	74.47	0.7940	0.6720
XGB + SVM	0.7822	71.28	0.7712	0.6363
XGB + RF	0.8235	74.47	0.7927	0.6743
SVM + RF	0.8070	73.19	0.7957	0.6478
XGB + RF + SVM	0.8105	73.62	0.8103	0.6342
Logistic regression	0.6620	84.76	0.9721	0.3519

Abbreviations: AUC = area under the curve; XGB = XGBoost; RF = random forest; SVM = support vector machine.

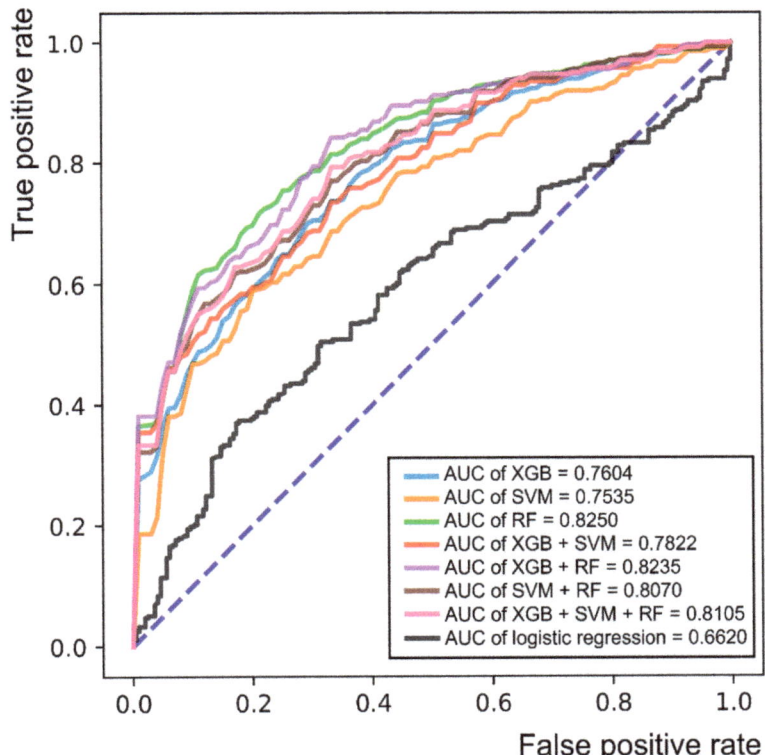

Figure 3. Receiver operating characteristic (ROC) curve for single or combinations of various machine learning algorithms and logistic regression analysis in the classification of the combination of the normal, possible, and probable groups versus the confirmed group. Abbreviations: AUC = area under the curve; XGB = XGBoost; RF = random forest; SVM = support vector machine.

3.4. Development of a Decision-Making Model Using Influential Features from the RF Algorithm

RF analysis using the classification of the combination of the normal, possible, and probable groups versus the confirmed group was used to derive influential features, which consisted of clinical data and methods 1 and 3 for laboratory data. When these features are accumulated in the order of the importance score, the AUC and accuracy increase and then reach a maximum value at a certain moment (Figure 4a,b). In the case of AUC, the maximum value was reached when the number of parameters reached 69 (0.8302), and in the case of accuracy, the maximum value was reached when the number of parameters was 38 (76.17%) (Figure 4a,b). From this classification, the average value of HbA1c was identified as the first single discriminator for group determination between the combination of the normal, possible, and probable groups and the confirmed group (Figure 4c). The top 69 influential features are shown in Table 5. The average serum glucose level during the follow-up period was the most important feature (importance score = 0.997768) for determining the group in the classification, and the average values of the International Federation of Clinical Chemistry (IFCC; 0.794161), HbA1c (0.789265), and albumin levels (0.731579) during the follow-up period are shown in order of importance score (Table 5).

Table 5. Top 69 influential features in the classification of the combination of the normal, possible, and probable groups versus the confirmed group.

Ranking	Feature Name	Importance Score	Ranking	Feature Name	Importance Score
1	Avg glucose	0.997768	36	Avg WBC	0.280162
2	Avg IFCC	0.794161	37	Avg PLT	0.262754
3	Avg HbA1c	0.789265	38	Avg chloride	0.250326
4	Avg albumin	0.731579	39	Avg uric acid	0.246706
5	Height	0.57069	40	CP IFCC	0.246499
6	Avg Diff count (lymphocyte %)	0.546759	41	CP creatinine (spot urine)	0.242497
7	Avg creatinine (spot urine)	0.493981	42	Avg MCV	0.240183
8	Avg Diff count (neutrophil %)	0.486409	43	Avg Diff count (eosinophil%)	0.237532
9	Disease duration	0.467576	44	Avg MCH	0.229848
10	Avg sodium	0.455435	45	Avg Diff count (monocyte %)	0.225926
11	Avg HCT	0.451166	46	CP HbA1c	0.225847
12	Avg ALT (GPT)	0.450865	47	Avg MCHC	0.222184
13	Avg RBC	0.417525	48	Avg bilirubin	0.217108
14	Avg Hb	0.383685	49	Avg free T4	0.208568
15	BMI	0.375055	50	CP urine SG	0.204239
16	Avg HDL	0.374211	51	Avg Diff count (basophil %)	0.201151
17	Avg BUN	0.351033	52	Diabetic retinopathy	0.176286
18	Avg AST (GOT)	0.348776	53	CP TG	0.155261
19	Avg ALP	0.342055	54	Use of insulin	0.14617
20	Avg BST	0.33438	55	CP HDL	0.146164
21	Avg creatinine	0.332449	56	CP cholesterol	0.127665
22	Age	0.319338	57	CP WBC	0.096003
23	Avg urine pH	0.31512	58	CP PLT	0.09567
24	Avg calcium	0.309396	59	Sex	0.084762
25	Avg TG	0.307935	60	CP BST	0.083089
26	Avg LDL	0.305571	61	CP ALP	0.080399
27	Avg TSH	0.303504	62	Smoking	0.068729
28	Avg protein	0.302998	63	CP creatinine	0.065407
29	CP glucose	0.297945	64	CP Diff count (lymphocyte %)	0.065285
30	CP urine pH	0.290718	65	CP bilirubin	0.060325
31	Avg cholesterol	0.287416	66	Use of sulfonylurea	0.05838
32	Avg potassium	0.286635	67	CP AST (GOT)	0.052956
33	Weight	0.285151	68	CP ALT (GPT)	0.050693
34	Avg urine SG	0.282845	69	Use of metformin	0.048544
35	CP LDL	0.280875			

Abbreviations: Avg = average; IFCC = International Federation of Clinical Chemistry; HbA1c = hemoglobin A1c; Diff = differential; HCT = hematocrit; ALT (GPT) = alanine aminotransferase (glutamic pyruvate transaminase); BST = blood sugar test; RBC = red blood cell; Hb = Hemoglobin; BMI= body mass index; HDL = high-density lipoprotein cholesterol; BUN = blood urea nitrogen; AST (GOT) = aspartate aminotransferase (glutamic oxaloacetic transaminase); ALP = alkaline phosphatase; TG = triglyceride; LDL = low-density lipoprotein cholesterol; TSH = thyroid-stimulating hormone; CP = change pattern; SG = specific gravity; WBC = white blood cell; PLT = platelet; MCV = mean cell volume; MCH = mean corpuscular hemoglobin; MCHC = mean corpuscular hemoglobin concentration; T4 = thyroxine.

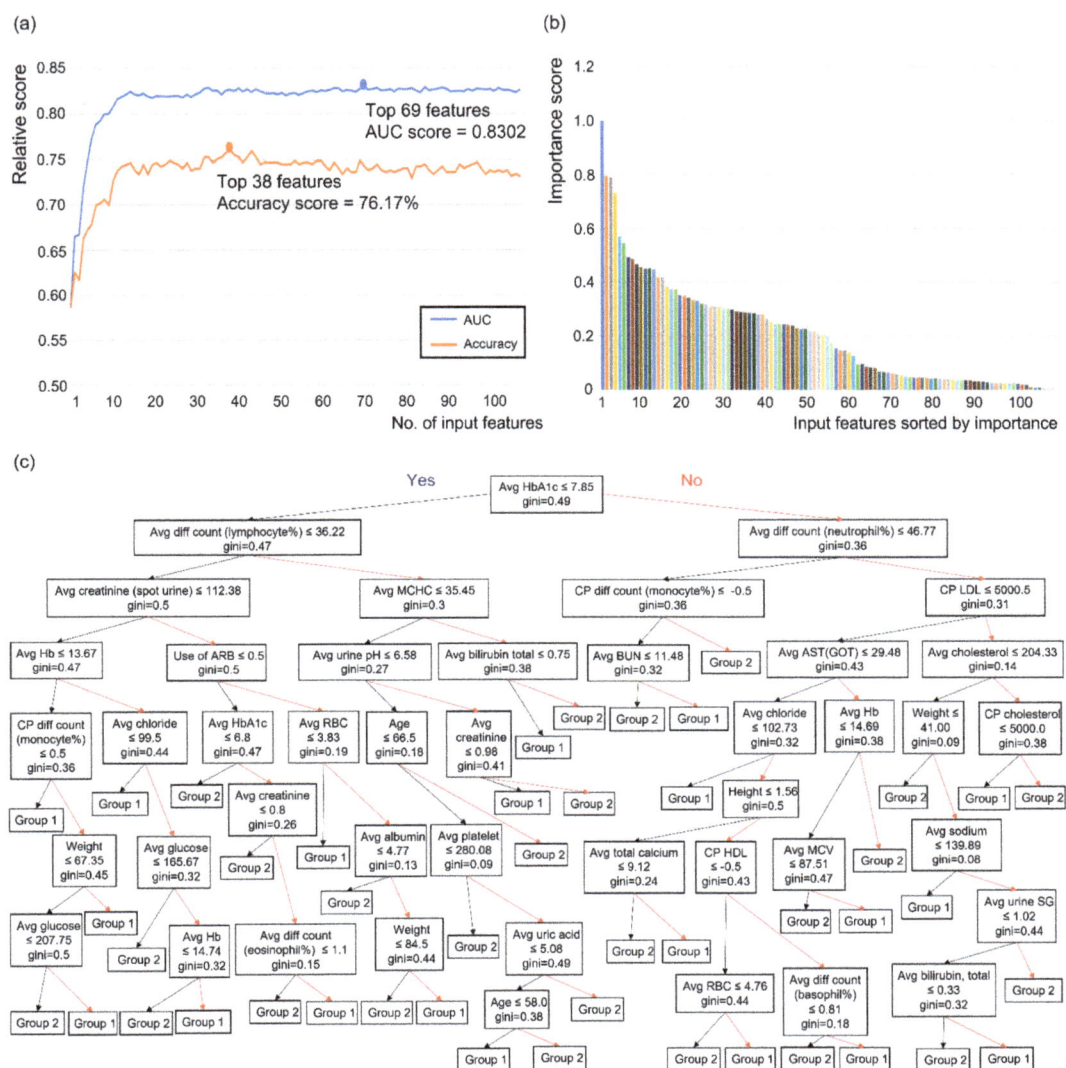

Figure 4. Application of random forest algorithm and process of extraction of important features in the classification of the combination of the normal, possible, and probable groups versus the confirmed group. (**a**) Model performance according to the number of input features sorted by importance, (**b**) the result of arranging input features in order of importance score, (**c**) a decision tree using the random forest algorithm with the classification of the combination of the normal, possible, and probable groups versus the confirmed group. Note: Group 1 = a group in which the normal, possible, and probable groups are combined, Group 2 = the confirmed group. Black arrow = positive results for the above features, red arrow = negative results for the above features, gini = gini index. Abbreviations: AUC = area under the curve; ALP = alkaline phosphatase; ALT (GPT) = alanine aminotransferase (glutamic pyruvate transaminase); AST (GOT) = aspartate aminotransferase (glutamic oxaloacetic transaminase); Avg = average; BST = blood sugar test; BUN = blood urea nitrogen; CP = change pattern; Diff = differential; T4 = thyroxine; Hb = hemoglobin; HbA1c = hemoglobin A1c; HCT = hematocrit; HDL = high-density lipoprotein cholesterol; IFCC = International Federation of Clinical Chemistry; LDL = low-density lipoprotein cholesterol; MCH = mean corpuscular hemoglobin; MCHC = mean corpuscular hemoglobin concentration; MCV = mean cell volume; PLT = platelet; RBC = red blood cell; TG = triglyceride; TSH = thyroid-stimulating hormone; SG = specific gravity; WBC = white blood cell.

3.5. ML Analysis of the Confirmed Group to Identify Demyelinated and Mixed Types of DSPN

We compared the demyelinated subgroup with the mixed subgroup, as shown in electrophysiological studies of the confirmed group, using various ML algorithms and logistic regression analysis (Table 6). ML analysis revealed that the combination of XGB and SVM models showed the highest AUC and accuracy values of 0.5698 and 67.78%, respectively, whereas the statistical method using logistic regression showed a higher AUC value (0.6350). However, the overall AUC values of all ML algorithms and logistic regression analysis were much lower than the AUC value (0.8250) when RF was used to compare the combination of the normal, possible, and probable groups versus the confirmed group, and the specificity was quite low (0 and 0.3889 for RF and logistic regression, respectively) to predict the two subgroups within the confirmed group (Table 6).

Table 6. Machine learning and logistic regression results analyzing the demyelinated type vs. mixed type.

Model	AUC	Accuracy (%)	Sensitivity	Specificity
XGB	0.5492	62.39	0.8329	0.1797
SVM	0.5105	68.15	1.0000	0.0000
RF	0.5426	64.25	0.9245	0.0436
XGB + SVM	0.5698	67.78	0.9947	0.0000
XGB + RF	0.5579	64.52	0.9317	0.0378
SVM + RF	0.5457	67.41	0.9889	0.0000
XGB + RF + SVM	0.5601	67.41	0.9897	0.0000
Logistic regression	0.6350	70.97	0.8812	0.3889

Abbreviations: AUC = area under the curve; XGB = XGBoost; RF = random forest; SVM = support vector machine.

4. Discussion

Interest in machine learning algorithms is widely increasing in the medical field because they can be used to predict disease development and generate semantic interpretations [36]. In the field of endocrinology, the prediction of diabetes is expected to be very useful for preventing disease progression and complications [37]. In this study, we have performed conventional statistics, as well as various ML algorithms to compare predictive power expressed in AUC and accuracy. Logistic regression analysis, a traditional statistical method, has an obvious limitation compared to the ML analysis. Only a small number of clinical and laboratory data (9 variables among over 400 data) were used during the statistical processing, which inevitably resulted in poor AUC whereas ML analysis could include over 100 meaningful data. Classical statistics usually draw population inferences, but become less precise when input variables that exceed the number of subjects, therefore appropriate ML method can help overcome this limitation [22].

As in all other fields, for the results of ML analysis to be more accurate, the input data must have extensive and accurate information. Laboratory data are usually obtained numerous times for a single subject during the follow-up period, and effective processing of meaningful data can have a significant impact on the establishment of predictive models. In this study, we tried various methods to optimize input data during the preprocessing step, especially for standardization of laboratory tests conducted at various time points. First, from the 432 types of laboratory data received for all patients, only 39 datapoints repeatedly obtained for more than half of all patients were filtered out. Then, depending on the timing of the laboratory data received, data were classified into average, initial, and change patterns of each value, and we found that average and changed patterns were meaningful parameters for ML analysis. Through these preprocesses, we are confident that we have increased the reliability of laboratory data and created a more accurate predictive model. When compared to previous studies that made predictive models of DSPN using ML algorithms in diabetic patients (Table 7), they did not explain what time point was used or whether there was any consideration of the amount of change in the laboratory data in addition to the data imputation process that handles missing data [24,25,27,38]. In addition, they did not provide any diagnostic tools, such as decision tree or nomogram, except Dagliati et al. [25].

Table 7. Comparison of previous studies that used machine learning algorithms to predict DPSN in type 2 diabetes mellitus patients.

References	Criteria to Diagnose DSPN	Suggested ML Models	AUC/Accuracy	Laboratory Data Processing	Providing Decision-Making Tool
Kazemi et al., 2016 [24]	clinical (T1DM and T2DM)	MSVM	UC/0.76	UC	N
Dagliati et al., 2018 [25]	UC	LR	0.726/0.746	UC	nomogram
Fan et al., 2021 [27]	UC	EM	0.847/0.783	UC	N
Maeda-Gutierrez et al., 2021 [38]	clinical	RF	0.65/UC	UC	N
Current study	electrophysiological	RF	0.825/0.7447	average/change pattern	decision tree

Abbreviations: ML = machine learning, AUC = area under the curve; MSVM = multicategory support vector machine; LR = logistic regression; EM = ensemble model; RF = random forest; UC = uncheckable; N = none.

Various criteria for defining DSPN have been developed, and many of them have been designed to classify the severity of DSPN based on clinical signs and symptoms alone [39] or in combination with physical examination [40,41] or electrophysiological findings [7,10]. Neurological signs, especially sensory abnormalities, are sensitive and specific findings for diagnosing DSPN and have been correlated with electrophysiological findings in previous studies [12,42,43]; however, we found that clinical data alone, which was categorized as normal, possible and probable groups defined in a previous study [7], was not effective in predicting DSPN in T2DM patients. Other studies have revealed that clinical symptoms and signs are too variable and inaccurate [44] and do not correlate well with the development of pathophysiological changes in the peripheral nervous system [13]. On the basis of our results, we confirmed that severity grading based on clinical symptoms and signs is not helpful and that electrophysiological assessment is essential in predicting DSPN. However, small fiber involvement, which is frequently occurs in early DSPN, is not identified by conventional NCS. Therefore, more specialized diagnostic tools such as quantitative sensory testing, skin biopsy, and corneal confocal microscopy are needed to identify small fiber damage [45,46].

We failed to classify the demyelinated and mixed types in the confirmed group in this study. Axonal involvement is frequently observed in DSPN, as is demyelination [17], and even axonal loss, which precedes demyelination, in sural nerves or plantar nerves of DSPN patients might be a primary finding [47,48]. Electrophysiological analysis, which shows decreased conduction velocity of sensory and motor nerves, decreased compound muscle action potential, and prolonged latency of F-wave, is considered to be highly sensitive for early diagnosis of DSPN [16,49], but NSC cannot be used to assess therapeutic effects in diabetic patients [49]. Electromyography can be useful for detecting abnormal spontaneous activities in distal muscles in moderate to severe DSPN [50], although this test is also useful for ruling out other neuropathies, such as radiculopathies, mononeuropathies, or myopathies. In this study, we could not find axonal involvement without demyelination within DSPN patients. In T2DM, segmental demyelination is prominent with a milder axonal involvement whereas axonal loss is more severe in T1DM [51,52]. Initially, we considered abnormal electromyographic findings with abnormal NCS (mixed type) to be advanced or severe type DSPN, and diabetic patients with mixed type DSPN might show abnormal clinical and laboratory findings more frequently than those with demyelinated type DSPN. However, ML analysis and logistic regression did not effectively suggest any difference between the demyelinated and mixed types. Therefore, electrophysiological analysis is necessary to differentiate these two types of diabetic patients.

Numerous ML algorithms have been used to predict DM and diabetic complications such as retinopathy, nephropathy, foot ulceration and DSPN [24–29]. XGB is a scalable end-to-end tree boosting system [32] and is more suitable for small sample sizes unless the data are not highly dispersed when predicting glucose variability in T2DM patients [53]. SVM was used for microarray or high-dimensional data and is suitable for predicting DSPN in DM patients with a clinical data-based classification [24] and distinguishing retinopathy between diabetic patients and normal controls [26]. RF is an ensemble of decision trees and can minimize the individual error of trees [23]. RF has shown good performance in predicting the development and classification of DSPN based on clinical symptoms and examinations of type 1 diabetic patients [29]. Logistic regression analysis is a common statistical method used to develop a model for binary outcomes in the medical field [54] and can also be used as a supervised learning technique in ML methods. Even though various ML algorithms have been successfully developed as predictive models for the purpose of preventing the occurrence of diseases or their complications, some recent studies have shown that logistic regression has similar results to ML analysis [55,56], and attempts to combine logistic regression and ML methods also appear to enhance the performance of statistical methods in an automated manner [57]. In our study, the AUC of RF was superior to that of logistic regression when subjects were classified into two groups: confirmed vs. other combinations (Table 4), but the AUC of logistic regression was higher than that of ML algorithms for comparison between the demyelinated and mixed subgroups within the confirmed group (Table 6). The development of proper hybrid models for statistical and ML algorithms might increase the power of DSPN prediction in future studies.

In previous studies, numerous predisposing factors have been associated with DSPN in diabetic patients, particularly, duration of diabetes and HbA1c in T2DM patients [21,58]; moreover, old age, increased height, obesity, higher body mass index, poor glucose control, alcohol abuse, smoking, hypertension, cardiovascular disease, low level of HDL, dyslipidemia, hypertriglyceridemia, and microalbuminuria have also been shown to be risk factors in previous studies [18–21,58–61]. We found that the average values of numerous laboratory datapoints during the follow-up period (serum glucose, IFCC, HbA1c, albumin, and differential counts of lymphocytes and neutrophils) were important predisposing factors, as were clinical data such as height and disease duration (Table 5). The albumin has important antioxidant and anti-inflammatory properties, and the lower level of serum albumin was associated with the prevalence of DSPN or peripheral nerve dysfunctions in T2DM patients in previous studies [62,63] In our study, average value of HbA1c is the most sensitive node of a decision tree among the influence features, and average differential counts of lymphocytes and neutrophils are the second node (Figure 4c). Although there is no standardized decision-making algorithm for DSPN diagnosis, HbA1c qualifies as an important diagnostic criterion for DPSN because HbA1c a major risk factor for microvascular complications and closely associated with DSPN in T2DM [64] The neutrophil-lymphocyte ratio is an inflammatory marker and an important factor that predicts cardiovascular disease [65] and foot ulcer infection [66] in diabetic patients. Neutrophil level was also the most sensitive node for decision making of DPSN prediction in a previous study [67], and higher neutrophil-lymphocyte ratio might be related to chronic inflammatory process and increase the risk of DSPN [68].

In this study, we analyzed a small-sized sample, especially the probable group ($n = 13$), which might cause problems for pattern recognition and poor accuracy [69]. Many studies in the medical field often have only a small number of patients. In this study, we tried to increase the accuracy by dividing the patients into ten groups for use as a test set and a tenfold stratified cross validation set to compensate for the small sample size [31], but a more accurate prediction might be achieved with a larger number of diabetic patients. We further plan to perform ML analysis to predict various complications in diabetic patients in a prospective multicenter study and develop an application attached to an existing electronic health record system for easier transfer of patient data that can assist in predicting complications in diabetic patients. In addition, it was difficult to use deep learning model because insufficient sample size can lead to overfitting. If sufficient data is accumulated, it is possible to build deep learning model using time-series laboratory data or to apply a method of transfer learning with DSPN patient using pre-trained models for all diabetic patients.

5. Conclusions

In this study, we revealed that the ML algorithms, whose AUC values were superior to logistic regression, can be applied to type 2 DM patients to predict DSPN and that the classification depending only on clinical symptoms and signs of suspected DSPN was not appropriate for the application of ML algorithms to develop prediction models. In addition, ML algorithms cannot predict the type of electrophysiological features in DSPN, namely, demyelinated and mixed subgroups. We concluded that ML techniques, especially RF, can predict DSPN effectively when comparing the combination of the normal, possible, and probable groups with the confirmed group of DM patients and that electrophysiological analysis is important for identifying DSPN.

Author Contributions: Conceptualization, J.K.H.; data curation, D.Y.S., W.S.Y. and J.W.P.; formal analysis, D.Y.S., B.L., W.S.Y., J.W.P. and J.K.H.; funding acquisition, J.K.H.; investigation, D.Y.S., B.L. and J.K.H.; methodology, D.Y.S., B.L. and J.K.H.; project administration, J.K.H.; resources, W.S.Y. and J.W.P.; software, D.Y.S. and B.L.; supervision, J.K.H.; validation, D.Y.S., B.L. and J.K.H.; visualization, B.L. and J.K.H.; writing—original draft, D.Y.S., B.L. and J.K.H.; writing—review and editing, D.Y.S. and J.K.H. All authors have read and agreed to the published version of the manuscript.

Funding: This study was supported by grants (2019R1A6A1A11034536, 2020R1A2C2004764) through the National Research Foundation (NRF) and Ministry of Science and ICT (MSIT) and a Korea Medical Device Development Fund grant (202017D01) funded by the Korean government (MSIT, the Ministry of Trade, Industry and Energy, the Ministry of Health & Welfare, and the Ministry of Food and Drug Safety).

Institutional Review Board Statement: The study was conducted according to the guidelines of the Declaration of Helsinki and approved by the Institutional Review Board of Dankook University Hospital (IRB No. 2019-12-009).

Informed Consent Statement: Not applicable.

Data Availability Statement: The data presented in this study are available from the corresponding author upon reasonable request.

Conflicts of Interest: Bora Lee is an employee of Deargen, Co., Ltd., Daejeon 34051, Korea.

References

1. Center for Disease Control and Prevention. National diabetes statistics report, 2020. In *Atlanta, GA: Centers for Disease Control and Prevention, US Department of Health and Human Services*; Center for Disease Control and Prevention: Atlanta, GA, USA, 2020; pp. 12–15.
2. Mohamadi, A.; Cooke, D.W. Type 2 diabetes mellitus in children and adolescents. *Adolesc. Med. State Art Rev.* **2010**, *21*, 103–119. [PubMed]
3. Russell, J.W.; Zilliox, L.A. Diabetic neuropathies. *Continuum* **2014**, *20*, 1226–1240. [CrossRef]
4. Feldman, E.L.; Callaghan, B.C.; Pop-Busui, R.; Zochodne, D.W.; Wright, D.E.; Bennett, D.L.; Bril, V.; Russell, J.W.; Viswanathan, V. Diabetic neuropathy. *Nat. Rev. Dis. Primers* **2019**, *5*, 41. [CrossRef] [PubMed]
5. Sloan, G.; Selvarajah, D.; Tesfaye, S. Pathogenesis, diagnosis and clinical management of diabetic sensorimotor peripheral neuropathy. *Nat. Rev. Endocrinol.* **2021**, *17*, 400–420. [CrossRef]
6. Kaku, M.; Vinik, A.; Simpson, D.M. Pathways in the diagnosis and management of diabetic polyneuropathy. *Curr. Diabetes Rep.* **2015**, *15*, 609. [CrossRef] [PubMed]
7. Tesfaye, S.; Boulton, A.J.; Dyck, P.J.; Freeman, R.; Horowitz, M.; Kempler, P.; Lauria, G.; Malik, R.A.; Spallone, V.; Vinik, A.; et al. Diabetic neuropathies: Update on definitions, diagnostic criteria, estimation of severity, and treatments. *Diabetes Care* **2010**, *33*, 2285–2293. [CrossRef]
8. Thomas, P.K. Classification, differential diagnosis, and staging of diabetic peripheral neuropathy. *Diabetes* **1997**, *46*, S54–S57. [CrossRef]
9. Boulton, A.J.; Vinik, A.I.; Arezzo, J.C.; Bril, V.; Feldman, E.L.; Freeman, R.; Malik, R.A.; Maser, R.E.; Sosenko, J.M.; Ziegler, D.; et al. Diabetic neuropathies: A statement by the American Diabetes Association. *Diabetes Care* **2005**, *28*, 956–962. [CrossRef]

10. England, J.D.; Gronseth, G.S.; Franklin, G.; Miller, R.G.; Asbury, A.K.; Carter, G.T.; Cohen, J.A.; Fisher, M.A.; Howard, J.F.; Kinsella, L.J.; et al. Distal symmetrical polyneuropathy: A definition for clinical research. A report of the American Academy of Neurology, the American Association of Electrodiagnostic Medicine, and the American Academy of Physical Medicine and Rehabilitation. *Arch. Phys. Med. Rehabil.* **2005**, *86*, 167–174. [CrossRef]
11. Dyck, P.J.; Kratz, K.M.; Karnes, J.L.; Litchy, W.J.; Klein, R.; Pach, J.M.; Wilson, D.M.; O'Brien, P.C.; Melton, L.J., 3rd. The prevalence by staged severity of various types of diabetic neuropathy, retinopathy, and nephropathy in a population-based cohort: The Rochester Diabetic Neuropathy Study. *Neurology* **1993**, *43*, 817–824. [CrossRef]
12. Meijer, J.W.; Bosma, E.; Lefrandt, J.D.; Links, T.P.; Smit, A.J.; Stewart, R.E.; van der Hoeven, J.H.; Hoogenberg, K. Clinical diagnosis of diabetic polyneuropathy with the diabetic neuropathy symptom and diabetic neuropathy examination scores. *Diabetes Care* **2003**, *26*, 697–701. [CrossRef]
13. Himeno, T.; Kamiya, H.; Nakamura, J. Lumos for the long trail: Strategies for clinical diagnosis and severity staging for diabetic polyneuropathy and future directions. *J. Diabetes Investig.* **2020**, *11*, 5–16. [CrossRef]
14. Bril, V.; Perkins, B.A. Validation of the Toronto clinical scoring system for diabetic polyneuropathy. *Diabetes Care* **2002**, *25*, 2048–2052. [CrossRef]
15. American Diabetes Association. Standards of medical care in diabetes—2016 abridged for primary care providers. *Clin. Diabetes A Publ. Am. Diabetes Assoc.* **2016**, *34*, 3. [CrossRef] [PubMed]
16. England, J.D.; Gronseth, G.S.; Franklin, G.; Miller, R.G.; Asbury, A.K.; Carter, G.T.; Cohen, J.A.; Fisher, M.A.; Howard, J.F.; Kinsella, L.J.; et al. Distal symmetric polyneuropathy: A definition for clinical research: Report of the American Academy of Neurology, the American Association of Electrodiagnostic Medicine, and the American Academy of Physical Medicine and Rehabilitation. *Neurology* **2005**, *64*, 199–207. [CrossRef] [PubMed]
17. Pasnoor, M.; Dimachkie, M.M.; Kluding, P.; Barohn, R.J. Diabetic neuropathy part 1: Overview and symmetric phenotypes. *Neurol. Clin.* **2013**, *31*, 425–445. [CrossRef] [PubMed]
18. Tesfaye, S.; Stevens, L.K.; Stephenson, J.M.; Fuller, J.H.; Plater, M.; Ionescu-Tirgoviste, C.; Nuber, A.; Pozza, G.; Ward, J.D. Prevalence of diabetic peripheral neuropathy and its relation to glycaemic control and potential risk factors: The EURODIAB IDDM Complications Study. *Diabetologia* **1996**, *39*, 1377–1384. [CrossRef] [PubMed]
19. Adler, A.I.; Boyko, E.J.; Ahroni, J.H.; Stensel, V.; Forsberg, R.C.; Smith, D.G. Risk factors for diabetic peripheral sensory neuropathy. Results of the Seattle Prospective Diabetic Foot Study. *Diabetes Care* **1997**, *20*, 1162–1167. [CrossRef] [PubMed]
20. Adler, A. Risk factors for diabetic neuropathy and foot ulceration. *Curr. Diabetes Rep.* **2001**, *1*, 202–207. [CrossRef]
21. Tesfaye, S.; Chaturvedi, N.; Eaton, S.E.; Ward, J.D.; Manes, C.; Ionescu-Tirgoviste, C.; Witte, D.R.; Fuller, J.H.; EURODIAB Prospective Complications Study Group. Vascular risk factors and diabetic neuropathy. *N. Engl. J. Med.* **2005**, *352*, 341–350. [CrossRef] [PubMed]
22. Bzdok, D.; Altman, N.; Krzywinski, M. Statistics versus machine learning. *Nat. Methods* **2018**, *15*, 233–234. [CrossRef]
23. Breiman, L. Random forests. *Mach. Learn.* **2001**, *45*, 5–32. [CrossRef]
24. Kazemi, M.; Moghimbeigi, A.; Kiani, J.; Mahjub, H.; Faradmal, J. Diabetic peripheral neuropathy class prediction by multicategory support vector machine model: A cross-sectional study. *Epidemiol. Health* **2016**, *38*, e2016011. [CrossRef] [PubMed]
25. Dagliati, A.; Marini, S.; Sacchi, L.; Cogni, G.; Teliti, M.; Tibollo, V.; de Cata, P.; Chiovato, L.; Bellazzi, R. Machine learning methods to predict diabetes complications. *J. Diabetes Sci. Technol.* **2018**, *12*, 295–302. [CrossRef]
26. Tsao, H.Y.; Chan, P.Y.; Su, E.C.Y. Predicting diabetic retinopathy and identifying interpretable biomedical features using machine learning algorithms. *BMC Bioinform.* **2018**, *19*, 283. [CrossRef]
27. Fan, Y.; Long, E.; Cai, L.; Cao, Q.; Wu, X.; Tong, R. Machine learning approaches to predict risks of diabetic complications and poor glycemic control in nonadherent type 2 diabetes. *Front. Pharmacol.* **2021**, *12*, 665951. [CrossRef] [PubMed]
28. Schafer, Z.; Mathisen, A.; Svendsen, K.; Engberg, S.; Rolighed Thomsen, T.; Kirketerp-Moller, K. Toward machine-learning-based decision support in diabetes care: A risk stratification study on diabetic foot ulcer and amputation. *Front. Med.* **2020**, *7*, 601602. [CrossRef] [PubMed]
29. Haque, F.; Bin Ibne Reaz, M.; Chowdhury, M.E.H.; Srivastava, G.; Md Ali, S.H.; Bakar, A.A.A.; Bhuiyan, M.A.S. Performance analysis of conventional machine learning algorithms for diabetic sensorimotor polyneuropathy severity classification. *Diagnostics* **2021**, *11*, 801. [CrossRef]
30. American Diabetes Association. Classification and diagnosis of diabetes: Standards of medical care in diabetes-2020. *Diabetes Care* **2020**, *43*, S14–S31. [CrossRef]
31. Kohavi, R. A study of cross-validation and bootstrap for accuracy estimation and model selection. In *IJCAI*; Morgan Kaufmann: Burlington, MA, USA, 1995; pp. 1137–1145.
32. Chen, T.; Guestrin, C. Xgboost: A scalable tree boosting system. In Proceedings of the 22nd ACM SIGKDD International Conference on Knowledge Discovery and Data Mining, San Francisco, CA, USA, 13–17 August 2016; Association for Computing Machinery: New York, NY, USA; pp. 785–794.
33. Hearst, M.A.; Dumais, S.T.; Osuna, E.; Platt, J.; Scholkopf, B. Support vector machines. *IEEE Intell. Syst. Appl.* **1998**, *13*, 18–28. [CrossRef]
34. Sagi, O.; Rokach, L. Ensemble learning: A survey. *Wiley Interdiscip. Rev. Data Min. Knowl. Discov.* **2018**, *8*, e1249. [CrossRef]
35. Drummond, C.; Holte, R.C. Severe class imbalance: Why better algorithms aren't the answer. In *European Conference on Machine Learning*; Springer: Berlin, Germany, 2005; pp. 539–546.

36. Ravi, D.; Wong, C.; Deligianni, F.; Berthelot, M.; Andreu-Perez, J.; Lo, B.; Yang, G.Z. Deep learning for health informatics. *IEEE J. Biomed. Health Inform.* **2017**, *21*, 4–21. [CrossRef]
37. Kavakiotis, I.; Tsave, O.; Salifoglou, A.; Maglaveras, N.; Vlahavas, I.; Chouvarda, I. Machine learning and data mining methods in diabetes research. *Comput. Struct. Biotechnol. J.* **2017**, *15*, 104–116. [CrossRef]
38. Maeda-Gutierrez, V.; Galvan-Tejada, C.E.; Cruz, M.; Valladares-Salgado, A.; Galvan-Tejada, J.I.; Gamboa-Rosales, H.; Garcia-Hernandez, A.; Luna-Garcia, H.; Gonzalez-Curiel, I.; Martinez-Acuna, M. Distal symmetric polyneuropathy identification in type 2 diabetes subjects: A random forest approach. *Healthcare* **2021**, *9*, 138. [CrossRef]
39. Meijer, J.W.; Smit, A.J.; Sonderen, E.V.; Groothoff, J.W.; Eisma, W.H.; Links, T.P. Symptom scoring systems to diagnose distal polyneuropathy in diabetes: The diabetic neuropathy symptom score. *Diabet. Med.* **2002**, *19*, 962–965. [CrossRef]
40. Feldman, E.L.; Stevens, M.J.; Thomas, P.K.; Brown, M.B.; Canal, N.; Greene, D.A. A practical two-step quantitative clinical and electrophysiological assessment for the diagnosis and staging of diabetic neuropathy. *Diabetes Care* **1994**, *17*, 1281–1289. [CrossRef]
41. Perkins, B.A.; Olaleye, D.; Zinman, B.; Bril, V. Simple screening tests for peripheral neuropathy in the diabetes clinic. *Diabetes Care* **2001**, *24*, 250–256. [CrossRef] [PubMed]
42. Abraham, A.; Alabdali, M.; Alsulaiman, A.; Albulaihe, H.; Breiner, A.; Katzberg, H.D.; Aljaafari, D.; Lovblom, L.E.; Bril, V. The sensitivity and specificity of the neurological examination in polyneuropathy patients with clinical and electrophysiological correlations. *PLoS ONE* **2017**, *12*, e0171597. [CrossRef] [PubMed]
43. Franse, L.V.; Valk, G.D.; Dekker, J.H.; Heine, R.J.; van Eijk, J.T. 'Numbness of the feet' is a poor indicator for polyneuropathy in Type 2 diabetic patients. *Diabet. Med.* **2000**, *17*, 105–110. [CrossRef] [PubMed]
44. Dyck, P.J.; Overland, C.J.; Low, P.A.; Litchy, W.J.; Davies, J.L.; Dyck, P.J.; O'Brien, P.C.; Cl vs. NPhys Trial Investigators; Albers, J.W.; Andersen, H.; et al. Signs and symptoms versus nerve conduction studies to diagnose diabetic sensorimotor polyneuropathy: Cl vs. NPhys. trial. *Muscle Nerve* **2010**, *42*, 157–164. [CrossRef]
45. Chen, X.; Graham, J.; Dabbah, M.A.; Petropoulos, I.N.; Ponirakis, G.; Asghar, O.; Alam, U.; Marshall, A.; Fadavi, H.; Ferdousi, M.; et al. Small nerve fiber quantification in the diagnosis of diabetic sensorimotor polyneuropathy: Comparing corneal confocal microscopy with intraepidermal nerve fiber density. *Diabetes Care* **2015**, *38*, 1138–1144. [CrossRef] [PubMed]
46. Javed, S.; Petropoulos, I.N.; Tavakoli, M.; Malik, R.A. Clinical and diagnostic features of small fiber damage in diabetic polyneuropathy. *Handb. Clin. Neurol.* **2014**, *126*, 275–290. [CrossRef] [PubMed]
47. Dyck, P.J.; Lais, A.; Karnes, J.L.; O'Brien, P.; Rizza, R. Fiber loss is primary and multifocal in sural nerves in diabetic polyneuropathy. *Ann. Neurol.* **1986**, *19*, 425–439. [CrossRef]
48. Galiero, R.; Ricciardi, D.; Pafundi, P.C.; Todisco, V.; Tedeschi, G.; Cirillo, G.; Sasso, F.C. Whole plantar nerve conduction study: A new tool for early diagnosis of peripheral diabetic neuropathy. *Diabetes Res. Clin. Pract.* **2021**, *176*, 108856. [CrossRef]
49. Petropoulos, I.N.; Ponirakis, G.; Khan, A.; Almuhannadi, H.; Gad, H.; Malik, R.A. Diagnosing diabetic neuropathy: Something old, something new. *Diabetes Metab. J.* **2018**, *42*, 255–269. [CrossRef]
50. Perkins, B.; Bril, V. Electrophysiologic testing in diabetic neuropathy. *Handb. Clin. Neurol.* **2014**, *126*, 235–248. [CrossRef]
51. Sima, A.A.; Zhang, W. Mechanisms of diabetic neuropathy: Axon dysfunction. *Handb. Clin. Neurol.* **2014**, *126*, 429–442. [CrossRef]
52. Sima, A.A.; Kamiya, H. Diabetic neuropathy differs in type 1 and type 2 diabetes. *Ann. N. Y. Acad. Sci.* **2006**, *1084*, 235–249. [CrossRef]
53. Elhadd, T.; Mall, R.; Bashir, M.; Palotti, J.; Fernandez-Luque, L.; Farooq, F.; Mohanadi, D.A.; Dabbous, Z.; Malik, R.A.; Abou-Samra, A.B.; et al. Artificial Intelligence (AI) based machine learning models predict glucose variability and hypoglycaemia risk in patients with type 2 diabetes on a multiple drug regimen who fast during ramadan (The PROFAST—IT Ramadan study). *Diabetes Res. Clin. Pract.* **2020**, *169*, 108388. [CrossRef]
54. Kleinbaum, D.G.; Klein, M. Introduction to logistic regression. In *Logistic Regression*; Springer: New York, NY, USA, 2010; pp. 1–39. [CrossRef]
55. Panesar, S.S.; D'Souza, R.N.; Yeh, F.C.; Fernandez-Miranda, J.C. Machine learning versus logistic regression methods for 2-year mortality prognostication in a small, heterogeneous glioma database. *World Neurosurg. X* **2019**, *2*, 100012. [CrossRef] [PubMed]
56. Lynam, A.L.; Dennis, J.M.; Owen, K.R.; Oram, R.A.; Jones, A.G.; Shields, B.M.; Ferrat, L.A. Logistic regression has similar performance to optimised machine learning algorithms in a clinical setting: Application to the discrimination between type 1 and type 2 diabetes in young adults. *Diagn. Progn. Res.* **2020**, *4*, 6. [CrossRef]
57. Levy, J.J.; O'Malley, A.J. Don't dismiss logistic regression: The case for sensible extraction of interactions in the era of machine learning. *BMC Med. Res. Methodol.* **2020**, *20*, 171. [CrossRef]
58. Liu, X.; Xu, Y.; An, M.; Zeng, Q. The risk factors for diabetic peripheral neuropathy: A meta-analysis. *PLoS ONE* **2019**, *14*, e0212574. [CrossRef]
59. Andersen, S.T.; Witte, D.R.; Dalsgaard, E.M.; Andersen, H.; Nawroth, P.; Fleming, T.; Jensen, T.M.; Finnerup, N.B.; Jensen, T.S.; Lauritzen, T.; et al. Risk factors for incident diabetic polyneuropathy in a cohort with screen-detected type 2 diabetes followed for 13 years: ADDITION-Denmark. *Diabetes Care* **2018**, *41*, 1068–1075. [CrossRef]
60. Callaghan, B.C.; Gao, L.; Li, Y.; Zhou, X.; Reynolds, E.; Banerjee, M.; Pop-Busui, R.; Feldman, E.L.; Ji, L. Diabetes and obesity are the main metabolic drivers of peripheral neuropathy. *Ann. Clin. Transl. Neurol.* **2018**, *5*, 397–405. [CrossRef]
61. Callaghan, B.C.; Price, R.S.; Feldman, E.L. Distal symmetric polyneuropathy: A review. *JAMA* **2015**, *314*, 2172–2181. [CrossRef]
62. Li, L.; Liu, B.; Lu, J.; Jiang, L.; Zhang, Y.; Shen, Y.; Wang, C.; Jia, W. Serum albumin is associated with peripheral nerve function in patients with type 2 diabetes. *Endocrine* **2015**, *50*, 397–404. [CrossRef] [PubMed]

63. Yan, P.; Tang, Q.; Wu, Y.; Wan, Q.; Zhang, Z.; Xu, Y.; Zhu, J.; Miao, Y. Serum albumin was negatively associated with diabetic peripheral neuropathy in Chinese population: A cross-sectional study. *Diabetol. Metab. Syndr.* **2021**, *13*, 100. [CrossRef] [PubMed]
64. Su, J.B.; Zhao, L.H.; Zhang, X.L.; Cai, H.L.; Huang, H.Y.; Xu, F.; Chen, T.; Wang, X.Q. HbA1c variability and diabetic peripheral neuropathy in type 2 diabetic patients. *Cardiovasc. Diabetol.* **2018**, *17*, 47. [CrossRef] [PubMed]
65. Azab, B.; Chainani, V.; Shah, N.; McGinn, J.T. Neutrophil-lymphocyte ratio as a predictor of major adverse cardiac events among diabetic population: A 4-year follow-up study. *Angiology* **2013**, *64*, 456–465. [CrossRef] [PubMed]
66. Altay, F.A.; Kuzi, S.; Altay, M.; Ates, I.; Gurbuz, Y.; Tutuncu, E.E.; Senturk, G.C.; Altin, N.; Sencan, I. Predicting diabetic foot ulcer infection using the neutrophil-to-lymphocyte ratio: A prospective study. *J. Wound Care* **2019**, *28*, 601–607. [CrossRef]
67. Metsker, O.; Magoev, K.; Yakovlev, A.; Yanishevskiy, S.; Kopanitsa, G.; Kovalchuk, S.; Krzhizhanovskaya, V.V. Identification of risk factors for patients with diabetes: Diabetic polyneuropathy case study. *BMC Med. Inform. Decis. Mak.* **2020**, *20*, 201. [CrossRef]
68. Liu, S.; Zheng, H.; Zhu, X.; Mao, F.; Zhang, S.; Shi, H.; Li, Y.; Lu, B. Neutrophil-to-lymphocyte ratio is associated with diabetic peripheral neuropathy in type 2 diabetes patients. *Diabetes Res. Clin. Pract.* **2017**, *130*, 90–97. [CrossRef]
69. Combrisson, E.; Jerbi, K. Exceeding chance level by chance: The caveat of theoretical chance levels in brain signal classification and statistical assessment of decoding accuracy. *J. Neurosci. Methods* **2015**, *250*, 126–136. [CrossRef]

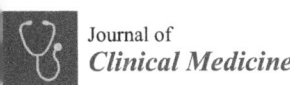

Article

Comparing Multiple Linear Regression and Machine Learning in Predicting Diabetic Urine Albumin–Creatinine Ratio in a 4-Year Follow-Up Study

Li-Ying Huang [1], Fang-Yu Chen [1], Mao-Jhen Jhou [2], Chun-Heng Kuo [1], Chung-Ze Wu [3,4], Chieh-Hua Lu [5], Yen-Lin Chen [6], Dee Pei [1], Yu-Fang Cheng [7] and Chi-Jie Lu [2,8,9,*]

1. Division of Endocrinology and Metabolism, Department of Internal Medicine, Department of Medical Education, Fu Jen Catholic University Hospital, School of Medicine, College of Medicine, Fu Jen Catholic University, New Taipei City 24352, Taiwan; liyinghuang@yahoo.com (L.-Y.H.); julia0770@yahoo.com.tw (F.-Y.C.); cpp0103@gmail.com (C.-H.K.); peidee@gmail.com (D.P.)
2. Graduate Institute of Business Administration, Fu Jen Catholic University, New Taipei City 242062, Taiwan; aaa73160@gmail.com
3. Division of Endocrinology, Department of Internal Medicine, Shuang Ho Hospital, New Taipei City 23561, Taiwan; chungze@yahoo.com.tw
4. Division of Endocrinology and Metabolism, Department of Internal Medicine, School of Medicine, College of Medicine, Taipei Medical University, Taipei 11031, Taiwan
5. Division of Endocrinology and Metabolism, Department of Internal Medicine, Tri-Service General Hospital, School of Medicine, National Defense Medical Center, Taipei 11490, Taiwan; undeca2001@gmail.com
6. Department of Pathology, Tri-Service General Hospital, National Defense Medical Center, Taipei 11490, Taiwan; anthonypatho@gmail.com
7. Department of Endocrinology and Metabolism, Changhua Christian Hospital, Changhua 50051, Taiwan; cch143989@gmail.com
8. Artificial Intelligence Development Center, Fu Jen Catholic University, New Taipei City 242062, Taiwan
9. Department of Information Management, Fu Jen Catholic University, New Taipei City 242062, Taiwan
* Correspondence: 059099@mail.fju.edu.tw; Tel.: +886-2-2905-2973

Abstract: The urine albumin–creatinine ratio (uACR) is a warning for the deterioration of renal function in type 2 diabetes (T2D). The early detection of ACR has become an important issue. Multiple linear regression (MLR) has traditionally been used to explore the relationships between risk factors and endpoints. Recently, machine learning (ML) methods have been widely applied in medicine. In the present study, four ML methods were used to predict the uACR in a T2D cohort. We hypothesized that (1) ML outperforms traditional MLR and (2) different ranks of the importance of the risk factors will be obtained. A total of 1147 patients with T2D were followed up for four years. MLR, classification and regression tree, random forest, stochastic gradient boosting, and eXtreme gradient boosting methods were used. Our findings show that the prediction errors of the ML methods are smaller than those of MLR, which indicates that ML is more accurate. The first six most important factors were baseline creatinine level, systolic and diastolic blood pressure, glycated hemoglobin, and fasting plasma glucose. In conclusion, ML might be more accurate in predicting uACR in a T2D cohort than the traditional MLR, and the baseline creatinine level is the most important predictor, which is followed by systolic and diastolic blood pressure, glycated hemoglobin, and fasting plasma glucose in Chinese patients with T2D.

Keywords: type 2 diabetes; nephropathy; urine albumin-creatinine ratio; machine learning

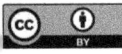

1. Introduction

Type 2 diabetes (T2D) has become a growing global issue in recent decades. According to the 2021 Atlas of the International Diabetes Federation, it is estimated that there are 5.37 billion patients worldwide, and this trend will further increase to 6.0 billion by 2045 [1]. Not surprisingly, a similar endemic was noted in Taiwan. According to the data bank of the

National Health Insurance Company, the total number of diabetic patients increased from 1.32 million to 2.2 million within 10 years (2005 to 2014). This represents an astonishing 66% increase [2]. It is now the 5th highest cause of death. In 2020, the cost spent on T2D was over 10 billion USD, which is approximately 4.66% of the budget of the National Health Insurance Company in one year. The accompanying complications, such as micro- and macrovascular diseases, impose heavy burdens on individuals and their families, as well as health providers and society [3,4]. It is important to note that this trend is particularly prominent among people aged <40 and ≥ 80 years [5].

Among all the complications, diabetic nephropathy is the leading cause of chronic kidney disease and end-stage renal disease (ESRD) [6], which are associated with high morbidity and mortality rate. According to the annual report of the US Renal Data System, Taiwan has the highest incidence (523 per million population) and prevalence of treated ESRD requiring renal replacement therapy [7]. In 2019, there were 84,615 dialysis patients and the National Health Insurance spent 1.54 billion, which is approximately 8.7–9.3% of the annual budget [8,9]. Therefore, its early detection and prevention are urgently required.

It is well known that urine albumin–creatinine ratio (uACR) is a strong predictor of the subsequent decline of the glomerular filtration rate in T2D, with an average of 0.93 mL per minute per month in approximately 35% of the subjects [10]. The underlying pathophysiology is due to the increased glomerular pressure, which is independent of hyperfiltration or hyperglycemia [11–13].

Traditionally, most studies have used multiple linear regression (MLR) to explore the relationships between risk factors and outcomes (complications) in medical research. Nevertheless, artificial intelligence using machine learning (ML), which enables machines to learn from past data or experiences without being explicitly programmed, has now become a new modality for data analysis that is competitive with MLR [14–16]. Because ML can capture nonlinear relationships in data and complex interactions among multiple predictors, it has the potential to outperform conventional MLR in disease prediction [17].

To our knowledge, only one study has attempted to predict the uACR in a T2D cohort. Thus, in the present study, we applied four different ML methods and attempted to answer the following questions in a diabetic cohort that was followed up for four years.

1. Compare the prediction accuracy between ML and traditional MLR.
2. Rank the importance of risk factors, such as demographic and biochemistry data.

2. Methods

2.1. Participant and Study Design

Data for this study were obtained from the diabetic outpatient clinic of the Cardinal Tien Hospital in Taiwan from 2013 to 2019. This study is a prospective study, as we have collected our patients from 2013 to 2016. We designated this cohort as the Cardinal Tien Diabetes Study Cohort. Informed consent was obtained from all participants, and data were collected anonymously. The study protocol was approved by the Institutional Review Board of the hospital. In total, 1682 T2D patients were enrolled. After excluding subjects with different causes, 1147 subjects remained for analysis (women: 608, men: 539), as shown in Figure 1. They were followed up for 4 years. The following were the criteria for inclusion: (1) type 2 diabetes; (2) age between 50 and 75 years; (3) body mass in the range of 22–30 kg/m^2; (4) glycated hemoglobin level between 6.5 and 10.5%; (5) the patients did not undergo regular dialysis. A flowchart of participant selection is displayed in Figure 1.

On the day of the study, senior nursing staff recorded the subject's medical history, including information on any current medications, and a physical examination was performed. The waist circumference was measured horizontally at the level of the natural waist. The body mass index (BMI) was calculated as the participant's body weight (kg) divided by the square of the participant's height (m). The systolic blood pressure (SBP) and diastolic blood pressure (DBP) were measured using standard mercury sphygmomanometers on the right arm of each subject while seated.

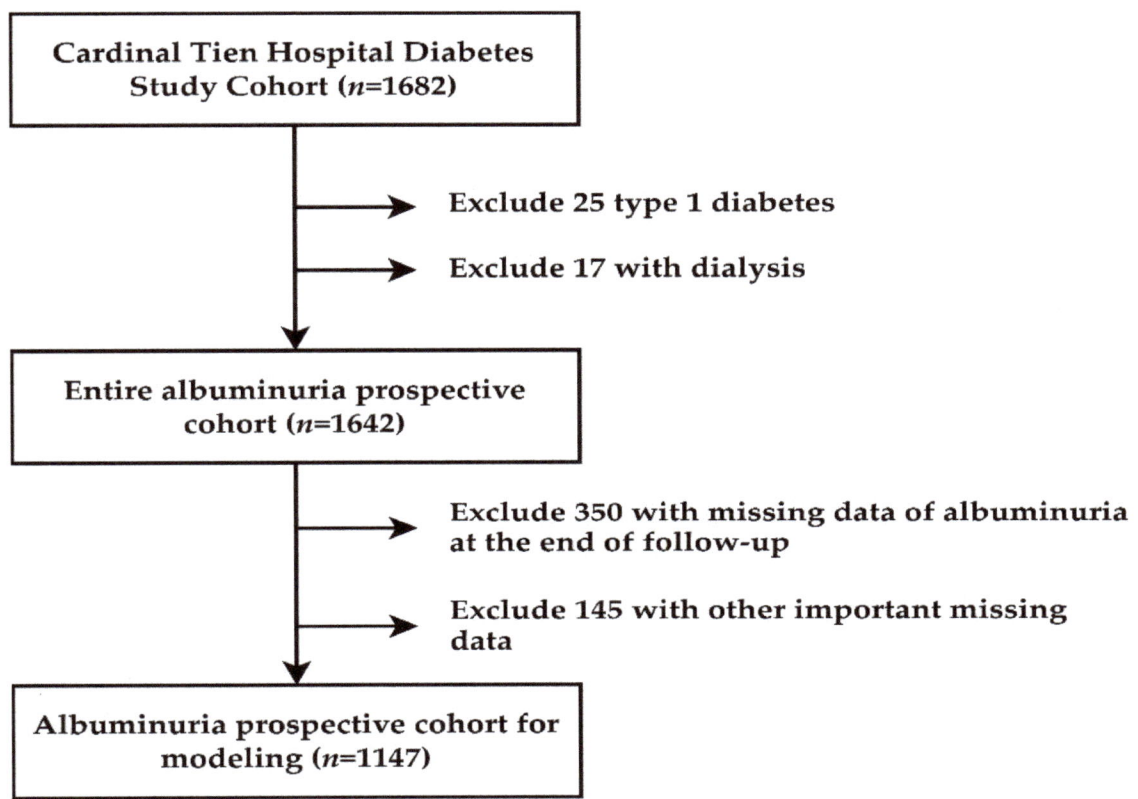

Figure 1. Flowchart of sample selection from the Cardinal Tien Hospital Diabetes Study Cohort.

As previously published, the procedures for collecting demographic and biochemical data are as follows [18]. After fasting for 10 h, blood samples were collected for biochemical analyses. Plasma was separated from the blood within 1 h of collection and stored at 30 °C until the analysis of fasting plasma glucose (FPG) and lipid profiles. FPG was measured using the glucose oxidase method (YSI 203 glucose analyzer; Yellow Springs Instruments, Yellow Springs, OH, USA). The total cholesterol and triglyceride (TG) levels were measured using the dry multilayer analytical slide method with a Fuji Dri-Chem 3000 analyzer (Fuji Photo Film, Tokyo, Japan). The serum high-density lipoprotein cholesterol (HDL-C) and low-density lipoprotein cholesterol (LDL-C) concentrations were analyzed using an enzymatic cholesterol assay, following dextran sulfate precipitation. A Beckman Coulter AU 5800 biochemical analyzer was used to determine the urine ACR by turbidimetry.

Table 1 lists the definitions of the 15 baseline clinical variables (independent variables, sex, age, BMI, duration of diabetes, smoking, alcohol use, FPG, glycated hemoglobin, triglyceride, HDL-C, LDL-C, alanine aminotransferase, creatinine (Cr), SBP, and DBP) used in this study. The uACR at the end of the follow-up was a numerical variable, which was used as a dependent (target) variable, while the remaining 15 variables were used as predictor variables in this study.

Table 1. Variable definition.

Variables	Description	Unit
Sex	Male/Female	-
Age	Patient age	year
Body mass index	Body mass index	Kg/m^2
Duration of diabetes	Duration of diabetes	year
Smoking	No/Yes	-
Alcohol	No/Yes	-
Baseline fasting plasma glucose	Fasting plasma glucose baseline	mg/dL
Baseline glycated hemoglobin	HbA1c (Glycated hemoglobin) baseline	%
Baseline triglyceride	Triglyceride baseline	mg/dL
Baseline high-density lipoprotein cholesterol	High-density lipoprotein cholesterol baseline	mg/dL
Baseline low-density lipoprotein cholesterol	Low-density lipoprotein cholesterol baseline	mg/dL
Baseline alanine aminotransferase baseline	Alanine aminotransferase baseline	U/L
Baseline creatinine	Creatinine baseline	mg/dL
Baseline systolic blood pressure	Systolic blood pressure baseline	mmHg
Baseline diastolic blood pressure	Diastolic blood pressure baseline	mmHg
uACR at the end of follow-up	Urine albumin to creatinine ratio = albumin (mg/dL)/urine creatinine (mg/dL) follow up 4 year	mg/g

uACR: urine albumin–creatinine ratio.

2.2. Proposed Scheme

This research proposed a scheme based on four machine learning methods, namely classification and regression tree (CART), random forest (RF), stochastic gradient boosting (SGB), and eXtreme gradient boosting (XGBoost), to construct predictive models for predicting diabetic uACR and to identify the importance of these risk factors. These ML methods have been applied in various healthcare applications and do not have prior assumptions regarding data distribution [19–28]. MLR was used as the benchmark for comparison.

The first method, CART, is a tree-structure method [29]. It is composed of root nodes, branches, and leaf nodes that grow recursively based on the tree structures from the root nodes and split at each node based on the Gini index to produce branches and leaf nodes with the rule. Then, the pruning node in the overgrown tree for optimal tree size using the cost-complexity criterion generates different decision rules to compose a complete structure tree [30,31].

RF, the second method in this study, is an ensemble learning decision tree algorithm that combines bootstrap resampling and bagging [32]. RF's principle entails randomly generating many different and unpruned CART decision trees, in which the decrease in Gini impurity is regarded as the splitting criterion, and all generated trees are combined into a forest. Then, all the trees in the forest are averaged or voted to generate output probabilities and a final model that generates a robust model [33].

The third method, SGB, is a tree-based gradient boosting learning algorithm that combines both bagging and boosting techniques to minimize the loss function to solve the overfitting problem of traditional decision trees [34,35]. In SGB, many stochastic weak learners of trees are sequentially generated through multiple iterations, in which each tree concentrates on correcting or explaining errors of the tree generated in the previous iteration, that is, the residual of the previous iteration tree is used as the input for the newly generated tree. This iterative process is repeated until the convergence condition or a stopping criterion is reached for the maximum number of iterations. Finally, the cumulative results of many trees are used to determine the final robust model.

XGBoost, the fourth method of this study, is a gradient boosting technology based on an SGB optimized extension [36]. Its principle is to train many weak models sequentially to ensemble them using the gradient boosting method of outputs, which achieves a better prediction performance. In XGBoost, Taylor binomial expansion is used to approximate the objective function and arbitrary differentiable loss functions to accelerate the model construction convergence process [37]. Then, XGBoost applies a regularized boosting technique to penalize the complexity of the model and correct overfitting, thus increasing model accuracy [36].

A flowchart of the proposed prediction and important variable identification scheme that combines the four ML methods is shown in Figure 2. First, patient data were collected using the proposed method to prepare the dataset. The dataset was then randomly divided into an 80% training dataset for model building and a 20% testing dataset for model testing. In the training process, each ML method has its hyperparameters that must be tuned to construct a relatively well-performed model. In this study, a 10-fold cross-validation (CV) technique for hyperparameter tuning was used. The training dataset was further randomly divided into a training dataset to build the model with a different set of hyperparameters and a validation dataset for model validation. All possible combinations of the hyperparameters were investigated using a grid search. The model with the lowest root mean square error for the validation dataset was viewed as the best model for each ML method. The best turned RF, SGB, CART, and XGBoost models were generated, and the corresponding variable importance ranking information was obtained.

During the testing process, the testing dataset was used to evaluate the predictive performance of the best RF, SGB, CART, and XGBoost models. As the target variable of the models built in this study is a numerical variable, the metrics used for model performance comparison are the mean absolute percentage error (MAPE), symmetric MAPE (SMAPE), and relative absolute error (RAE), which are shown in Table 2.

Table 2. Equation of Performance Metrics.

Metrics	Description	Calculation
MAPE	Mean Absolute Percentage Error	$MAPE = \frac{1}{n} \sum_{i=1}^{n} \left| \frac{y_i - \hat{y}_i}{y_i} \right| \times 100$
SMAPE	Symmetric Mean Absolute Percentage Error	$SMAPE = \frac{1}{n} \sum_{i=1}^{n} \frac{|y_i - \hat{y}_i|}{(|y_i| + |\hat{y}_i|)/2} \times 100$
RAE	Relative Absolute Error	$RAE = \sqrt{\frac{\sum_{i=1}^{n}(y_i - \hat{y}_i)^2}{\sum_{i=1}^{n}(y_i)^2}}$

where $\hat{y}_i$ and y_i represent predicted and actual values, respectively; n stands the number of instances.

To provide a more robust comparison, the training and testing processes mentioned above were randomly repeated 10 times. The averaged metrics of the RF, SGB, CART, and XGBoost models were used to compare the model performance of the benchmark MLR model that used the same training and testing dataset as the ML methods. An ML model with an average metric lower than that of MLR was considered a convincing model.

Because all of the ML methods used can produce the importance ranking of each predictor variable, we defined that the priority demonstrated in each model ranked 1 as the most critical risk factor and 15 as the last selected risk factor. The different ML methods may produce different variable importance rankings because they have different modeling characteristics; therefore, we integrated the variable importance ranking of the convincing ML models to enhance the stability and integrity of re-ranking the importance of risk factors. In the final stage of the proposed scheme, we summarize and discuss our significant findings regarding the convincing ML models and identify important variables.

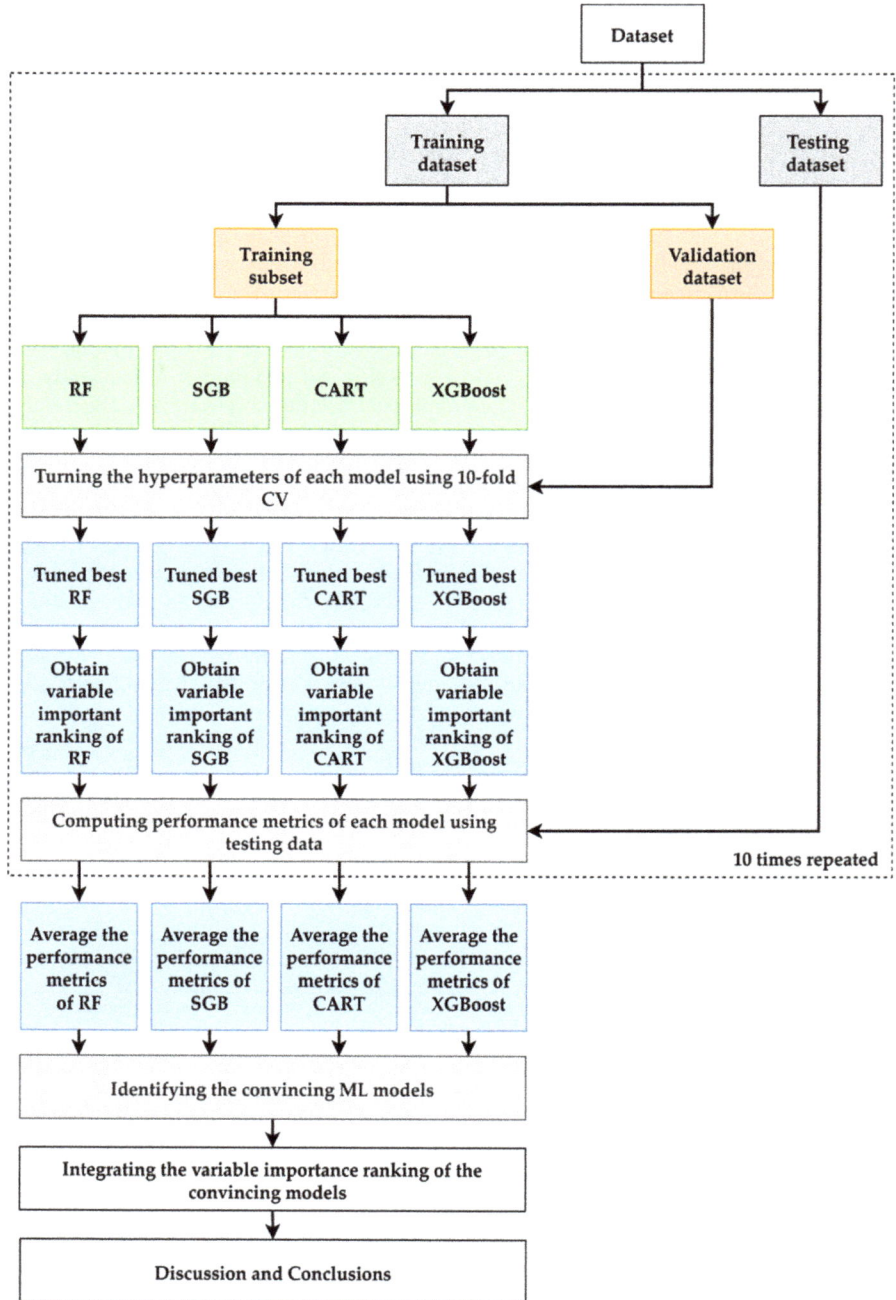

Figure 2. Proposed ML prediction scheme.

In this study, all methods were performed using R software version 4.0.5 and RStudio version 1.1.453 with the required packages installed (http://www.R-project.org, accessed on 1 February 2022; https://www.rstudio.com/products/rstudio/, accessed on 1 February 2022). The implementations of RF, SGB, CART, and XGBoost were the "randomForest" R package version 4.6-14 [38], "gbm" R package version 2.1.8 [39], "rpart" R package version 4.1-15 [40], and "XGBoost" R package version 1.5.0.2, respectively [41]. In addition, to estimate the best hyperparameter set for the developed effective CART, RF, SGB, and XGBoost methods, the "caret" R package version 6.0–90 was used [42]. The MLR was implemented using the "stats" R package version 4.0.5, and the default setting was used to construct the models.

3. Results

A total of 1147 participants were enrolled in the study (men: 539, women: 608). The demographic data are shown in Table 3 (mean ± standard deviation). The results of the comparison between the traditional MLR and the four ML methods (i.e., RF, SGB, CART, and XGBoost) in predicting diabetic uACR in a 4-year follow-up cohort are shown in Table 4. From the table, it can be seen that all four ML methods yielded lower prediction errors than the MLR method and were all convincing ML models. To determine whether the four ML methods significantly outperformed the MLR method, the Wilcoxon signed-rank test was used. The Wilcoxon signed-rank test is one of the most popular distribution-free, non-parametric statistical tests for evaluating the performance of two prediction models [43]. Table 5 shows the test results of the four ML methods and the MLR method. It can be observed from the table that the prediction error values of all ML methods were significantly different from those of the MLR method. Therefore, it can be determined that the ML methods used in this study significantly outperformed traditional MLR in predicting uACR at the end of the follow-up in terms of prediction error.

Table 3. Participant demographics.

Variables	Mean ± SD	N
Age	63.82 ± 11.49	1123
BMI	26.45 ± 3.95	1134
Duration of diabetes	14.13 ± 7.65	1137
Baseline fasting plasma glucose	149.84 ± 42.80	1146
Baseline glycated hemoglobin	7.74 ± 1.49	1140
Baseline triglyceride	142.99 ± 94.55	1144
Baseline high-density lipoprotein cholesterol	44.87 ± 12.00	845
Baseline low-density lipoprotein cholesterol	98.82 ± 27.73	1129
Baseline alanine aminotransferase baseline	29.38 ± 21.48	1134
Baseline creatinine	0.90 ± 0.37	1093
Baseline systolic blood pressure	131.13 ± 14.07	969
Baseline diastolic blood pressure	75.91 ± 11.66	969
uACR at the end of follow-up	195.30 ± 711.98	1147
	N (%)	N
Sex		1147
Male	608 (53.01%)	
Female	539 (46.99%)	
Smoking		716
No	430 (60.06%)	
Yes	286 (39.94%)	
Alcohol		789
No	715 (90.62%)	
Yes	74 (9.38%)	

BMI: body mass index. uACR: urine albumin–creatinine ratio.

Table 4. The average performance of the MLR, RF, SGB, CART, and XGBoost methods.

	MAPE	SMAPE	RAE
MLR	18.245 (4.79)	1.545 (0.04)	1.126 (0.17)
RF	16.174 (4.82)	1.266 (0.05)	1.072 (0.19)
SGB	14.850 (3.09)	1.522 (0.07)	1.040 (0.16)
CART	9.528 (1.76)	1.312 (0.06)	0.841 (0.10)
XGBoost	11.872 (2.80)	1.274 (0.06)	0.915 (0.11)

MLR: multiple linear regression; RF: random forest; SGB: stochastic gradient boosting; CART: classification and regression tree; XGBoost: eXtreme gradient boosting; MAPE: mean absolute percentage error; SMAPE: symmetric mean absolute percentage error; RAE: relative absolute error.

Table 5. Wilcoxon sign-rank test between four ML methods and MLR method.

	RF	SGB	CART	XGBoost
MLR	41.736 (0.001) **	20.814 (0.001) **	30.680 (0.001) **	44.489 (0.001) **

The numbers in parentheses are the corresponding p-value; **: $p < 0.05$.

Table 6 presents the average importance ranking of each factor generated by the RF, SGB, CART, and XGBoost methods. It can be observed from the figure that the different ML methods generated different relative importance rankings for each factor. The darkness of the blue color indicates the importance of risk factors. The darker the blue color, the more important the risk factor. For instance, in the RF method, the first three important factors were baseline Cr, age, and baseline SBP. The most important feature of the SGB method was baseline Cr, which was followed by baseline HDL-C and baseline DBP. To fully integrate the importance rankings of each factor in all the four ML methods, the average importance ranking of each risk factor was obtained by averaging the ranking values of each variable in each method.

Table 6. Importance ranking of each risk factor using the four convincing methods.

Variables	RF	SGB	CART	XGBoost	Average	
Sex	11.3	14.9	15.0	13.7	13.7	
Age	4.8	9.0	9.5	5.4	7.2	
Body mass index	14.9	11.8	12.0	9.8	12.1	
Duration of diabetes	8.8	7.0	10.7	8.4	8.7	Rank value
Smoking	10.8	14.4	15.0	14.7	13.7	1.0~1.4
Alcohol	11.6	13.6	15.0	14.6	13.7	1.5~2.4
Baseline fasting plasma glucose	5.4	6.3	10.9	5.3	7.0	2.5~3.4
Baseline glycated hemoglobin	5.8	5.0	10.3	6.1	6.8	3.5~4.4
Baseline triglyceride	11.9	10.2	12.7	13.1	12.0	4.5~5.4
Baseline high-density lipoprotein cholesterol	7.7	2.8	5.8	6.8	5.8	5.5~
Baseline low-density lipoprotein cholesterol	5.8	10.9	11.2	7.5	8.9	
Baseline alanine aminotransferase baseline	9.6	8.3	12.4	12.6	10.7	
Baseline creatinine	1.3	1.1	1.8	1.1	1.3	
Baseline systolic blood pressure	5.0	4.9	4.3	3.9	4.5	
Baseline diastolic blood pressure	5.3	4.1	4.1	4.7	4.6	

Note: Different blue colors indicate different rank values of risk factors. The darker the blue color, the more important the risk factor.

Figure 3 depicts the risk factors based on the increasing order of the averaged ranking values. It can be noted from the figure that the first six important risk factors in predicting diabetic uACR in a 4-year follow-up cohort are baseline Cr, baseline SBP, baseline DBP, baseline HDL-C, baseline glycated hemoglobin, and baseline FPG.

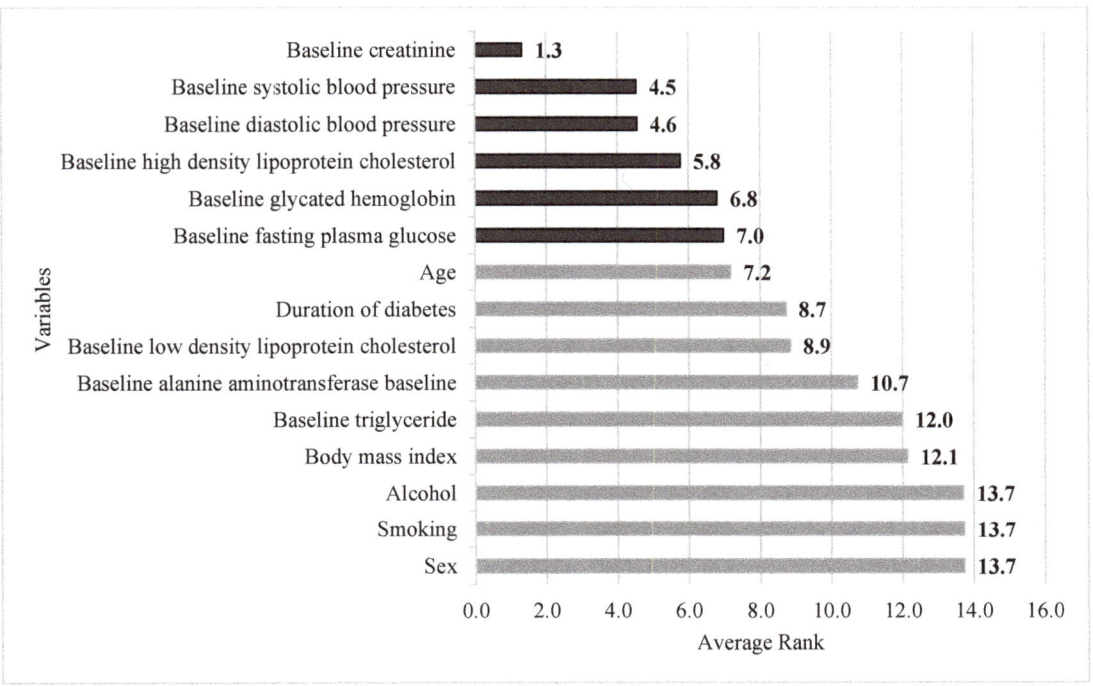

Figure 3. Integrated importance ranking of all risk factors. Note: The darker color indicates the first six important risk factors of this study.

4. Discussion

As mentioned in the Introduction, the present study has two goals. The first was to compare the accuracy between ML methods and MLR, and the second was to identify the rank of different risk factors for predicting uACR. Our study showed that all four ML methods outperformed the MLR. We also found that baseline Cr, blood pressure, HDL-C, glycated hemoglobin, and FPG were the most important factors.

Traditionally, MLR has been widely used to analyze medical research to deal with continuous variables. However, it is difficult to describe the nonlinear data patterns of MLR, and the effective use of MLR requires fitting its strong assumptions during modeling. Unlike MLR, ML does not require strong model assumptions and can capture the delicate underlying nonlinear relationships contained in empirical data [19]. Our present data showed that all four ML methods are superior to MLR because the MAPE and RAE of the ML methods all have lower values (Table 4). Our results suggest that ML might have a great potential for medical studies and applications.

Because diabetic nephropathy causes a serious burden on individuals and consumes a large portion of the government health budget, extensive studies have focused on this topic [6,44–47]. From these previous studies, it could be concluded that sex, high blood glucose and blood pressure, smoking, dyslipidemia, decreased glomerular filtration rate, BMI, and uACR are common risk factors for future uACR. However, in the present study, our data showed that baseline Cr, DBP, SBP, HDL-C, glycated hemoglobin, and FPG were the most important risks. Additionally, the roles of diabetes duration, glycated hemoglobin, BMI, HDL-cholesterol, triglyceride, sex, smoking, and alcohol use were less important.

Our data suggest that the most important predictor of albuminuria is baseline Cr. This is not surprising because albuminuria occurs early in the course of diabetic nephropathy [48]. According to the majority of previous studies, a summary of this relationship could be depicted as follows: diabetic patients with albuminuria are at a higher risk of end-stage renal and cardiovascular diseases [49,50]. This indicates that albuminuria is the cause of end-stage renal disease, which differs from the findings of the present study. Our results show that an increase in serum Cr level could predict albuminuria four years later, which is an opposite cause–effect relationship to the majority of the other studies. However, our finding can be supported by the cornerstone study conducted by Gansevoort et al. [51]. This meta-analysis clearly showed that there are independent, continuous, and negative associations between serum Cr and albuminuria. Thus, it could be postulated that each of these factors could affect the other at the same time. Further research is required to explore this area.

Both diastolic and systolic blood pressures were identified as the second and third important factors for predicting albuminuria. Their relationships are well known and have been extensively studied [52]. Similar to the role of increased serum Cr levels, kidney disease causes an increase in BP, which could further deteriorate renal function. More specifically, the change in BP is in concordance with and even precedes albuminuria [53]. By controlling BP, the speed of end-stage renal disease progression can be slowed down [54].

Interestingly, HDL cholesterol level was the only lipid found to be correlated with albuminuria. However, few studies have focused on this topic. Most previous studies have demonstrated that different stages of diabetic kidney disease (DKD) have different influences on blood lipid levels [55,56]. Other studies measured apolipoproteins and the size of LDL-cholesterol, which all showed positive correlations with DKD, including albuminuria [57]. To our knowledge, only two studies are relatively close to the present findings. The first study was performed by Sacks et al. In a group of 2535 T2D patients, they evaluated the impact of HDL-C levels on uACR. Furthermore, kidney disease was defined as albuminuria, proteinuria, or decreased eGFR. The data showed that the odds ratio of having kidney disease decreased by 0.86 (0.82–0.91) for every 0.2 mmol/L (approximately 1 quintile) increase in HDL-C [58]. The second study was conducted on a cohort of 524 Chinese patients. Using multiple logistic regression, after adjusting for the available confounding factors, they suggested that subjects with the highest quartile HDL-C had a lower odds ratio (OR = 0.17, 95% confidence interval 0.15–0.52) of having uACR than the lowest quartile. However, a limitation of this study was that it was cross-sectional. Thus, it was unable to infer the causation or directionality of this relationship [59]. This study responds to this limitation in its longitudinal design. The causative influence of HDL-C level can be explained by several assumptions. First, the glomerular and renal tubules could be injured by impaired HDL-C function, which hinders the reversal of the cholesterol transport process [60]. Second, the antioxidative ability of the HDL-C is reduced and oxidative stress is increased, which further influences the immune-mediated diabetic nephropathy [61]. Finally, it is well known that low HDL-C levels are associated with insulin resistance, hyperinsulinemia, and hyperglycemia. All these untoward derangements can damage endothelial cells in the glomerulus [62,63].

The last two factors affecting albuminuria are glycated hemoglobin and FPG levels. This finding is compatible with the results of the Diabetes Control and Complication Trial (DCCT) [64]. The data showed positive relationships between glucose control and albuminuria. Moreover, after controlling for blood glucose levels, albuminuria also improved [65]. Because DCCT enrolled patients with type 1 diabetes, its pathophysiology is different from that of the present study. Regarding T2D, few studies have been conducted in this area. A comprehensive meta-analysis conducted by Lo et al. [66] showed that for intensive control (glycated hemoglobin < 7% and FPG < 6.6 mmol/L), the relative risk of having uACR was 0.59 (confidence interval: 0.38–0.93). As this study enrolled 11 studies (29,141 subjects) and follow-ups were conducted for an average of 56.7 months, their conclusion is convincing. The underlying pathophysiology to support this result is that high blood glucose concentration could involve mesangial cell damage in nephrons [67]. However, it is worth noting that both A1c and FPG were classified as important predictors. This might indicate that because FPG is only one blood glucose measurement within 90 days compared to A1c, it is less accurate than A1c. Our results show that they are 'independent' of each other.

Interestingly, in the present study, the duration of diabetes, body mass index, sex, smoking, and alcohol use were less important. This finding could be attributed to the nature of the ML. ML methods are data-driven, non-parametric models. They can map any nonlinear function without an a priori assumption about the properties of the data and have the ability to capture subtle functional relationships among the empirical data, even though the underlying relationships are unknown or difficult to describe [68–70]. These factors may contain richer linear pattern information and less important nonlinear information than baseline creatinine, blood pressure, albuminuria level, and age. Thus, they were ranked as less important risk factors using ML methods.

This study had some limitations. First, the smoking and alcohol details need to be more defined because some other reports have shown that they have an important impact on the occurrence of diabetic nephropathy. Second, we did not collect information on the use of angiotensin-converting enzyme inhibitors, angiotensin receptor blockers, sodium-glucose cotransporter 2 inhibitors, and glucagon-like peptide-1 agonists. All these medications would have beneficial effects on DKD. Third, some of the data, such as uACR and blood pressure, were collected only once. For some of the participants, we did have data more than once. However, because the number is less than the present number, we still chose to enroll subjects with only one value. Even though these drawbacks do exist, our large n number and the characteristics of ML (alleviating the effects of extremes) could at least partially adjust.

5. Conclusions

ML might be more accurate in predicting uACR in T2D than the traditional MLR, and the baseline creatinine level is the most important factor to predict uACR in a T2D cohort, which is followed by systolic and diastolic blood pressure, glycated hemoglobin, and fasting plasma glucose.

Author Contributions: Developed the theory and wrote the draft, L.-Y.H.; Conceived and planned the experiment, F.-Y.C.; perform the machine learning analysis, M.-J.J.; helped to do the figures and tables, C.-H.K.; supervised the project, C.-Z.W.; discuss the results and contributed to the final manuscript, C.-H.L.; discuss the results and contributed to the final manuscript, Y.-L.C. and Y.-F.C.; collecting the medical records, D.P.; designed the data analysis scheme and wrote the draft, C.-J.L. All authors have read and agreed to the published version of the manuscript.

Funding: This research received no external funding.

Institutional Review Board Statement: The study was approved by the Research Ethics Review Committee at the Cardinal Tien Hospital (IRB No. CTH-100-2-5-036).

Informed Consent Statement: This manuscript contains no person's details, images, or videos.

Data Availability Statement: Data available on request due to privacy/ethical restrictions.

Conflicts of Interest: The authors declare no conflict of interest.

References

1. International Diabetes Federation. *IDF Diabetes Atlas*, 10th ed.; International Diabetes Federation: Brussels, Belgium, 2021; Available online: http://www.diabetesatlas.org/ (accessed on 22 March 2022).
2. Sheen, Y.-J.; Hsu, C.-C.; Jiang, Y.-D.; Huang, C.-N.; Liu, J.-S.; Sheu, W.H.-H. Trends in prevalence and incidence of diabetes mellitus from 2005 to 2014 in Taiwan. *J. Formos. Med. Assoc.* **2019**, *118*, S66–S73. [CrossRef] [PubMed]
3. Tseng, C.H.; Chong, C.K.; Heng, L.T.; Tseng, C.P.; Tai, T.Y. The incidence of type 2 diabetes mellitus in Taiwan. *Diabetes Res. Clin. Pract.* **2000**, *50*, S61–S64. [CrossRef]
4. Chang, C.-J.; Lu, F.-H.; Yang, Y.-C.; Wu, J.-S.; Wu, T.-J.; Chen, M.-S.; Chuang, L.-M.; Tai, T.Y. Epidemiologic study of type 2 diabetes in Taiwan. *Diabetes Res. Clin. Pract.* **2000**, *50*, S49–S59. [CrossRef]
5. Chang, C.H.; Shau, W.Y.; Jiang, Y.D.; Li, H.Y.; Chang, T.J.; Sheu, W.H.; Kwok, C.F.; Ho, L.T.; Chuang, L.M. Type 2 diabetes prevalence and incidence among adults in Taiwan during 1999–2004: A national health insurance data set study. *Diabet. Med.* **2010**, *27*, 636–643. [CrossRef]

6. Alicic, R.Z.; Rooney, M.T.; Tuttle, K.R. Diabetic Kidney Disease: Challenges, Progress, and Possibilities. *Clin. J. Am. Soc. Nephrol.* **2017**, *12*, 2032–2045. [CrossRef]
7. United States Renal Data System. *2020 Usrds Annual Data Report: Epidemiology of Kidney Disease in the United States*; National Institutes of Health; National Institute of Diabetes and Digestive and Kidney Diseases: Bethesda, MD, USA, 2020.
8. Chiang, J.K.; Chen, J.S.; Kao, Y.H. Comparison of medical outcomes and health care costs at the end of life between dialysis patients with and without cancer: A national population-based study. *BMC Nephrol.* **2019**, *20*, 265. [CrossRef]
9. Taiwan Society of Nephrology. National Health Research Institutes, Taiwan Annual Report on Kidney Disease in Taiwan. 2020. Available online: https://www.tsn.org.tw/UI/L/L002.aspx (accessed on 22 March 2022).
10. Nelson, R.G.; Bennett, P.H.; Beck, G.J.; Tan, M.; Knowler, W.C.; Mitch, W.E.; Hirschman, G.H.; Myers, B.D. Development and progression of renal disease in Pima Indians with non-insulin-dependent diabetes mellitus. Diabetic Renal Disease Study Group. *N. Engl. J. Med.* **1996**, *335*, 1636–1642. [CrossRef]
11. Anderson, S.; Meyer, T.W.; Rennke, H.G.; Brenner, B.M. Control of glomerular hypertension limits glomerular injury in rats with reduced renal mass. *J. Clin. Investig.* **1985**, *76*, 612–619. [CrossRef]
12. Anderson, S.; Rennke, H.G.; Brenner, B.M. Therapeutic advantage of converting enzyme inhibitors in arresting progressive renal disease associated with systemic hypertension in the rat. *J. Clin. Investig.* **1986**, *77*, 1993–2000. [CrossRef]
13. Zatz, R.; Dunn, B.R.; Meyer, T.W.; Anderson, S.; Rennke, H.G.; Brenner, B.M. Prevention of diabetic glomerulopathy by pharmacological amelioration of glomerular capillary hypertension. *J. Clin. Investig.* **1986**, *77*, 1925–1930. [CrossRef]
14. Marateb, H.R.; Mansourian, M.; Faghihimani, E.; Amini, M.; Farina, D. A hybrid intelligent system for diagnosing microalbuminuria in type 2 diabetes patients without having to measure urinary albumin. *Comput. Biol. Med.* **2014**, *45*, 34–42. [CrossRef] [PubMed]
15. Ye, Y.; Xiong, Y.; Zhou, Q.; Wu, J.; Li, X.; Xiao, X. Comparison of Machine Learning Methods and Conventional Logistic Regressions for Predicting Gestational Diabetes Using Routine Clinical Data: A Retrospective Cohort Study. *J. Diabetes Res.* **2020**, *2020*, 4168340. [CrossRef] [PubMed]
16. Nusinovici, S.; Tham, Y.C.; Yan, M.Y.C.; Ting, D.S.W.; Li, J.; Sabanayagam, C.; Wong, T.Y.; Cheng, C.Y. Logistic regression was as good as machine learning for predicting major chronic diseases. *J. Clin. Epidemiol.* **2020**, *122*, 56–69. [CrossRef] [PubMed]
17. Miller, D.D.; Brown, E.W. Artificial Intelligence in Medical Practice: The Question to the Answer? *Am. J. Med.* **2018**, *131*, 129–133. [CrossRef]
18. Lu, C.-H.; Pei, D.; Wu, C.-Z.; Kua, H.-C.; Liang, Y.-J.; Chen, Y.-L.; Lin, J.-D. Predictors of abnormality in thallium myocardial perfusion scans for type 2 diabetes. *Heart Vessel.* **2021**, *36*, 180–188. [CrossRef]
19. Tseng, C.-J.; Lu, C.-J.; Chang, C.-C.; Chen, G.-D.; Cheewakriangkrai, C. Integration of data mining classification techniques and ensemble learning to identify risk factors and diagnose ovarian cancer recurrence. *Artif. Intell. Med.* **2017**, *78*, 47–54. [CrossRef]
20. Ting, W.-C.; Chang, H.-R.; Chang, C.-C.; Lu, C.-J. Developing a Novel Machine Learning-Based Classification Scheme for Predicting SPCs in Colorectal Cancer Survivors. *Appl. Sci.* **2020**, *10*, 1355. [CrossRef]
21. Shih, C.-C.; Lu, C.-J.; Chen, G.-D.; Chang, C.-C. Risk Prediction for Early Chronic Kidney Disease: Results from an Adult Health Examination Program of 19,270 Individuals. *Int. J. Environ. Res. Public Health* **2020**, *17*, 4973. [CrossRef]
22. Lee, T.-S.; Chen, I.-F.; Chang, T.-J.; Lu, C.-J. Forecasting Weekly Influenza Outpatient Visits Using a Two-Dimensional Hierarchical Decision Tree Scheme. *Int. J. Environ. Res. Public Health* **2020**, *17*, 4743. [CrossRef]
23. Chang, C.-C.; Yeh, J.-H.; Chen, Y.-M.; Jhou, M.-J.; Lu, C.-J. Clinical Predictors of Prolonged Hospital Stay in Patients with Myasthenia Gravis: A Study Using Machine Learning Algorithms. *J. Clin. Med.* **2021**, *10*, 4393. [CrossRef]
24. Chang, C.-C.; Huang, T.-H.; Shueng, P.-W.; Chen, S.-H.; Chen, C.-C.; Lu, C.-J.; Tseng, Y.-J. Developing a Stacked Ensemble-Based Classification Scheme to Predict Second Primary Cancers in Head and Neck Cancer Survivors. *Int. J. Environ. Res. Public Health* **2021**, *18*, 12499. [CrossRef] [PubMed]
25. Chiu, Y.-L.; Jhou, M.-J.; Lee, T.-S.; Lu, C.-J.; Chen, M.-S. Health Data-Driven Machine Learning Algorithms Applied to Risk Indicators Assessment for Chronic Kidney Disease. *Risk Manag. Healthc. Policy* **2021**, *14*, 4401–4412. [CrossRef] [PubMed]
26. Wu, T.-E.; Chen, H.-A.; Jhou, M.-J.; Chen, Y.-N.; Chang, T.-J.; Lu, C.-J. Evaluating the Effect of Topical Atropine Use for Myopia Control on Intraocular Pressure by Using Machine Learning. *J. Clin. Med.* **2021**, *10*, 111. [CrossRef]
27. Wu, C.-W.; Shen, H.-L.; Lu, C.-J.; Chen, S.-H.; Chen, H.-Y. Comparison of Different Machine Learning Classifiers for Glaucoma Diagnosis Based on Spectralis OCT. *Diagnostics* **2021**, *11*, 1718. [CrossRef]
28. Chang, C.-C.; Yeh, J.-H.; Chiu, H.-C.; Chen, Y.-M.; Jhou, M.-J.; Liu, T.-C.; Lu, C.-J. Utilization of Decision Tree Algorithms for Supporting the Prediction of Intensive Care Unit Admission of Myasthenia Gravis: A Machine Learning-Based Approach. *J. Pers. Med.* **2022**, *12*, 32. [CrossRef] [PubMed]
29. Breiman, L.; Friedman, J.H.; Olshen, R.A.; Stone, C.J. Classification and Regression Trees. *Biometrics* **1984**, *40*, 874. [CrossRef]
30. Patel, N.; Upadhyay, S. Study of various decision tree pruning methods with their empirical comparison in WEKA. *Int. J. Comput. Appl.* **2012**, *60*, 20–25. [CrossRef]
31. Tierney, N.J.; Harden, F.A.; Harden, M.J.; Mengersen, K.L. Using decision trees to understand structure in missing data. *BMJ Open* **2015**, *5*, e007450. [CrossRef]
32. Breiman, L. Random forests. *Mach. Learn.* **2001**, *45*, 5–32. [CrossRef]
33. Calle, M.; Urrea, V. Letter to the editor: Stability of random forest importance measures. *Brief. Bioinform.* **2011**, *12*, 86–89. [CrossRef]

34. Friedman, J. Greedy function approximation: A gradient boosting machine. *Ann. Stat.* **2001**, *29*, 1189–1232. [CrossRef]
35. Friedman, J. Stochastic gradient boosting. *Comput. Stat. Data Anal.* **2002**, *38*, 367–378. [CrossRef]
36. Chen, T.; Guestrin, C. XGBoost: A Scalable Tree Boosting System. In Proceedings of the 22nd ACM SIGKDD International Conference on Knowledge Discovery and Data Mining, San Francisco, CA, USA, 13–17 August 2016; pp. 785–794.
37. Torlay, L.; Perrone-Bertolotti, M.; Thomas, E.; Baciu, M. Machine learning–XGBoost analysis of language networks to classify patients with epilepsy. *Brain Inform.* **2017**, *4*, 159–169. [CrossRef]
38. Breiman, L.; Cutler, A.; Liaw, A.; Wiener, M. randomForest: Breiman and Cutler's Random Forests for Classification and Regression. R Package Version, 4.6-14. 2022. Available online: https://CRAN.R-project.org/package=randomForest (accessed on 1 January 2022).
39. Greenwell, B.; Boehmke, B.; Cunningham, J. Gbm: Generalized Boosted Regression Models. R Package Version, 2.1.8. 2020. Available online: https://CRAN.R-project.org/package=gbm (accessed on 1 January 2022).
40. Therneau, T.; Atkinson, B. Rpart: Recursive Partitioning and Regression Trees. R Package Version, 4.1.15. 2022. Available online: https://CRAN.R-project.org/package=rpart (accessed on 1 January 2022).
41. Chen, T.; He, T.; Benesty, M.; Khotilovich, V.; Tang, Y.; Cho, H.; Chen, K.; Mitchell, R.; Cano, I.; Zhou, T.; et al. Xgboost: Extreme Gradient Boosting. R Package Version, 1.5.0.2. 2022. Available online: https://CRAN.R-project.org/package=xgboost (accessed on 1 January 2022).
42. Kuhn, M. Caret: Classification and Regression Training. R Package Version, 6.0-90. 2022. Available online: https://CRAN.R-project.org/package=caret (accessed on 1 January 2022).
43. Diebold, F.X.; Mariano, R.S. Comparing Predictive Accuracy. *J. Bus. Econ. Stat.* **1995**, *20*, 134–144. [CrossRef]
44. Gross, J.L.; De Azevedo, M.J.; Silveiro, S.P.; Canani, L.H.; Caramori, M.L.; Zelmanovitz, T. Diabetic nephropathy: Diagnosis, prevention, and treatment. *Diabetes Care* **2005**, *28*, 164–176. [CrossRef] [PubMed]
45. Harjutsalo, V.; Groop, P.-H. Epidemiology and risk factors for diabetic kidney disease. *Adv. Chronic Kidney Dis.* **2014**, *21*, 260–266. [CrossRef]
46. Duan, J.; Wang, C. Prevalence and risk factors of chronic kidney disease and diabetic kidney disease in Chinese rural residents: A cross-sectional survey. *Sci. Rep.* **2019**, *9*, 10408. [CrossRef]
47. Hussain, S.; Jamali, M.C.; Habib, A.; Hussain, M.S.; Akhtar, M.; Najmi, A.K. Diabetic kidney disease: An overview of prevalence, risk factors, and biomarkers. *Clin. Epidemiol. Glob. Health* **2021**, *9*, 2–6. [CrossRef]
48. Wu, X.Q.; Zhang, D.D.; Wang, Y.N.; Tan, Y.Q.; Yu, X.Y.; Zhao, Y.Y. AGE/RAGE in diabetic kidney disease and ageing kidney. *Free Radic. Biol. Med.* **2021**, *171*, 260–271. [CrossRef]
49. Newman, D.J.; Mattock, M.B.; Dawnay, A.B.; Kerry, S.; McGuire, A.; Yaqoob, M.; Hitman, G.A.; Hawke, C. Systematic review on urine albumin testing for early detection of diabetic complications. *Health Technol. Assess.* **2005**, *9*, 1–122. [CrossRef]
50. Hong, J.W.; Ku, C.R.; Noh, J.H.; Ko, K.S.; Rhee, B.D.; Kim, D.-J. Association between low-grade albuminuria and cardiovascular risk in Korean adults: The 2011–2012 Korea National Health and Nutrition Examination Survey. *PLoS ONE* **2015**, *10*, e0118866. [CrossRef] [PubMed]
51. Gansevoort, R.T.; Matsushita, K.; Van Der Velde, M.; Astor, B.C.; Woodward, M.; Levey, A.S.; De Jong, P.E.; Coresh, J. Lower estimated GFR and higher albuminuria are associated with adverse kidney outcomes. A collaborative meta-analysis of general and high-risk population cohorts. *Kidney Int.* **2011**, *80*, 93–104. [CrossRef] [PubMed]
52. Hsu, C.C.; Brancati, F.L.; Astor, B.C.; Kao, W.H.; Steffes, M.W.; Folsom, A.R.; Coresh, J. Blood pressure, atherosclerosis, and albuminuria in 10,113 participants in the atherosclerosis risk in communities study. *J. Hypertens.* **2009**, *27*, 397–409. [CrossRef] [PubMed]
53. Fagerudd, J.A.; Tarnow, L.; Jacobsen, P.; Stenman, S.; Nielsen, F.S.; Pettersson-Fernholm, K.J.; Grönhagen-Riska, C.; Parving, H.H.; Groop, P.H. Predisposition to essential hypertension and development of diabetic nephropathy in NIDDM. *Diabetes* **1998**, *47*, 439–444. [CrossRef]
54. Ruggenenti, P.; Fassi, A.; Ilieva, A.P.; Bruno, S.; Iliev, I.P.; Brusegan, V.; Rubis, N.; Gherardi, G.; Arnoldi, F.; Ganeva, M.; et al. Preventing microalbuminuria in type 2 diabetes. *N. Engl. J. Med.* **2004**, *351*, 1941–1951. [CrossRef]
55. Shoji, T.; Emoto, M.; Kawagishi, T.; Kimoto, E.; Yamada, A.; Tabata, T.; Ishimura, E.; Inaba, M.; Okuno, Y.; Nishizawa, Y. Atherogenic lipoprotein changes in diabetic nephropathy. *Atherosclerosis* **2001**, *156*, 425–433. [CrossRef]
56. Jenkins, A.J.; Lyons, T.J.; Zheng, D.; Otvos, J.D.; Lackland, D.T.; Mcgee, D.; Garvey, W.T.; Klein, R.L.; The DCCT/EDIC Research Group. Lipoproteins in the dcct/edic cohort: Associations with diabetic nephropathy. *Kidney Int.* **2003**, *64*, 817–828. [CrossRef]
57. Tolonen, N.; Forsblom, C.; Thorn, L.; Wadén, J.; Rosengård-Bärlund, M.; Saraheimo, M.; Feodoroff, M.; Mäkinen, V.P.; Gordin, D.; Taskinen, M.R.; et al. Lipid abnormalities predict progression of renal disease in patients with type 1 diabetes. *Diabetologia* **2009**, *52*, 2522–2530. [CrossRef]
58. Sacks, F.M.; Hermans, M.P.; Fioretto, P.; Valensi, P.; Davis, T.; Horton, E.; Wanner, C.; Al-Rubeaan, K.; Aronson, R.; Barzon, I.; et al. Association between plasma triglycerides and high-density lipoprotein cholesterol and microvascular kidney disease and retinopathy in type 2 diabetes mellitus: A global case-control study in 13 countries. *Circulation* **2014**, *129*, 999–1008. [CrossRef]
59. Sun, X.; Xiao, Y.; Li, P.M.; Ma, X.Y.; Sun, X.J.; Lv, W.S.; Wu, Y.L.; Liu, P.; Wang, Y.G. Association of serum high-density lipoprotein cholesterol with microalbuminuria in type 2 diabetes patients. *Lipids Health Dis.* **2018**, *17*, 229. [CrossRef]
60. Vaziri, N.D. Lipotoxicity and impaired high density lipoprotein-mediated reverse cholesterol transport in chronic kidney disease. *J. Ren. Nutr.* **2010**, *20*, S35–S43. [CrossRef] [PubMed]

61. Li, C.; Gu, Q. Protective effect of paraoxonase 1 of high-density lipoprotein in type 2 diabetic patients with nephropathy. *Nephrology* **2009**, *14*, 514–520. [CrossRef] [PubMed]
62. Drew, B.G.; Duffy, S.J.; Formosa, M.F.; Natoli, A.K.; Henstridge, D.C.; Penfold, S.A.; Thomas, W.G.; Mukhamedova, N.; de Courten, B.; Forbes, J.M.; et al. High-density lipoprotein modulates glucose metabolism in patients with type 2 diabetes mellitus. *Circulation* **2009**, *119*, 2103–2111. [CrossRef] [PubMed]
63. Brunham, L.R.; Kruit, J.K.; Hayden, M.R.; Verchere, C.B. Cholesterol in β-cell dysfunction: The emerging connection between HDL cholesterol and Type 2 diabetes. *Curr. Diabetes Rep.* **2010**, *10*, 55–60. [CrossRef]
64. Bilous, R. Microvascular disease: What does the UKPDS tell us about diabetic nephropathy? *Diabet Med.* **2003**, *20*, 25–29. [CrossRef]
65. The Diabetes Control and Complications (DCCT) Research Group. Effect of intensive therapy on the development and progression of diabetic nephropathy in the Diabetes Control and Complications Trial. *Kidney Int.* **1995**, *47*, 1703–1720. [CrossRef]
66. Lo, C.; Zoungas, S. Intensive glucose control in patients with diabetes prevents onset and progression of microalbuminuria, but effects on end-stage kidney disease are still uncertain. *Evid. Based Med.* **2017**, *22*, 219–220. [CrossRef]
67. Genuth, S.; Eastman, R.; Kahn, R.; Klein, R.; Lachin, J.; Lebovitz, H.; Nathan, D.; Vinicor, F.; American Diabetes Association. Implications of the United Kingdom prospective diabetes study. *Diabetes Care* **2003**, *26*, S28–S32. [CrossRef]
68. Chen, I.-F.; Lu, C.-J. Sales forecasting by combining clustering and machine-learning techniques for computer retailing. *Neural Comput. Appl.* **2017**, *28*, 2633–2647. [CrossRef]
69. Jiang, F.; Jiang, Y.; Zhi, H.; Dong, Y.; Li, H.; Ma, S.; Wang, Y.; Dong, Q.; Shen, H.; Wang, Y. Artificial intelligence in healthcare: Past, present and future. *Stroke Vasc. Neurol.* **2017**, *2*, 230. [CrossRef]
70. Koteluk, O.; Wartecki, A.; Mazurek, S.; Kołodziejczak, I.; Mackiewicz, A. How Do Machines Learn? Artificial Intelligence as a New Era in Medicine. *J. Pers. Med.* **2021**, *11*, 32. [CrossRef] [PubMed]

Article

Measuring of Advanced Glycation End Products in Acute Stroke Care: Skin Autofluorescence as a Predictor of Ischemic Stroke Outcome in Patients with Diabetes Mellitus

Alexandra Filipov *, Heike Fuchshuber, Josephine Kraus, Anne D. Ebert, Vesile Sandikci and Angelika Alonso

Department of Neurology, Medical Faculty Mannheim, University of Heidelberg, 68167 Mannheim, Germany; heike_fuchshuber@web.de (H.F.); josephine.kraus@umm.de (J.K.); anne.ebert@umm.de (A.D.E.); vesile.sandikci@umm.de (V.S.); angelika.alonso@umm.de (A.A.)
* Correspondence: alexandra.filipov@umm.de; Tel.: +49-621-383-3628; Fax: +49-621-383-3807

Abstract: *Background:* Patients with diabetes mellitus (DM) are known to show poor recovery after stroke. This specific burden might be due to acute and chronic hyperglycemic effects. Meanwhile, the underlying mechanisms are a cause of discussion, and the best measure to predict the outcome is unclear. Skin autofluorescence (SAF) reflects the in-patient load of so-called advanced glycation end products (AGEs) beyond HbA1c and represents a valid and quickly accessible marker of chronic hyperglycemia. We investigated the predictive potential of SAF in comparison to HbA1c and acute hyperglycemia on the functional outcome at 90 days after ischemic stroke in a cohort of patients with DM. *Methods:* We prospectively included 113 patients with DM type 2 hospitalized for acute ischemic stroke. SAF was measured on each patient's forearm by a mobile AGE-Reader mu© in arbitrary units. HbA1c and the area under the curve (AUC) of the blood sugar profile after admission were assessed. Functional outcome was assessed via phone interview after 90 days. A poor outcome was defined as a deterioration to a modified Rankin Scale score ≥ 3. A good outcome was defined as a modified Rankin Scale score < 3 or as no deterioration from premorbid level. *Results:* Patients with a poor outcome presented with higher values of SAF (mean 3.38 (SD 0.55)) than patients with a good outcome (mean 3.13 (SD 0.61), $p = 0.023$), but did not differ in HbA1c and acute glycemia. In logistic regression analysis, age ($p = 0.021$, OR 1.24 [1.12–1.37]) and SAF ($p = 0.021$, OR 2.74 [1.16–6.46]) significantly predicted a poor outcome, whereas HbA1c and acute glycemia did not. Patients with a poor 90-day outcome and higher SAF experienced more infections (4.2% vs. 33.3% ($p < 0.01$)) and other various in-hospital complications (21.0% vs. 66.7% ($p < 0.01$)) than patients with a good outcome and lower SAF levels. *Conclusions:* SAF offers an insight into glycemic memory and appears to be a significant predictor of poor stroke outcomes in patients with DM exceeding HbA1c and acute glycemia. Measuring SAF could be useful to identify specifically vulnerable patients at high risk of complications and poor outcomes.

Keywords: stroke outcome; diabetes mellitus; hyperglycemia; skin autofluorescence; advanced glycation end products; poststroke complications

1. Introduction

Around 30% of patients in ischemic stroke care suffer from diabetes mellitus (DM). Concomitantly, due to acute and chronic hyperglycemic effects, patients with DM show poor recovery after stroke [1]. HbA1c from nonenzymatic glycation of hemoglobin represents the best-established marker of chronic hyperglycemia regarding the last three months. Meanwhile, different long-lasting molecules underlie similar transformations and form the group of advanced glycation end products (AGEs), also known as glycemic memory [2]. Skin autofluorescence (SAF) represents a valid, quick and noninvasive approach to measure AGEs in vivo [3] and is a marker of vasculopathy in DM type 2 [4]. We aimed to investigate the predictive potential of SAF as a surrogate of long-term hyperglycemia in comparison to

HbA1c as marker of intermediate glycemia and acute hyperglycemia on stroke outcome in a cohort of patients with DM.

2. Materials and Methods

From December 2018 to September 2020, patients were prospectively recruited at the University Hospital of Mannheim, Germany. Our assessments were based on the most prevalent scoring scales in stroke medicine [5]. The modified Rankin scale (mRS) is a 7-item scale indicating functional dependency. A score of 0 is considered no disability, 5 is disability requiring constant care for all needs and 6 is death. A score of more than 2 is the hallmark of functional dependency. The Barthel Index (BI) is a scale used to measure performance in activities of daily living according to 10 different variables. The National Institutes of Health Stroke Scale (NIHSS) is a 15-item neurologic examination scale evaluating the effect of cerebral infarction on the levels of consciousness, language, neglect, visual field, extraocular movement, motor strength, ataxia, dysarthria and sensory loss. We included adult patients with known DM type 2 or HbA1c $\geq 6.5\%$ at admission hospitalized for ischemic stroke (according to World Health Organisation definition [6]) presenting within 3 days after symptom onset with a persistent deficit ((mRS) score ≥ 1). Written consent was obtained from the patient or their legal representative. Patients necessitating hemodialysis were excluded [7]. SAF was measured bedside on the patient's volar forearm by a mobile AGE-Reader mu© (DiagnOptics Technologies B.V., Groningen, The Netherlands). According to usage instructions, the patient placed their volar forearm on the measurement window where light was radiated on the previously degreased skin. The reflected light was registered to measure SAF that was displayed within 12 s in arbitrary units (AU) (for validation study and technical details, see Meerwaldt et al., 2004 and 2005 [8,9]). Three measurements were performed bedside with a slight change in the forearm's position. The mean value was calculated for further analysis as intraindividual variance in same-day measurement ranges around 5% according to reference data [8] without relevant postprandial changes [10]. A routine blood analysis included HbA1c. From routine capillary blood sugar profiling, we calculated the area under the curve (AUC) in mg/mL × 24 h, representing acute glycemia with respect to the first two days after admission, standardized in 24 h. Insulin was administered after blood sugar measuring, as clinically required. Baseline parameters from medical history including preexisting functional deficit (pre-mRS) were registered, as well as severity of stroke by NIHSS. If indicated, acute revascularization therapy was performed according to local standards. We recorded in-hospital complications such as (symptomatic) intracranial hemorrhage ((S)ICH) [11] in follow-up cranial imaging, as well as infectious complications [12]. Other complications (recurrent stroke, epileptic seizures, delirium, acute renal failure, thrombosis, pulmonary embolism, myocardial infarction and others) were recorded if they required diagnostic or therapeutic measures. For follow-up, we performed a phone interview after 90 (± 3) days poststroke and determined mRS and BI. A poor functional outcome whilst taking into account prior deficit was defined as a deterioration from premorbid mRS to mRS ≥ 3 at 90 days poststroke. A good outcome was defined as a mRS < 3 or as no deterioration from premorbid mRS.

Statistical analysis was performed with SPSS® 27.0 (IBM, Armonk, New York, NY, USA). p values < 0.05 were considered statistically significant. We compared baseline and clinical characteristics, in-hospital complications and 90 days of BI between patients with a poor and a good 90-day outcome. Intergroup differences were assessed using t-test for metric variables, Mann–Whitney U test for ordinal variables and Chi^2 test/Fisher's exact test for categorical variables as appropriate. We further performed a multiple logistic regression analysis, including the preliminarily defined predictors SAF, HbA1c and AUC as glycemic variables adjusted for age and NIHSS at admission as the strongest known predictors of a poor 90-day outcome [13].

3. Results

A total of 113 patients (mean age 71.4 years, SD 10.29; 59.3% male) were included. There was no significant correlation either between SAF and HbA1c (Pearson's correlation coefficient, r = 0.02) or between SAF and age (r = 0.17). Furthermore, we did not find a correlation between NIHSS at admission and either glucose at admission (Spearman's rank correlation coefficient, ρ = 0.041) or glycemic AUC (ρ = 0.029). After three months, we were unable to follow up on six patients (5.3%). The premorbid deficit was low in our cohort: before the index stroke, 86.7% of the patients were functionally independent, as indicated by mRS $\leq$ 2. On day 90, this was the case for only 52.3% (see Figure 1). Additionally, 90 days poststroke, 62 (57.9%) patients showed a good outcome, while 45 (42.1%) showed a poor outcome according to our definition.

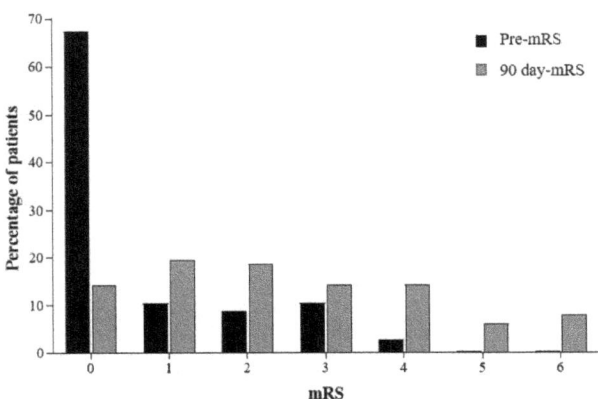

Figure 1. Shift in functional outcome after 90 days: premorbid modified Rankin scale (Pre-mRS; n = 113), modified Rankin Scale on day 90 (90 d-mRS; n = 107).

When comparing patients with good versus poor outcome, (see in Table 1) patients with poor outcomes were older (mean age 69.0 years (SD 9.57) vs. 76.3 years (SD 9.10), p < 0.001) and had a higher level of premorbid functional deficit (pre-mRS: median 0 (IQR 0; 0) vs. 1 (IQR 0; 3), p < 0.001; pre-BI: median 100 (IQR 100; 100) vs. 100 (IQR 85; 100), p < 0.001). Male patients were more likely to achieve a good outcome (72.6% vs. 40.0%, p < 0.001). Patients with a poor outcome exhibited more often known macrovascular disease (32.3% vs. 60.0%, p = 0.004) and renal failure (29.0% vs. 48.9%, p = 0.036) and were more often under antithrombotic treatment (27.4% vs. 48.9%, p = 0.023). Instead, patients with a good outcome were more often under a combination of basal insulin and oral antidiabetic treatment (BOT) (27.4% vs. 4.4%, p = 0.002). Considering stroke characteristics, patients with a good outcome showed more frequently infratententorial strokes (30.6% vs. 11.1%, p = 0.017). There was no difference considering stroke outcome and stroke etiology in our cohort.

Table 1. Baseline characteristics.

Population	Good Outcome (90 d mRS < 3 or No Deterioration)	Poor Outcome (90 d mRs $\geq$ 3 and Deterioration)	p
n	62	45	
Age, mean (sd) [years]	69.0 (9.57)	76.3 (9.10)	<0.001 *
Male, n (%)	45 (72.6)	18 (40.0)	0.001 *
Premorbid-mRS, median (IQR)	0 (0; 0)	1 (0; 3)	<0.001 *
Premorbid-BI, median (IQR)	100(100; 100)	100 (85; 100)	<0.001 *

Table 1. Cont.

Population	Good Outcome (90 d mRS < 3 or No Deterioration)	Poor Outcome (90 d mRs ≥ 3 and Deterioration)	p
Risk factors			
Hypertension, n (%)	54 (87.1)	40 (88.9)	0.779
Hyperlipidemia, n (%)	20 (32.3)	21 (46.7)	0.130
Atrial fibrillation, n (%)	13 (21.0)	17 (37.8)	0.056
Macrovascular disease, n (%)	20 (32.3)	27 (60.0)	0.004 *
Renal failure, n (%)	18 (29.0)	22 (48.9)	0.036 *
Previous stroke, n (%)	10 (16.1)	7 (15.6)	0.936
Smoking, n (%)	11 (17.7)	4 (8.9)	0.263
Alcohol abuse, n (%)	3 (4.8)	1 (2.2)	0.637
Premedication			
Oral anticoagulation, n (%)	10 (16.1)	7 (15.6)	0.936
Antithrombotic agent, n (%)	17 (27.4)	22 (48.9)	0.023 *
Statin, n (%)	28 (45.2)	27 (60.0)	0.130
Antihypertensive medication, n (%)	46 (74.2)	39 (86.7)	0.115
BOT, n (%)	17 (27.4)	2 (4.4)	0.002 *
Insulin, n (%)	22 (35.5)	14 (31.1)	0.637
Oral antidiabetic, n (%)	45 (72.6)	25 (55.6)	0.068
Glycemia			
SAF, mean (sd) [AU]	3.13 (0.61)	3.38 (0.55)	0.023 *
AUC, mean (sd) [mg/(mL × 24 h)]	40.38 (10.58)	41.49 (14.16)	0.647
HbA1c, mean (sd) [%]	7.57 (1.29)	7.67 (1.58)	0.718
Admission variables			
NIHSS, median (IQR)	4 (2; 6)	10 (5; 16)	<0.001 *
Systolic blood pressure, mean (sd) [mmHg]	170.51 (32.35)	163.81 (24.48)	0.285
Plasma glucose, mean (sd) [mg/dL]	191.2 (65.01)	197.84 (79.48)	0.637
Acute revasculating therapy, n (%)	21 (33.9)	25 (55.6)	0.025 *
Intravenous thrombolysis, n (%)	19 (30.6)	20 (44.4)	0.143
Mechanical thrombectomy, n (%)	6 (9.7)	11 (24.4)	0.039
Complications in stay			
ICH, n (%)	13 (21.0)	11 (24.4)	0.670
SICH, n (%)	0 (0.0)	1 (2.2)	0.421
Poststroke infection, n (%)	3 (4.8)	15 (33.3)	<0.001 *
Death, n (%)	0 (0.0)	4 (8.9)	0.029 *
Other complications, n (%)	13 (21.0)	30 (66.7)	<0.001 *
90 d Outcome			
90 d mRS, median (IQR)	1 (0; 2)	4 (3; 5)	<0.001 *
90 d Barthel, median (IQR)	100 (100; 100)	35 (0; 65)	<0.001 *
Stroke characteristics			
Supratentorial, n (%)	48 (77.4)	40 (88.9)	0.125
Infratentorial, n (%)	19 (30.6)	5 (11.1)	0.017
Supratent. and Infratent., n (%)	6 (9.7)	0 (0.0)	0.039
Large artery disease, n (%)	6 (9.7)	9 (20.0)	0.129
Small artery disease, n (%)	15 (24.2)	10 (22.2)	0.812
Proximal embolism, n (%)	41 (66.1)	28 (62.2)	0.677

p-values < 0.005 are considered statistically significant; * significant, (%) percentage of outcome quality, day (d), number (n), skin autofluorescence (SAF), arbitrary unit (AU), basal insulin and oral antidiabetic treatment (BOT), area under the curve (AUC), modified Rankin Scale (mRS), National Institutes of Health Stroke Scale (NIHSS), Barthel Index (BI), intracerebral hemorrhage (ICH), symptomatic intracerebral hemorrhage (SICH), standard deviation (SD), interquartile range (IQR).

Considering the severity of stroke, patients with a poor outcome showed higher NIHSS scores at admission (median 10 (IQR 5; 16) vs. median 4 (IQR 2; 6), $p < 0.001$), and they received more frequently revascularization therapy (55.6% vs. 33.9%, *p* = 0.025). There was no significant group difference concerning intravenous thrombolysis, but a higher frequency of mechanical thrombectomy in patients with poor outcome (24.4% vs. 9.7%, *p* = 0.039). Complications during the hospital stay did not differ between patients with poor outcome and good outcome in terms of hemorrhagic complications, whereas the rate of intracerebral hemorrhage was generally low in our sample. Poststroke infection occurred more often in patients with poor outcome (33.3% vs. 4.8%, *p* < 0.001) as well as other complications during hospital care (66.7% vs. 21.0%, *p* < 0.001). The total in-patient mortality rate amounted to 3.5%. Among patients with a poor outcome, 8.9% died during the initial hospital stay.

Patients with a poor versus good outcome did not differ in admission glucose, in glycemic AUC, or in HbA1c. However, patients with a poor outcome showed higher SAF (mean 3.13 (SD 0.61) vs. mean 3.38 (SD 0.55), *p* = 0.023) (see Figure 2).

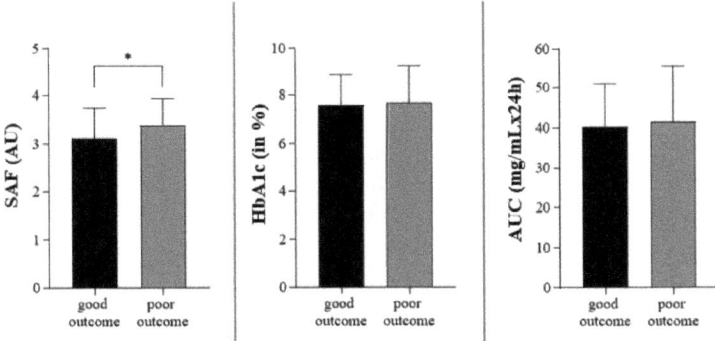

Figure 2. Differences in glycemic variables according to 90-day outcome: mean and standard deviation of SAF, HbA1c and AUC. * Significant difference, skin autofluorescence (SAF), area under the curve (AUC), arbitrary units (AU).

Logistic regression analysis revealed rising age (*p* = 0.021; odds ratio (OR) 1.07 [1.01–1.12]) and rising NIHSS at admission (*p* < 0.001, OR 1.24 [1.12–1.37]) as predictors being significantly associated with a poor outcome. Regarding glycemic variables, rising SAF turned out to be significantly associated with a poor outcome (*p* = 0.021, OR 2.74 [1.16–6.46]). Meanwhile, HbA1c and AUC did not add significant prediction to the model (see in Table 2).

Table 2. Predictors of outcome.

Predictor	*p*	OR [CI]
Age [years]	0.021 *	1.07 [1.01–1.12]
NIHSS [/]	<0.001 *	1.24 [1.12–1.37]
HbA1c [%]	0.520	-
AUC [mg/mL × 24 h]	0.397	-
SAF [AU]	0.021 *	2.74 [1.16–6.46]

p-values < 0.05 are considered statistically significant; * significant; OR: odds ratio; CI: confidence interval, skin autofluorescence (SAF), area under the curve (AUC), National Institutes of Health Stroke Scale (NIHSS).

4. Discussion

The mechanisms mediating poor stroke outcome in patients with DM might consist of acute and chronic hyperglycemic effects, although the best measure of hyperglycemia to predict outcome is largely unknown [1].

4.1. Troubled Water: Acute Hyperglycemia

Patients with DM are specifically prone to stress hyperglycemia in the context of a severe illness such as stroke [14]. Acute hyperglycemia has been associated with poor stroke outcome, as it was supposed to drive ischemic damage [15]. On the other hand, interventions with aggressive insulin therapy in acute stroke care were not beneficial [16,17]. So, given a connection between hyperglycemia and poor outcome, cause and effect are not clearly attributable. Most prior studies investigating the impact of acute hyperglycemia on stroke outcome have referred to admission glucose and used different arbitrary cut-off values to define hyperglycemia [18]. In this regard, Fuentes et al., (2009) performed blood sugar profiling for 48 h postadmission and confirmed hyperglycemia exceeding 155 mg/dL to be a significant predictor of a poor outcome. In our study, we did not focus on a cut-off value, as we expected expansive glycemic variations in our cohort. In an attempt to meet and objectify the glycemic ups and downs as a dynamic value, we operationalized acute glycemia as the AUC of the blood sugar profile postadmission. Interestingly, patients with a poor and a good outcome did not differ in acute glycemia, neither in admission glucose nor in glycemic AUC. Additionally, AUC was not significantly associated with a poor outcome in logistic regression analysis. In our cohort, neither admission glucose nor AUC correlated with the NIHSS at admission. Accordingly, our data do not support the theory of hyperglycemic derailment in the context of severe stroke in patients with DM. It must be considered that revascularization therapy can result in a reversal of initially severe stroke symptoms. Nevertheless, in our cohort, patients with a poor outcome more frequently underwent acute therapy and thrombectomy, implying only moderate success. On the other hand, in lacunar stroke, mild hyperglycemia might be even favorable [19]. However, according to our results, we cannot attribute a poor stroke outcome to acute hyperglycemia.

4.2. The Foot of the Iceberg: Chronic Hyperglycemia

Meanwhile pre-stroke glycemic control might predict stroke outcome [20–23]. In our study, patients with good and poor outcomes differed only in SAF regarding glycemic variables, and SAF was the only glycemic predictor significantly associated with a poor outcome, even when adjusting for age and NIHSS. An increase in SAF in one AU was associated with an approximately three-fold risk of a poor outcome on day 90 (OR 2.74). The SAF values we measured lay slightly above the range of age-adapted reference values for patients with DM [4], reflecting the specific vascular risk in our cohort of acute stroke patients. We deduce that SAF reflecting long-term glycemic control is supposed to have a higher impact on stroke outcome than HbA1c or acute glycemia. Possible mechanisms by which chronic hyperglycemia affects stroke outcome include preexisting vascular damage on the macro- and microvascular level impairing collateral flow. Regarding the molecular level, accumulated AGEs are supposed to mediate a self-perpetuating chronic vascular inflammation [24], mainly by interaction with their receptor RAGE (receptor for advanced glycation end products), leading to endothelial dysfunction and arterial stiffness [25], hypercoagulation, diminished fibrinolysis and vasoconstriction [26]. An excess of AGE-RAGE interaction-related downstream inflammatory markers is likely to increase poststroke inflammation, which is known to increase ischemic damage within the brain but also leads to systemic effects such as cardiac injury [27]. This effect seems to be most important in cardioembolic stroke, which was the most frequent subtype in our sample without having a statistical effect on outcome, likely due to a limited sample size. Additionally, AGE-RAGE-mediated effects may promote ICH by blood–brain-barrier disruptions [28] and may increase susceptibility to infectious complications [29]. In our sample, patients with a poor outcome and with higher SAF levels showed more infectious [30] and other in-hospital complications, which are known to impair long-term outcome poststroke [13] on a sensorimotor but also on a cognitive level, especially when combined with renal failure [31]. It seems reasonable that patients with a good outcome and lower SAF benefitted from a better long-term metabolic control prior to the index stroke. Our cohort reflects this point, as patients with a good outcome were more often under BOT, implying a more sophisticated antidiabetic treatment.

We can assume that SAF offers an insight to the extent of the diabetic burden being predictive for stroke outcome in DM, and HbA1c remains the "tip of the iceberg".

5. Limitations

This was a monocentric study in a local urban population, and a certain selection bias concerning standards of acute stroke treatment and further rehabilitation can be expected. The limited number of included patients a priori impeded an exhaustive prediction model with respect to additional potential predictors. The follow-up interviewer was not blinded for glycemic values, allowing a certain rater bias. The measuring of acute glycemia was not continuous but based on blood sugar profile. Still, we found SAF to have the highest predictive value on stroke outcome amongst glycemic variables when controlling for age and severity of stroke. An unexpected finding from our cohort was an important sex-dependent difference in stroke outcome. A possible explanation could be higher age and higher premorbid dependency in female patients [32].

6. Conclusions and Future Perspectives

According to our results, SAF, representing long-term glycemic memory, is a significant predictor of a poor functional outcome after ischemic stroke in patients with DM and exceeds HbA1c and acute hyperglycemia in its predictive value. SAF might be a useful tool to identify patients at high risk of complications and poor outcome requiring special attention (for example, preventive antibiotics, prolonged monitoring, adapted antithrombotic treatment). Our study must be considered preliminary. Larger neurovascular patient populations need to be investigated for SAF in the form of registries to create a more exhaustive prediction model and to establish a sensitive and specific cut-off value to distinguish patients at high risk of a poor outcome.

Regarding potential specific therapeutic interventions in the context of acute stroke, it might not be possible to reverse the weight of an iceberg that has accumulated over the years. However, to remain with the allegory, investigating water for potentially assailable key point biomarkers along the RAGE axis could offer future opportunities. For example, soluble RAGE showed a promising ability to counterbalance endothelial dysfunction in a mouse model in the short term [33]. Along these lines, future research is needed.

Author Contributions: A.F. developed the theory, conceptualized and organized the study, screened and included patients, helped with data acquisition and data curation and wrote the manuscript with input from all authors. H.F. is a doctoral student who mainly acquired and curated the data. J.K. supported with patient screening and inclusion. A.D.E. prepared the raw data and performed the statistical analysis. She was supported by V.S. who mainly designed the figures. A.A. is the supervising senior professor. All authors have read and agreed to the published version of the manuscript.

Funding: This research received no external funding.

Institutional Review Board Statement: The study was conducted in accordance with the Declaration of Helsinki, and approved by the Institutional Review Board of the Ethikkommission II der Universität Heidelberg. (2018-574N-MA, 26 June 2018).

Informed Consent Statement: Informed consent was obtained from all subjects involved in the study.

Data Availability Statement: The data that support the findings of this study are available on reasonable request from the corresponding author. The data are not publicly available due to containing information that could compromise the privacy of research participants.

Conflicts of Interest: The authors have no conflict of interest to declare.

References

1. Lau, L.H.; Lew, J.; Borschmann, K.; Thijs, V.; Ekinci, E.I. Prevalence of diabetes and its effects on stroke outcomes: A meta-analysis and literature review. *J. Diabetes Investig.* **2019**, *10*, 780–792. [CrossRef] [PubMed]
2. Lachin, J.M.; Genuth, S.; Nathan, D.M.; Zinman, B.; Rutledge, B.N. Effect of glycemic exposure on the risk of microvascular compli-cations in the diabetes control and complications trial–revisited. *Diabetes* **2008**, *57*, 995–1001. [CrossRef] [PubMed]
3. Smit, A.J.; Gerrits, E.G. Skin autofluorescence as a measure of advanced glycation endproduct deposition: A novel risk marker in chronic kidney disease. *Curr. Opin. Nephrol. Hypertens.* **2010**, *19*, 527–533. [CrossRef]
4. Lutgers, H.L.; Graaff, R.; Links, T.P.; Ubink-Veltmaat, L.J.; Bilo, H.J.; Gans, R.O.; Smit, A.J. Skin autofluorescence as a noninvasive marker of vascular damage in patients with type 2 diabetes. *Diabetes Care* **2006**, *29*, 2654–2659. [CrossRef] [PubMed]
5. Quinn, T.J.; Dawson, J.; Walters, M.R.; Lees, K.R. Functional outcome measures in contemporary stroke trials. *Int. J. Stroke Off. J. Int. Stroke Soc.* **2009**, *4*, 200–205. [CrossRef]
6. Coupland, A.P.; Thapar, A.; Qureshi, M.I.; Jenkins, H.; Davies, A.H. The definition of stroke. *J. R. Soc. Med.* **2017**, *110*, 9–12. [CrossRef] [PubMed]
7. Meerwaldt, R.; Zeebregts, C.J.; Navis, G.; Hillebrands, J.L.; Lefrandt, J.D.; Smit, A.J. Accumulation of advanced glycation end prod-ucts and chronic complications in ESRD treated by dialysis. *Am. J. Kidney Dis. Off. J. Natl. Kidney Found.* **2009**, *53*, 138–150. [CrossRef]
8. Meerwaldt, R.; Graaff, R.; Oomen, P.H.N.; Links, T.P.; Jager, J.J.; Alderson, N.L.; Thorpe, S.R.; Baynes, J.W.; Gans, R.O.B.; Smit, A.J. Simple non-invasive assessment of advanced gly-cation endproduct accumulation. *Diabetologia* **2004**, *47*, 1324–1330. [CrossRef]
9. Meerwaldt, R.; Links, T.; Graaff, R.; Thorpe, S.R.; Baynes, J.W.; Hartog, J.; Gans, R.; Smit, A. Simple noninvasive measurement of skin autofluores-cence. *Ann. N. Y. Acad. Sci.* **2005**, *1043*, 290–298. [CrossRef]
10. Stirban, A.; Pop, A.; Fischer, A.; Heckermann, S.; Tschoepe, D. Variability of skin autofluorescence measurement over 6 and 12 weeks and the influence of benfotiamine treatment. *Diabetes Technol. Ther.* **2013**, *15*, 733–737. [CrossRef]
11. Wahlgren, N.; Ahmed, N.; Dávalos, A.; A Ford, G.; Grond, M.; Hacke, W.; Hennerici, M.G.; Kaste, M.; Kuelkens, S.; Larrue, V.; et al. Thrombolysis with alteplase for acute ischaemic stroke in the Safe Implementation of Thrombolysis in Stroke-Monitoring Study (SITS-MOST): An observational study. *Lancet* **2007**, *369*, 275–282. [CrossRef]
12. Nationales Referenzzentrum für Surveillance von nosokomialen Infektionen. *Definitionen nosokomialer Infektionen für die Surveil-lance im Krankenhaus-Infektions-Surveillance-System (KISS-Definitionen)*; Robert Koch-Institut: Berlin, Germany, 2017; 80p.
13. Grube, M.M.; Koennecke, H.-C.; Walter, G.; Meisel, A.; Sobesky, J.; Nolte, C.H.; Wellwood, I.; Heuschmann, P.U.; on behalf of the Berlin Stroke Register (BSR). Influence of acute complications on outcome 3 months after ischemic stroke. *PLoS ONE* **2013**, *8*, e75719. [CrossRef] [PubMed]
14. Capes, S.E.; Hunt, D.; Malmberg, K.; Pathak, P.; Gerstein, H.C. Stress Hyperglycemia and Prognosis of Stroke in Nondiabetic and Diabetic Patients: A Systematic Overview. *Stroke* **2001**, *32*, 2426–2432. [CrossRef] [PubMed]
15. Luitse, M.J.; Biessels, G.J.; Rutten, G.; Kappelle, L.J. Diabetes, hyperglycaemia, and acute ischaemic stroke. *Lancet Neurol.* **2012**, *11*, 261–271. [CrossRef]
16. Johnston, K.C.; Bruno, A.; Pauls, Q.; Hall, C.E.; Barrett, K.M.; Barsan, W.; Fansler, A.; Van De Bruinhorst, K.; Janis, S.; Durkalski-Mauldin, V.L.; et al. Intensive vs Standard Treatment of Hyperglycemia and Functional Outcome in Patients With Acute Ischemic Stroke: The SHINE Randomized Clinical Trial. *JAMA* **2019**, *322*, 326–335. [CrossRef]
17. Bellolio, M.F.; Gilmore, R.M.; Ganti, L. Insulin for glycaemic control in acute ischaemic stroke. *Cochrane Libr.* **2014**, *23*, CD005346. [CrossRef]
18. Fuentes, B.; Castillo, J.; José, B.S.; Leira, R.; Serena, J.; Vivancos, J.; Dávalos, A.; Gil Nuñez, A.; Egido, J.; Díez-Tejedor, E. The prognostic value of capillary glucose levels in acute stroke: The GLycemia in Acute Stroke (GLIAS) study. *Stroke A J. Cereb. Circ.* **2009**, *40*, 562–568. [CrossRef]
19. Uyttenboogaart, M.; Koch, M.W.; Stewart, R.E.; Vroomen, P.C.; Luijckx, G.-J.; De Keyser, J. Moderate hyperglycaemia is associated with favourable outcome in acute lacunar stroke. *Brain A J. Neurol.* **2007**, *130*, 1626–1630. [CrossRef]
20. Lattanzi, S.; Bartolini, M.; Provinciali, L.; Silvestrini, M. Glycosylated Hemoglobin and Functional Outcome after Acute Ischemic Stroke. *J. Stroke Cerebrovasc. Dis. Off. J. Natl. Stroke Assoc.* **2016**, *25*, 1786–1791. [CrossRef]
21. Kamouchi, M.; Matsuki, T.; Hata, J.; Kuwashiro, T.; Ago, T.; Sambongi, Y.; Fukushima, Y.; Sugimori, H.; Kitazono, T.; for the FSR Investigators. Prestroke glycemic control is associated with the functional outcome in acute ischemic stroke: The Fukuoka Stroke Registry. *Stroke* **2011**, *42*, 2788–2794. [CrossRef]
22. Luitse, M.J.; Velthuis, B.K.; Kappelle, L.J.; van der Graaf, Y.; Biessels, G.J.; on behalf of the DUST Study Group. Chronic hyperglycemia is related to poor functional out-come after acute ischemic stroke. *Int. J. Stroke Off. J. Int. Stroke Soc.* **2017**, *12*, 180–186. [CrossRef] [PubMed]
23. Wang, H.; Cheng, Y.; Chen, S.; Li, X.; Zhu, Z.; Zhang, W. Impact of Elevated Hemoglobin A1c Levels on Functional Outcome in Patients with Acute Ischemic Stroke. *J. Stroke Cerebrovasc. Dis. Off. J. Natl. Stroke Assoc.* **2019**, *28*, 470–476. [CrossRef] [PubMed]
24. Stirban, A.; Gawlowski, T.; Roden, M. Vascular effects of advanced glycation endproducts: Clinical effects and molecular mech-anisms. *Mol. Metab.* **2014**, *3*, 94–108. [CrossRef] [PubMed]
25. Corte, V.D.; Tuttolomondo, A.; Pecoraro, R.; Di Raimondo, D.; Vassallo, V.; Pinto, A. Inflammation, Endothelial Dysfunction and Arterial Stiffness as Therapeutic Targets in Cardiovascular Medicine. *Curr. Pharm. Des.* **2016**, *22*, 4658–4668. [CrossRef] [PubMed]

26. Domingueti, C.P.; Dusse, L.M.; Carvalho, M.; Sousa, L.; Gomes, K.B.; Fernandes, A.P. Diabetes mellitus: The linkage between oxida-tive stress, inflammation, hypercoagulability and vascular complications. *J. Diabetes Its Complicat.* **2016**, *30*, 738–745. [CrossRef]
27. Maida, C.D.; Norrito, R.L.; Daidone, M.; Tuttolomondo, A.; Pinto, A. Neuroinflammatory Mechanisms in Ischemic Stroke: Focus on Cardioembolic Stroke, Background, and Therapeutic Approaches. *Int. J. Mol. Sci.* **2020**, *21*, 6454. [CrossRef]
28. Hussain, M.; Bork, K.; Gnanapragassam, V.S.; Bennmann, D.; Jacobs, K.; Navarette-Santos, A.; Hofmann, B.; Simm, A.; Danker, K.; Horstkorte, R. Novel insights in the dysfunc-tion of human blood-brain barrier after glycation. *Mech. Ageing Dev.* **2016**, *155*, 48–54. [CrossRef]
29. Liesz, A.; Dalpke, A.; Mracsko, E.; Roth, S.; Zhou, W.; Yang, H.; Tatjana, E.; Akhisaroglu, M.; Fleming, T.; Eigenbrod, T.; et al. DAMP Signaling is a Key Pathway Inducing Immune Modulation after Brain Injury. *J. Neurosci.* **2015**, *35*, 583–598. [CrossRef]
30. Filipov, A.; Fuchshuber, H.; Kraus, J.; Ebert, A.D.; Sandikci, V.; Alonso, A. Skin Autofluorescence is an Independent Predictor of Post Stroke Infection in Diabetes. *J. Stroke Cerebrovasc. Dis. Off. J. Natl. Stroke Assoc.* **2021**, *30*, 105949. [CrossRef]
31. Ben Assayag, E.; Eldor, R.; Korczyn, A.; Kliper, E.; Shenhar-Tsarfaty, S.; Tene, O.; Molad, J.; Shapira, I.; Berliner, S.; Volfson, V.; et al. Type 2 Diabetes Mellitus and Impaired Renal Function Are Associated With Brain Alterations and Poststroke Cognitive Decline. *Stroke* **2017**, *48*, 2368–2374. [CrossRef]
32. Eriksson, M.; Glader, E.-L.; Norrving, B.; Terént, A.; Stegmayr, B. Sex differences in stroke care and outcome in the Swedish nation-al quality register for stroke care. *Stroke* **2009**, *40*, 909–914. [CrossRef] [PubMed]
33. Jeong, J.; Lee, J.; Lim, J.; Cho, S.; An, S.; Lee, M.; Yoon, N.; Seo, M.; Lim, S.; Park, S. Soluble RAGE attenuates AngII-induced endothelial hyperpermeability by disrupting HMGB1-mediated crosstalk between, AT1R and RAGE. *Exp. Mol. Med.* **2019**, *51*, 1–15. [CrossRef] [PubMed]

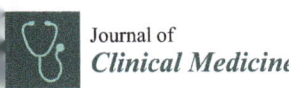

Article

Simple Predictors for Cardiac Fibrosis in Patients with Type 2 Diabetes Mellitus: The Role of Circulating Biomarkers and Pulse Wave Velocity

Ekaterina B. Luneva *, Anastasia A. Vasileva, Elena V. Karelkina, Maria A. Boyarinova, Evgeny N. Mikhaylov, Anton V. Ryzhkov, Alina Y. Babenko, Alexandra O. Konradi and Olga M. Moiseeva

Almazov National Medical Research Centre, 197341 Saint-Petersburg, Russia; vasileva_aa@almazovcentre.ru (A.A.V.); karelkina_ev@almazovcentre.ru (E.V.K.); boyarinova_ma@almazovcentre.ru (M.A.B.); e.mikhaylov@almazovcentre.ru (E.N.M.); ryzhkov_av@almazovcentre.ru (A.V.R.); babenko_ayu@almazovcentre.ru (A.Y.B.); konradi_ao@almazovcentre.ru (A.O.K.); moiseeva_om@almazovcentre.ru (O.M.M.)
* Correspondence: elunyova@gmail.com; Tel.: +7-(812)-702-3716

Abstract: Cardiac fibrosis is the basis of structural and functional disorders in patients with diabetes mellitus (T2DM). A wide range of laboratory and instrumental methods is used for its prediction. The study aimed to identify simple predictors of cardiac fibrosis in patients with T2DM based on the analysis of circulating fibrosis biomarkers and arterial stiffness. The study included patients with T2DM ($n = 37$) and cardiovascular risk factors (RF, $n = 27$) who underwent ECHO, cardiac magnetic resonance imaging (MRI), pulse wave analysis (PWV), reactive hyperemia (RH), peripheral arterial tonometry, carotid ultrasonography, and assessment of serum fibrosis biomarkers. As a control group, 15 healthy subjects were examined. Left ventricular concentric hypertrophy was accompanied by an increased serum galectin-3 level in T2DM patients. There was a relationship between the PICP and HbA1c levels in both main groups ($R2 = 0.309$; $p = 0.014$). A negative correlation between PICP level and the global longitudinal strain (GLS) was found ($r = -0.467$; $p = 0.004$). The RH index had a negative correlation with the duration of diabetes ($r = -0.356$; $p = 0.03$), the carotid-femoral PWV ($r = -0.371$; $p = 0.024$), and the carotid intima-media thickness ($r = -0.622$; $p < 0.001$). The late gadolinium-enhanced (LGE) cardiac MRI was detected in 22 (59.5%) T2DM and in 4 (14.85%) RF patients. Diabetes, its baseline treatment with metformin, HbA1c and serum TIMP-1 levels, and left ventricle hypertrophy had moderate positive correlations with LGE findings ($p < 0.05$). Using the multivariate regression analysis, increased TIMP-1 level was identified as an independent factor associated with cardiac fibrosis.

Keywords: cardiac fibrosis; diabetes mellitus; pulse wave velocity

1. Introduction

Cardiovascular (CV) complications remain the leading cause of premature death and disability in type 2 diabetes mellitus (T2DM) [1]. According to the population-based studies, patients with T2DM have a 2–5-fold increased CV risk when combined with traditional risk factors such as hypertension, dyslipidemia, advanced age, obesity, and smoking [2]. At the same time, obesity is among the strongest predictors of T2DM development. T2DM promotes pro-inflammatory and prothrombotic signaling, resulting in endothelial dysfunction and atherogenesis acceleration associated with CV events [3].

Heart failure seems to become one of the most prevalent and serious T2DM consequences, being considered either manifestation of diabetic cardiomyopathy or macrovascular ischemic heart disease or both [4]. Left ventricular (LV) hypertrophy with myocardial fibrosis is a typical sign of diabetic cardiomyopathy. Echocardiographic (ECHO) parameters of LV diastolic function and global longitudinal strain (GLS) are widely used as nonspecific surrogate markers of myocardial fibrosis in clinical practice [5,6]. Unlike ECHO as a screening tool for functional LV assessment, cardiac magnetic resonance imaging (MRI) is a robust non-invasive method for myocardial fibrosis detection and quantification. Despite cardiac MRI's potential benefits, its real implementation is limited by low availability and high cost [7]. Plasma-circulating biomarkers are also widely used for indirect cardiac fibrosis assessment; however, their diagnostic value is still a matter of debate [8,9]. T2DM is one of the major determinants of accelerated arterial stiffening along with hypertension and age. It is suggested that cardiac fibrosis in T2DM patients is associated with increased arterial wall stiffness as well. The increased arterial stiffness has been shown significantly impact LV afterload and, therefore, is crucial for the development of heart failure with preserved ejection fraction (HFpEF) [10,11].

The elaboration of non-invasive markers predicting cardiac fibrosis is of essential importance since fibrosis is strongly associated with CV events and may require more aggressive treatment.

The present study aimed at identifying simple predictors of cardiac fibrosis in patients with T2DM based on the analysis of circulating fibrosis biomarkers and arterial stiffness. T2DM has been shown to be associated with tissue fibrosis in general and cardiac fibrosis in particular [12]. Plasma concentrations of circulating biomarkers that may characterize the presence and extent of fibrosis are associated with other morbidity and risk factors, such as obesity and hypertension. Moreover, their reference level should be evaluated in healthy subjects for the assessment of their significance when changed. Therefore, along with T2DM patients, we included two more subgroups: subjects without T2DM but with cardiovascular risk factors and healthy controls.

2. Materials and Methods

2.1. Study Population

The cross-sectional study recruited subjects from the outpatient clinic of the Almazov National Medical Research Centre between August 2019 and July 2020. Subjects fulfilling inclusion criteria were invited into the study by a treating physician (screening) and referred to an investigator. The subjects were divided into three groups: T2DM patients, patients with CV risk factors (RF), and healthy control (HC) subjects.

The inclusion criteria for the T2DM group were the following: glycated hemoglobin (HbA1c) level > 6.5% at screening and T2DM diagnosed >1 year ago. The RF group inclusion criteria were the combination of two common risk factors: obesity (BMI > 30.0 kg/m^2) and hypertension (office blood pressure level > 140/90 mm Hg) or dyslipidemia (the history of LDL cholesterol > 3 mmol/L). The HC group comprised blood donors without a history of CV disease.

The exclusion criteria were changes in pharmacological treatment (drugs and/or doses) within 1 month; inadequate blood pressure control ($\geq$140/80 mm Hg at office visits); a history of coronary artery disease, myocardial infarction, or TIA/stroke; LV ejection fraction < 50%; an implanted pacemaker or cardioverter-defibrillator; ongoing infectious or neoplastic diseases; documented osteoporosis or osteopenia; pregnancy or breastfeeding; any intervention or surgery within 6 months. The study was approved by the Ethics Committee of the Almazov Centre (No. 05072019 dated 8 July 2019), and all participants signed an informed consent form before the inclusion. The baseline evaluation included medical history and physical examination, routine laboratory tests, circulating fibrosis biomarkers, endothelial function assessment, pulse wave analysis, carotid intima-media thickness, and echocardiography. Contrast-enhanced cardiac MRI was performed in the T2DM and RF groups. The HC group underwent biomarker analysis only.

The primary study assessment measure included the evaluation of a possible association between cardiac fibrosis as detected by cardiac MRI, artery stiffness, and circulating biomarkers. The secondary study analysis was the evaluation of factors independently associated with the presence of cardiac fibrosis.

This observational study was registered as a part of an umbrella project #075-15-2020-800 by the Ministry of Science and Higher Education. The local legislation does not require observational studies registration in public databases.

2.2. Blood Assays

Peripheral venous blood samples were obtained at the first visit. Serum samples were obtained following centrifugation at 2500× g for 10 min at 4 °C. Samples were aliquoted and stored at −80 °C until required. Lab parameters included HbA1c (Tina-Quant Hemoglobin A1c Gen.3, Cobas Integra 400+, Roche Diagnostics GmbH, Mannheim, Germany), creatinine, lipids (Cobas Integra 400+, Roche Diagnostics GmbH, Mannheim, Germany), high-sensitivity C-reactive protein by the immunoturbidimetric CRP-Latex assay (Tina-quant® CRP latex, Cobas Integra 400+, Roche Diagnostics GmbH, Mannheim, Germany), NT-proBNP (Elecsys, Roche Diagnostics GmbH, Mannheim, Germany), and soluble suppression of tumorigenicity 2 sST2 (Presage ST2 kit, Critical Diagnostics, CA, USA). Carboxy-terminal propeptide of collagen 1 (PICP, USCN Life Science, Wuhan, China), amino-terminal propeptide of collagen 3 (PIIINP, USCN Life Science, Wuhan, China), carboxy-terminal telopeptide of collagen 1 (ICTP, MyBioSource, San Diego, CA, USA), transforming growth factor β-1 (TGFβ1, R&D systems Inc., Minneapolis, MN, USA), matrix metalloproteinase 9 (MMP9, R&D systems Inc., Minneapolis, MN, USA), tissue inhibitor of metalloproteinase 1 (TIMP1, R&D systems Inc., Minneapolis, MN, USA), and galectin-3 (R&D systems Inc., Minneapolis, MN, USA) were quantified using a specific enzyme-linked immunosorbent assay (ELISA, microplate reader "Bio-Rad 680", Bio-Rad Laboratories Inc, Hercules, California, USA) as a serum biomarker of fibrosis. These biomarkers were selected based on previous publications demonstrating their role in cardiac fibrosis [8].

2.3. Blood Pressure Measurement

Office blood pressure (BP) was measured with a calibrated automatic sphygmomanometer (OMRON M3 Expert, Omron Dalian, Kioto, Japan). We used a BP cuff that fits the participants' arm circumference. Three measurements were performed in a seated position after a 5-min rest with a 5-min interval. The average value of the two last measurements was calculated.

2.4. Pulse Wave Analysis

BP waveforms were recorded on the carotid and femoral arteries using applanation tonometry (SphygmoCor, AtCor Medical, Sidney, Australia) in standardized conditions (supine position, quiet atmosphere, and temperature 24 °C). Caffeine and smoking were not allowed within 3 h before evaluation. Pulse wave velocity (PWV) was calculated automatically according to the patient's height, weight, and brachial BP assessed before the procedure. The cut-off value for carotid-femoral PWV was 10 m/s [13].

2.5. Reactive Hyperemia Peripheral Arterial Tonometry

Endothelial function was assessed using peripheral arterial tonometry with the EndoPAT2000 device (Itamar Medical, Caesarea, Israel). Reactive hyperemia index (RHI) was evaluated according to the previously reported protocol [14]. RHI < 1.67 was considered a sign of peripheral arterial endothelial dysfunction [14].

2.6. Echocardiography

Echocardiography was performed using the Vivid 7 system (GE Healthcare, Chicago, IL, USA) according to a standard protocol with an assessment of global longitudinal strain (GLS) and the ratio of early diastolic transmitral flow velocity to the average peak early diastolic mitral annular velocity (E/e') as a measure of filling pressures [14,15]. LV mass/body surface area >115 g/m^2 in men and >95 g/m^2 in women was defined as LV hypertrophy [15,16].

2.7. Cardiac MRI

Cardiac MRI was carried out using a high-field 3 T MRI scanner MAGNETOM Trio A Tim System 3T (Siemens Healthineers, Erlangen, Germany) in an ECG-synchronized mode. The procedure was performed according to the standard protocol, which included late gadolinium enhancement (LGE) sequences using PSIR (Phase-sensitive Inversion Recovery) sequences with an inversion time of 200 ms, a repetition time of 8.5 ms, and an echo time of 3.5 ms, after 10 min gadopentetate dimeglumine (0.2 mmol/kg, Gadovist, BayerHealthcare, Berlin, Germany) administration. All analyses were performed by an independent reader. Left ventricular function was evaluated semi-automatically using commercially available software (Syngo Via, Siemens Healthineers, Erlangen, Germany) according to ACCF/ACR/AHA/NASCI/SCMR recommendations [17]. Following automatic contour detection of the LV endocardium, all borders were corrected manually. The extent of LGE was calculated semi-quantitatively by counting the number of LV segments showing visually-determined LGE. LGE volume was calculated by summation of the LGE areas in all short-axis slices, which was expressed as a volumetric proportion of the total LV myocardium using a similar approach previously described [18]. Analysis of LGE was performed visually in a short-axis stack and a four-chamber view for the presence of LGE using the 17-segment model of the American Heart Association (AHA) [19].

2.8. Carotid Ultrasonography

Carotid ultrasound studies were performed by high-resolution B-mode ultrasonography (Vivid7, GE Healthcare, Chicago, IL, USA) with a linear array broadband transducer 7 MHz. The standard protocol included bilateral measurements at a distance of 1 cm from the bifurcation of the common carotid artery along its posterior wall in three positions (anterior, middle, and posterior longitudinal). The intima-media thickness (IMT) was defined as the distance between the first and second echogenic lines of the artery. Then, the mean IMT on both sides was calculated as an arithmetic mean of three dimensions. The subclinical vascular damage was detected if IMT ≥ 0.9 mm.

2.9. Statistical Analysis

Data are presented as mean ($\pm$standard deviation) or median (interquartile range) for normal and abnormal distributed continuous variables, respectively, whereas categorical data were expressed as frequencies and percentages. Differences in baseline characteristics were evaluated using Student's t-test, Mann–Whitney U test, or Chi-square test, depending on the variable category. The one-way ANOVA and post hoc (Tukey–Kramer test) were also used for the comparison of parameters in three groups. Spearman correlation was used to evaluate relationships involving ordinal variables. Statistical significance was considered at $p < 0.05$. A correlation matrix incorporating all evaluated clinical, laboratory parameters, and serum biomarkers was created. Those factors that had a statistically significant correlation with MRI-LGE-positive findings were studied using logistic regression. When factors had a significant cross-correlation ($\rho > 0.65$), one of them was selected for the multivariate regression analysis based on a higher correlation coefficient with LGE positivity. Factors independently associated with MRI-detected fibrosis were evaluated using two multivariate binary logistic regression models: the first aimed at the inclusion of all factors significantly correlated with MRI-detected fibrosis and incorporated a combination of clinical, echocardiography, and biochemical markers; the second model aimed at the inclusion of only additional factors with moderate-to-significant correlation (serum biomarkers and pulse wave velocity). We suggested that the latter model would be practically applicable for the identification of cardiac-fibrosis-positive serum biomarkers in the mixed population. The regression analysis was performed for the total study population and for T2DM patients separately. IBM software SPSS Version 23 (SPSS, Inc., Chicago, IL, USA) and Statistica 13.0 (Statsoft, Tulsa, OK, USA) were applied for statistical analysis.

3. Results

3.1. Patient Baseline Characteristics

The study population comprised 79 subjects: 37 subjects in the T2DM group (age ranging between 44 and 70 years), 27 subjects in the risk factors (RF) group (age 40–68 years), and 15 subjects in the healthy control (HC) group (age 50–65 years). The baseline subjects' characteristics are summarized in Table 1. There were no differences in age, sex, blood pressure (BP) level, and smoking status between the T2DM and RF groups. Patients without diabetes tended to have a higher body mass index (BMI) with the same waist circumference, but statistically it was not significant. All hypertensive patients were receiving angiotensin-converting enzyme inhibitors (ACEI) or angiotensin II receptor blockers (ARB). Although statistically borderline, the prevalence of carotid intima-media thickness (IMT) ≥ 0.9 mm tended to be higher in T2DM patients (19% vs. 3.7% in the RF group, $p = 0.052$), whereas the carotid-femoral PWV ≥ 10 m/s was significantly more prevalent in the T2DM group (32% vs. 3.7%, respectively; $\chi 2 = 8.65$; $p = 0{,}003$). Despite a significantly lower reactive hyperemia index in the diabetic patients, the percentage of patients with reactive hyperemia index (RHI) < 1.67 did not differ between the T2DM and RF groups: 65% vs. 52%, respectively ($p = 0.296$). The RHI had a negative correlation with the duration of diabetes (r = −0.356; $p = 0.03$), the carotid-femoral PWV (r = −0.371; $p = 0.024$), and the carotid IMT (r = −0.622; $p < 0.001$). A negative correlation between the RHI and carotid IMT was observed in the RF group (r = −0.558; $p = 0.002$). There was no difference in the estimated glomerular filtration rate (eGFR) between the groups.

Table 1. Baseline characteristics of study subjects.

Variables	T2DM Group $n = 37$	RF Group $n = 27$	HC Group $n = 15$	p [1,2]-Value	p [2,3]-Value
	1	2	3		
Age, years	57.5 ± 8.4	54.0 ± 8.9	55.6 ± 3.6	0.122	0.378
Male, n (%)	17 (46)	12 (44)	7 (47)	0.905	0.735
BMI, kg/m	32.9 ± 6.5	35.6 ± 2.7	23.8 ± 2.0	0.051	<0.001
Waist circumference, cm	109.4 ± 14.0	113.6 ± 8.9		0.186	
Male	111.5 ± 14.3	118.2 ± 8.7		0.166	
Female	107.8 ± 14.0	109.9 ± 7.4		0.598	
T2DM duration, years	9.0 [5.0–12.0]	-			
Hypertension, n (%)	21 (57)	19 (70)	0	0.058	
Current smoker, n (%)	12 (32)	11 (41)	3 (20)	0.792	0.071
Office systolic BP, mm Hg	131 ± 17	130 ± 17	118 ± 9	0.673	0.002
Office diastolic BP, mm Hg	77 ± 10	81 ± 14	75 ± 8	0.415	0.130
Carotid-femoral PWV, m/s	9.9 ± 2.2	7.9 ± 1.7		0.0002	
Carotid IMT, mm	0.715 ± 0.374	0.618 ± 0.113	0.535 ± 0.114	0.010	<0.001
RHI	1.50 ± 0.35	1.70 ± 0.31		0.019	
eGFR, mL/min/1.73 m^2	88.4 ± 15.8	90.1 ± 15.9		0.550	
Echocardiography					
LA volume index, mL/m^2	36.7 ± 6.8	32.7 ± 6.0		0.016	
LV mass index, g/m^2	120.8 ± 32.0	102.0 ± 23.3		0.008	
Male	131.9 ± 38.6	111.8 ± 24.1	90.3 ± 13.4	0.170	0.002
Female	111.3 ± 21.9	93.6 ± 19.7		0.014	
Relative wall thickness	0.448 ± 0.050	0.434 ± 0.048		0.813	
LV EF, %	60.6 ± 5.5	60.9 ± 3.3		0.603	
E/e'	8.2 ± 1.9	7.3 ± 1.2		0.021	
GLS, %	−18.0 ± 3.0	−19.1 ± 2.1		0.110	

Table 1. Cont.

Variables	T2DM Group n = 37	RF Group n = 27	HC Group n = 15	$p^{1,2}$-Value	$p^{2,3}$-Value
	1	2	3		
Medication					
Metformin, n (%)	22(59)	1(4)	–	<0.001	
DPP-4 inhibitors, n (%)	5(13.5)	–	–		
Sulphonylureas, n (%)	2(5.4)	–	–		
Insulin, n (%)	8 (21.6)	–	–		
ACEI or ARB, n (%)	21 (56.8)	19 (70)	–	0.058	
Low-dose aspirin, n (%)	13 (48.1)	4 (14.8)	–	0.002	
Statins, n (%)	18 (48.6)	4 (14.8)	–	<0.01	

Data are presented as mean ± SD or median (interquartile range, IQR) for normal and abnormal distributed continuous variables. Categorical data were expressed as numbers of subjects and percentages. RF—risk factors; HC—healthy control; BMI—body mass index; BP—blood pressure; IMT—intima-media thickness; RHI—reactive hyperemia index; eGFR—estimated glomerular filtration rate (MDRD derived); LA—left atrium; LV—left ventricle; EF—ejection fraction; E/e'—the ratio of mitral inflow early diastolic velocity to the average peak early diastolic mitral annular velocity; GLS—global longitudinal strain; DPP-4—dipeptidylpeptidase-4; ACEI—angiotensin-converting enzyme inhibitor; ARB—angiotensin II receptor blocker; BMI—body mass index; PWV—pulse wave velocity; $p^{1,2}$—comparison between T2DM and RF groups; $p^{2,3}$—comparison with healthy controls.

3.2. Laboratory Measurements

There was a significant difference in serum lipid levels between the groups. Thus, RF patients were characterized by higher mean low-density cholesterol (LDL-C) intima-media thickness and triglyceride levels (Table 2). Surprisingly, the HC subjects had similar lipid levels when compared with the RF group. Serum Carboxy-terminal propeptide of collagen 1 (PICP) and amino-terminal propeptide of collagen 3 (PIIINP) levels as the collagen metabolism markers were significantly increased in the T2DM and RF groups compared to the HC subjects. Among T2DM patients, statin therapy was associated with a lower PICP level: 129 ng/mL [QIR: 115–146] vs. 192 ng/mL [QIR: 169–195] in patients without statins ($p < 0.001$). Interestingly, there were no differences in PIIINP levels between the T2DM and RF groups. Concentrations of matrix metalloproteinase 9 (MMP9), tissue inhibitor of metalloproteinase 1 (TIMP1), and carboxy-terminal telopeptide of collagen 1 (ICTP) were the lowest in the HC group. However, T2DM patients had higher TIMP1 and ICTP levels. The increased soluble suppression of tumorigenicity 2 (sST2) level was associated with an increase in IMT in both T2DM ($r = 0.361$; $p = 0.028$) and RF patients ($r = 0.499$; $p = 0.008$), presumably due to negative effects on endothelial function and RHI as its marker ($R^2 = 0.357$; $p = 0.004$). Higher serum TGFβ1 levels were revealed in T2DM and RF groups compared to the HC subjects, but serum TGFβ1 had a significant positive correlation with BMI (body mass index) ($r = 0.564$; $p = 0.0002$), waist circumference ($r = 0.432$; $p = 0.008$) and a negative correlation with eGFR ($r = -0.471$; $p = 0.008$) only in the T2DM group. Serum galectin-3 level, as well as TGF, was predominantly increased in T2DM patients. There were no gender differences in the profile of serum fibrosis biomarkers.

3.3. Echocardiography and Cardiac MRI Analysis

Left ventricle (LV) hypertrophy was revealed in 30 diabetic (81%) and 9 (33%) RF patients ($\chi 2 = 15.4$; $p = 0.0005$), including 25 (67.6%) and 5 (18.5%) patients ($p = 0.0005$) with concentric LV hypertrophy, respectively. The LV concentric hypertrophy was accompanied by an increased serum galectin-3 level in T2DM patients: 9.92 ng/mL [QIR: 8.38–12.96] vs. 8.14 ng/mL [QIR: 6.58–9.85], $p = 0.039$. Left atrial (LA) enlargement (index LA volume ≥ 34 mL/m^2) was noted in 21 (56.8%) T2DM and 8 (29.6%) RF patients ($p = 0.094$). In T2DM patients, LA enlargement was associated with a higher serum PIIINP level ($r = 0.434$; $p = 0.007$). A negative correlation between PICP level and the global longitudinal strain (GLS) was found ($r = -0.467$; $p = 0.004$). This fact is especially interesting since we revealed the relationship between PICP and HbA1c levels in both main groups ($R2 = 0.309$; $p = 0.014$).

Another marker of diastolic dysfunction such as the E/e' ratio correlated with HbA1c (r = 0.426; p = 0.029) and TIMP1 (r = 0.543; p = 0.004) levels only in RF patients.

Table 2. Lab tests and fibrosis biomarkers.

Variables	T2DM Group n = 37	RF Group n = 27	HC Group n = 15	$p^{1,2}$-Value	$p^{2,3}$-Value
	1	2	3		
Total cholesterol, mmol/L	4.84 ± 0.97	5.40 ± 1,11	4.52 ± 1,24	0.056	0.095
HDL-C, mmol/L	1.11 ± 0.26	1.15 ± 0.28	1.16 ± 0.31	0.757	0.62
LDL-C, mmol/L	2.67 ± 0.91	3.49 ± 0.92	2.62 ± 0.98	0.002	0.017
Triglycerides, mmol/L	2.58 ± 1.07	1.88 ± 0.78	1.67 ± 0.93	0.007	0.22
hsCRP, mg/L	2.55 [1.21–4.78]	3.84 [1.99–5.70]	1.67 [0.73–2.96]	0.185	0.11
HbA1c, %	8.9 ± 1.4	5.74 ± 0.85	-	<0.001	-
NT-proBNP, pg/mL	91 [16–148]	27.5 [15.7–47.6]	-	<0.001	-
PICP, ng/mL	136.0 [117.2–166.0]	108.4 [93.2–148.8]	84.0 [69.0–98.3]	0.006	0.001
PIIINP, ng/mL	5.74 [4.43–6.77]	5.09 [4.44–5.96]	3.99 [3.27–4.27]	0.265	0.002
sST2, ng/mL	19.1 [14.9–26.7]	13.2 [10.2–21.8]	12.6 [10.3–16.2]	0.016	0.912
MMP-9, ng/mL	794 [497–1015]	490 [341–911]	277 [253–319]	0.084	0.002
TIMP-1, ng/mL	188 [171–237]	152 [137–185]	141 [120–164]	0.004	0.023
TGF-β1, ng/mL	35.7 [24.5–48.6]	29.6 [15.3–42.2]	12.8 [11.9–18.6]	0.067	<0.001
galectin-3, ng/mL	9.5 [7.8–12.5]	7.8 [6.8–9.9]	6.9 [6.0–7.2]	0.029	0.010
ICTP, ng/mL	5,25 [3.5–6.8]	3.49 [3.03–5.89]	2.98 [2.68–3.97]	0.046	0.030

Data are presented as mean ± SD or median (interquartile range, IQR) for normal and abnormal distributed continuous variables. Categorical data were expressed as numbers of subjects and percentages. HDL-C—high-density lipoproteins; LDL-C—low-density lipoproteins; hsCRP—high-sensitive C-reactive protein; HbA1c—glycated hemoglobin A1c; NT-proBNP; RF—risk factors; HC—healthy control; PICP—carboxy-terminal propeptide of collagen 1; PIIINP—amino-terminal propeptide of collagen 3; sST2—soluble suppression of tumorigenicity 2; MMP-9—matrix metalloproteinase 9; TIMP-1—tissue inhibitor of metalloproteinase 1; TGF-β1—transforming growth factor β-1; ICTP—carboxy-terminal telopeptide of collagen 1. $p^{1,2}$ and $p^{2,3}$—compression between groups.

LGE was detected in 22 (59.5%) T2DM patients and in 4 (14.85%) RF patients. LGE was found predominantly in the anteroseptal and inferior mid-wall and basal segments (Figure 1). By semi-quantitative assessment, LGE volume was 13% [QIR: 9–14%] in T2DM patients, while among RF patients only 4% [QIR: 2–4%] (p = 0.002).

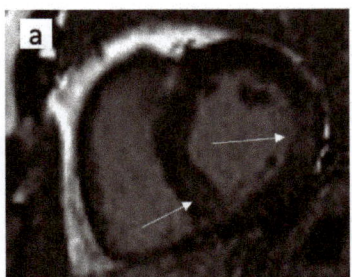 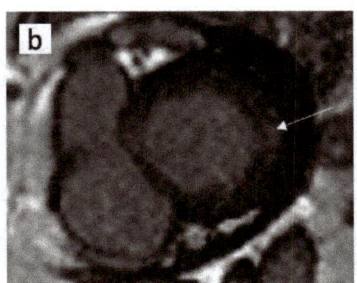 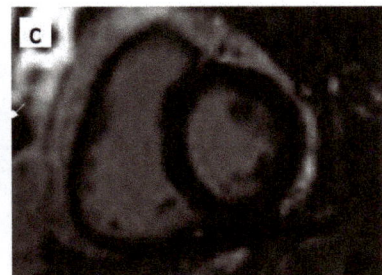

Figure 1. Examples of cardiac MRI with and without LGE: (a) a T2DM patient with positive LGE; (b) RF patient with positive LGE; (c) RF patient without LGE; the white arrows indicate LGE areas in the septum; (a) left lateral LV wall (a,b).

Diabetes, its baseline treatment with metformin, HbA1c, and serum TIMP-1 levels, and LV hypertrophy had moderate positive correlations with LGE-MRI findings (p < 0.05). Although statistically significant, statin treatment, BMI, PWV, and galectin-3 serum level had a weak positive correlation with LGE positivity. LDL-C level had a weak negative correlation with cardiac MRI-detected fibrosis. Univariate logistic regression coefficients are presented in Table 3. The multivariate regression analysis identified that in the first model, TIMP-1 level was the only independent factor associated with cardiac fibrosis. The second model identified TIMP-1 levels and galectin-3 levels as factors independently associated with cardiac fibrosis (Tables 4 and 5). In T2DM patients, the regression analysis confirmed significant associations of TIMP-1 and PWV with cardiac fibrosis, and the multivariate model identified TIMP-1 as the only factor independently associated with LGE-positive findings (Tables 3 and 4).

Table 3. Univariate logistic regression analysis of factors associated with cardiac fibrosis as detected by MRI.

	Estimate	Standard Error	Wald Stat.	Lower CL—95. %	Upper CL—95. %	p
			All subjects (T2DM+RF+HC groups)			
T2DM: Yes	1.101	0.32	11.807	0.473	1.728	<0.001
BMI, kg/m^2	−0.104	0.053	3.832	−0.209	0.0001	0.05
Metformin baseline therapy: Yes	1.06	0.305	12.042	0.461	1.659	<0.001
Statins: Yes	0.785	0.281	7.794	0.234	1.335	0.005
PWV, m/s	0.327	0.135	5.898	0.063	0.591	0.015
RHI	−1.398	0.8	3.053	−2.966	0.17	0.081
LV hypertrophy	0.799	0.299	7.161	0.214	1.384	0.008
HbA1c, %	0.52	0.167	9.682	0.192	0.848	0.002
LDL-C, mM/L	−0.534	0.294	3.306	−1.109	0.042	0.069
TIMP-1, ng/mL	0.018	0.006	8.438	0.006	0.03	0.004
Galectin-3, ng/mL	0.225	0.09	6.159	0.047	0.403	0.013
			T2DM patients only			
PWV, m/s	−0.351	0.194	3.261	−0.73	0.03	0.042
TIMP-1, ng/mL	−0.02	0.008	5.187	0.036	−0.003	0.05

Table 4. General multivariate regression model of cardiac fibrosis predictors (as detected by MRI).

	Estimate	Standard Error	Wald Stat.	Lower CL—95, %	Upper CL—95, %	p
			All subjects (T2DM+RF+HC groups)			
Intercept	−5.596	2.189	6.533	−9.887	−1.304	0.01
PWV, m/s	0.12	0.175	0.471	−0.223	0.464	0.492
TIMP-1, ng/mL	0.014	0.007	4.042	0.0003	0.028	0.044
Galectin-3, ng/mL	0.136	0.109	1.57	−0.077	0.349	0.21
T2DM: Yes	0.67	0.426	2.466	−0.166	1.506	0.116
LV hypertrophy: Yes	0.524	0.412	1.623	−0.282	1.331	0.203
			T2DM patients only			
Intercept	6.607	2.778	5.657	1.163	12.052	0.02
PWV, m/s	−0.353	0.218	2.623	−0.780	0.074	0.12
TIMP-1, ng/mL	−0.018	0.009	4.596	−0.035	−0.002	0.03

Table 5. Multivariate model with additional factors only that predicted cardiac fibrosis in all subjects (as detected by MRI).

	Estimate	Standard Error	Wald Stat.	Lower CL—95, %	Upper CL—95, %	p
			All subjects (T2DM+RF+HC groups)			
Intercept	−7.128	1.996	12.749	−11.04	−3.215	0.0004
PWV, m/s	0.208	0.155	1.796	−0.096	0.512	0.18
TIMP-1, ng/mL	0.017	0.007	6.265	0.004	0.029	0.01
Galectin-3, ng/mL	0.189	0.099	3.648	−0.005	0.384	0.049

4. Discussion

Myocardial fibrosis is usually assessed by an easy scoring system using late gadolinium-enhanced cardiac magnetic resonance (LGE-MRI) imaging. This method is widely used for the risk stratification of patients with cardiovascular disease, yet it is the most accurate method to reveal replacement myocardial fibrosis; however, it is less sensitive in interstitial fibrosis detection. LGE has been reported to predict death and myocardial infarction in a cohort of 1969 patients with and without T2DM [20].

The univariate logistic regression identified the association of T2DM, glycated hemoglobin level, and metformin intake with LGE-positive MRI findings, emphasizing the important role of impaired glucose metabolism in the development of myocardial fibrosis. Previously, an in vitro study has shown that hyperglycemia is a powerful stimulator of fibroblast proliferation, myofibroblast differentiation, and extracellular matrix proteins' secretion [21].

T2DM patients have a higher prevalence of increased LV mass index, concentric LV hypertrophy in combination with LA enlargement, and increased E/e' ratio compared with the RF group. This confirms a link between LV hypertrophy with positive LGE and might be associated with poorly controlled T2DM and higher HbA1c levels. LV hypertrophy with diastolic dysfunction is typical for diabetic cardiomyopathy but is also widely prevalent in the elderly population, females, and patients with hypertension and obesity [22,23]. Importantly, we have not found any association between cardiac remodeling and the above-mentioned risk factors in T2DM patients and suggest that this could be explained in part by limited sample size and previous antihypertensive therapy. Moreover, T2DM and RF groups included obese patients, and obesity is one of the pivotal contributors to myocardial fibrosis [24]. This fact is confirmed by the results of the large Multi-Ethnic Study of Atherosclerosis study, where an increased BMI has been shown to be associated with the concentric hypertrophy by cardiac MRI [25].

Pulse wave velocity (PWV) is widely used for arterial stiffness measurement [26]. According to the univariate analysis, cardiac fibrosis is associated with TIMP and galectin-3 levels, as well as with the carotid-femoral PWV. Adjusted for age and blood pressure, T2DM duration appears to be the most important contributor to arterial stiffness [27]. The relationship between arterial stiffness and the severity of LV diastolic dysfunction has been confirmed in a wide variety of cardiovascular diseases [28,29]. Recently, PWV has been linked to different cardiovascular events, including CV mortality [30]. The association between obesity and arterial stiffness confirms the results of the previous study by Desamericq et al. [31]. The correlation between positive LGE and PWV observed in our study supports the conception of common pathophysiological mechanisms of cardiac and vascular remodeling in T2DM. However, according to the multivariate analysis, PWV is not an independent predictor of cardiac fibrosis, while circulating TIMP1 and galectin-3 are strongly associated with cardiac fibrosis being active participants in the pathophysiology of heart and vascular remodeling.

Studies on galectin-3, a protein of the lectin family secreted by activated macrophages and fibroblasts, open novel opportunities for non-invasive cardiac remodeling monitoring in T2DM patients. Previous studies have identified higher circulating galectin-3 levels predicting the onset of HFpEF [32,33]. In addition to LGE-MRI, galectin-3 seems to play an important role in the sudden death risk stratification of heart failure patients [34]. Our study confirms the predictive value of galectin-3 in the diagnosis of cardiac fibrosis.

The circulating serum biomarkers of collagen synthesis and degradation are used for indirect myocardial fibrosis assessment [8]. A distinctive feature of T2DM and RF patients included in this study is the high PIIINP level (as a marker of III collagen synthesis activation) [35]. Circulating PIIINP can serve as a marker of large vessel remodeling [36]. Histological studies have shown increased PICP and PIIINP levels associated with interstitial and perivascular cardiac fibrosis in T2DM, regardless of the presence of coronary atherosclerosis and hypertension [37]. In our study, elevated serum PIIINP levels were associated with LA enlargement as a marker of LV diastolic dysfunction. Opposite, a decrease in the GLS as an early marker of LV systolic dysfunction was related to the circulating PICP level. An interesting finding is a reduction in PICP level as a marker of type I collagen synthesis during statin therapy. We speculate that low adherence to statin therapy might be associated with an increase in heart failure and chronic kidney disease risk among T2DM patients [38,39].

The presence of a positive correlation between BMI and serum TGF-β1 level, a paracrine regulator of extracellular matrix synthesis, supports the consideration of obesity as a myocardial fibrosis accelerator. A significant increase in TIMP1 and ICTP levels has been identified in both groups. Previously, direct relations between plasma TIMP-1 levels and all major CVD risk factors, including male gender, have been demonstrated in the Framingham heart study [40]. It should be noted that obese patients in our study are characterized by an increased HbA1c level, and the higher serum TIMP1 concentration is associated with elevated E/e' rati, as a marker of LV diastolic dysfunction. In a recent study, TIMP1 has been shown to activate adipogenesis by accelerating lipid accumulation, adipocyte differentiation, and pro-inflammatory cytokine production [41]. Thus, in T2DM patients, TIMP1 may be involved in the target organ damage due to its role in adipogenesis, systemic inflammation, and fibrosis. We suggest this is a major reason why among the numerous factors, TIMP1 is an independent predictor of cardiac fibrosis.

Study Limitations

The study was performed on a limited non-random patient group who were referred to the Almazov Centre due to poor glycemic control. Both cardiovascular (antihypertensive and hypolipidemic) and antidiabetic therapy were not standardized before patient inclusion. There was a significant overlap of CV risk factors between the groups, and all of them may influence CV remodeling. Myocardial fibrosis was assessed with LGE-MRI imaging, which is less informative when diffuse myocardial fibrosis is present.

5. Conclusions

Our cross-sectional study demonstrates that T2DM patients have elevated levels of circulating fibrosis markers and a high prevalence of LGE-MRI. Galectin-3 and TIMP1 serum levels are strongly associated with LGE-MRI in T2DM patients and patients with cardiovascular risk factors. Serum TIMP1 level is an independent predictor of cardiac fibrosis.

Author Contributions: Conceptualization, E.B.L., A.Y.B., A.O.K. and O.M.M.; methodology, E.B.L., M.A.B., A.A.V., E.V.K., E.N.M., A.Y.B. and O.M.M.; validation, E.B.L., E.N.M. and O.M.M.; formal analysis, O.M.M. and E.B.L.; investigation, E.B.L., M.A.B., A.A.V., E.V.K., A.V.R. and O.M.M.; resources, E.N.M., A.O.K. and O.M.M.; data curation, O.M.M.; writing—original draft preparation, E.B.L., E.N.M. and O.M.M.; writing—review and editing, all authors; visualization, A.V.R.; supervision, A.O.K. and O.M.M.; project administration, E.B.L.; funding acquisition, E.N.M. and O.M.M. All authors have read and agreed to the published version of the manuscript.

Funding: This research was funded by the Ministry of Science and Higher Education, grant number 075-15-2020-800.

Institutional Review Board Statement: The study was conducted in accordance with the Declaration of Helsinki and approved by the Ethics Committee of the Almazov Centre (No. 05072019 dated 8 July 2019).

Informed Consent Statement: Informed consent was obtained from all subjects involved in the study.

Data Availability Statement: All relevant data are included in the manuscript.

Conflicts of Interest: The authors declare no conflict of interest. The funder had no role in the design of the study; in the collection, analyses, or interpretation of data; in the writing of the manuscript, or in the decision to publish the results.

References

1. Rawshani, A.; Rawshani, A.; Franzén, S.; Sattar, N.; Eliasson, B.; Svensson, A.M.; Zethelius, B.; Miftaraj, M.; McGuire, D.K.; Rosengren, A.; et al. Risk factors, mortality, and cardiovascular outcomes in patients with type 2 diabetes. *N. Engl. J. Med.* **2018**, *379*, 633–644. [CrossRef] [PubMed]
2. Di Cesare, M.; Bentham, J.; Stevens, G.A.; Zhou, B.; Danaei, G.; Lu, Y.; Bixby, H.; Cowan, M.J.; Riley, L.M.; Hajifathalian, K.; et al. Trends in adult body-mass index in 200 countries from 1975 to 2014: A pooled analysis of 1698 population-based measurement studies with 19·2 million participants. *Lancet* **2016**, *387*, 1377–1396. [CrossRef]
3. Beckman, J.A.; Creager, M.A.; Libby, P. Diabetes and atherosclerosis: Epidemiology, pathophysiology, and management. *JAMA* **2002**, *287*, 2570–2581. [CrossRef] [PubMed]
4. Kenny, H.C.; Abel, E.D. Heart Failure in Type 2 Diabetes Mellitus. *Circ. Res.* **2019**, *124*, 121–141. [CrossRef] [PubMed]
5. Burlew, B.S.; Weber, K.T. Cardiac fibrosis as a cause of diastolic dysfunction. *Herz* **2002**, *27*, 92–98. [CrossRef]
6. Karamitsos, T.D.; Arvanitaki, A.; Karvounis, H.; Neubauer, S.; Ferreira, V.M. Myocardial tissue characterization and fibrosis by imaging. *JACC Cardiovasc. Imaging* **2020**, *13*, 1221–1234. [CrossRef] [PubMed]
7. Tadic, M.; Cuspidi, C.; Calicchio, F.; Grassi, G.; Mancia, G. Diabetic cardiomyopathy: How can cardiac magnetic resonance help? *Acta Diabetol.* **2020**, *57*, 1027–1034. [CrossRef]
8. López, B.; González, A.; Ravassa, S.; Beaumont, J.; Moreno, M.U.; San José, G.; Querejeta, R.; Díez, J. Circulating biomarkers of myocardial fibrosis: The need for a reappraisal. *J. Am. Coll. Cardiol.* **2015**, *65*, 2449–2456. [CrossRef]
9. Richards, A.M. Circulating biomarkers of cardiac fibrosis: Do we have any and what use are they? *Circ. Heart Fail.* **2017**, *10*, e003936. [CrossRef]
10. Shim, C.Y.; Hong, G.R.; Ha, J.W. Ventricular stiffness and ventricular-arterial coupling in heart failure: What is it, how to assess, and why? *Heart Fail. Clin.* **2019**, *15*, 267–274. [CrossRef]
11. Yoshida, Y.; Nakanishi, K.; Daimon, M.; Ishiwata, J.; Sawada, N.; Hirokawa, M.; Kaneko, H.; Nakao, T.; Mizuno, Y.; Morita, H.; et al. Sex-specific difference in the association between arterial stiffness and subclinical left ventricular dysfunction. *Eur. Heart J. Cardiovasc. Imaging* **2020**, *28*, jeaa156. [CrossRef]
12. Ban, C.R.; Twigg, S.M. Fibrosis in diabetes complications: Pathogenic mechanisms and circulating and urinary markers. *Vasc. Health Risk Manag.* **2008**, *4*, 575–596. [CrossRef] [PubMed]
13. Van Bortel, L.M.; Laurent, S.; Boutouyrie, P.; Chowienczyk, P.; Cruickshank, J.K.; De Backer, T.; Filipovsky, J.; Huybrechts, S.; Mattace-Raso, F.U.; Protogerou, A.D.; et al. Artery Society; European Society of Hypertension working group on vascular structure and function; European Network for Noninvasive Investigation of Large Arteries. Expert consensus document on the measurement of aortic stiffness in daily practice using carotid-femoral pulse wave velocity. *J. Hypertens.* **2012**, *30*, 445–448. [CrossRef] [PubMed]
14. Michelsen, M.M.; Mygind, N.D.; Pena, A.; Aziz, A.; Frestad, D.; Host, N.; Prescott, E. Steering committee of the iPOWER study. Peripheral reactive hyperemia index and coronary microvascular function in women with no obstructive CAD: The iPOWER study. *JACC Cardiovasc. Imaging* **2016**, *9*, 411–417. [CrossRef]
15. Nagueh, S.F.; Smiseth, O.A.; Appleton, C.P.; Byrd, B.F., 3rd; Dokainish, H.; Edvardsen, T.; Flachskampf, F.A.; Gillebert, T.C.; Klein, A.L.; Lancellotti, P.; et al. Recommendations for the evaluation of left ventricular diastolic function by echocardiography: An update from the American Society of Echocardiography and the European Association of Cardiovascular Imaging. *J. Am. Soc. Echocardiogr* **2016**, *29*, 277–314. [CrossRef]
16. Lang, R.M.; Badano, L.P.; Mor-Avi, V.; Afilalo, J.; Armstrong, A.; Ernande, L.; Flachskampf, F.A.; Foster, E.; Goldstein, S.A.; Kuznetsova, T.; et al. Recommendations for cardiac chamber quantification by echocardiography in adults: An update from the American Society of Echocardiography and the European Association of Cardiovascular Imaging. *J. Am. Soc. Echocardiogr* **2015**, *28*, 1–39.e14. [CrossRef]
17. Hundley, W.G.; Bluemke, D.A.; Finn, J.P.; Flamm, S.D.; Fogel, M.A.; Friedman, M.G.; Ho, V.B.; Jerosch-Herold, M.; Kramer, C.M.; Manning, W.J.; et al. ACCF/ACR/AHA/NASCI/SCMR 2010 expert consensus document on cardiovascular magnetic resonance: A report of the American College of Cardiology Foundation Task Force on Expert Consensus Documents. *Circulation* **2010**, *121*, 2462–2508. [CrossRef]
18. Kim, E.K.; Lee, S.C.; Hwang, J.W.; Chang, S.A.; Park, S.J.; On, Y.K.; Park, K.M.; Choe, Y.H.; Kim, S.M.; Park, S.W.; et al. Differences in apical and non-apical types of hypertrophic cardiomyopathy: A prospective analysis of clinical, echocardiographic, and cardiac magnetic resonance findings and outcome from 350 patients. *Eur. Heart J. Cardiovasc. Imaging* **2016**, *17*, 678–686. [CrossRef]
19. Cerqueira, M.D.; Weissman, N.J.; Dilsizian, V.; Jacobs, A.K.; Kaul, S.; Laskey, W.K.; Pennell, D.J.; Rumberger, J.A.; Ryan, T.; Verani, M.S.; et al. Standardized myocardial segmentation and nomenclature for tomographic imaging of the heart: A statement for healthcare professionals from the Cardiac Imaging Committee of the Council on Clinical Cardiology of the American Heart Association. *Circulation* **2002**, *105*, 539–542. [CrossRef]
20. Giusca, S.; Kelle, S.; Nagel, E.; Buss, S.J.; Voss, A.; Puntmann, V.; Fleck, E.; Katus, H.A.; Korosoglou, G. Differences in the prognostic relevance of myocardial ischaemia and scar by cardiac magnetic resonance in patients with and without diabetes mellitus. *Eur. Heart J. Cardiovasc. Imaging* **2016**, *17*, 812–820. [CrossRef]
21. Tuleta, I.; Frangogiannis, N.G. Diabetic fibrosis. *Biochim. Biophys. Acta Mol. Basis Dis.* **2021**, *1867*, 166044. [CrossRef] [PubMed]

22. Paolillo, S.; Marsico, F.; Prastaro, M.; Renga, F.; Esposito, L.; De Martino, F.; Di Napoli, P.; Esposito, I.; Ambrosio, A.; Ianniruberto, M.; et al. Diabetic cardiomyopathy: Definition, diagnosis, and therapeutic implications. *Heart Fail. Clin.* **2019**, *15*, 341–347. [CrossRef] [PubMed]
23. Hogg, K.; Swedberg, K.; McMurray, J. Heart failure with preserved left ventricular systolic function; epidemiology, clinical characteristics, and prognosis. *J. Am. Coll. Cardiol.* **2004**, *43*, 317–327. [CrossRef] [PubMed]
24. Di Bello, V.; Santini, F.; Di Cori, A.; Pucci, A.; Palagi, C.; Delle Donne, M.G.; Fierabracci, P.; Marsili, A.; Talini, E.; Giannetti, M.; et al. Obesity cardiomyopathy: Is it a reality? An ultrasonic tissue characterization study. *J. Am. Soc. Echocardiogr.* **2006**, *19*, 1063–1071. [CrossRef] [PubMed]
25. Turkbey, E.B.; McClelland, R.L.; Kronmal, R.A.; Burke, G.L.; Bild, D.E.; Tracy, R.P.; Arai, A.E.; Lima, J.A.; Bluemke, D.A. The impact of obesity on the left ventricle: The Multi-Ethnic Study of Atherosclerosis (MESA). *JACC Cardiovasc. Imaging* **2010**, *3*, 266–274. [CrossRef] [PubMed]
26. Milan, A.; Zocaro, G.; Leone, D.; Tosello, F.; Buraioli, I.; Schiavone, D.; Veglio, F. Current assessment of pulse wave velocity: Comprehensive review of validation studies. *J. Hypertens.* **2019**, *37*, 1547–1557. [CrossRef] [PubMed]
27. Coutinho, T.; Borlaug, B.A.; Pellikka, P.A.; Turner, S.T.; Kullo, I.J. Sex differences in arterial stiffness and ventricular-arterial interactions. *J. Am. Coll. Cardiol.* **2013**, *61*, 96–103. [CrossRef]
28. Smulyan, H.; Lieber, A.; Safar, M.E. Hypertension, diabetes type II, and their association: Role of arterial stiffness. *Am. J. Hypertens.* **2016**, *29*, 5–13. [CrossRef]
29. Mottram, P.M.; Haluska, B.A.; Leano, R.; Carlier, S.; Case, C.; Marwick, T.H. Relation of arterial stiffness to diastolic dysfunction in hypertensive heart disease. *Heart* **2005**, *91*, 1551–1556. [CrossRef]
30. Sharif, S.; Visseren, F.L.J.; Spiering, W.; de Jong, P.A.; Bots, M.L.; Westerink, J. SMART study group. Arterial stiffness as a risk factor for cardiovascular events and all-cause mortality in people with Type 2 diabetes. *Diabet. Med.* **2019**, *36*, 1125–1132. [CrossRef]
31. Desamericq, G.; Tissot, C.M.; Akakpo, S.; Tropeano, A.I.; Millasseau, S.; Macquin-Mavier, I. Carotid-femoral pulse wave velocity is not increased in obesity. *Am. J. Hypertens.* **2015**, *28*, 546–551. [CrossRef] [PubMed]
32. Alonso, N.; Lupón, J.; Barallat, J.; de Antonio, M.; Domingo, M.; Zamora, E.; Moliner, P.; Galán, A.; Santesmases, J.; Pastor, C.; et al. Impact of diabetes on the predictive value of heart failure biomarkers. *Cardiovasc. Diabetol.* **2016**, *15*, 151. [CrossRef] [PubMed]
33. Vora, A.; de Lemos, J.A.; Ayers, C.; Grodin, J.L.; Lingvay, I. Association of galectin-3 with diabetes mellitus in the Dallas Heart Study. *J. Clin. Endocrinol. Metab.* **2019**, *104*, 4449–4458. [CrossRef] [PubMed]
34. Shah, N.N.; Ayyadurai, P.; Saad, M.; Kosmas, C.E.; Dogar, M.U.; Patel, U.; Vittorio, T.J. Galactin-3 and soluble ST2 as complementary tools to cardiac MRI for sudden cardiac death risk stratification in heart failure: A review. *JRSM Cardiovasc. Dis.* **2020**, *9*, 2048004020957840. [CrossRef] [PubMed]
35. Barchetta, I.; Cimini, F.A.; De Gioannis, R.; Ciccarelli, G.; Bertoccini, L.; Lenzi, A.; Baroni, M.G.; Cavallo, M.G. Procollagen-III peptide identifies adipose tissue-associated inflammation in type 2 diabetes with or without nonalcoholic liver disease. *Diabetes Metab. Res. Rev.* **2018**, *34*, e2998. [CrossRef]
36. Agarwal, I.; Arnold, A.; Glazer, N.L.; Barasch, E.; Djousse, L.; Fitzpatrick, A.L.; Gottdiener, J.S.; Ix, J.H.; Jensen, R.A.; Kizer, J.R.; et al. Fibrosis-related biomarkers and large and small vessel disease: The Cardiovascular Health Study. *Atherosclerosis* **2015**, *239*, 539–546. [CrossRef]
37. Russo, I.; Frangogiannis, N.G. Diabetes-associated cardiac fibrosis: Cellular effectors, molecular mechanisms and therapeutic opportunities. *J. Mol. Cell. Cardiol.* **2016**, *90*, 84–93. [CrossRef]
38. Hermida, N.; Markl, A.; Hamelet, J.; Van Assche, T.; Vanderper, A.; Herijgers, P.; van Bilsen, M.; Hilfiker-Kleiner, D.; Noppe, G.; Beauloye, C.; et al. HMGCoA reductase inhibition reverses myocardial fibrosis and diastolic dysfunction through AMP-activated protein kinase activation in a mouse model of metabolic syndrome. *Cardiovasc. Res.* **2013**, *99*, 44–54. [CrossRef]
39. Mach, F.; Baigent, C.; Catapano, A.L.; Koskinas, K.C.; Casula, M.; Badimon, L.; Chapman, M.J.; De Backer, G.G.; Delgado, V.; Ference, B.A.; et al. 2019 ESC/EAS Guidelines for the management of dyslipidaemias: Lipid modification to reduce cardiovascular risk. *Eur. Heart J.* **2020**, *41*, 111–188. [CrossRef]
40. Sundström, J.; Evans, J.C.; Benjamin, E.J.; Levy, D.; Larson, M.G.; Sawyer, D.B.; Siwik, D.A.; Colucci, W.S.; Wilson, P.W.; Vasan, R.S. Relations of plasma total TIMP-1 levels to cardiovascular risk factors and echocardiographic measures: The Framingham heart study. *Eur. Heart J.* **2004**, *25*, 1509–1516. [CrossRef]
41. Wang, Y.; Yuan, J.M.; Pan, A.; Koh, W.P. Tissue inhibitor matrix metalloproteinase 1 and risk of type 2 diabetes in a Chinese population. *BMJ Open Diabetes Res. Care* **2020**, *8*, e001051. [CrossRef] [PubMed]

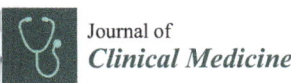

Article

Fasting Glucose Variability as a Risk Indicator for End-Stage Kidney Disease in Patients with Diabetes: A Nationwide Population-Based Study

Da Young Lee [1,†], Jaeyoung Kim [2,3,†], Sanghyun Park [4], So Young Park [1], Ji Hee Yu [1], Ji A. Seo [1], Nam Hoon Kim [1], Hye Jin Yoo [1], Sin Gon Kim [1], Kyung Mook Choi [1], Sei Hyun Baik [1], Kyungdo Han [5,*] and Nan Hee Kim [1,6,*]

1. Division of Endocrinology and Metabolism, Department of Internal Medicine, Korea University College of Medicine, Seoul 02841, Korea; ddkristin412@gmail.com (D.Y.L.); psyou0623@gmail.com (S.Y.P.); dniw99@gmail.com (J.H.Y.); seojia@korea.ac.kr (J.A.S.); pourlife@naver.com (N.H.K.); deisy21@naver.com (H.J.Y.); k50367@korea.ac.kr (S.G.K.); medica7@gmail.com (K.M.C.); 103hyun@gmail.com (S.H.B)
2. Research Institute for Skin Image, Korea University College of Medicine, Seoul 08308, Korea; jaykim830@gmail.com
3. Core Research & Development Center, Korea University Ansan Hospital, Ansan 15355, Korea
4. Division of Endocrinology and Metabolism, Department of Internal Medicine, Seoul St. Mary's Hospital, College of Medicine, The Catholic University of Korea, Seoul 06591, Korea; ujk8774@naver.com
5. Department of Statistics and Actuarial Science, Soongsil University, Seoul 06978, Korea
6. BK21 FOUR R&E Center for Learning Health Systems, Korea University, Seoul 02841, Korea
* Correspondence: hkd917@naver.com (K.H.); nhkendo@gmail.com (N.H.K.); Tel.: +82-2-820-7025 (K.H.); +82-31-412-4274 (N.H.K.); Fax: +82-2-823-1746 (K.H.); +82-31-412-6770 (N.H.K.)
† Da Young Lee and Jaeyoung Kim contributed equally to this article.

Abstract: Given the fact that diabetes remains a leading cause of end-stage kidney disease (ESKD), multi-aspect approaches anticipating the risk for ESKD and timely correction are crucial. We investigated whether fasting glucose variability (FGV) could anticipate the development of ESKD and identify the population prone to the harmful effects of GV. We included 777,192 Koreans with diabetes who had undergone health examinations more than three times in 2005–2010. We evaluated the risk of the first diagnosis of ESKD until 2017, according to the quartile of variability independent of the mean (VIM) of FG using multivariate-adjusted Cox proportional hazards analyses. During the 8-year follow-up, a total of 7290 incidents of ESKD were found. Subjects in the FG VIM quartile 4 had a 27% higher risk for ESKD compared to quartile 1, with adjustment for cardiovascular risk factors and the characteristics of diabetes. This effect was more distinct in patients aged < 65 years; those with a long duration of diabetes; the presence of hypertension or dyslipidemia; and prescribed angiotensin-converting enzyme inhibitors, metformin, sulfonylurea, α-glucosidase inhibitors, and insulin. In contrast, the relationship between baseline FG status and ESKD risk showed a U-shaped association. FGV is an independent risk factor for kidney failure regardless of FG.

Keywords: diabetes mellitus; glucose variability; end-stage kidney disease; Korean National Health Insurance Corporation

1. Introduction

Diabetes remains a leading cause of end-stage kidney disease (ESKD) globally and accounts for 35–50% of these cases [1].

Although several medications, such as sodium-glucose cotransporter 2 inhibitors (SGLT2 inhibitors), angiotensin-converting enzyme inhibitors (ACE inhibitors), and angiotensin-receptor blockers (ARBs), have some protective mechanism against deterioration of renal function, their prevention capacity for ESKD is only 22–40% [2,3]. Therefore, to reduce the burden of ESKD, multi-aspect approaches exploring new biomarkers for anticipating the risk for ESKD and timely correction are crucial in patients with diabetes.

The variability of cardio-metabolic parameters has been an interesting issue because of its predictive value for numerous clinical outcomes [4,5]. Glucose variability (GV) consists of short-term, intraday GV derived from the continuous glucose monitoring system and long-term fasting glucose (FG) variability over several months to years, reflecting the stability of the medication's effect, adherence, and residual insulin secretion [6]. Several studies have reported that high GV is associated with an increased risk of diabetic vascular complications [7,8], heart failure [9], and poor prognosis for acute lung diseases [10].

Regarding kidney outcomes, long-term variability in comprehensive cardio-metabolic risk factors showed a positive association with the future risk of ESKD in the general population, but not in diabetes [4,11]. Furthermore, in patients with diabetes, most evidence adopted glycated hemoglobin (HbA1c) variability rather than GV, and study outcomes were the development of macroalbuminuria or kidney function decline, rather than the development of ESKD [12–15]. This is attributed to the lower incidence rates of ESKD compared to other diabetic vascular complications, such as cardiovascular disease (CVD) [16]. To overcome this limitation, large-scale epidemiologic studies are essential to explore ESKD outcomes.

Therefore, we investigated whether FGV could predict the risk of ESKD using nationally representative population-based cohort data in Korea. We also compared the impact of FGV with FG on future ESKD risk and verified the specific population prone to the detrimental effect of higher FGV.

2. Materials and Methods

2.1. Study Design and Subjects

This was a retrospective observational study (Figures S1 and S2). We extracted the data of the participants who had undergone health examinations supported by the National Health Insurance Corporation (NHIC) at least twice from 2005 to 2008, and simultaneously at least once between 1 January 2009 and 31 December 2010 (referred to as "baseline exam"). That is, the study subjects underwent at least three health examinations during the five years between 2005 and 2010 (referred to as the FGV assessment period). Among them, we excluded 16,736,363 participants without diabetes, aged < 40 years; those with previous histories of ESKD and missing data in the inclusion criteria; and those who were diagnosed with ESKD within one year after baseline. A total of 777,192 participants were included in the study.

The NHIC is a nationally operating health insurance system in Korea and covers approximately 97% of Koreans. The NHIC database contains eligibility information; health examination results, including questionnaires on lifestyle; and a medical care institution database [17,18]. Enrollees of the NHIC are encouraged to perform a standardized medical examination annually or biannually. Information about medical treatments was recognized by the medical bills charged by healthcare providers with the International Classification of Diseases, 10th Revision (ICD-10).

This research was approved by the NHIC and the Institutional Review Board of the Korea University Ansan Hospital (2019AS0138) and followed the Helsinki Declaration of 1975.

2.2. Anthropometric and Laboratory Measurements

Demographic characteristics, lifestyle habits, and medical history were identified using questionnaires during medical examinations. Alcohol consumption was categorized as near abstinence, moderate (<30 g/day), or severe ($\geq$30 g/day). Smoking history was stratified into never, ex-, and current smokers. Regular exercise was defined as >30 min of moderate-intensity exercise or >20 min of vigorous-intensity exercise $\geq$1 per week [19].

Body mass index was calculated as weight (kg) divided by the square of height (m). Blood pressure (BP) was checked after $\geq$5 min of rest.

Venous blood sampling was conducted in the morning after an overnight fast of $\geq$8 h to measure the concentrations of hemoglobin, plasma glucose, creatinine, high-density lipoprotein cholesterol, low-density lipoprotein cholesterol, triglycerides, and total cholesterol.

Midstream urine samples were collected to measure urine protein using a urine dipstick with the following grades: absent, trace (±), 1+, 2+, 3+, and 4+, which correspond to the amount of urine protein of undetectable, 10, 30, 100, 300, and 1000 mg/dL, respectively [4].

Quality control of laboratory tests was performed, followed by the Korean Association of Laboratory Quality Control.

2.3. Definition of Glucose Variability

Using FG concentrations measured at least three times during the five years prior to and including the baseline, the variability independent of the mean (VIM) of FG was calculated as a primary variability indicator (Figure S2). The equation is as follows:

$$\text{VIM} = 100 \times \frac{\text{SD}}{\text{mean}^\beta}$$

Standard deviation (SD), coefficient of variation (CV, SD/mean), and average real variability (ARV) were estimated [20].

$$\text{ARV} = \frac{1}{n-1} \sum_{k=1}^{n-1} \times |\text{BP}_{k+1} - \text{BP}_K|$$

where n is the number of FG measurements, and k ranges from 1 to n − 1.

2.4. Operational Definition of Diseases

Diabetes was defined as a fasting plasma glucose level ≥ 126 mg/dL or at least one prescription of glucose-lowering medicine (GLM) per year with ICD-10 codes E10–14. We defined type 1 diabetes in patients if they had both an ICD-10 code E10 and at least one prescription history of insulin, while the remaining patients were referred to as having type 2 diabetes.

The study outcome was a new diagnosis of ESKD, identified by the initiation of renal replacement therapy or kidney transplantation under ICD-10 codes N18–19, Z49, Z90, Z94, or Z99.2 [21]. Because dialysis is reimbursed when registered in Korea, we could discern all cases of renal replacement therapy under the claim codes for peritoneal dialysis (O7071–O7075 or V003), hemodialysis (O7011–O7020 or V001), and kidney transplantation (R3280) [21]. We excluded acute renal failure events, which were defined as individuals with transient renal replacement therapy or continuous renal replacement therapy without a previous history of CKD. Deceased cases, identified by the nationwide death certificate data of the Korea National Statistical Office, were censored at the time of their death. The follow-up period was calculated from the time interval between the baseline exam and incident ESKD, date of death, or 31 December 2017, whichever came first (Figure S2).

Hypertension was defined as systolic BP ≥ 140 mmHg, diastolic BP ≥ 90 mmHg, or at least one prescription of antihypertensive drugs per year under ICD-10 codes I10–I15. The presence of malignancy was defined by registration in the Korea Central Cancer Registry with ICD-10 C00–C96 before the baseline examination. Low-income status was defined as the lowest 20% income identified by the amount of health insurance premium or eligibility as medical care [17,18]. Dyslipidemia was determined by total cholesterol concentration ≥6.21 mmol/L or at least one prescription of antihyperlipidemic medications under ICD-10 code E78. The estimated glomerular filtration rate (eGFR) < 60 mL/min/1.73 m^2, estimated by the Modification of Diet in Renal Disease formula [22], was stratified according to the presence of chronic kidney disease (CKD) [23].

The prescription of ACE inhibitors or ARBs, oral GLM among metformin, sulfonylurea, meglitinide, thiazolidinedione, inhibitors of dipeptidyl peptidase 4 (DPP-4 inhibitors), α-glucosidase inhibitor (AGI), and insulin in the 12 months before baseline was identified. History of heart disease or stroke was estimated using self-reports.

2.5. Statistical Analysis

Data are shown as mean ± SD, median (interquartile range), or number (%). After stratifying the subjects according to the FG VIM quartile, we compared baseline features using chi-squared tests and analysis of variance for continuous variables. Triglyceride concentrations were log-transformed for the analysis.

Multivariable regression analyses were conducted using the Cox proportional hazards model to estimate the time-dependent risk of ESKD according to FG VIM quartiles, with quartile 1 as the reference group. In model 1, age, sex, body mass index, alcohol drinking, smoking, exercise, presence of CKD, hypertension, dyslipidemia, and low-income status were adjusted. In model 2, the duration of diabetes as continuous variable, insulin prescription, the number of classes of oral GLM during 12 months prior to baseline exam, mean FG measured for the five years preceding the baseline exam, and the number of exams were additionally adjusted. To evaluate the change in significance according to the cutoff value of VIM, we further divided the study population into deciles and reiterated the above-mentioned regression analysis with decile 1 as a reference. In addition, we explored whether the main findings would change after replacing the parameters of FGV with SD, CV, and ARV instead of VIM.

For subgroup analyses, we determined the hazard ratios (HRs) and 95% confidence intervals (CIs) of FG VIM quartile 4 versus quartile 1–3 for ESKD after dividing the subjects according to clinically relevant factors and the characteristics of diabetes. Regression analysis was performed using the same adjustment strategy.

To evaluate the association of a single FG concentration with the risk of ESKD, we repeated the analysis according to baseline FG concentration, with 100–119 mg/dL as a reference group. The mean FG was excluded as a confounder in this analysis.

We found a variable inflation factor for all covariates of less than 2.0, and there was no multicollinearity in the covariates. Statistical analysis was performed using SAS version 9.3 (SAS Institute Inc., Cary, NC, USA). Statistical significance was set at $p < 0.05$.

3. Results

Compared with participants in the FG VIM quartile 1, those in the FG VIM quartile 4 were younger, had a higher proportion of males, were current smokers, and had higher fasting glucose and triglyceride levels (Table 1). Among comorbidities, they had more CKD but less hypertension, dyslipidemia, ischemic heart disease, and stroke. In the case of the characteristics of diabetes, people in FG VIM quartile 4 had a higher proportion of insulin users, individuals prescribed with ≥2 GLM during one year before baseline, and those with a duration of diabetes of at least five years.

Table 1. Baseline characteristics of the study subjects according to quartiles of fasting glucose variability [a].

Characteristics	VIM Q1 (n = 194,302)	VIM Q2 (n = 194,291)	VIM Q3 (n = 194,301)	VIM Q4 (n = 194,298)	p-Value
Age (years)	61.2 ± 9.8	60.2 ± 10.0	59.7 ± 10.2	59.4 ± 10.5	<0.001
Sex, male (%)	109,509 (56.4)	116,074 (59.7)	120,274 (61.9)	125,355 (64.5)	<0.001
BMI (kg/m^2)	24.7 ± 3	24.9 ± 3.1	24.9 ± 3.1	24.8 ± 3.2	<0.001
Systolic BP (mmHg)	128.3 ± 15.2	128.7 ± 15.2	128.8 ± 15.3	128.5 ± 15.3	<0.001
Fasting glucose (mg/dL)	125.0 ± 33.9	130.1 ± 35.5	135.7 ± 39.0	146.0 ± 53.4	<0.001
Total cholesterol (mg/dL)	193.6 ± 39.1	194.9 ± 39.9	195.6 ± 40.7	194.4 ± 41.5	<0.001
Triglyceride (mg/dL)	132.9 (132.5–133.2)	138.4 (138.1–138.8)	143 (142.6–143.4)	146.3 (146.0–146.7)	<0.001
HDL-C (mg/dL)	52.7 ± 22.8	52.3 ± 21.5	52 ± 21.8	51.5 ± 21.3	<0.001
LDL-C (mg/dL)	111.6 ± 43.0	111.6 ± 42.7	111.2 ± 43.4	109.5 ± 44.5	<0.001
GLU_VIM (%)	8.2 ± 3	16.6 ± 2.2	25.5 ± 3	43.5 ± 11.1	<0.001
GLU_SD (mg/dL)	8.1 ± 5.3	16.8 ± 8.5	26.7 ± 13.1	49.0 ± 25.2	<0.001
GLU_CV (%)	6.2 ± 2.6	12.7 ± 2.9	19.9 ± 4.3	35 ± 11.2	<0.001
GLU_ARV (mg/dL)	10 ± 7.2	20.3 ± 11.9	31.6 ± 18.3	56.5 ± 34.3	<0.001

Table 1. Cont.

Characteristics	VIM Q1 (n = 194,302)	VIM Q2 (n = 194,291)	VIM Q3 (n = 194,301)	VIM Q4 (n = 194,298)	p-Value
Current smoker (%)	31,644 (16.3)	36,873 (19.0)	42,614 (21.9)	50,137 (25.8)	<0.001
Heavy drinking (%)	12,395 (6.4)	13,844 (7.1)	14,670 (7.6)	14,289 (7.4)	<0.001
Regular exercise (%)	49,893 (25.7)	48,442 (24.9)	46,317 (23.8)	43,246 (22.3)	<0.001
eGFR (mL/minute/1.73 m^2)	79.6 (68.5–92.6)	79.9 (68.5–92.9)	80.1 (68.5–93.3)	79.6 (67.7–92.9)	<0.001
Chronic kidney disease (%) [b]	23,041 (11.9)	22,930 (11.8)	23,569 (12.1)	26,133 (13.5)	
Dipstick proteinuria (%)					<0.001
Absence (%)	178,444 (91.8)	177,043 (91.1)	175,837 (90.5)	173,973 (89.5)	
Trace (%)	6065 (3.1)	6380 (3.3)	6777 (3.5)	6723 (3.5)	
1 + (%)	5939 (3.1)	6580 (3.4)	6999 (3.6)	7742 (4)	
2 + (%)	2841 (1.5)	3149 (1.6)	3450 (1.8)	4205 (2.2)	
3 + (%)	841 (0.4)	924 (0.5)	1064 (0.6)	1378 (0.7)	
4 + (%)	172 (0.1)	215 (0.1)	174 (0.1)	277 (0.1)	
Comorbidities					
Hypertension (%)	119,605 (61.6)	117,761 (60.6)	115,704 (59.6)	112,881 (58.1)	<0.001
Dyslipidemia (%)	102,627 (52.8)	98,666 (50.8)	95,100 (48.9)	90,667 (46.7)	<0.001
IHD (%)	28,614 (14.7)	26,445 (13.6)	24,879 (12.8)	23,758 (12.2)	<0.001
Stroke (%)	10,979 (5.7)	10,286 (5.3)	9961 (5.1)	9996 (5.1)	<0.001
Income (lower 20%, %)	34,931 (18.0)	36,804 (18.9)	39,098 (20.1)	43,447 (22.4)	<0.001
ACE inhibitors or ARBs (%)	71,197 (36.6)	69,355 (35.7)	67,950 (35.0)	67,800 (34.9)	<0.001
Oral GLM					
Metformin	72,551 (37.3)	75,633 (38.9)	79,615 (41.0)	85,739 (44.1)	<0.001
Sulfonylurea	70,505 (36.3)	76,924 (39.6)	84,825 (43.7)	92,837 (47.8)	<0.001
Meglitinide	3960 (2)	4286 (2.2)	4821 (2.5)	5950 (3.1)	<0.001
Thiazolidinedione	11,624 (6)	12,466 (6.4)	13,402 (6.9)	14,708 (7.6)	<0.001
DPP-4 inhibitor	7602 (3.9)	7871 (4.1)	8300 (4.3)	8531 (4.4)	<0.001
a-Glucosidase inhibitor	18,941 (9.8)	21,134 (10.9)	24,274 (12.5)	28,984 (14.9)	<0.001
Number of oral GLM					<0.001
0	96,962 (49.9)	93,619 (48.2)	88,878 (45.7)	82,779 (42.6)	
1	34,341 (17.7)	31,949 (16.4)	29,574 (15.2)	26,813 (13.8)	
2	42,096 (21.7)	44,622 (23.0)	47,759 (24.6)	51,446 (26.5)	
3	17,310 (8.9)	19,723 (10.2)	22,828 (11.8)	26,763 (13.8)	
≥4	3593 (1.9)	4378 (2.3)	5262 (2.7)	6497 (3.3)	
Insulin	8125 (4.2)	9515 (4.9)	11,928 (6.1)	19,582 (10.1)	<0.001
Duration of diabetes	2.7 ± 3.1	2.8 ± 3.1	3 ± 3.2	3.3 ± 3.2	<0.001
≥5 years (%)	56,944 (29.3)	59,454 (30.6)	63,309 (32.6)	68,451 (35.2)	<0.001
Type 1 diabetes (%)	1274 (0.7)	1537 (0.8)	2106 (1.1)	4153 (2.1)	<0.001
Number of exams					<0.001
3	167,018 (86.0)	152,379 (78.4)	146,220 (75.3)	142,455 (73.3)	
4	13,832 (7.1)	19,418 (10.0)	22,307 (11.5)	24,566 (12.6)	
5	13,452 (6.9)	22,494 (11.6)	25,774 (13.3)	27,277 (14)	
Time interval between adjacent exams (years)	1.87 (1.3–2.1)	1.8 (1.1–2.1)	1.76 (1.1–2.1)	1.71 (1.1–2.1)	<0.001

[a] Q1: 0–12.7; Q2: 12.8–20.6; Q3: 20.7–31.2; Q4: ≥31.3. [b] Presence of chronic kidney disease represents estimated glomerular filtration rate < 60 mL/minute/1.73 m^2. Data are presented as mean ± standard deviation, median (interquartile range), or number (%). One-way analysis of variance and the chi-squared test were used to compare the characteristics of the study subjects at baseline. Post hoc multiple comparison analysis was performed with Bonferroni correction, and triglyceride levels were log-transformed for analysis. p-values were <0.001 for all variables because of the large sample size. Abbreviations: VIM, variability independent of mean; BMI, body mass index; BP, blood pressure; HDL-C, high-density lipoprotein-cholesterol; LDL-C, low-density lipoprotein-cholesterol; SD, standard deviation; CV, coefficient of variation; ARV, average real variability; eGFR, estimated glomerular filtration rate; IHD, ischemic heart disease; ACE inhibitor, angiotensin-converting enzyme inhibitor; ARB, angiotensin-receptor blocker; GLM, glucose-lowering medicine; DPP-4 inhibitor, inhibitors of dipeptidyl peptidase 4; ICD-10, International Classification of Diseases, 10th Revision.

During 8.0 (7.4–8.4) years of median (interquartile range) follow-up period, a total of 7290 cases of ESKD were identified (Table 2). Age- and sex-adjusted HRs for ESKD serially increased as the FG VIM quartile increased. In model 2, the HR (95% CI) for ESKD of participants in FG VIM quartile 4 was 1.27 (1.19–1.36), with adjustment for clinically relevant factors, duration of diabetes, history of CKD, mean FG, and the number of exams.

When the participants were divided into deciles in more detail, significantly higher risks for ESKD were found in D9 and D10 with a cutoff value of D9 of 34.4 (Table S1). A similar association was observed when FGV parameters were changed to SD, CV, and ARV (Table S2).

Table 2. Hazard ratios and 95% confidence intervals for the incidence of end-stage of kidney disease by quartiles of fasting glucose variability [a].

	Events (n)	Follow-Up Duration (Person-Years)	Incidence Rate (Per 1000 Person-Years)	Age- and Sex- Adjusted HR (95% CI)	Multivariate-Adjusted HR (95% CI)	
					Model 1	Model 2
Q1 (n = 194,302)	1412	1,478,422.2	0.96	1 (Ref.)	1 (Ref.)	1 (Ref.)
Q2 (n = 194,291)	1487	1,483,681.0	1.00	1.07 (0.99–1.15)	1.05 (0.97–1.13)	0.99 (0.92–1.06)
Q3 (n = 194,301)	1721	1,482,829.3	1.16	1.25 (1.16–1.34)	1.21 (1.12–1.3)	1.03 (0.96–1.1)
Q4 (n = 194,298)	2670	1,468,254.3	1.82	1.96 (1.84–2.10)	1.79 (1.68–1.91)	1.27 (1.19–1.36)

[a] Q1: 0–12.7; Q2: 12.8–20.5; Q3: 20.6–31.2; Q4: ≥31.3. Model 1 is adjusted for age, sex, body mass index, smoking, alcohol drinking, exercise, presence of chronic kidney disease, dyslipidemia, hypertension, and low-income status. Model 2 is the same as model 1, plus an adjustment for duration of diabetes as continuous variable, the number of classes of oral glucose-lowering medicine, the presence of prescription history of insulin, the mean of fasting glucose, and the number of exams.

In subgroup analyses, increased risk for ESKD in VIM quartile 4 versus quartile 1–3 was more evident in individuals aged 40–64 years, with a prescription history of ACE inhibitors or ARBs, hypertension, and dyslipidemia (Table 3). Among the various characteristics of diabetes, the impact of higher FGV was more distinct in patients with a long duration of diabetes and the prescription of metformin, sulfonylurea, AGI, and insulin (Table 4).

Table 3. Subgroup analysis according to clinically relevant factors in the fasting glucose variability quartile 4 versus quartiles 1–3.

	IR per 1000	HR (95% CI)	p for Interaction
Age (years)			0.000
40–64 (n = 521,902)	1.50	1.36 (1.28–1.45)	
≥65 (n = 255,290)	2.61	1.14 (1.06–1.23)	
Sex			0.849
Male (n = 471,212)	2.02	1.26 (1.19–1.33)	
Female (n = 305,980)	1.46	1.27 (1.16–1.39)	
BMI			0.325
<25 kg/m^2 (n = 425,481)	1.94	1.24 (1.16–1.32)	
≥25 kg/m^2 (n = 351,711)	1.68	1.3 (1.2–1.4)	
Current smoking			0.215
No (n = 615,924)	1.88	1.28 (1.21–1.35)	
Yes (n = 161,268)	1.63	1.19 (1.08–1.32)	
Hypertension			0.004
No (n = 311,241)	0.51	1.05 (0.92–1.2)	
Yes (n = 465,951)	2.80	1.3 (1.23–1.37)	
ACE inhibitor or ARB			0.001
No (n = 500,890)	0.70	1.11 (1.01–1.21)	
Yes (n = 276,302)	3.99	1.33 (1.25–1.4)	
Chronic kidney disease			0.988
No (n = 681,519)	0.75	1.26 (1.17–1.36)	
Yes (n = 95,673)	9.33	1.26 (1.19–1.34)	
Dyslipidemia			0.035
No (n = 390,132)	1.15	1.18 (1.09–1.28)	
Yes (n = 387,060)	2.58	1.31 (1.23–1.39)	
Income lower 20%			0.636
No (n = 622,912)	1.79	1.27 (1.2–1.34)	
Yes (n = 154,280)	1.92	1.23 (1.12–1.37)	

Adjusted for age, sex, body mass index, smoking, alcohol drinking, exercise, presence of dyslipidemia, hypertension, chronic kidney disease, low-income status, duration of diabetes as continuous variable, the number of classes of oral glucose-lowering medicine, presence of prescription history of insulin, mean fasting, and the number of exams. Each variable used to stratify the participants was excluded from the adjustment.

Table 4. Subgroup analysis according to the characteristics of diabetes in the fasting glucose variability quartile 4 versus quartiles 1–3.

	IR per 1000	HR (95% CI)	p for Interaction
Baseline fasting glucose			0.305
<126 mg/dL (n = 349,855)	2.67	1.16 (1.08–1.25)	
≥126 mg/dL (n = 427,337)	1.34	1.23 (1.15–1.31)	
Duration of diabetes			<0001
<5 years (n = 529,034)	0.63	1.01 (0.92–1.11)	
≥5 years (n = 248,158)	4.11	1.38 (1.3–1.46)	
Type of diabetes			0.348
Type 2 diabetes (n = 768,122)	1.65	1.26 (1.19–1.32)	
Type 1 diabetes (n = 9070)	10.06	1.16 (0.98–1.36)	
Metformin			0.002
No (n = 463,634)	1.34	1.16 (1.08–1.25)	
Yes (n = 313,538)	2.43	1.35 (1.26–1.44)	
Sulfonylurea			0.011
No (n = 452,101)	1.24	1.16 (1.07–1.26)	
Yes (n = 325,091)	2.46	1.32 (1.25–1.41)	
Meglitinide			0.276
No (n = 758,175)	1.69	1.27 (1.21–1.34)	
Yes (n = 19,017)	5.99	1.16 (0.99–1.36)	
Thiazolidinedione			0.174
No (n = 724,992)	1.74	1.25 (1.18–1.31)	
Yes (n = 52,200)	2.73	1.39 (1.2–1.61)	
DPP-4 inhibitor			0.182
No (n = 744,888)	1.80	1.25 (1.19–1.31)	
Yes (n = 32,304)	2.31	1.45 (1.17–1.78)	
α-Glucosidase inhibitor			0.003
No (n = 683,859)	1.42	1.2 (1.13–1.27)	
Yes (n = 93,333)	4.20	1.4 (1.29–1.53)	
Insulin			0.001
No (n = 728,042)	1.14	1.19 (1.12–1.26)	
Yes (n = 49,150)	8.38	1.42 (1.31–1.54)	

Adjusted for age, sex, body mass index, smoking, alcohol drinking, exercise, presence of dyslipidemia, hypertension, chronic kidney disease, low-income status, duration of diabetes as continuous variable, the number of classes of oral glucose-lowering medicine, presence of prescription history of insulin, mean fasting, and the number of exams. Each variable used to stratify the participants was excluded from the adjustment.

On the other hand, baseline FG levels showed a U-shaped association with the risk of ESKD (Table S3). Compared to participants whose FG concentrations were in the range of 100–119 mg/dL, individuals with FG < 100 mg/dL or ≥180 mg/dL had a higher risk of ESKD.

4. Discussion

4.1. Significant Findings of the Present Study

These results confirmed the hypothesis that FGV is significantly associated with an increased risk of ESKD among patients with diabetes. The risk for ESKD was 27% higher in the group with the highest FGV than in the lowest FGV group. The predictive value of high FGV on the incident ESKD was more prominent in patients with young age; hypertension; dyslipidemia; a long duration of diabetes; and who were treated with ACE inhibitors or ARBs, metformin, sulfonylurea, AGI, and insulin. In contrast, the association between FG and the risk of ESKD was U-shaped.

4.2. Kidney Outcomes and Long-Term Glucose Variability

Most previous studies have chosen HbA1c variability rather than FG variability for glucose variability assessment, and their study outcomes were renal function decline or development of albuminuria, not ESKD [17–19,21]. In the Action in Diabetes and Vascular Disease: Preterax and Diamicron MR Controlled Evaluation (ADVANCE) trial, SD of FG over 24 months exhibited a positive association with the risk of nephropathy combined with retinopathy [8]. Recently, a meta-analysis of three well-known clinical trials, the U.K. Prospective Diabetes Study, the Action to Control Cardiovascular Risk in Diabetes trial, and the Veteran Affairs Diabetes Trial, showed that FGV was associated with a 30–40% increase in the risk of incident moderate to severe nephropathy, defined by eGFR < 45 mL/min/1.73 m^2 [24].

Only one study has evaluated the impact of FGV on the development of ESKD using a population-based study [25,26]. The Taiwan Diabetes Study reported that FG-CV and HbA1c-CV could predict the development of diabetic nephropathy [27] and ESKD [28] in patients with type 2 diabetes. In the present study, compared to the previous one, we included more patients with diabetes (n = 777,192 vs. 31,841) and calculated the FGV for a longer period (5 vs. 1 year). Although ESKD is a hard outcome of diabetic renal complications, it is hard to study ESKD as an outcome due to the lower incidence. The incidence rate of ESKD in 2018 was 374.7 cases per million [16], lower than that of CVD, at 8980 cases per million in 2017 [29]. To overcome this limitation, a large population-based study is necessary. Because the NHIC entirely operates the health insurance system in Korea, we could use almost all Koreans with diabetes and subsequently obtained 777,192 individuals eligible for this study, making it possible to perform a more detailed subgroup analysis.

In patients with diabetes, oscillation in the FG level during a long follow-up period might reflect poor self-care, overall poor compliance, and suboptimal strategy for GLMs [30]. Because HbA1c is the average plasma glucose during 2–3 months, HbA1c variability implies a change in glycemic status rather than glucose fluctuation itself. In other words, FG might be better at capturing real-time glucose variations than HbA1c levels [7]. Therefore, FGV in our study was derived from yearly or biannually measured FG levels over five years, allowing for a comprehensive evaluation of a patient over a long period of time. In addition, this simple strategy for estimating FGV could be helpful for public health policy makers to select high-risk populations and support active prevention.

On the other hand, a high risk for ESKD was observed in individuals whose baseline FG levels were <100mg/dL or ≥180 mg/dL. These findings were consistent with another nationwide cohort study of Koreans with diabetes using GLMs [31], suggesting that intensive glucose control might not necessarily diminish the progression of established diabetic kidney disease.

4.3. Interpretation for the Impact of Glucose Variability

There is little data available to explain the mechanism linking glucose variability and ESKD risk directly. Cha et al. demonstrated the negative association of plasma adiponectin and glypican-4 levels with eGFR and positive association with urinary albumin levels [32]. The findings that transient glucose spikes could induce oxidative stress and impair endothelial function more than sustained hyperglycemia [33,34] and that glomerular permeability, mesangial lipid accumulation, and collagen synthesis are increased after intermittent exposure to high glucose levels [25,26] could be a pathophysiologic explanation of this association.

The results of the subgroup analysis provide a chance to identify the population more vulnerable to FGV (Table 3). It is possible that individuals with a long duration of diabetes are sensitive to oxidative stress because their enzymatic antioxidant defense systems are less efficient [29,35]. The presence of hypertension or dyslipidemia itself is an already proven risk factor for ESKD [36]. Its significant interaction with the harmful effect of high FGV on the risk of ESKD suggests a synergic relationship.

Interestingly, a significant effect of FGV was not observed in individuals aged ≥ 65 years. This may be due to the competing risk of death in patients with diabetic ESKD [37]. A Finnish nationwide cohort study showed that the cumulative risk of ESKD decreased with increasing age [38]. At the same time, mortality increased among the older age groups, with a 100-fold higher incidence of death than the ESKD cases throughout the

20-year-of follow-up [38]. Therefore, we theorize that the deceased cases ahead of ESKD might diminish the ESKD cases, weakening the effect of FGV.

The valid interaction with the prescription of ACE inhibitors or ARB, metformin, sulfonylurea, AGI, and insulin should be interpreted cautiously. There have been no previous studies exploring the interaction between GLM and the impact of FGV on ESKD, but only showed that sulfonylurea increases the glucose variability [39], whereas DPP-4 inhibitors and degludec reduced it [40,41]. Subjects with higher FGV might be treated with more GLMs due to their clinical condition. If they were not prescribed more GLMs, their FGV would be higher, and the association with ESKD risk might be stronger than in the present study.

SGLT2 inhibitors and glucagon-like peptide-1 receptor agonists, which have been known to prevent CKD progression, have been reimbursable for patients with diabetes in Korea since 2014 and 2015, respectively [2,3]. Because the prescriptions of these GLMs were negligible during the glucose variability assessment period (2005–2010), their impact on the incidence of ESKD until 2017 was expected to be minimal.

4.4. Parameters for Estimating Glycemic Variability

There is no consensus on a standardized index for glucose variability with distinct characteristics [42]. SD refers to the dispersion of measurements around the mean, and CV reflects a standardized variation that provides direct comparison among study groups. ARV is the average of the absolute differences of successive measurements and might be a reliable index for time series variability [20,43]. However, we chose VIM as the primary parameter of FGV because VIM is a measure of variability designed not to correlate with mean levels which is appropriate for the purpose of this study [44]. SD, CV, and ASV are partially dependent on mean despite of adjustment for mean value [45]. When we analyzed SD or CV again, a similar trend was observed (Table S2).

4.5. Limitations

This nationwide population-based study clearly showed the influence of long-term FG variability on incident ESKD with a long-term follow-up period. The 5-year FGV levels used in the present study were much longer than those used in previous studies. However, several limitations of this study should be considered.

First, given that we extracted study subjects according to the times of health check-ups to calculate long-term glucose variability, those with healthier lifestyle and slightly elevated glucose concentrations could be included, which might be a source of selection bias. Moreover, it is not available for complete information of hypoglycemia events. Second, postprandial glucose, HbA1c, serum c-peptide, and autoantibody levels were not included in this database. To enhance the accuracy of diagnosis of diabetes and subtype, we used ICD-10 codes with prescription histories of GLM and FG levels. Although we could not use HbA1c variability, the variability of FG was a stronger predictor of microvascular and macrovascular events than HbA1c variability in the ADVANCE trial [8]. Third, health examinations provided by the NHIC measure only dipstick proteinuria, not urine albuminuria. Finally, given the retrospective design of this study, reverse causation and undetected exposure of the risk factors of ESKD were possible [46]. We excluded incident ESKD cases developed one year after the baseline to minimize this issue. Additionally, the fasting period was not standardized fasting period could influence the FG levels.

Despite those limitations, a large-sized population-based cohort study covering almost entire Koreans is still the most suitable design for investigating rare outcomes such as ESKD possible [46].

5. Conclusions

This large-scale nationwide population-based study demonstrated that FG variability was independently associated with an increased risk of ESKD among patients with diabetes, especially in those with young age, long duration of diabetes, and comorbidities who need more GLM and RAS inhibitors. These findings highlight that reducing FGV is a vital strategy to reduce the incidence of ESKD in diabetes, especially in high-risk populations.

Supplementary Materials: The following are available online at https://www.mdpi.com/article/10.3390/jcm10245948/s1, Figure S1: Selection of study subjects. Figure S2: Study design showing the period estimating glucose variability and the risk of incident end-stage kidney disease (ESKD). Table S1: Hazard ratios (HRs) and 95% confidence intervals (CIs) for the incidence of end-stage kidney disease by deciles of fasting glucose variability. Table S2: Hazard ratios (HRs) and 95% confidence intervals (CIs) for the incidence of end-stage kidney disease by quartiles of fasting glucose variability, assessed by standard deviation, coefficient of variation, and average real variability. Table S3: Hazard ratios and 95% confidence intervals for the incidence of end-stage of renal disease according to baseline fasting glucose concentration.

Author Contributions: Conception and design: D.Y.L., J.K., S.Y.P., K.H. and N.H.K. (Nan Hee Kim); analysis and interpretation of the data: D.Y.L., J.K., S.P., J.A.S., N.H.K. (Nam Hoon Kim), H.J.Y. and N.H.K. (Nan Hee Kim); drafting of the article: D.Y.L., J.K. and S.Y.P.; critical revision for important intellectual content: J.H.Y., J.A.S., N.H.K. (Nam Hoon Kim), H.J.Y., S.G.K., K.M.C. and S.H.B.; final approval of the article: K.H. and N.H.K. (Nan Hee Kim); statistical expertise, collection and assembly of data: S.P. and K.H.; obtaining of funding: D.Y.L. and N.H.K. (Nan Hee Kim); administrative, technical, or logistical support: J.K., S.P. and K.H. All authors have read and agreed to the published version of the manuscript.

Funding: This research was supported Visit-to-Visit Glucose Variability Predicts the Development of End-Stage Renal Disease in Type 2 Diabetes by the Bio and Medical Technology Development Program of the National Research Foundation (NRF) funded by the Korean government (MSIT) (NRF-2019M3E5D3073102 and NRF-2019R1H1A2039682), a Korea University Grant (K1810951), and the Basic Science Research Program through NRF funded by the Ministry of Education (NRF-2020R1I1A1A0107166512).

Institutional Review Board Statement: The study was conducted according to the guidelines of the Declaration of Helsinki and approved by the Institutional Review Board of the Korea University Ansan Hospital (No. 2019AS0138; date of approval is 18 June 2019).

Informed Consent Statement: Not applicable.

Data Availability Statement: The data that support the findings of this study are available from the National Health Insurance Corporation, but restrictions apply to the availability of these data, which were used under license for the current study, and thus are not publicly available. Data are, however, available from the authors upon reasonable request and with permission of the National Health Insurance Corporation.

Conflicts of Interest: The authors declare no conflict of interest.

References

1. Saran, R.; Li, Y.; Robinson, B.; Ayanian, J.; Balkrishnan, R.; Bragg-Gresham, J.; Chen, J.T.; Cope, E.; Gipson, D.; He, K.; et al. US Renal Data System 2014 Annual Data Report: Epidemiology of Kidney Disease in the United States. *Am. J. Kidney Dis.* **2015**, *66*, S1–S305. [CrossRef] [PubMed]
2. Kidney Disease: Improving Global Outcomes (KDIGO) Diabetes Work Group. KDIGO 2020 Clinical Practice Guideline for Diabetes Management in Chronic Kidney Disease. *Kidney Int.* **2020**, *98*, S1–S115. [CrossRef] [PubMed]
3. De Bhailís, Á.M.; Azmi, S.; Kalra, P.A. Diabetic kidney disease: Update on clinical management and non-glycaemic effects of newer medications for type 2 diabetes. *Ther. Adv. Endocrinol. Metab.* **2021**, *12*, 20420188211020664. [CrossRef] [PubMed]
4. Kim, M.K.; Han, K.; Kim, H.S.; Park, Y.M.; Kwon, H.S.; Yoon, K.H.; Lee, S.H. Effects of Variability in Blood Pressure, Glucose, and Cholesterol Concentrations, and Body Mass Index on End-Stage Renal Disease in the General Population of Korea. *J. Clin. Med.* **2019**, *8*, 755. [CrossRef]
5. Kwon, S.; Lee, S.R.; Choi, E.K.; Lee, S.H.; Han, K.D.; Lee, S.Y.; Yang, S.; Park, J.; Choi, Y.J.; Lee, H.J.; et al. Visit-to-visit variability of metabolic parameters and risk of heart failure: A nationwide population-based study. *Int. J. Cardiol.* **2019**, *293*, 153–158. [CrossRef]
6. Lee, S.-H.; Kim, M.K.; Rhee, E.-J. Effects of Cardiovascular Risk Factor Variability on Health Outcomes. *Endocrinol. Metab.* **2020**, *35*, 217–226. [CrossRef]
7. Zhou, J.J.; Schwenke, D.C.; Bahn, G.; Reaven, P. Glycemic variation and cardiovascular risk in the Veterans Affairs Diabetes trial. *Diabetes Care* **2018**, *41*, 2187–2194. [CrossRef]

8. Hirakawa, Y.; Arima, H.; Zoungas, S.; Ninomiya, T.; Cooper, M.; Hamet, P.; Mancia, G.; Poulter, N.; Harrap, S.; Woodward, M.; et al. Impact of visit-to-visit glycemic variability on the risks of macrovascular and microvascular events and all-cause mortality in type 2 diabetes: The ADVANCE trial. *Diabetes Care* **2014**, *37*, 2359–2365. [CrossRef]
9. Yokota, S.; Tanaka, H.; Mochizuki, Y.; Soga, F.; Yamashita, K.; Tanaka, Y.; Shono, A.; Suzuki, M.; Sumimoto, K.; Mukai, J.; et al. Association of glycemic variability with left ventricular diastolic function in type 2 diabetes mellitus. *Cardiovasc. Diabetol.* **2019**, *18*, 166. [CrossRef]
10. Ferreira, L.; Moniz, A.C.; Carneiro, A.S.; Miranda, A.S.; Fangueiro, C.; Fernandes, D.; Silva, I.; Palhinhas, I.; Lemos, J.; Antunes, J.; et al. The impact of glycemic variability on length of stay and mortality in diabetic patients admitted with community-acquired pneumonia or chronic obstructive pulmonary disease. *Diabetes Metab. Syndr.* **2019**, *13*, 149–153. [CrossRef]
11. Lee, D.Y.; Han, K.; Yu, J.H.; Park, S.; Heo, J.I.; Seo, J.A.; Kim, N.H.; Yoo, H.J.; Kim, S.G.; Kim, S.M.; et al. Gamma-glutamyl transferase variability can predict the development of end-stage of renal disease: A nationwide population-based study. *Sci. Rep.* **2020**, *10*, 11668. [CrossRef]
12. Yang, C.Y.; Su, P.F.; Hung, J.Y.; Ou, H.T.; Kuo, S. Comparative predictive ability of visit-to-visit HbA1c variability measures for microvascular disease risk in type 2 diabetes. *Cardiovasc. Diabetol.* **2020**, *19*, 105. [CrossRef]
13. Chiu, W.C.; Lai, Y.R.; Cheng, B.C.; Huang, C.C.; Chen, J.F.; Lu, C.H. HbA1C Variability Is Strongly Associated with Development of Macroalbuminuria in Normal or Microalbuminuria in Patients with Type 2 Diabetes Mellitus: A Six-Year Follow-Up Study. *BioMed Res. Int.* **2020**, *2020*, 7462158. [CrossRef]
14. Lee, C.L.; Chen, C.H.; Wu, M.J.; Tsai, S.F. The variability of glycated hemoglobin is associated with renal function decline in patients with type 2 diabetes. *Ther. Adv. Chronic. Dis.* **2020**, *11*, 2040622319898370. [CrossRef]
15. Penno, G.; Solini, A.; Bonora, E.; Fondelli, C.; Orsi, E.; Zerbini, G.; Morano, S.; Cavalot, F.; Lamacchia, O.; Laviola, L.; et al. HbA1c variability as an independent correlate of nephropathy, but not retinopathy, in patients with type 2 diabetes: The Renal Insufficiency And Cardiovascular Events (RIACE) Italian multicenter study. *Diabetes Care* **2013**, *36*, 2301–2310. [CrossRef]
16. United States Renal Data System. 2020 USRDS Annual Data Report: End Stage Renal Disease: 11 International Comparisions. Available online: https://adr.usrds.org/2020/end-stage-renal-disease/11-international-comparisons (accessed on 1 July 2021).
17. Lee, Y.H.; Han, K.; Ko, S.H.; Ko, K.S.; Lee, K.U.; Taskforce Team of Diabetes Fact Sheet of the Korean Diabetes Association. Data Analytic Process of a Nationwide Population-Based Study Using National Health Information Database Established by National Health Insurance Service. *Diabetes Metab. J.* **2016**, *40*, 79–82. [CrossRef]
18. Song, S.O.; Jung, C.H.; Song, Y.D.; Park, C.Y.; Kwon, H.S.; Cha, B.S.; Park, J.Y.; Lee, K.U.; Ko, K.S.; Lee, B.W. Background and data configuration process of a nationwide population-based study using the Korean National Health Insurance System. *Diabetes Metab. J.* **2014**, *38*, 395–403. [CrossRef]
19. Oh, J.Y.; Yang, Y.J.; Kim, B.S.; Kang, J.H. Validity and reliability of Korean version of International Physical Activity Questionnaire (IPAQ) short form. *J. Korean Acad. Fam. Med.* **2007**, *28*, 532–541.
20. Mena, L.; Pintos, S.; Queipo, N.V.; Aizpúrua, J.A.; Maestre, G.; Sulbarán, T. A reliable index for the prognostic significance of blood pressure variability. *J. Hypertens.* **2005**, *23*, 505–511. [CrossRef]
21. Kim, M.K.; Han, K.; Koh, E.S.; Kim, H.S.; Kwon, H.S.; Park, Y.M.; Yoon, K.H.; Lee, S.H. Variability in Total Cholesterol Is Associated With the Risk of End-Stage Renal Disease: A Nationwide Population-Based Study. *Arterioscler. Thromb. Vasc. Biol.* **2017**, *37*, 1963–1970. [CrossRef]
22. Levey, A.S.; Coresh, J.; Greene, T.; Stevens, L.A.; Zhang, Y.L.; Hendriksen, S.; Kusek, J.W.; Van Lente, F. Using standardized serum creatinine values in the modification of diet in renal disease study equation for estimating glomerular filtration rate. *Ann. Intern. Med.* **2006**, *145*, 247–254. [CrossRef] [PubMed]
23. Kidney Disease: Improving Global Outcomes (KDIGO). KDIGO 2012 clinical practice guideline for the evaluation and management of chronic kidney disease: Chapter 1: Definition and classification of CKD. *Kidney Int. Suppl.* **2013**, *3*, 19–62. [CrossRef] [PubMed]
24. Zhou, J.J.; Coleman, R.; Holman, R.R.; Reaven, P. Long-term glucose variability and risk of nephropathy complication in UKPDS, ACCORD and VADT trials. *Diabetologia* **2020**, *63*, 2482–2485. [CrossRef] [PubMed]
25. Jones, S.C.; Saunders, H.J.; Qi, W.; Pollock, C.A. Intermittent high glucose enhances cell growth and collagen synthesis in cultured human tubulointerstitial cells. *Diabetologia* **1999**, *42*, 1113–1119. [CrossRef] [PubMed]
26. Song, K.H.; Park, J.; Ha, H. High glucose increases mesangial lipid accumulation via impaired cholesterol transporters. *Transpl. Proc.* **2012**, *44*, 1021–1025. [CrossRef]
27. Lin, C.C.; Chen, C.C.; Chen, F.N.; Li, C.I.; Liu, C.S.; Lin, W.Y.; Yang, S.Y.; Lee, C.C.; Li, T.C. Risks of diabetic nephropathy with variation in hemoglobin A1c and fasting plasma glucose. *Am. J. Med.* **2013**, *126*, 1017.e1–1017.e10. [CrossRef] [PubMed]
28. Yang, Y.F.; Li, T.C.; Li, C.I.; Liu, C.S.; Lin, W.Y.; Yang, S.Y.; Chiang, J.H.; Huang, C.C.; Sung, F.C.; Lin, C.C. Visit-to-Visit Glucose Variability Predicts the Development of End-Stage Renal Disease in Type 2 Diabetes. *Medicine* **2015**, *94*, e1804. [CrossRef]
29. Bigagli, E.; Lodovici, M. Circulating Oxidative Stress Biomarkers in Clinical Studies on Type 2 Diabetes and Its Complications. *Oxidative Med. Cell. Longev.* **2019**, *2019*, 5953685. [CrossRef]
30. Ceriello, A.; Rossi, M.C.; De Cosmo, S.; Lucisano, G.; Pontremoli, R.; Fioretto, P.; Giorda, C.; Pacilli, A.; Viazzi, F.; Russo, G.; et al. Overall Quality of Care Predicts the Variability of Key Risk Factors for Complications in Type 2 Diabetes: An Observational, Longitudinal Retrospective Study. *Diabetes Care* **2019**, *42*, 514–519. [CrossRef]

31. Jung, H.H. Evaluation of Serum Glucose and Kidney Disease Progression Among Patients With Diabetes. *JAMA Netw. Open* **2021**, *4*, e2127387. [CrossRef]
32. Cha, J.J.; Min, H.S.; Kim, K.; Lee, M.J.; Lee, M.H.; Kim, J.E.; Song, H.K.; Cha, D.R.; Kang, Y.S. Long-term study of the association of adipokines and glucose variability with diabetic complications. *Korean J. Intern. Med.* **2018**, *33*, 367–382. [CrossRef] [PubMed]
33. Salisbury, D.; Bronas, U. Reactive oxygen and nitrogen species: Impact on endothelial dysfunction. *Nurs. Res.* **2015**, *64*, 53–66. [CrossRef] [PubMed]
34. El-Osta, A.; Brasacchio, D.; Yao, D.; Pocai, A.; Jones, P.L.; Roeder, R.G.; Cooper, M.E.; Brownlee, M. Transient high glucose causes persistent epigenetic changes and altered gene expression during subsequent normoglycemia. *J. Exp. Med.* **2008**, *205*, 2409–2417. [CrossRef] [PubMed]
35. Rizvi, S.I.; Maurya, P.K. Markers of oxidative stress in erythrocytes during aging in humans. *Ann. N. Y. Acad. Sci. USA* **2007**, *1100*, 373–382. [CrossRef]
36. Kidney Disease: Improving Global Outcomes (KDIGO) Diabetes Work Group. KDIGO 2012 Clinical Practice Guideline for the Evaluation and Management of Chronic Kidney Disease. *Kidney Int.* **2013**, *3*, 81–90. [CrossRef]
37. Jiang, Y.; Fine, J.P.; Mottl, A.K. Competing Risk of Death With End-Stage Renal Disease in Diabetic Kidney Disease. *Adv. Chronic. Kidney Dis.* **2018**, *25*, 133–140. [CrossRef]
38. Finne, P.; Groop, P.H.; Arffman, M.; Kervinen, M.; Helve, J.; Grönhagen-Riska, C.; Sund, R. Cumulative Risk of End-Stage Renal Disease Among Patients With Type 2 Diabetes: A Nationwide Inception Cohort Study. *Diabetes Care* **2019**, *42*, 539–544. [CrossRef]
39. Yamazaki, M.; Hasegawa, G.; Majima, S.; Mitsuhashi, K.; Fukuda, T.; Iwase, H.; Kadono, M.; Asano, M.; Senmaru, T.; Tanaka, M.; et al. Effect of repaglinide versus glimepiride on daily blood glucose variability and changes in blood inflammatory and oxidative stress markers. *Diabetol. Metab. Syndr.* **2014**, *6*, 54. [CrossRef]
40. Vora, J.; Cariou, B.; Evans, M.; Gross, J.L.; Harris, S.; Landstedt-Hallin, L.; Mithal, A.; Rodriguez, M.R.; Meneghini, L. Clinical use of insulin degludec. *Diabetes Res. Clin. Pract.* **2015**, *109*, 19–31. [CrossRef]
41. Lee, S.; Lee, H.; Kim, Y.; Kim, E. Effect of DPP-IV Inhibitors on Glycemic Variability in Patients with T2DM: A Systematic Review and Meta-Analysis. *Sci. Rep.* **2019**, *9*, 13296. [CrossRef]
42. Inzucchi, S.E.; Umpierrez, G.; DiGenio, A.; Zhou, R.; Kovatchev, B. How well do glucose variability measures predict patient glycaemic outcomes during treatment intensification in type 2 diabetes? *Diabetes Res. Clin. Pract.* **2015**, *108*, 179–186. [CrossRef]
43. Hansen, T.W.; Thijs, L.; Li, Y.; Boggia, J.; Kikuya, M.; Björklund-Bodegård, K.; Richart, T.; Ohkubo, T.; Jeppesen, J.; Torp-Pedersen, C.; et al. Prognostic value of reading-to-reading blood pressure variability over 24 hours in 8938 subjects from 11 populations. *Hypertension* **2010**, *55*, 1049–1057. [CrossRef]
44. Rothwell, P.M.; Howard, S.C.; Dolan, E.; O'Brien, E.; Dobson, J.E.; Dahlöf, B.; Sever, P.S.; Poulter, N.R. Prognostic significance of visit-to-visit variability, maximum systolic blood pressure, and episodic hypertension. *Lancet* **2010**, *375*, 895–905. [CrossRef]
45. Lee, H.J.; Choi, E.K.; Han, K.D.; Lee, E.; Moon, I.; Lee, S.R.; Cha, M.J.; Oh, S.; Lip, G.Y.H. Bodyweight fluctuation is associated with increased risk of incident atrial fibrillation. *Heart Rhythm* **2020**, *17*, 365–371. [CrossRef]
46. Sedgwick, P. Retrospective cohort studies: Advantages and disadvantages. *BMJ Br. Med. J.* **2014**, *348*, g1072. [CrossRef]

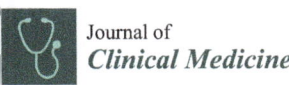

Review

Evaluation of Quality and Bone Microstructure Alterations in Patients with Type 2 Diabetes: A Narrative Review

José Ignacio Martínez-Montoro [1], Beatriz García-Fontana [2,3,4,*], Cristina García-Fontana [2,3,4,*] and Manuel Muñoz-Torres [2,3,4,5,*]

1. Department of Endocrinology and Nutrition, Virgen de la Victoria University Hospital, Instituto de Investigación Biomédica de Málaga (IBIMA), Faculty of Medicine, University of Malaga, 29010 Malaga, Spain; joseimartinezmontoro@gmail.com
2. Bone Metabolic Unit, Endocrinology and Nutrition Division, University Hospital Clínico San Cecilio, 18016 Granada, Spain
3. Instituto de Investigación Biosanitaria de Granada (Ibs. GRANADA), 18012 Granada, Spain
4. Centro de Investigación Biomédica en Red Fragilidad y Envejecimiento Saludable (CIBERFES), Instituto de Salud Carlos III, 28029 Madrid, Spain
5. Department of Medicine, University of Granada, 18016 Granada, Spain
* Correspondence: bgfontana@fibao.es (B.G.-F.); cgfontana@hotmail.com (C.G.-F.); mmt@mamuto.es (M.M.-T.)

Abstract: Bone fragility is a common complication in subjects with type 2 diabetes mellitus (T2DM). However, traditional techniques for the evaluation of bone fragility, such as dual-energy X-ray absorptiometry (DXA), do not perform well in this population. Moreover, the Fracture Risk Assessment Tool (FRAX) usually underestimates fracture risk in T2DM. Importantly, novel technologies for the assessment of one microarchitecture in patients with T2DM, such as the trabecular bone score (TBS), high-resolution peripheral quantitative computed tomography (HR-pQCT), and microindentation, are emerging. Furthermore, different serum and urine bone biomarkers may also be useful for the evaluation of bone quality in T2DM. Hence, in this article, we summarize the limitations of conventional tools for the evaluation of bone fragility and review the current evidence on novel approaches for the assessment of quality and bone microstructure alterations in patients with T2DM.

Keywords: type 2 diabetes mellitus; bone fragility; fracture risk; bone structure; bone quality

1. Introduction

In the last few decades, type 2 diabetes mellitus (T2DM) has dramatically increased in prevalence worldwide, resulting in significant burdens on patients suffering from this condition and healthcare systems [1]. Of note, the rising prevalence of this disease is associated with the development of a wide range of complications, including retinopathy, nephropathy, neuropathy, and cardiovascular disease [1,2]. These complications often affect the quality of life of patients with T2DM, including their physical and psychological functioning [3]. Although some of these comorbidities have a well-known impact on the quality of life [4,5], others have received less attention [6].

Mounting evidence reveals that bone fragility is common in T2DM [7]. Several studies have shown that T2DM constitutes an independent risk factor for osteoporotic fractures, presenting a particularly strong association with hip fractures [8–11]. Indeed, a number of meta-analyses have confirmed that T2DM is associated with an increased risk of incident hip, vertebral, and non-vertebral fractures [12–14]. Since T2DM has a strong relationship with hip fractures that need replacement surgery using total hip arthroplasty, new techniques have been developed in this field [15,16]. Importantly, increases in the incidence of fractures lead to greater costs and healthcare resource utilization in this population [17]. Moreover, fractures are associated with functional impairment and reduction of health-related quality of life [18,19]. Given the important health and socioeconomic impact of skeletal fragility and fractures, individuals with T2DM, especially those with major diabetes-related determinants and other conventional risk factors for osteoporosis, should be assessed for the presence of bone fragility and their fracture risk [20]. However, traditional imaging techniques and fracture risk assessment tools may not be accurate for this purpose in patients with T2DM [21].

In this review, we summarize the main limitations of commonly used methods to evaluate bone fragility and estimate fracture risk in patients with T2DM, and we also discuss the potential role of novel strategies in the evaluation of quality and bone microstructure alterations in this population. Although some of these issues have been addressed in previous works [22], the current knowledge on novel techniques and biomarkers for the evaluation of bone fragility in T2DM is still limited. We have updated all the information available on the pathogenic mechanisms that explain bone fragility in patients with T2DM. In addition, we have reviewed the role of new technologies and biomarkers in the assessment of bone fragility in T2DM, considering the main clinical studies currently available.

2. Search Strategy and Limitations of the Review

We conducted a comprehensive literature search of articles published in PubMed until March 2022. Peer-reviewed articles related to T2DM and bone fragility published in English were selected, with special attention to clinical studies evaluating bone mineral density (BMD) by dual energy X-ray absorptiometry (DXA) in patients with T2DM, as well as clinical studies assessing bone microstructure through the trabecular bone score (TBS), high-resolution peripheral quantitative computed tomography (HR-pQCT), and microindentation in this population. Finally, we included clinical studies related to the evaluation of novel non-invasive biomarkers of bone quality and fracture risk prediction in T2DM. Original human research articles, including randomized controlled trials, prospective and retrospective observational studies, and cross-sectional studies were considered. The largest studies, as well as the most recent and solid available evidence, were prioritized. Remarkably, a considerable number of the available studies were conducted in postmenopausal women with T2DM; therefore, these results have to be considered cautiously in subjects with T2DM and different characteristics. Moreover, several studies included in this review had a cross-sectional design; thus, further large-scale long-term prospective studies are needed in this field.

3. Determinants of Skeletal Fragility and Increased Risk of Fracture in T2DM

Several determinants have been identified in the pathogenesis of bone fragility and increased fracture risk in subjects with T2DM [23] (Figure 1). Notably, a longer duration of T2DM was reported to be an independent risk factor for major osteoporotic fractures in women aged ≥ 40 and with ≥ 10 years of diabetes duration [24], and a recent meta-analysis showed a greater increase in the risk of both hip and non-vertebral fractures in subjects with longer diabetes duration [13]. Besides this, poor glycemic control is closely linked to fracture risk, as several large-scale population-based cohort studies have demonstrated [25–27]. In this regard, the generation of advanced glycation end-products (AGEs) resulting from chronic exposure to hyperglycemia is one of the key mechanisms in the pathophysiology of bone fragility in T2DM [23]. As such, non-enzymatic glycosylation of collagen leads to the formation of collagen-AGEs, which are involved in the development of impaired bone mineralization and quality through different alterations of the extracellular matrix, a reduction of alkaline phosphatase activity in osteoblasts, and an overactivation of the receptor for AGEs (the latter associated with the release of pro-inflammatory cytokines and reactive oxygen species—ROS—by osteoclasts) [23,28]. On the other hand, it is also postulated that the main event related to bone fragility in T2DM is an overall inhibition of bone cells function and decreased bone turnover [23,29]. This effect may be driven in part by insulin resistance [30].

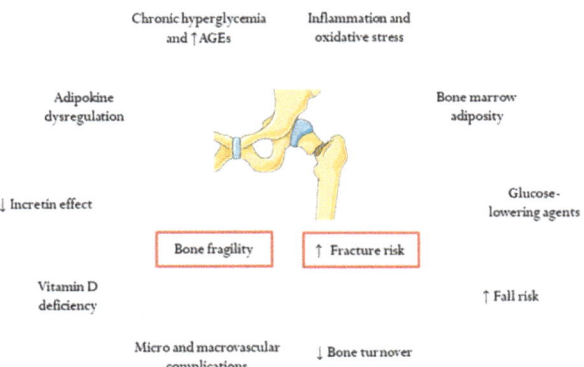

Figure 1. Determinants of bone fragility and increased fracture risk in type 2 diabetes. AGEs, advanced glycation end products.

In addition to chronic hyperglycemia and AGE formation, other mechanisms play a role in bone fragility in T2DM, as previously reviewed [7,23,31]. Among them, a proinflammatory state and oxidative stress, along with adipokine dysregulation and marrow adiposity, have a strong influence on bone metabolism [7,31]. Loss of incretin effect has also been implicated in the pathogenesis of skeletal fragility in T2DM [31,32]. Microvascular disease and impaired vascular bone intercommunication determine alterations of bone quality and microarchitecture [7,31]. Ischemic heart disease has also been reported to be associated with an increased risk of vertebral fractures in T2DM [33]. Vitamin D deficiency, commonly found in patients with T2DM, could play a role in both T2DM development and bone fragility [34]. Pathological changes in gut microbiota composition in T2DM may also trigger bone alterations in this population [35].

Further to this, glucose-lowering agents may also be crucial contributors to the reported associations between T2DM and bone fragility [36,37]. The potential benefits of some drugs for bone density and fracture risk (i.e., metformin, glucagon-like peptide 1 receptors agonists and dipeptidyl peptidase-4 inhibitors) [38–40] remain to be confirmed in specifically designed studies. Conversely, the long-term use of thiazolidinediones has been independently associated with fracture risk [41], and sodium-glucose cotransporter-2 inhibitors could also have this effect [42,43]. Remarkably, both insulin and sulfonylureas significantly increase fall-related fractures due to episodes of hypoglycemia [44]. In this vein, other prevalent factors in T2DM (i.e., visual impairment, peripheral neuropathy, autonomic dysfunction/postural hypotension, foot ulcers/amputation, and sarcopenia) also lead to an increased risk of fall-related fractures [31,45].

4. Bone Density and Fracture Risk Prediction in T2DM

Despite skeletal fragility and fracture risk being greater in subjects with T2DM, this condition is usually associated with normal or even increased BMD measured by DXA [46]. Thus, women with T2DM in the Women's Health Initiative Observational Study presented higher hip and spine BMD scores compared to those without T2DM [47]. Similarly, in a cross-sectional study including two Swedish cohorts, both men and women exhibited a progressively higher hip BMD according to normal fasting plasma glucose/impaired fasting plasma glucose/T2DM subgroups [48]. In the prospective population-based cohort from the Rotterdam Study, inadequate glycemic control was associated with both higher BMD and increased fracture risk in participants with T2DM [27]. Furthermore, a meta-analysis of 15 observational studies (3473 subjects with T2DM and 19,139 healthy controls) showed that participants with T2DM had significantly higher BMD at the femoral neck, hip, and spine [49].

It is noteworthy that these results contrast with those reported by studies assessing BMD in type 1 diabetes mellitus (T1DM), in which BMD is generally low [50]. Although the mechanisms involved in the association between T2DM and normal/high BMD are not fully understood, some data suggest that these findings might be related to chronic hyperinsulinemia and insulin resistance [51], as well as the effect of some adipokines, such as leptin, on bone metabolism [52]. Excess weight/obesity, which are often encountered in patients with T2DM, could also play a role in increased BMD, although some studies have reported that this relationship remains after adjusting for the body mass index (BMI) [49]. Since T2DM is associated with increased fracture risk, regardless of whether there is a normal/high BMD, a fact known as "the diabetic paradox of bone fragility" [53], the diagnosis of osteoporosis based on BMD measured by DXA, should be cautiously considered [21].

On the other hand, the Fracture Risk Assessment Tool (FRAX), which is widely used to estimate 10-year absolute fracture risk, has been demonstrated to underestimate the risk for both hip and major osteoporotic fractures in patients with T2DM [54]. These results are influenced, in part, by the higher BMD observed in patients with T2DM [49]. Indeed, contrary to T1DM, T2DM is not included in the FRAX tool as a secondary cause of osteoporosis [55]. In this regard, some authors have proposed a correction factor with the use of glycated hemoglobin in order to improve the predictive ability of this algorithm for fracture risk [56]. Recently, adjustment of FRAX for T2DM has been suggested in order to create a useful alternative [57,58], although further research is warranted to confirm these results. Alternatively, certain methods (i.e., inputting rheumatoid arthritis, adjusting FRAX by TBS, reducing the femoral T-score by 0.5, and increasing the age by 10 years) have been proposed to improve the performance of FRAX in T2DM, although no single method appears to be optimal in all settings [59]. In light of the above, new approaches to the evaluation of bone fragility in patients with T2DM are needed.

5. Bone Microstructure in T2DM

As previously discussed, patients with T2DM have normal or elevated BMD; however, bone microarchitecture alterations may be present in this group, resulting in an increased fracture risk [60]. In this context, the trabecular bone score, high-resolution peripheral quantitative computed tomography, and microindentation are useful techniques for the evaluation of the bone microstructure in T2DM.

5.1. Trabecular Bone Score

The TBS is a non-invasive, indirect index of trabecular microarchitecture [61]. It is derived from experimental variograms of the projected two-dimensional lumbar spine DXA image and can assess pixel gray-level variations of this area, which translate into a bone microstructure-related score [61]. Accordingly, a high TBS is related to numerous, well-connected and less sparse trabeculae (i.e., normal bone microarchitecture), whereas a low TBS indicates a reduced number of trabeculae and less connectivity, as well as trabecular separation (i.e., altered bone microarchitecture) [61], as shown in Figure 2. In this regard, the proposed TBS cut-off values are as follows: TBS > 1.31 (normal microarchitecture), TBS between 1.23 and 1.31 (partially degraded microarchitecture), and TBS < 1.23 (degraded microarchitecture) [62].

TBS has been demonstrated to be an independent predictor for osteoporotic fractures [62–64]. In addition to this, TBS can detect differences between DXA images with similar BMDs [61] and helps to improve the performance of BMD assessed by DXA in the prediction of osteoporotic fractures [65,66]. Indeed, TBS has been incorporated into the FRAX algorithm (FRAX adjusted for TBS), although the clinical impact of this adjustment is yet to be properly evaluated [62].

In patients with T2DM, TBS has been reported to be significantly decreased compared to subjects without diabetes, which suggests that this index could be a useful tool for the diagnosis of bone fragility in this population [67]. TBS may be decreased even in prediabetes, indicating that the degradation of bone microarchitecture may occur in early stages of the disease [68]. Interestingly, in a recent cross-sectional study including 137 patients with T2DM aged 49–85 and 300 healthy controls, the presence of T2DM was associated with significantly lower TBS values despite higher lumbar spine BMD; adiposity (estimated by the relative fat mass) and insulin resistance could play a role in these results [69]. Accordingly, visceral fat reduction may increase TBS values [70]. Furthermore, higher glycated hemoglobin levels and a longer disease duration in patients with T2DM are related to lower TBS values, although the interference of abdominal soft tissue thickness should be considered when interpreting these findings [68,71–73]. Moreover, diabetic microvascular disease may be linked to lower TBS [74].

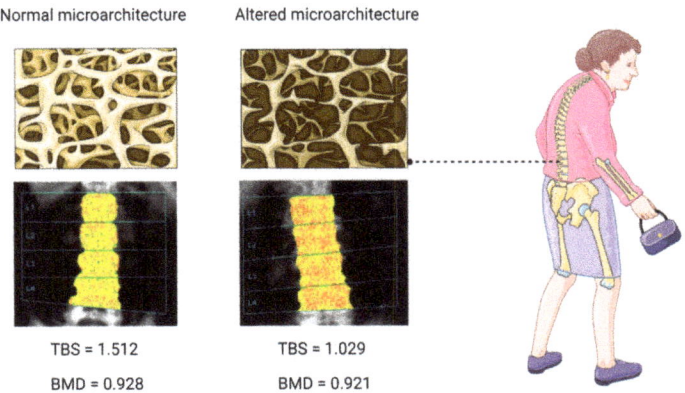

Figure 2. Trabecular bone score (TBS) as a useful technology for the assessment of the trabecular microarchitecture. TBS > 1.31 (**left**) denotes a normal microarchitecture, whereas TBS < 1.23 (**right**) indicates an altered microarchitecture. TBS can detect differences between similar values of lumbar spine bone mineral density (BMD) estimated by dual-energy X-ray absorptiometry (DXA) (g/cm^2).

Notably, several studies have shown that TBS can predict incident/prevalent osteoporotic fractures independent of BMD [75–78] (Table 1). In a retrospective cohort study from the Manitoba Bone Density Program (29,407 women ≥ 50 years, 2356 with diagnosed T2DM), lumbar spine TBS was a BMD-independent predictor of major osteoporotic fractures in both participants with and without T2DM [75]. In a study including 206 postmenopausal women with/without T2DM, TBS values ≤1.130 presented an adequate diagnostic accuracy for vertebral fractures in the former [76], whereas, in a cross-sectional study conducted on 548 patients with T2DM, TBS correlated with prevalent vertebral fractures [77]. Finally, in a study including 285 postmenopausal women with T2DM, TBS had the strongest association with vertebral fractures [78]. Considering all these findings together, TBS may constitute a useful approach for the diagnosis of bone fragility and the evaluation of fracture risk in T2DM, although further prospective studies are needed to corroborate these data.

Table 1. Clinical studies showing an independent association between the trabecular bone score (TBS) and osteoporotic fractures in patients with type 2 diabetes mellitus.

Study	Design	Study Population	Results
Leslie et al., 2013 [75]	Retrospective cohort (mean follow-up 4.7 years)	29,407 women ≥ 50 years (2356 with diagnosed T2DM)	TBS predicted major osteoporotic fractures (hip, spine, forearm and humerus) in T2DM (HR 1.27, CI 1.10–1.46)
Zhukouskaya et al., 2015 [76]	Cross-sectional	99 postmenopausal women with T2DM/107 healthy controls	TBS was associated with VF (AUC 0.69, cut-off value 1.130 in ROC curve analysis)
Yamamoto et al., 2019 [77]	Cross-sectional	584 patients with T2DM (257 postmenopausal women and 291 men > 50 years)	TBS correlated with prevalent VF in multivariate logistic regression analysis
Lin et al., 2019 [78]	Cross-sectional	285 postmenopausal women with T2DM	TBS had the strongest association with VF (AUC 0.775)

T2DM, type 2 diabetes mellitus; TBS, trabecular bone score; VF, vertebral fractures; HR, hazard ratio; CI, confidence interval; ROC, receiver operating characteristic; AUC, area under the curve.

5.2. High-Resolution, Peripheral, Quantitative Computed Tomography

HR-pQCT is a non-invasive three-dimensional imaging modality that permits the assessment of bone microarchitecture, including the measurement of volumetric cortical and trabecular bone mineral density (vBMD), cortical thickness/porosity, bone strength, and other parameters in the appendicular skeleton (i.e., distal radius and tibia) [79]. In recent years, HR-pQCT has emerged as a promising technique that could become widely used for the diagnosis of osteoporosis and for clinical fragility fracture prediction [80,81].

In a pilot study conducted on 19 postmenopausal women with T2DM matched to 19 controls, Burghardt et al. showed for the first time that T2DM may be associated with bone microarchitecture alterations, as assessed by HR-pQCT [82]. It was observed that, although participants with T2DM had higher trabecular vBMD and trabecular thickness, they also presented higher cortical porosity and impaired bone strength, measured by micro-finite element analysis [82]. Similarly, Patsh et al. reported increased cortical porosity at the ultradistal and distal radio and tibia in 80 postmenopausal women with T2DM [83], while Yu and colleagues also found defects in cortical bone microarchitecture (i.e., higher cortical porosity and lower cortical vBMD) in African American women with T2DM compared to healthy controls [84]. Data from the Framingham Study (a total of 1069 subjects underwent HR-pQCT, 129 subjects with T2DM) showed that patients with T2DM had lower vBMD and higher cortical porosity compared to controls [85]. Interestingly, in a prospective exploratory study that involved postmenopausal women with T2DM with/without a history of fragility fractures and controls, patients with T2DM and a history of fractures exhibited the highest cortical porosity [86]. Cortical porosity increased over time similarly in the three groups, although patients with T2DM and a history of fractures presented the greatest decreases in bone strength indices in the follow-up period, a fact that suggests that cortical porosity may develop early, followed by small increases in this parameter along with significant material strength impairment [86]. Of note, cortical bone deficits assessed by HR-pQCT in T2DM may be driven by the presence of microvascular disease and/or poor metabolic control [87,88].

Conversely, other studies did not find significant differences in bone microarchitecture determined by HR-pQCT between subjects with and without T2DM [89]. Intriguingly, in a population-based sample of women aged 75–80 (99 women with T2DM and 954 controls), T2DM was associated with better bone microarchitecture (including higher trabecular and cortical vBMD in several regions and lower cortical porosity) [90]. In this context, large-scale clinical studies on the topic are required to evaluate the role of HR-pQCT in the diagnosis of bone fragility in T2DM. Moreover, the impacts of cortical porosity and other parameters, as estimated by HR-pQCT, on the prediction of fractures in T2DM are yet to be elucidated.

5.3. Microindentation

Microindentation is an invasive technique that enables percutaneous evaluation of the resistance of bone to indentation in vivo [91]. By indenting a probe tip through the skin covering the tibia and measuring the depth that it penetrates the bone after the generation of an impact force, impact microindentation measurement directly assesses the mechanical characteristics of cortical bone, which are estimated by the bone material strength index (BMSi) [92]. This technique may be particularly useful in populations presenting discrepancies between BMD and increased fracture risk, such as those with T2DM [93]. Accordingly, some studies have reported decreased BMSi in postmenopausal women with T2DM [89,90,94]. Moreover, altered matrix bone properties evaluated by microindentation were confirmed in this population, even though BMD assessed by DXA and/or bone microarchitecture assessed by HR-pQCT showed no differences between subjects with T2DM and healthy controls [89,90]. Remarkably, in a cross-sectional study including 340 men aged 33–96, participants with T2DM exhibited lower mean BMSi compared to subjects with normoglycemia/impaired fasting glucose [95]. However, it should be noted that further work is needed with regard to this technique for the assessment of bone fragility in patients with T2DM.

6. Bone Quality in T2DM: The Role of Biomarkers of Bone Fragility

In addition to bone mineralization and microarchitecture, skeletal material properties are also influenced by bone turnover and the quality of collagen, which may be affected by the accumulation of AGEs, leading to the alteration of collagen crosslinks and function as discussed in previous sections [23]. In this regard, it has been stated that bone turnover is decreased in T2DM, which results in reduced serum levels of bone remodeling markers [23,96–98]. However, it remains unknown whether these biochemical markers may be helpful for the diagnosis of bone fragility or the prediction of fracture risk in patients with T2DM. On the one hand, decreased circulating levels of parathyroid hormone (PTH) along with osteocalcin were shown to be associated with a higher risk of vertebral fracture in postmenopausal women with T2DM [99]. On the contrary, in a recent study, Napoli et al. showed that serum bone turnover markers (terminal telopeptide of type 1 collagen-CTX, osteocalcin, and procollagen type 1 N-terminal propeptide-P1NP) were not able to predict fracture risk in T2DM [100].

On the other hand, AGES related to collagen, such as pentosidine and N-carboxymethyl lysine (CML), are increased in bone biopsy specimens from subjects with T2DM [60,101,102]. Therefore, circulating/urinary levels of these AGEs may become attractive surrogate markers of bone quality in subjects with T2DM. Besides this, other novel biomarkers could play a role in the evaluation of bone fragility in T2DM.

6.1. Pentosidine

Pentosidine is a well-characterized AGE derived from the non-enzymatic reaction of pentoses with lysine and arginine residues [103]. Pentosidine levels are increased in T2DM [104]; moreover, circulating levels of pentosidine appear to be higher in patients with T2DM and poor metabolic control, and they are also related to T2DM-associated cardiovascular disease and microvascular complications [104–106].

Higher concentrations of pentosidine can also be found in the cancellous bone of patients with T2DM, and this accumulation may be associated with bone fragility via reduced post-yield strain and toughness due to alterations of the bone matrix [60,107,108]. These disturbances may be related to a decreased bone turnover induced by this AGE [109]. Of note, serum/urinary levels of pentosidine may also be applicable markers of bone fragility in T2DM. Thus, serum levels of pentosidine have been reported to be linked to the presence of vertebral fractures in postmenopausal women with T2DM, who presented similar BMD values/bone turnover markers to controls [110]. Furthermore, in a cross-sectional study, urine pentosidine levels were higher in patients with T2DM and vertebral fractures, and were negatively correlated with TBS [111]. In an observational cohort study (501 participants with T2DM and 427 without T2DM), Schwartz et al. showed that urine pentosidine was able to predict incident clinical fractures only in adults with T2DM, while prevalent vertebral fractures were also associated with urine pentosidine in this population [112].

6.2. N-carboxymethyl Lysine

The AGE N-carboxymethyl lysine (CML) may also play an important role in bone fragility in patients with T2DM [102]. In this regard, CML content in human cortical bone has been reported to be higher in subjects with T2DM, which may affect collagen properties [102]. In a large cohort from the Cardiovascular Health Study (3373 participants), serum levels of CML were associated with increased risk of incident hip fracture, independent of the BMD, with no differences in the hazard ratio between participants with and without T2DM [113]. Recently, in a cohort study including 712 participants with T2DM and 2332 subjects without, Dhaliwal et al. showed that circulating levels of CML were higher in patients with T2DM, and higher levels of this AGE were related to an increased risk of incident clinical fractures in this group, independent of the BMD [114]. Indeed, in this study, no relationship was found between hip BMD and CML, which reinforces the notion that bone quality is a major determinant of the pathophysiology of increased fracture risk in T2DM [114].

6.3. Sclerostin

Sclerostin is an inhibitor of the pro-osteogenic Wnt signaling pathway, which results in decreased bone turnover [23,115]. Hence, some studies have found that higher levels of this protein could be associated with a higher risk of osteoporotic fractures [116,117].

Increased circulating levels of sclerostin have been observed in patients with T2DM and may be involved in low bone turnover and a greater risk of fracture found in this population [118]. Thus, higher serum levels of sclerostin have been reported in postmenopausal women with T2DM and fragility fractures, compared to those without fragility fractures [119,120]. In addition to this, in a cross-sectional study including postmenopausal women and men aged >50 years with T2DM, elevated sclerostin levels correlated with the presence of vertebral fractures [121].

6.4. MicroRNAs

MicroRNAs (miRNAs) are epigenetic regulators of different cellular processes, including bone development, homeostasis, and healing [122]. Although evidence regarding the role of these elements in bone fragility in T2DM is still limited, some studies have shed light on their potential utility [123–125]. In a study conducted on 168 postmenopausal women with T2DM, three different miRNAs, including senescent miR-31-5p, were significantly associated with incident fragility fractures [123]. In previous analyses, Heilmeier et al. also reported that individual miRNAs or miRNA combinations were able to discriminate the fracture status in postmenopausal women with T2DM [124]. Chen et al. also described several miRNAs with potential implications for fracture prediction in postmenopausal women with T2DM [125].

6.5. Other Biomarkers

Aside from in the serum and urine, AGE deposition can be measured in other tissues, such as the skin. Therefore, skin autofluorescence (SAF), which is based on the non-invasive measurement of AGE accumulation in the human skin, has emerged as a promising technique [126]. However, little evidence is available concerning bone fragility/fracture risk estimation through this tool. In two cross-sectional studies, SAF was inversely correlated with BMSi in patients with T2DM [94,127]. Interestingly, SAF was associated with prevalent vertebral and major osteoporotic fractures in participants from the Rotterdam Study [128]. However, these data must be assessed specifically in individuals with T2DM.

In another area, the fingernail quality may serve as a non-invasive marker of the bone quality in T2DM [129,130]. Nevertheless, further investigation is needed.

7. Conclusions

Since traditional methods for the evaluation of BMD and fracture risk in individuals with T2DM can lead to significant errors, additional techniques are needed. TBS may be considered as a useful non-invasive index of bone microarchitecture, which is often altered in patients with T2DM. Since TBS is derived from DXA images, it may represent an applicable tool for the diagnosis of bone fragility in T2DM. In addition, it could facilitate follow-up and the evaluation of response to treatment in these patients, and may help to unravel the role of certain glucose-lowering agents in bone fragility. HR-pQCT also permits the evaluation of bone microstructure; however, this technique involves significant costs and exposure to radiation, which should be considered. Future opportunities in this area include the evaluation of bone microstructure by DXA-3D, which has shown remarkable results in several conditions other than T2DM and may provide accurate estimations of bone structure and strength, thus offering additional information with regard to fracture risk. Despite the fact that microindentation is a promising method for the evaluation of bone matrix properties, it requires an invasive procedure, which may limit its application in clinical practice. On the other hand, some biochemical markers may represent interesting non-invasive alternatives for the evaluation of skeletal fragility/fracture risk prediction in patients with T2DM, although it is noteworthy that the current evidence regarding some of these alternatives is still limited; therefore, further research (e.g., validation studies) is needed before these biomarkers may be included in routine practice. Further large-scale, long-term prospective studies are needed in the evaluation of quality and bone microstructure alterations in patients with T2DM.

Author Contributions: Conceptualization, J.I.M.-M. and M.M.-T.; writing—original draft preparation, J.I.M.-M.; writing—review and editing, J.I.M.-M., B.G.-F., C.G.-F. and M.M.-T.; supervision, B.G.-F., C.G.-F. and M.M.-T.; funding acquisition, B.G.-F., C.G.-F. and M.M.-T. All authors have read and agreed to the published version of the manuscript.

Funding: This research was funded by Instituto de Salud Carlos III grants (PI18–00803, PI21–01069, and PI18–01235), co-funded by the European Regional Development Fund (FEDER) and by a Junta de Andalucía grant (PI-0268–2019). In addition, C.G-F. was funded by a postdoctoral fellowship from the Instituto de Salud Carlos III (CD20/00022).

Institutional Review Board Statement: Not applicable.

Informed Consent Statement: Not applicable.

Data Availability Statement: Not applicable.

Acknowledgments: The images in Figures 1 and 2 were obtained from smart.servier.com (accessed on 26 February 2022).

Conflicts of Interest: The authors declare no conflict of interest. The funders played no role in the writing of the manuscript or in the decision to publish the results.

References

1. Zheng, Y.; Ley, S.H.; Hu, F.B. Global aetiology and epidemiology of type 2 diabetes mellitus and its complications. *Nat. Rev. Endocrinol.* **2018**, *14*, 88–98. [CrossRef] [PubMed]
2. Dal Canto, E.; Ceriello, A.; Rydén, L.; Ferrini, M.; Hansen, T.B.; Schnell, O.; Standl, E.; Beulens, J.W. Diabetes as a cardiovascular risk factor: An overview of global trends of macro and micro vascular complications. *Eur. J. Prev. Cardiol.* **2019**, *26* (Suppl. 2), 25–32. [CrossRef] [PubMed]
3. Alaofè, H.; Amoussa Hounkpatin, W.; Djrolo, F.; Ehiri, J.; Rosales, C. Factors Associated with Quality of Life in Patients with Type 2 Diabetes of South Benin: A Cross-Sectional Study. *Int. J. Environ. Res. Public Health* **2022**, *19*, 2360. [CrossRef] [PubMed]
4. Fenwick, E.K.; Pesudovs, K.; Khadka, J.; Dirani, M.; Rees, G.; Wong, T.Y.; Lamoureux, E.L. The impact of diabetic retinopathy on quality of life: Qualitative findings from an item bank development project. *Qual. Life Res.* **2012**, *21*, 1771–1782. [CrossRef] [PubMed]
5. Degu, H.; Wondimagegnehu, A.; Yifru, Y.M.; Belachew, A. Is health related quality of life influenced by diabetic neuropathic pain among type II diabetes mellitus patients in Ethiopia? *PLoS ONE* **2019**, *14*, e0211449. [CrossRef] [PubMed]
6. Sinjari, B.; Feragalli, B.; Cornelli, U.; Belcaro, G.; Vitacolonna, E.; Santilli, M.; Rexhepi, I.; D'Addazio, G.; Zuccari, F.; Caputi, S. Artificial Saliva in Diabetic Xerostomia (ASDIX): Double Blind Trial of Aldiamed® Versus Placebo. *J. Clin. Med.* **2020**, *9*, 2196. [CrossRef]
7. Khosla, S.; Samakkarnthai, P.; Monroe, D.G.; Farr, J.N. Update on the pathogenesis and treatment of skeletal fragility in type 2 diabetes mellitus. *Nat. Rev. Endocrinol.* **2021**, *17*, 685–697. [CrossRef]
8. Schousboe, J.T.; Morin, S.N.; Kline, G.A.; Lix, L.M.; Leslie, W.D. Differential risk of fracture attributable to type 2 diabetes mellitus according to skeletal site. *Bone* **2021**, *154*, 116220. [CrossRef]
9. Wang, B.; Wang, Z.; Poundarik, A.A.; Zaki, M.J.; Bockman, R.S.; Glicksberg, B.S.; Nadkarni, G.N.; Vashishth, D. Unmasking Fracture Risk in Type 2 Diabetes: The Association of Longitudinal Glycemic Hemoglobin Level and Medications. *J. Clin. Endocrinol. Metab.* **2021**, *107*, e1390–e1401. [CrossRef]
10. Schwartz, A.V. Epidemiology of fractures in type 2 diabetes. *Bone* **2016**, *82*, 2–8. [CrossRef]
11. Koromani, F.; Ghatan, S.; van Hoek, M.; Zillikens, M.C.; Oei, E.H.G.; Rivadeneira, F.; Oei, L. Type 2 Diabetes Mellitus and Vertebral Fracture Risk. *Curr. Osteoporos. Rep.* **2021**, *19*, 50–57. [CrossRef] [PubMed]
12. Koromani, F.; Oei, L.; Shevroja, E.; Trajanoska, K.; Schoufour, J.; Muka, T.; Franco, O.H.; Ikram, M.A.; Zillikens, M.C.; Uitterlinden, A.G.; et al. Vertebral Fractures in Individuals with Type 2 Diabetes: More Than Skeletal Complications Alone. *Diabetes Care* **2020**, *43*, 137–144. [CrossRef] [PubMed]

13. Vilaca, T.; Schini, M.; Harnan, S.; Sutton, A.; Poku, E.; Allen, I.E.; Cummings, S.R.; Eastell, R. The risk of hip and non-vertebral fractures in type 1 and type 2 diabetes: A systematic review and meta-analysis update. *Bone* **2020**, *137*, 115457. [CrossRef] [PubMed]
14. Janghorbani, M.; van Dam, R.M.; Willett, W.C.; Hu, F.B. Systematic Review of Type 1 and Type 2 Diabetes Mellitus and Risk of Fracture. *Am. J. Epidemiol.* **2007**, *166*, 495–505. [CrossRef]
15. Ammarullah, M.I.; Afif, I.Y.; Maula, M.I.; Winarni, T.I.; Tauviqirrahman, M.; Akbar, I.; Basri, H.; van der Heide, E.; Jamari, J. Tresca Stress Simulation of Metal-on-Metal Total Hip Arthroplasty during Normal Walking Activity. *Materials* **2021**, *14*, 7554. [CrossRef]
16. Jamari, J.; Ammarullah, M.; Saad, A.P.M.; Syahrom, A.; Uddin, M.; van der Heide, E.; Basri, H. The Effect of Bottom Profile Dimples on the Femoral Head on Wear in Metal-on-Metal Total Hip Arthroplasty. *J. Funct. Biomater.* **2021**, *12*, 38. [CrossRef]
17. Sato, M.; Ye, W.; Sugihara, T.; Isaka, Y. Fracture risk and healthcare resource utilization and costs among osteoporosis patients with type 2 diabetes mellitus and without diabetes mellitus in Japan: Retrospective analysis of a hospital claims database. *BMC Musculoskelet. Disord.* **2016**, *17*, 489. [CrossRef]
18. Shah, A.; Wu, F.; Jones, G.; Cicuttini, F.; Toh, L.S.; Laslett, L.L. The association between incident vertebral deformities, health-related quality of life and functional impairment: A 10.7-year cohort study. *Osteoporos. Int.* **2021**, *32*, 2247–2255. [CrossRef]
19. Peeters, C.M.M.; Visser, E.; Van de Ree, C.L.P.; Gosens, T.; Den Oudsten, B.L.; De Vries, J. Quality of life after hip fracture in the elderly: A systematic literature review. *Injury* **2016**, *47*, 1369–1382. [CrossRef]
20. Ferrari, S.L.; Abrahamsen, B.; Napoli, N.; Akesson, K.; Chandran, M.; Eastell, R.; El-Hajj Fuleihan, G.; Josse, R.; Kendler, D.L.; Kraenzlin, M.; et al. Diagnosis and management of bone fragility in diabetes: An emerging challenge. *Osteoporos. Int.* **2018**, *29*, 2585–2596. [CrossRef]
21. de Waard, E.A.C.; van Geel, T.A.C.M.; Savelberg, H.H.C.M.; Koster, A.; Geusens, P.P.M.M.; van den Bergh, J.P.W. Increased fracture risk in patients with type 2 diabetes mellitus: An overview of the underlying mechanisms and the usefulness of imaging modalities and fracture risk assessment tools. *Maturitas* **2014**, *79*, 265–274. [CrossRef] [PubMed]
22. Walsh, J.S.; Vilaca, T. Obesity, Type 2 Diabetes and Bone in Adults. *Calcif. Tissue Int.* **2017**, *100*, 528–535. [CrossRef] [PubMed]
23. Hofbauer, L.C.; Busse, B.; Eastell, R.; Ferrari, S.; Frost, M.; Müller, R.; Burden, A.M.; Rivadeneira, F.; Napoli, N.; Rauner, M. Bone fragility in diabetes: Novel concepts and clinical implications. *Lancet Diabetes Endocrinol.* **2022**, *10*, 207–220. [CrossRef]
24. Majumdar, S.R.; Leslie, W.D.; Lix, L.M.; Morin, S.N.; Johansson, H.; Oden, A.; McCloskey, E.V.; Kanis, J.A. Longer Duration of Diabetes Strongly Impacts Fracture Risk Assessment: The Manitoba BMD Cohort. *J. Clin. Endocrinol. Metab.* **2016**, *101*, 4489–4496. [CrossRef] [PubMed]
25. Dufour, A.B.; Kiel, D.P.; Williams, S.A.; Weiss, R.J.; Samelson, E.J. Risk Factors for Incident Fracture in Older Adults with Type 2 Diabetes: The Framingham Heart Study. *Diabetes Care* **2021**, *44*, 1547–1555. [CrossRef] [PubMed]
26. Li, C.-I.; Liu, C.-S.; Lin, W.-Y.; Meng, N.-H.; Chen, C.-C.; Yang, S.-Y.; Chen, H.-J.; Lin, C.-C.; Li, T.-C. Glycated Hemoglobin Level and Risk of Hip Fracture in Older People with Type 2 Diabetes: A Competing Risk Analysis of Taiwan Diabetes Cohort Study. *J. Bone Miner. Res.* **2015**, *30*, 1338–1346. [CrossRef]
27. Oei, L.; Zillikens, M.C.; Dehghan, A.; Buitendijk, G.H.S.; Castaño-Betancourt, M.C.; Estrada, K.; Stolk, L.; Oei, E.H.G.; van Meurs, J.B.J.; Janssen, J.A.M.J.L.; et al. High Bone Mineral Density and Fracture Risk in Type 2 Diabetes as Skeletal Complications of Inadequate Glucose Control: The Rotterdam Study. *Diabetes Care* **2013**, *36*, 1619–1628. [CrossRef]
28. Romero-Díaz, C.; Duarte-Montero, D.; Gutiérrez-Romero, S.A.; Mendivil, C.O. Diabetes and Bone Fragility. *Diabetes Ther.* **2020**, *12*, 71–86. [CrossRef]
29. Starup-Linde, J.; Vestergaard, P. Biochemical bone turnover markers in diabetes mellitus—A systematic review. *Bone* **2016**, *82*, 69–78. [CrossRef]
30. Tonks, K.T.; White, C.; Center, J.R.; Samocha-Bonet, D.; Greenfield, J. Bone Turnover Is Suppressed in Insulin Resistance, Independent of Adiposity. *J. Clin. Endocrinol. Metab.* **2017**, *102*, 1112–1121. [CrossRef]
31. Napoli, N.; Chandran, M.; Pierroz, D.D.; Abrahamsen, B.; Schwartz, A.V.; Ferrari, S.L. Mechanisms of diabetes mellitus-induced bone fragility. *Nat. Rev. Endocrinol.* **2017**, *13*, 208–219. [CrossRef] [PubMed]
32. Nuche-Berenguer, B.; Portal-Núñez, S.; Moreno, P.; González, N.; Acitores, A.; López-Herradón, A.; Esbrit, P.; Valverde, I.; Villanueva-Peñacarrillo, M.L. Presence of a functional receptor for GLP-1 in osteoblastic cells, independent of the cAMP-linked GLP-1 receptor. *J. Cell. Physiol.* **2010**, *225*, 585–592. [CrossRef] [PubMed]
33. Muñoz-Torres, M.; Reyes-García, R.; García-Martin, A.; Jiménez-Moleón, J.J.; Gonzalez-Ramírez, A.R.; Lara-Villoslada, M.J.; Moreno, P.R. Ischemic heart disease is associated with vertebral fractures in patients with type 2 diabetes mellitus. *J. Diabetes Investig.* **2013**, *4*, 310–315. [CrossRef] [PubMed]
34. Mitri, J.; Pittas, A.G. Vitamin D and Diabetes. *Endocrinol. Metab. Clin. N. Am.* **2014**, *43*, 205–232. [CrossRef]
35. Knudsen, J.K.; Leutscher, P.; Sørensen, S. Gut Microbiota in Bone Health and Diabetes. *Curr. Osteoporos. Rep.* **2021**, *19*, 462–479. [CrossRef]
36. Shanbhogue, V.V.; Mitchell, D.M.; Rosen, C.J.; Bouxsein, M.L. Type 2 diabetes and the skeleton: New insights into sweet bones. *Lancet Diabetes Endocrinol.* **2016**, *4*, 159–173. [CrossRef]
37. Rozas-Moreno, P.; Reyes-García, R.; Jódar-Gimeno, E.; Varsavsky, M.; Luque-Fernández, I.; Cortés-Berdonces, M.; Muñoz-Torres, M. Recomendaciones sobre el efecto de los fármacos antidiabéticos en el hueso. *Endocrinol. Diabetes Nutr.* **2017**, *64*, 1–6. [CrossRef]

38. Molinuevo, M.S.; Schurman, L.; McCarthy, A.D.; Cortizo, A.M.; Tolosa, M.J.; Gangoiti, M.V.; Arnol, V.; Sedlinsky, C. Effect of metformin on bone marrow progenitor cell differentiation: In vivo and in vitro studies. *J. Bone Miner. Res.* **2010**, *25*, 211–221. [CrossRef]
39. Monami, M.; Dicembrini, I.; Antenore, A.; Mannucci, E. Dipeptidyl Peptidase-4 Inhibitors and Bone Fractures: A meta-analysis of randomized clinical trials. *Diabetes Care* **2011**, *34*, 2474–2476. [CrossRef]
40. Su, B.; Sheng, H.; Zhang, M.; Bu, L.; Yang, P.; Li, L.; Li, F.; Sheng, C.; Han, Y.; Qu, S.; et al. Risk of bone fractures associated with glucagon-like peptide-1 receptor agonists' treatment: A meta-analysis of randomized controlled trials. *Endocrine* **2014**, *48*, 107–115. [CrossRef]
41. Zhu, Z.-N.; Jiang, Y.-F.; Ding, T. Risk of fracture with thiazolidinediones: An updated meta-analysis of randomized clinical trials. *Bone* **2014**, *68*, 115–123. [CrossRef] [PubMed]
42. Kohan, D.E.; Fioretto, P.; Tang, W.; List, J.F. Long-term study of patients with type 2 diabetes and moderate renal impairment shows that dapagliflozin reduces weight and blood pressure but does not improve glycemic control. *Kidney Int.* **2014**, *85*, 962–971. [CrossRef]
43. Neal, B.; Perkovic, V.; Mahaffey, K.W.; de Zeeuw, D.; Fulcher, G.; Erondu, N.; Shaw, W.; Law, G.; Desai, M.; Matthews, D.R.; et al. Canagliflozin and Cardiovascular and Renal Events in Type 2 Diabetes. *N. Engl. J. Med.* **2017**, *377*, 644–657. [CrossRef] [PubMed]
44. Johnston, S.S.; Conner, C.; Aagren, M.; Ruiz, K.; Bouchard, J. Association between hypoglycaemic events and fall-related fractures in Medicare-covered patients with type 2 diabetes. *Diabetes Obes. Metab.* **2012**, *14*, 634–643. [CrossRef] [PubMed]
45. Mayne, D.; Stout, N.R.; Aspray, T.J. Diabetes, falls and fractures. *Age Ageing* **2010**, *39*, 522–525. [CrossRef] [PubMed]
46. Dennison, E.M.; Syddall, H.E.; Aihie Sayer, A.; Craighead, S.; Phillips, D.I.W.; Cooper, C. Type 2 diabetes mellitus is associated with increased axial bone density in men and women from the Hertfordshire Cohort Study: Evidence for an indirect effect of insulin resistance? *Diabetologia* **2004**, *47*, 1963–1968. [CrossRef]
47. Bonds, D.E.; Larson, J.C.; Schwartz, A.V.; Strotmeyer, E.S.; Robbins, J.; Rodriguez, B.L.; Johnson, K.C.; Margolis, K. Risk of Fracture in Women with Type 2 Diabetes: The Women's Health Initiative Observational Study. *J. Clin. Endocrinol. Metab.* **2006**, *91*, 3404–3410. [CrossRef]
48. Mitchell, A.; Fall, T.; Melhus, H.; Wolk, A.; Michaëlsson, K.; Byberg, L. Type 2 Diabetes in Relation to Hip Bone Density, Area, and Bone Turnover in Swedish Men and Women: A Cross-Sectional Study. *Calcif. Tissue Int.* **2018**, *103*, 501–511. [CrossRef]
49. Ma, L.; Oei, L.; Jiang, L.; Estrada, K.; Chen, H.; Wang, Z.; Yu, Q.; Zillikens, M.C.; Gao, X.; Rivadeneira, F. Association between bone mineral density and type 2 diabetes mellitus: A meta-analysis of observational studies. *Eur. J. Epidemiol.* **2012**, *27*, 319–332. [CrossRef]
50. Pan, H.; Wu, N.; Yang, T.; He, W. Association between bone mineral density and type 1 diabetes mellitus: A meta-analysis of cross-sectional studies. *Diabetes Metab. Res. Rev.* **2014**, *30*, 531–542. [CrossRef]
51. Srikanthan, P.; Crandall, C.J.; Miller-Martinez, D.; Seeman, T.E.; Greendale, G.A.; Binkley, N.; Karlamangla, A.S. Insulin Resistance and Bone Strength: Findings From the Study of Midlife in the United States. *J. Bone Miner. Res.* **2014**, *29*, 796–803. [CrossRef] [PubMed]
52. Upadhyay, J.; Farr, O.M.; Mantzoros, C.S. The role of leptin in regulating bone metabolism. *Metabolism* **2015**, *64*, 105–113. [CrossRef] [PubMed]
53. Botella Martínez, S.; Varo Cenarruzabeitia, N.; Escalada San Martin, J.; Calleja Canelas, A. The diabetic paradox: Bone mineral density and fracture in type 2 diabetes. *Endocrinol. Nutr.* **2016**, *63*, 495–501. [CrossRef] [PubMed]
54. Giangregorio, L.M.; Leslie, W.D.; Lix, L.M.; Johansson, H.; Oden, A.; McCloskey, E.; Kanis, J.A. FRAX underestimates fracture risk in patients with diabetes. *J. Bone Miner. Res.* **2012**, *27*, 301–308. [CrossRef] [PubMed]
55. El Miedany, Y. FRAX: Re-adjust or re-think. *Arch. Osteoporos.* **2020**, *15*, 150. [CrossRef]
56. Valentini, A.; Cianfarani, M.A.; De Meo, L.; Morabito, P.; Romanello, D.; Tarantino, U.; Federici, M.; Bertoli, A. FRAX tool in type 2 diabetic subjects: The use of HbA1c in estimating fracture risk. *Acta Diabetol.* **2018**, *55*, 1043–1050. [CrossRef]
57. Wen, Z.; Ding, N.; Chen, R.; Liu, S.; Wang, Q.; Sheng, Z.; Liu, H. Comparison of methods to improve fracture risk assessment in chinese diabetic postmenopausal women: A case-control study. *Endocrine* **2021**, *73*, 209–216. [CrossRef]
58. Hu, L.; Li, T.; Zou, Y.; Yin, X.-L.; Gan, H. The Clinical Value of the RA-Adjusted Fracture Risk Assessment Tool in the Fracture Risk Prediction of Patients with Type 2 Diabetes Mellitus in China. *Int. J. Gen. Med.* **2021**, *14*, 327–333. [CrossRef]
59. Leslie, W.D.; Johansson, H.; McCloskey, E.V.; Harvey, N.C.; Kanis, J.A.; Hans, D. Comparison of Methods for Improving Fracture Risk Assessment in Diabetes: The Manitoba BMD Registry. *J. Bone Miner. Res.* **2018**, *33*, 1923–1930. [CrossRef]
60. Hunt, H.B.; Torres, A.M.; Palomino, P.M.; Marty, E.; Saiyed, R.; Cohn, M.; Jo, J.; Warner, S.; Sroga, G.E.; King, K.B.; et al. Altered Tissue Composition, Microarchitecture, and Mechanical Performance in Cancellous Bone From Men With Type 2 Diabetes Mellitus. *J. Bone Miner. Res.* **2019**, *34*, 1191–1206. [CrossRef]
61. Silva, B.C.; Leslie, W.D.; Resch, H.; Lamy, O.; Lesnyak, O.; Binkley, N.; McCloskey, E.V.; Kanis, J.A.; Bilezikian, J.P. Trabecular Bone Score: A Noninvasive Analytical Method Based Upon the DXA Image. *J. Bone Miner. Res.* **2014**, *29*, 518–530. [CrossRef] [PubMed]
62. McCloskey, E.V.; Oden, A.; Harvey, N.C.; Leslie, W.D.; Hans, D.; Johansson, H.; Barkmann, R.; Boutroy, S.; Brown, J.; Chapurlat, R.; et al. A meta-analysis of trabecular bone score in fracture risk prediction and its relationship to FRAX. *J. Bone Miner. Res.* **2016**, *31*, 940–948. [CrossRef] [PubMed]
63. Hans, D.; Goertzen, A.L.; Krieg, M.-A.; Leslie, W.D. Bone microarchitecture assessed by TBS predicts osteoporotic fractures independent of bone density: The Manitoba study. *J. Bone Miner. Res.* **2011**, *26*, 2762–2769. [CrossRef] [PubMed]

64. Leslie, W.D.; Aubry-Rozier, B.; Lix, L.M.; Morin, S.N.; Majumdar, S.R.; Hans, D. Spine bone texture assessed by trabecular bone score (TBS) predicts osteoporotic fractures in men: The Manitoba Bone Density Program. *Bone* **2014**, *67*, 10–14. [CrossRef] [PubMed]
65. Briot, K.; Paternotte, S.; Kolta, S.; Eastell, R.; Reid, D.M.; Felsenberg, D.; Glüer, C.C.; Roux, C. Added value of trabecular bone score to bone mineral density for prediction of osteoporotic fractures in postmenopausal women: The OPUS study. *Bone* **2013**, *57*, 232–236. [CrossRef]
66. Boutroy, S.; Hans, D.; Sornay-Rendu, E.; Vilayphiou, N.; Winzenrieth, R.; Chapurlat, R. Trabecular bone score improves fracture risk prediction in non-osteoporotic women: The OFELY study. *Osteoporos. Int.* **2013**, *24*, 77–85. [CrossRef]
67. Ho-Pham, L.T.; Nguyen, T.V. Association between trabecular bone score and type 2 diabetes: A quantitative update of evidence. *Osteoporos. Int.* **2019**, *30*, 2079–2085. [CrossRef]
68. Ho-Pham, L.T.; Tran, B.; Do, A.T.; Nguyen, T.V. Association between pre-diabetes, type 2 diabetes and trabecular bone score: The Vietnam Osteoporosis Study. *Diabetes Res. Clin. Pract.* **2019**, *155*, 107790. [CrossRef]
69. Hayón-Ponce, M.; García-Fontana, B.; Avilés-Pérez, M.D.; González-Salvatierra, S.; Andújar-Vera, F.; Moratalla-Aranda, E.; Muñoz-Torres, M. Lower trabecular bone score in type 2 diabetes mellitus: A role for fat mass and insulin resistance beyond hyperglycaemia. *Diabetes Metab.* **2021**, *47*, 101276. [CrossRef]
70. Moon, H.U.; Lee, N.; Chung, Y.-S.; Choi, Y.J. Reduction of visceral fat could be related to the improvement of TBS in diabetes mellitus. *J. Bone Miner. Metab.* **2020**, *38*, 702–709. [CrossRef]
71. Palomo, T.; Dreyer, P.; Muszkat, P.; Weiler, F.G.; Bonansea, T.C.P.; Domingues, F.C.; Vieira, J.G.H.; Silva, B.C.; Brandão, C.M.A. Effect of soft tissue noise on trabecular bone score in postmenopausal women with diabetes: A cross sectional study. *Bone* **2022**, *157*, 116339. [CrossRef] [PubMed]
72. Depczynski, B.; Liew, P.Y.; White, C. Association of glycaemic variables with trabecular bone score in post-menopausal women with type 2 diabetes mellitus. *Diabet. Med.* **2020**, *37*, 1545–1552. [CrossRef] [PubMed]
73. Iki, M.; Fujita, Y.; Kouda, K.; Yura, A.; Tachiki, T.; Tamaki, J.; Winzenrieth, R.; Sato, Y.; Moon, J.-S.; Okamoto, N.; et al. Hyperglycemia is associated with increased bone mineral density and decreased trabecular bone score in elderly Japanese men: The Fujiwara-kyo osteoporosis risk in men (FORMEN) study. *Bone* **2017**, *105*, 18–25. [CrossRef] [PubMed]
74. El Asri, M.M.; Rodrigo, E.P.; de la Flor, S.D.-S.; Valdivieso, S.P.; Barrón, M.C.R.; Martínez, J.M.O.; Hernández, J.L.H. Índice trabecular óseo y niveles de 25-hidroxivitamina D en las complicaciones microvasculares de la diabetes mellitus tipo 2. *Med. Clin.* **2021**, in press. [CrossRef]
75. Leslie, W.D.; Aubry-Rozier, B.; Lamy, O.; Hans, D.; Manitoba Bone Density Program. TBS (Trabecular Bone Score) and Diabetes-Related Fracture Risk. *J. Clin. Endocrinol. Metab.* **2013**, *98*, 602–609. [CrossRef]
76. Zhukouskaya, V.V.; Ellen-Vainicher, C.; Gaudio, A.; Privitera, F.; Cairoli, E.; Ulivieri, F.M.; Palmieri, S.; Morelli, V.; Grancini, V.; Orsi, E.; et al. The utility of lumbar spine trabecular bone score and femoral neck bone mineral density for identifying asymptomatic vertebral fractures in well-compensated type 2 diabetic patients. *Osteoporos. Int.* **2016**, *27*, 49–56. [CrossRef]
77. Yamamoto, M.; Yamauchi, M.; Sugimoto, T. Prevalent vertebral fracture is dominantly associated with spinal microstructural deterioration rather than bone mineral density in patients with type 2 diabetes mellitus. *PLoS ONE* **2019**, *14*, e0222571. [CrossRef]
78. Lin, Y.-C.; Wu, J.; Kuo, S.-F.; Cheung, Y.-C.; Sung, C.-M.; Fan, C.-M.; Chen, F.-P.; Mhuircheartaigh, J.N. Vertebral Fractures in Type 2 Diabetes Patients: Utility of Trabecular Bone Score and Relationship with Serum Bone Turnover Biomarkers. *J. Clin. Densitom.* **2020**, *23*, 37–43. [CrossRef]
79. Nishiyama, K.K.; Shane, E. Clinical Imaging of Bone Microarchitecture with HR-pQCT. *Curr. Osteoporos. Rep.* **2013**, *11*, 147–155. [CrossRef]
80. Mikolajewicz, N.; Bishop, N.; Burghardt, A.J.; Folkestad, L.; Hall, A.; Kozloff, K.M.; Lukey, P.T.; Molloy-Bland, M.; Morin, S.N.; Offiah, A.; et al. HR-pQCT Measures of Bone Microarchitecture Predict Fracture: Systematic Review and Meta-Analysis. *J. Bone Miner. Res.* **2019**, *35*, 446–459. [CrossRef]
81. Cheung, W.; Hung, V.W.; Cheuk, K.; Chau, W.; Tsoi, K.K.; Wong, R.M.; Chow, S.K.; Lam, T.; Yung, P.S.; Law, S.; et al. Best Performance Parameters of HR-pQCT to Predict Fragility Fracture: Systematic Review and Meta-Analysis. *J. Bone Miner. Res.* **2021**, *36*, 2381–2398. [CrossRef] [PubMed]
82. Burghardt, A.J.; Issever, A.S.; Schwartz, A.V.; Davis, K.A.; Masharani, U.; Majumdar, S.; Link, T.M. High-Resolution Peripheral Quantitative Computed Tomographic Imaging of Cortical and Trabecular Bone Microarchitecture in Patients with Type 2 Diabetes Mellitus. *J. Clin. Endocrinol. Metab.* **2010**, *95*, 5045–5055. [CrossRef] [PubMed]
83. Patsch, J.M.; Burghardt, A.J.; Yap, S.P.; Baum, T.; Schwartz, A.V.; Joseph, G.B.; Link, T.M. Increased cortical porosity in type 2 diabetic postmenopausal women with fragility fractures. *J. Bone Miner. Res.* **2013**, *28*, 313–324. [CrossRef] [PubMed]
84. Yu, E.W.; Putman, M.S.; Derrico, N.; Abrishamanian-Garcia, G.; Finkelstein, J.S.; Bouxsein, M.L. Defects in cortical microarchitecture among African-American women with type 2 diabetes. *Osteoporos. Int.* **2015**, *26*, 673–679. [CrossRef] [PubMed]
85. Samelson, E.J.; Demissie, S.; Cupples, L.A.; Zhang, X.; Xu, H.; Liu, C.-T.; Boyd, S.K.; McLean, R.R.; Broe, K.E.; Kiel, D.P.; et al. Diabetes and Deficits in Cortical Bone Density, Microarchitecture, and Bone Size: Framingham HR-pQCT Study. *J. Bone Miner. Res.* **2018**, *33*, 54–62. [CrossRef]

86. Heilmeier, U.; Joseph, G.B.; Pasco, C.; Dinh, N.; Torabi, S.; Darakananda, K.; Youm, J.; Carballido-Gamio, J.; Burghardt, A.J.; Link, T.M.; et al. Longitudinal Evolution of Bone Microarchitecture and Bone Strength in Type 2 Diabetic Postmenopausal Women with and without History of Fragility Fractures—A 5-Year Follow-Up Study Using High Resolution Peripheral Quantitative Computed Tomography. *Front. Endocrinol.* **2021**, *12*, 599316. [CrossRef]
87. Shanbhogue, V.V.; Hansen, S.; Frost, M.; Jørgensen, N.R.; Hermann, A.P.; Henriksen, J.E.; Brixen, K. Compromised cortical bone compartment in type 2 diabetes mellitus patients with microvascular disease. *Eur. J. Endocrinol.* **2016**, *174*, 115–124. [CrossRef]
88. De Waard, E.A.C.; De Jong, J.J.A.; Koster, A.; Savelberg, H.H.C.M.; Van Geel, T.A.; Houben, A.J.H.M.; Schram, M.T.; Dagnelie, P.C.; Van Der Kallen, C.J.; Sep, S.J.S.; et al. The association between diabetes status, HbA1c, diabetes duration, microvascular disease, and bone quality of the distal radius and tibia as measured with high-resolution peripheral quantitative computed tomography—The Maastricht Study. *Osteoporos. Int.* **2018**, *29*, 2725–2738. [CrossRef]
89. Farr, J.N.; Drake, M.T.; Amin, S.; Melton, L.J., 3rd; McCready, L.K.; Khosla, S. In Vivo Assessment of Bone Quality in Postmenopausal Women with Type 2 Diabetes. *J. Bone Miner. Res.* **2014**, *29*, 787–795. [CrossRef]
90. Nilsson, A.G.; Sundh, D.; Johansson, L.; Nilsson, M.; Mellström, D.; Rudäng, R.; Zoulakis, M.; Wallander, M.; Darelid, A.; Lorentzon, M. Type 2 Diabetes Mellitus Is Associated with Better Bone Microarchitecture But Lower Bone Material Strength and Poorer Physical Function in Elderly Women: A Population-Based Study. *J. Bone Miner. Res.* **2017**, *32*, 1062–1071. [CrossRef]
91. Randall, C.; Bridges, D.; Guerri, R.; Nogues, X.; Puig, L.; Torres, E.; Mellibovsky, L.; Hoffseth, K.; Stalbaum, T.; Srikanth, A.; et al. Applications of a New Handheld Reference Point Indentation Instrument Measuring Bone Material Strength. *J. Med. Devices* **2013**, *7*, 041005. [CrossRef] [PubMed]
92. Bridges, D.; Randall, C.; Hansma, P.K. A new device for performing reference point indentation without a reference probe. *Rev. Sci. Instrum.* **2012**, *83*, 044301. [CrossRef] [PubMed]
93. Herrera, S.; Diez-Perez, A. Clinical experience with microindentation in vivo in humans. *Bone* **2017**, *95*, 175–182. [CrossRef] [PubMed]
94. Furst, J.R.; Bandeira, L.C.; Fan, W.-W.; Agarwal, S.; Nishiyama, K.K.; McMahon, D.J.; Dworakowski, E.; Jiang, H.; Silverberg, S.J.; Rubin, M.R. Advanced Glycation Endproducts and Bone Material Strength in Type 2 Diabetes. *J. Clin. Endocrinol. Metab.* **2016**, *101*, 2502–2510. [CrossRef]
95. Holloway-Kew, K.L.; Betson, A.; Rufus-Membere, P.G.; Gaston, J.; Diez-Perez, A.; Kotowicz, M.A.; Pasco, J.A. Impact microindentation in men with impaired fasting glucose and type 2 diabetes. *Bone* **2021**, *142*, 115685. [CrossRef]
96. Starup-Linde, J.; Lykkeboe, S.; Handberg, A.; Vestergaard, P.; Høyem, P.; Fleischer, J.; Hansen, T.K.; Poulsen, P.L.; Laugesen, E. Glucose variability and low bone turnover in people with type 2 diabetes. *Bone* **2021**, *153*, 116159. [CrossRef]
97. Starup-Linde, J.; Eriksen, S.A.; Lykkeboe, S.; Handberg, A.; Vestergaard, P. Biochemical markers of bone turnover in diabetes patients—A meta-analysis, and a methodological study on the effects of glucose on bone markers. *Osteoporos. Int.* **2014**, *25*, 1697–1708. [CrossRef]
98. Reyes-Garcia, R.; Rozas-Moreno, P.; López-Gallardo, G.; Garcia-Martin, A.; Varsavsky, M.; Avilés-Pérez, M.D.; Muñoz-Torres, M. Serum levels of bone resorption markers are decreased in patients with type 2 diabetes. *Acta Diabetol.* **2013**, *50*, 47–52. [CrossRef]
99. Yamamoto, M.; Yamaguchi, T.; Nawata, K.; Yamauchi, M.; Sugimoto, T. Decreased PTH Levels Accompanied by Low Bone Formation Are Associated with Vertebral Fractures in Postmenopausal Women with Type 2 Diabetes. *J. Clin. Endocrinol. Metab.* **2012**, *97*, 1277–1284. [CrossRef]
100. Napoli, N.; Conte, C.; Eastell, R.; Ewing, S.K.; Bauer, D.C.; Strotmeyer, E.S.; Black, D.M.; Samelson, E.J.; Vittinghoff, E.; Schwartz, A.V. Bone Turnover Markers Do Not Predict Fracture Risk in Type 2 Diabetes. *J. Bone Miner. Res.* **2020**, *35*, 2363–2371. [CrossRef]
101. Karim, L.; Moulton, J.; Van Vliet, M.; Velie, K.; Robbins, A.; Malekipour, F.; Abdeen, A.; Ayres, D.; Bouxsein, M.L. Bone microarchitecture, biomechanical properties, and advanced glycation end-products in the proximal femur of adults with type 2 diabetes. *Bone* **2018**, *114*, 32–39. [CrossRef] [PubMed]
102. Wölfel, E.M.; Jähn-Rickert, K.; Schmidt, F.N.; Wulff, B.; Mushumba, H.; Sroga, G.E.; Püschel, K.; Milovanovic, P.; Amling, M.; Campbell, G.M.; et al. Individuals with type 2 diabetes mellitus show dimorphic and heterogeneous patterns of loss in femoral bone quality. *Bone* **2020**, *140*, 115556. [CrossRef] [PubMed]
103. Sell, D.R.; Monnier, V.M. Structure elucidation of a senescence cross-link from human extracellular matrix. Implication of pentoses in the aging process. *J. Biol. Chem.* **1989**, *264*, 21597–21602. [CrossRef]
104. Sugiyama, S.; Miyata, T.; Ueda, Y.; Tanaka, H.; Maeda, K.; Kawashima, S.; Strihou, C.V.Y.D.; Kurokawa, K. Plasma levels of pentosidine in diabetic patients: An advanced glycation end product. *J. Am. Soc. Nephrol.* **1998**, *9*, 1681–1688. [CrossRef] [PubMed]
105. Yoshida, N.; Okumura, K.-I.; Aso, Y. High serum pentosidine concentrations are associated with increased arterial stiffness and thickness in patients with type 2 diabetes. *Metabolism* **2005**, *54*, 345–350. [CrossRef] [PubMed]
106. Kerkeni, M.; Saïdi, A.; Bouzidi, H.; Letaief, A.; Ben Yahia, S.; Hammami, M. Pentosidine as a biomarker for microvascular complications in type 2 diabetic patients. *Diabetes Vasc. Dis. Res.* **2013**, *10*, 239–245. [CrossRef] [PubMed]
107. Yamamoto, M.; Sugimoto, T. Advanced Glycation End Products, Diabetes, and Bone Strength. *Curr. Osteoporos. Rep.* **2016**, *14*, 320–326. [CrossRef]
108. Viguet-Carrin, S.; Roux, J.P.; Arlot, M.E.; Merabet, Z.; Leeming, D.; Byrjalsen, I.; Delmas, P.D.; Bouxsein, M.L. Contribution of the advanced glycation end product pentosidine and of maturation of type I collagen to compressive biomechanical properties of human lumbar vertebrae. *Bone* **2006**, *39*, 1073–1079. [CrossRef]

109. Valcourt, U.; Merle, B.; Gineyts, E.; Viguet-Carrin, S.; Delmas, P.D.; Garnero, P. Non-enzymatic Glycation of Bone Collagen Modifies Osteoclastic Activity and Differentiation. *J. Biol. Chem.* **2007**, *282*, 5691–5703. [CrossRef]
110. Yamamoto, M.; Yamaguchi, T.; Yamauchi, M.; Yano, S.; Sugimoto, T. Serum Pentosidine Levels Are Positively Associated with the Presence of Vertebral Fractures in Postmenopausal Women with Type 2 Diabetes. *J. Clin. Endocrinol. Metab.* **2008**, *93*, 1013–1019. [CrossRef]
111. Choi, Y.J.; Ock, S.Y.; Jin, Y.; Lee, J.S.; Kim, S.H.; Chung, Y.-S. Urinary Pentosidine levels negatively associates with trabecular bone scores in patients with type 2 diabetes mellitus. *Osteoporos. Int.* **2018**, *29*, 907–915. [CrossRef] [PubMed]
112. Schwartz, A.V.; Garnero, P.; Hillier, T.A.; Sellmeyer, D.E.; Strotmeyer, E.S.; Feingold, K.R.; Resnick, H.E.; Tylavsky, F.A.; Black, D.M.; Cummings, S.R.; et al. Pentosidine and Increased Fracture Risk in Older Adults with Type 2 Diabetes. *J. Clin. Endocrinol. Metab.* **2009**, *94*, 2380–2386. [CrossRef] [PubMed]
113. Barzilay, J.I.; Bůžková, P.; Zieman, S.J.; Kizer, J.R.; Djoussé, L.; Ix, J.H.; Tracy, R.P.; Siscovick, D.S.; Cauley, J.A.; Mukamal, K.J. Circulating Levels of Carboxy-Methyl-Lysine (CML) Are Associated with Hip Fracture Risk: The Cardiovascular Health Study. *J. Bone Miner. Res.* **2014**, *29*, 1061–1066. [CrossRef] [PubMed]
114. Dhaliwal, R.; Ewing, S.K.; Vashishth, D.; Semba, R.D.; Schwartz, A.V. Greater Carboxy-Methyl-Lysine Is Associated with Increased Fracture Risk in Type 2 Diabetes. *J. Bone Miner. Res.* **2022**, *37*, 265–272. [CrossRef] [PubMed]
115. Delgado-Calle, J.; Sato, A.Y.; Bellido, T. Role and mechanism of action of sclerostin in bone. *Bone* **2017**, *96*, 29–37. [CrossRef]
116. Ardawi, M.-S.M.; Rouzi, A.A.; Al-Sibiani, S.A.; Al-Senani, N.S.; Qari, M.H.; Mousa, S.A. High serum sclerostin predicts the occurrence of osteoporotic fractures in postmenopausal women: The center of excellence for osteoporosis research study. *J. Bone Miner. Res.* **2012**, *27*, 2592–2602. [CrossRef]
117. Arasu, A.; Cawthon, P.M.; Lui, L.-Y.; Do, T.P.; Arora, P.S.; Cauley, J.A.; Ensrud, K.E.; Cummings, S.R. The Study of Osteoporotic Fractures Research Group Serum Sclerostin and Risk of Hip Fracture in Older Caucasian Women. *J. Clin. Endocrinol. Metab.* **2012**, *97*, 2027–2032. [CrossRef]
118. García-Martín, A.; Rozas-Moreno, P.; Reyes-Garcia, R.; Morales-Santana, S.; García-Fontana, B.; Garcia-Salcedo, J.A.; Muñoz-Torres, M. Circulating Levels of Sclerostin Are Increased in Patients with Type 2 Diabetes Mellitus. *J. Clin. Endocrinol. Metab.* **2012**, *97*, 234–241. [CrossRef]
119. Heilmeier, U.; Carpenter, D.R.; Patsch, J.M.; Harnish, R.; Joseph, G.B.; Burghardt, A.J.; Baum, T.; Schwartz, A.V.; Lang, T.F.; Link, T.M. Volumetric femoral BMD, bone geometry, and serum sclerostin levels differ between type 2 diabetic postmenopausal women with and without fragility fractures. *Osteoporos. Int.* **2015**, *26*, 1283–1293. [CrossRef]
120. Ardawi, M.-S.M.; Akhbar, D.H.; AlShaikh, A.; Ahmed, M.M.; Qari, M.H.; Rouzi, A.A.; Ali, A.Y.; Abdulrafee, A.A.; Saeda, M.Y. Increased serum sclerostin and decreased serum IGF-1 are associated with vertebral fractures among postmenopausal women with type-2 diabetes. *Bone* **2013**, *56*, 355–362. [CrossRef]
121. Yamamoto, M.; Yamauchi, M.; Sugimoto, T. Elevated Sclerostin Levels Are Associated with Vertebral Fractures in Patients with Type 2 Diabetes Mellitus. *J. Clin. Endocrinol. Metab.* **2013**, *98*, 4030–4037. [CrossRef] [PubMed]
122. Hensley, A.P.; McAlinden, A. The role of microRNAs in bone development. *Bone* **2021**, *143*, 115760. [CrossRef] [PubMed]
123. Heilmeier, U.; Hackl, M.; Schroeder, F.; Torabi, S.; Kapoor, P.; Vierlinger, K.; Eiriksdottir, G.; Gudmundsson, E.F.; Harris, T.B.; Gudnason, V.; et al. Circulating serum microRNAs including senescent miR-31-5p are associated with incident fragility fractures in older postmenopausal women with type 2 diabetes mellitus. *Bone* **2022**, *158*, 116308. [CrossRef] [PubMed]
124. Heilmeier, U.; Hackl, M.; Skalicky, S.; Weilner, S.; Schroeder, F.; Vierlinger, K.; Patsch, J.M.; Baum, T.; Oberbauer, E.; Lobach, I.; et al. Serum miRNA Signatures Are Indicative of Skeletal Fractures in Postmenopausal Women with and without Type 2 Diabetes and Influence Osteogenic and Adipogenic Differentiation of Adipose Tissue-Derived Mesenchymal Stem Cells In Vitro. *J. Bone Miner. Res.* **2016**, *31*, 2173–2192. [CrossRef]
125. Chen, Y.-S.; Kang, X.-R.; Zhou, Z.-H.; Yang, J.; Xin, Q.; Ying, C.-T.; Zhang, Y.-P.; Tao, J. MiR-1908/EXO1 and MiR-203a/FOS, regulated by scd1, are associated with fracture risk and bone health in postmenopausal diabetic women. *Aging* **2020**, *12*, 9549–9584. [CrossRef]
126. Mulder, D.J.; Van De Water, T.; Lutgers, H.L.; Graaff, R.; Gans, R.O.; Zijlstra, F.; Smit, A.J. Skin Autofluorescence, a Novel Marker for Glycemic and Oxidative Stress-Derived Advanced Glycation Endproducts: An Overview of Current Clinical Studies, Evidence, and Limitations. *Diabetes Technol. Ther.* **2006**, *8*, 523–535. [CrossRef]
127. Samakkarnthai, P.; Sfeir, J.G.; Atkinson, E.J.; Achenbach, S.J.; Wennberg, P.W.; Dyck, P.J.; Tweed, A.J.; Volkman, T.L.; Amin, S.; Farr, J.N.; et al. Determinants of Bone Material Strength and Cortical Porosity in Patients with Type 2 Diabetes Mellitus. *J. Clin. Endocrinol. Metab.* **2020**, *105*, e3718–e3729. [CrossRef]
128. Waqas, K.; Chen, J.; Koromani, F.; Trajanoska, K.; Van Der Eerden, B.C.J.; Uitterlinden, A.G.; Rivadeneira, F.; Zillikens, M.C. Skin Autofluorescence, a Noninvasive Biomarker for Advanced Glycation End-Products, Is Associated with Prevalent Vertebral and Major Osteoporotic Fractures: The Rotterdam Study. *J. Bone Miner. Res.* **2020**, *35*, 1904–1913. [CrossRef]
129. Sihota, P.; Pal, R.; Yadav, R.N.; Neradi, D.; Karn, S.; Goni, V.G.; Sharma, S.; Mehandia, V.; Bhadada, S.K.; Kumar, N.; et al. Can fingernail quality predict bone damage in Type 2 diabetes mellitus? A pilot study. *PLoS ONE* **2021**, *16*, e0257955. [CrossRef]
130. Sihota, P.; Yadav, R.N.; Dhiman, V.; Bhadada, S.K.; Mehandia, V.; Kumar, N. Investigation of diabetic patient's fingernail quality to monitor type 2 diabetes induced tissue damage. *Sci. Rep.* **2019**, *9*, 3193. [CrossRef]

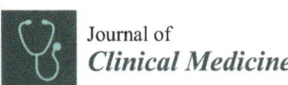

Review

Non-Alcoholic Fatty Liver Disease and Risk of Macro- and Microvascular Complications in Patients with Type 2 Diabetes

Alessandro Mantovani [1,*], Andrea Dalbeni [2], Giorgia Beatrice [1], Davide Cappelli [1] and Fernando Gomez-Peralta [3,*]

[1] Section of Endocrinology, Diabetes and Metabolism, Department of Medicine, University and Azienda Ospedaliera Universitaria Integrata of Verona, 37126 Verona, Italy; giorgiabeatricejb@gmail.com (G.B.); davide.cappelli3@gmail.com (D.C.)
[2] Section of General Medicine C and Liver Unit, University and Azienda Ospedaliera Universitaria Integrata of Verona, 37126 Verona, Italy; andrea.dalbeni@aovr.veneto.it
[3] Endocrinology and Nutrition Unit, Segovia General Hospital, 40002 Segovia, Spain
* Correspondence: alessandro.mantovani@univr.it (A.M.); fgomezperalta@gmail.com (F.G.-P.)

Abstract: Non-alcoholic fatty liver disease (NAFLD) is considered the hepatic manifestation of metabolic syndrome. To date, NAFLD is the most frequent chronic liver disease seen day by day in clinical practice across most high-income countries, affecting nearly 25–30% of adults in the general population and up to 70% of patients with T2DM. Over the last few decades, it clearly emerged that NAFLD is a "multisystemic disease" and that the leading cause of death among patients with NAFLD is cardiovascular disease (CVD). Indeed, several observational studies and some meta-analyses have documented that NAFLD, especially its advanced forms, is strongly associated with fatal and non-fatal cardiovascular events, as well as with specific cardiac complications, including sub-clinical myocardial alteration and dysfunction, heart valve diseases and cardiac arrhythmias. Importantly, across various studies, these associations remained significant after adjustment for established cardiovascular risk factors and other confounders. Additionally, several observational studies and some meta-analyses have also reported that NAFLD is independently associated with specific microvascular conditions, such as chronic kidney disease and distal or autonomic neuropathy. Conversely, data regarding a potential association between NAFLD and retinopathy are scarce and often conflicting. This narrative review will describe the current evidence about the association between NAFLD and the risk of macro- and microvascular manifestations of CVD, especially in patients with T2DM. We will also briefly discuss the biological mechanisms underpinning the association between NAFLD and its advanced forms and macro- and microvascular CVD.

Keywords: non-alcoholic fatty liver disease; NAFLD; non-alcoholic steatohepatitis; NASH; type 2 diabetes; cardiovascular disease; cardiovascular complications; CVD

1. Introduction

Non-alcoholic fatty liver disease (NAFLD) is a metabolic liver disease, which classically includes a spectrum of progressive pathological conditions, ranging from simple steatosis to non-alcoholic steatohepatitis (NASH) with different grades of fibrosis and cirrhosis (Figure 1) [1,2]. At present, NAFLD is the most common chronic liver disease seen day by day in clinical practice, as it affects roughly 25–30% of adults in the general population across various high-income countries [3], up to 70% of patients with type 2 diabetes (T2DM) [4] and all patients with obesity [5]. On the other side, most NAFLD patients have relevant metabolic comorbidities, including atherogenic dyslipidemia (~70%), obesity (~50%), hypertension (~40%) and T2DM (~30%) [6]. In this regard, alongside the increasing prevalence of metabolic syndrome worldwide, the overall prevalence of NAFLD is believed to rise further in the coming years.

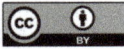

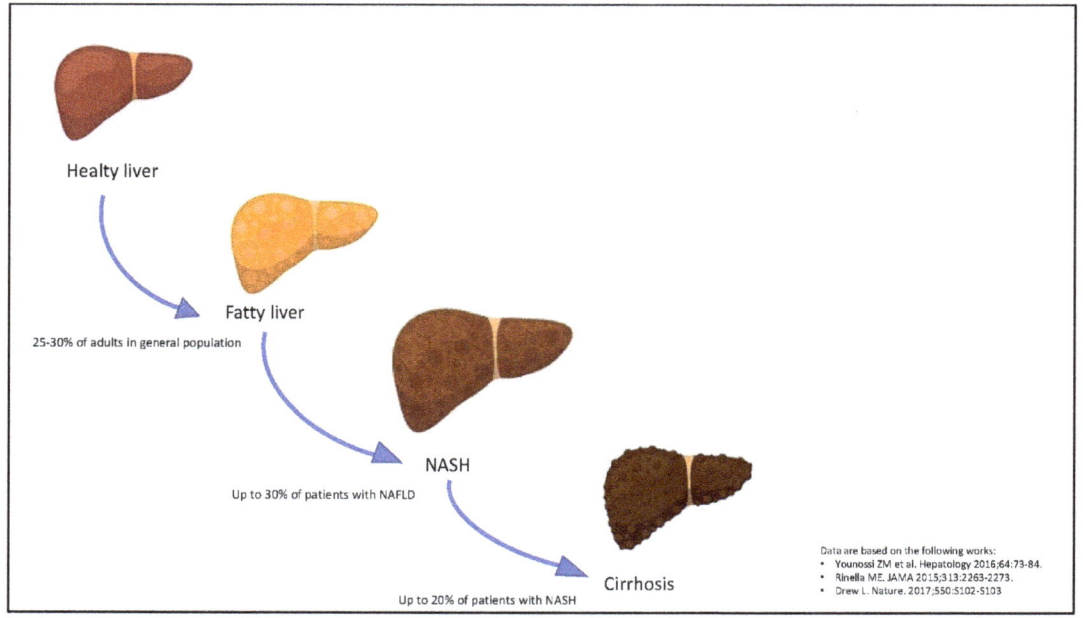

Figure 1. Progression of non-alcoholic fatty liver disease (NAFLD). The stages of NAFLD development classically are simple steatosis, non-alcoholic steatohepatitis (NASH) and cirrhosis.

The diagnosis of NAFLD is a diagnosis of exclusion [7]. It is essentially based on the following criteria: (a) presence of hepatic steatosis, as detected by specific serum biomarker scores (e.g., fatty liver index [FLI]), imaging techniques or liver histology, (b) no alcohol consumption (<20 g/day for women and <30 g/day for men), and (c) no other secondary causes of liver steatosis (e.g., virus, hepatotoxic drugs, hemochromatosis, autoimmune hepatitis) [7]. In the last two years, several experts in the field and many scientific societies have proposed a revision of the terminology, switching from NAFLD to metabolic-associated fatty liver disease (MAFLD) [8,9]. In this regard, the diagnosis of MAFLD can be undertaken from the presence of hepatic steatosis and at least one of the following criteria: (a) overweight/obesity, (b) T2DM, and (c) metabolic dysregulation (i.e., two or more factors among increased waist circumference, hypertriglyceridemia, low serum HDL-cholesterol levels, hypertension, impaired fasting glucose, insulin resistance and chronic inflammation) [8,9]. Several studies and some meta-analyses have recently indicated that the MAFLD criteria can identify more individuals with liver damage than NAFLD criteria [10]. However, given that there is still an intense debate about which term should be used [11,12], we have preferred to use still NAFLD term in this manuscript.

Importantly, in the last decades, it has also become clear that NAFLD is a "multi-systemic" disease [13]. Indeed, several observational studies and some meta-analyses have clearly documented that NAFLD is independently associated with serious hepatic complications (e.g., hepatic decompensation, hepatocellular carcinoma [HCC]) [5], but also with an increased risk of developing cardiovascular disease (CVD) [14], T2DM [15], chronic kidney disease (CKD) [16] and some extra-hepatic cancers [17]. Notably, among the various hepatic and extra-hepatic complications related to NAFLD, CVD is the leading cause of death among NAFLD patients.

This narrative review will discuss the current evidence regarding the association between NAFLD and the risk of macro- and microvascular CVD (Figure 2). In particular, it will describe the association between NAFLD and the risk of sub-clinical myocardial remodelling and dysfunction, heart valve diseases, cardiac arrhythmias, chronic kidney disease, distal or autonomic neuropathy, retinopathy and fatal and non-fatal cardiovascular events. A brief insight into the biological mechanisms underpinning the association between NAFLD and macro- and microvascular complications has been also given.

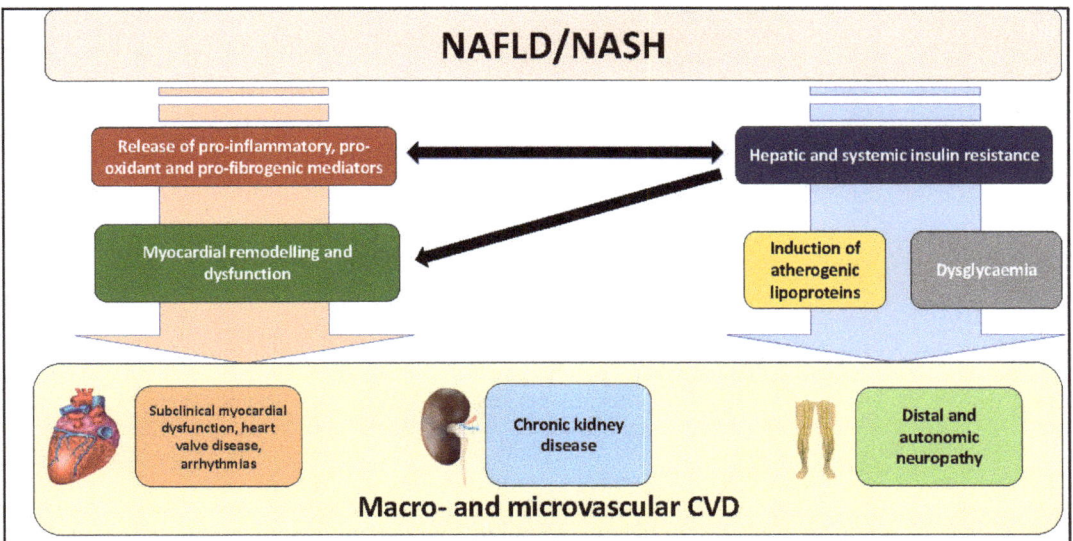

Figure 2. Macro- and microvascular manifestations of cardiovascular disease (CVD) linked to NAFLD and its advanced forms. Several observational studies and meta-analyses have clearly reported that NAFLD, mainly in its advanced forms, is strongly associated with an increased risk of sub-clinical myocardial remodelling and dysfunction, heart valve diseases, cardiac arrhythmias, chronic kidney disease, and distal or autonomic neuropathy. See text for details.

2. Biological Link between Non-Alcoholic Fatty Liver Disease (NAFLD) and Cardiovascular Disease (CVD)

The underlying biological mechanisms responsible for the association between NAFLD and the risk of specific cardiac complications are not completely established to date. It is beyond the scope of this narrative review to illustrate in detail the current evidence suggesting a specific role of NAFLD in the development and progression of various cardiac complications. That said, in brief, accumulating evidence now indicates that NAFLD, especially its severe forms, may play a part in the pathophysiology of cardiac complications through different mechanisms, such as:

(a) hepatic lipid accumulation (e.g., di-acyl glycerol [DAG]) in NAFLD patients impairs insulin signalling, thereby conditioning insulin resistance (IR) through different mechanisms, including the inhibition of phosphorylation of insulin receptor substrate-1 (IRS-1) [18] and the activation of protein kinase C (PKC)-e that can inhibit the action of insulin receptor and promote the lipid accumulation [19]. In particular, hepatic and systemic insulin resistance is one of the primary mechanisms for inducing atherogenic lipoproteins and dysglycaemia. Notably, both atherogenic dyslipidemia and dysglycaemia mediate CVD risk in NAFLD patients with T2DM;

(b) the release into the bloodstream of several pro-inflammatory (e.g., tumour necrosis factor-a [TNF-a], interleukin-6 [IL-6]), pro-oxidant and pro-coagulant factors (e.g., fibrinogen, factor VIII, plasminogen activator inhibitor-1) as well as pro-fibrogenic mediators. In particular, the synthesis of lipids, including DAG, may also contribute to the hepatic production of inflammatory cytokines and pro-coagulant factors [13,20–22];

(c) the bidirectional relationship between NAFLD and hypertension [23]. Several observational studies and some meta-analyses have reported that patients with NAFLD have an increased risk of developing hypertension [24], thus suggesting that this association may partly mediate the relationship between NAFLD and cardiac complications and that that NAFLD may be a consequence, but also a cause of hypertension [23];

(d) patients with NAFLD have early changes in myocardial substrate metabolism inducing cardiac functional disturbances, probably conditioning a higher risk of heart failure [25] and arrhythmias [22,26];

(e) chronic hyperglycemia induces an inflammatory and osteoblastic phenotype in valvular interstitial cells in experimental models of aortic valve sclerosis [27]. Increased valvular inflammation, through a systemic inflammatory state, could also mediate the increased cardiac valve sclerosis in NAFLD patients, independent of the presence of T2DM;

(f) experimental data also indicate that NAFLD, mainly when advanced stages occur, may contribute to the activation of multiple pathways involved in the pathophysiology of CKD [10,28]. In this regard, atherogenic dyslipidaemia, hypertension, insulin resistance, oxidative stress and pro-inflammatory factors that, as mentioned above, are promoted and exacerbated by NAFLD status, may directly contribute to the vascular and renal damage [28]. Moreover, impaired activation of the renin-angiotensin system (RAS) may also contribute to the renovascular injury by inflammation pathways [28]. Finally, accumulating evidence also suggests a potential and independent association between *PNPLA3* (patatin like phospholipase domain containing-3) rs738409, which is the most important polymorphism associated with NAFLD and its advanced forms [29], and kidney dysfunction [28].

All these factors can promote myocardial remodelling and dysfunction, thereby predisposing to the development of various cardiac complications [13,20–22].

3. Risk of Microvascular Complications

3.1. Chronic Kidney Disease (CKD)

Several observational studies and some meta-analyses have reported that NAFLD, as detected by indirect biomarkers of steatosis, ultrasonography or liver biopsy, is associated with an increased risk of prevalent and incident chronic kidney disease (CKD) in patients with and without T2DM, independent of established cardio-metabolic risk factors, diabetes-related variables and other potential confounders [28,30]. In a recent 2022 meta-analysis of 13 longitudinal studies for a total of 1,222,032 patients (~28% with NAFLD as detected by biomarkers, International Classification of Diseases [ICD] codes, imaging techniques or biopsy) and 33,840 new cases of incident CKD stage (defined as CKD stage ≥3 and/or overt proteinuria) over a median follow-up of nearly 10 years, our research group reported that NAFLD was associated with a 43% increased risk of incident CKD (random-effects hazard ratio 1.43, 95% confidence interval 1.33 to 1.54; I^2 = 60.7%), independent of age, sex, obesity, hypertension, T2DM and other CKD risk factors [16]. In a 2018 meta-analysis, the same research group documented that such association was slightly higher when the analysis was restricted to cohort studies involving exclusively patients with diabetes mellitus (random-effects hazard ratio 1.56, 95% confidence interval 1.07–2.05; I^2 = 0%) [31]. Interestingly, accumulating observational studies using vibration controlled transient elastography (VCTE), as non-invasive method to evaluate the degree of liver fibrosis, also reported an independent association between liver stiffness and renal dysfunction. In this regard, for instance, in a 2022 systematic review and meta-analysis of seven cross-sectional studies for a total of 7736 individuals with NAFLD, Ciarduillo et al. showed that liver fibrosis (as assessed by VCTE) was associated with an increased risk of prevalent CKD (defined as eGFR < 60 mL/min/1.73 m^2 and urinary albumin to creatinine ratio ≥30 mg/g) (random-effects odds ratio 2.49, 95% confidence interval 1.89–3.29; I^2 = 46.5%), as well as with an increased risk of prevalent albuminuria (random-effects odds ratio 1.98, 95% confidence interval 1.29–3.05; I^2 = 46.5%) [32]. However, it should be noted that, at present, only few observational studies on this topic have used liver biopsy for the diagnosis of NAFLD, which is the reference standard for diagnosing and staging NAFLD [1,2]. Conversely, most available studies on this topic have used liver ultrasonography, which is to date the recommended first-line imaging method for detecting NAFLD in clinical practice [1,2], able to accurately detect mild-to-moderate hepatic steatosis, as assessed by liver biopsy [7].

Notably, the presence of NAFLD may be even associated with CKD progression [33]. In a cohort study of nearly 1500 CKD patients who underwent periodic health check-ups, Jang et al. showed that age- and sex-adjusted decline in eGFR values was higher in patients with NAFLD (as detected by ultrasonography) when compared with those without NAFLD [34]. In that study, interestingly, the decline in estimated eGFR related to NAFLD was even higher in patients with higher NAFLD fibrosis score (which is an indirect marker of advanced liver fibrosis), in those with proteinuria and/or low eGFR values at baseline and in those who were active smokers or had hypertension at baseline [34]. Although additional studies are needed, preliminary evidence also indicates that the improvement in liver histology in NAFLD patients is associated with improved kidney function [33,35].

Observational studies involving patients with and without T2DM have reported that the presence of the G allele of rs738409 in the *PNPLA3* gene is associated with lower eGFR values and/or higher prevalence of CKD, even after adjustment for the presence of NAFLD and other cardio-renal risk factors [28,30,33,36–39]. In a cross-sectional study including 157 Italian patients with T2DM, who underwent liver ultrasonography and kidney function assessment, our research group reported that the presence of the G allele of rs738409 in the *PNPLA3* gene was associated with an increased risk of CKD (defined as <60 mL/min/1.73 m^2 and/or abnormal albuminuria), independent of liver disease severity, cardiorenal risk factors and other potential confounders [37]. Interestingly and notably, in that study, the authors also found that PNPLA3 mRNA expression was greatest in the liver and renal cortex, thereby suggesting that the *PNPLA3* rs738409 variant might contribute, at least in part, to the impaired kidney function in these patients [37]. These findings have also been confirmed in some cohorts of children and adolescents [40–42].

Taken together, these data strongly indicate that patients with NAFLD, especially those with severe forms, have an increased risk of developing CKD, independent of several cardio-renal risk factors and other confounders [28,33]. Interestingly, novel data also suggest that MAFLD criteria might identify patients with CKD better than NAFLD criteria [43]. However, seeing the observational nature of all studies available so far, it is essential to underline that a causal relationship between NAFLD and incident CKD cannot be proven yet [28,33].

3.2. Distal Symmetric Polyneuropathy and Autonomic Neuropathy

Some observational studies [44–46], although not all [47,48], have documented an association between NAFLD and the risk of prevalent distal symmetric polyneuropathy in T2DM patients, independent of multiple cardio-metabolic risk factors and diabetes-related variables. In a cross-sectional study involving roughly 400 outpatients with T2DM attending five Italian diabetes centers, who underwent liver ultrasonography, vibration controlled transient elastography (by FibroScan®) and evaluation of microvascular diabetic complications, Lombardi et al. documented that significant liver fibrosis (i.e., liver stiffness measurement [LSM] ≥ 7.0 and 6.2 kPa with M and XL probes, respectively) was independently associated with higher prevalence of microvascular diabetic complications (28% in patients with LSM < 7.0/6.2 kPa vs. 50% in patients with LSM ≥ 7.0/6.2 kPa, $p < 0.001$), including distal symmetric polyneuropathy (3% in patients with LSM < 7.0/6.2 kPa vs. 14% in patients with LSM ≥ 7.0/6.2 kPa, $p < 0.05$) [46]. Accumulating evidence also suggests the existence of an association between hepatic steatosis (as detected by imaging techniques) and cardiac autonomic dysfunction in patients with and without T2DM [49,50]. For instance, in a recent cross-sectional study including 173 individuals with T2DM and 183 age- and sex-matched nondiabetic controls from the Cooperative Health Research in South Tyrol (CHRIS) study, Targher et al. reported that individuals with T2DM and NAFLD (on ultrasonography) and individuals with NAFLD alone, but not those with T2DM alone, had an increased risk of cardiac sympathetic/parasympathetic imbalance (as assessed by low- to high-frequency power ratio and other heart rate variability measures obtained by a 20 min resting electrocardiogram), when compared with those without NAFLD and T2DM [50].

However, although this evidence is interesting, additional research is needed to corroborate these findings in larger populations and, more willingly, in longitudinal studies.

3.3. Diabetic Retinopathy

Some cross-sectional studies have investigated the relationship between NAFLD (as detected by imaging techniques) and the risk of prevalent diabetic retinopathy in patients with T2DM, reporting inconsistent results [44,51]. In this regard, a 2021 meta-analysis of nine cross-sectional studies for a total of 7170 patients with T2DM (57% with NAFLD on ultrasonography) reported no association between NAFLD and risk of prevalent diabetic retinopathy (random-effects odds ratio 0.94, 95% confidence interval 0.51–1.71; $I^2 = 96\%$) [52]. In addition, in that meta-analysis, subgroup analyses suggested that in China, Korea and Iran, T2DM patients with NAFLD had a decreased risk of diabetic retinopathy when compared with those without NAFLD, whereas in Italy and India, T2DM patients with NAFLD had an increased risk [52]. As suggested by the authors of that meta-analysis, the aforementioned results should be interpreted with caution, because of the high heterogeneity observed and the differences in the results seen across various countries. Hence, additional research is needed to better explore this issue [52].

4. Risk of Macrovascular Complications

4.1. Sub-Clinical Myocardial Remodelling and Dysfunction, Heart Valve Diseases and Cardiac Arrhythmias

A large body of evidence now supports the existence of a strong and independent association between NAFLD and sub-clinical myocardial remodelling and dysfunction, heart valve diseases (i.e., aortic-valve sclerosis and mitral annulus calcification) and cardiac arrhythmias (mainly atrial fibrillation) in patients with and without T2DM (Table 1) [13,22,23,53–56]. For instance, in a cross-sectional study involving 222 outpatients with T2DM (~70% with NAFLD on ultrasonography), our research group showed that NAFLD was associated with increased risk of left ventricular diastolic dysfunction (as evaluated by trans-thoracic echocardiography), independent of established CVD risk factors, diabetes-related covariates and other confounders [57]. Some recent observational studies using biopsy or vibration-controlled transient elastography (by FibroScan®) also observed a graded relationship between functional and structural myocardial abnormalities and NAFLD severity in patients with and without T2DM [22]. A 2019 meta-analysis of 16 observational studies further confirmed that NAFLD (as detected by imaging techniques or liver biopsy) was independently associated with many functional and structural myocardial abnormalities, including higher left ventricle mass, higher left ventricular end diastolic diameter, higher left atrium diameter and the ratio between left atrial volume and body surface area, higher posterior wall and septum thickness, lower E/A wave ratio, higher E/E' ratio, longer deceleration time and longer relaxation time [58]. Interestingly, recent observational studies also indicated that NAFLD (as detected by ultrasonography) was associated with a reduction in global longitudinal strain, which is a relatively novel echocardiographic parameter strongly associated with adverse cardiovascular outcomes [59–61].

Table 1. Main meta-analyses of observational studies assessing the relationship between NAFLD and macro- and microvascular complications in patients with and without type 2 diabetes.

Author, Ref.	Main Study Characteristics	Main Results
Fatal and non-fatal cardiovascular events		
Targher G et al. *J. Hepatol.* 2016; 65: 589–600.	16 observational studies were included for a total of 34,043 individuals with and without T2DM	NAFLD was associated with an increased risk of fatal and/or non-fatal CVD (random-effects odds ratio 1.64, 95% confidence interval 1.26–2.13). Patients with more severe forms of NAFLD were also more likely to develop fatal and non-fatal CVD events (random-effects odds ratio 2.58; 95% confidence interval 1.78–3.75)
Morrison AE et al. *Liver Int.* 2019; 39: 557–567.	13 observational studies were included	NAFLD was not associated with an increased risk of CVD (random-effects risks ratio 1.48, 95% confidence interval 0.96–2.29)
Liu Y et al. *Sci Rep.* 2019; 9: 11124	14 observational studies were included for a total of 498,501 individuals with and without T2DM	NAFLD was associated with an increased risk of all-cause mortality (random-effects hazard ratio 1.34; 95% confidence interval 1.17–1.54), but not with an increased risk of CVD (random-effects hazard ratio 1.13; 95% confidence interval 0.92–1.38)
Mantovani A et al. *Lancet Gastroenterol Hepatol.* 2021; 6: 903–913	36 longitudinal studies were included for a total of 5,802,226 middle-aged individuals with and without T2DM	NAFLD was associated with an increased risk of fatal or non-fatal CVD events (random-effects hazard ratio 1.45, 95% confidence interval 1.31–1.61). This risk increased progressively across the severity of NAFLD, especially the stage of fibrosis (random-effects hazard ratio 2.50, 95% confidence interval 1.68–3.72)
Alon L et al. *Eur J Prev Cardiol.* 2021 Dec 22: zwab212. doi: 10.1093/eurjpc/zwab212.	20 observational studies were included	NAFLD was associated with an increased risk of myocardial infarction (random-effects odds ratio 1.66, 95% confidence interval 1.39–1.99), ischemic stroke (random-effects odds ratio 1.41, 95% confidence interval 1.29–1.55), atrial fibrillation (random-effects odds ratio 1.27, 95% confidence interval 1.18–1.37), and heart failure (random-effects odds ratio 1.62, 95% confidence interval 1.43–1.84)
Cardiac function and structure		
Borges-Canha M et al. *Endocrine* 2019; 66: 467–476.	16 observational studies were included	NAFLD was associated with increased risk of (a) higher left ventricle mass and ratios between left ventricle mass and both height and body surface area; (b) higher left ventricular end diastolic diameter; (c) higher left atrium diameter and ratio between left atrial volume and body surface area; (d) higher posterior wall and septum thickness; (e) lower E/A wave ratio; (f) higher E/E′ ratio; (g) longer deceleration time and (h) longer relaxation time

Table 1. *Cont.*

Author, Ref.	Main Study Characteristics	Main Results
	Cardiac arrhythmias	
Minhas AM et al. *Cureus* 2017; 9: e1142.	3 observational studies were included for a total of 1,044 with NAFLD and 1,016 without NAFLD	Patients with NAFLD had a higher risk of AF (random-effects odds ratio 2.47, 95% confidence interval 1.30–4.66)
Wijarnpreecha K et al. *Clin Res Hepatol Gastroenterol.* 2017; 41: 525–532	5 observational studies (2 cross-sectional ones and 3 cohort ones) were included for a total of 238,129 participants with and without T2DM	Patients with NAFLD had a higher risk of AF (random-effects risks ratio 2.06, 95% confidence interval 1.10–3.85)
Mantovani A. et al. *Liver Int.* 2019; 39: 758–769	9 observational studies (5 cross-sectional ones and 4 cohort ones) were included for a total of 364,919 individuals with and without T2DM	NAFLD was associated with an increased risk of prevalent AF (random-effects odds ratio 2.07, 95% confidence interval 1.38–3.10). Conversely, NAFLD was associated with increased risk of incident AF only in T2DM patients (random-effects hazard ratio 4.96, 95% confidence interval 1.42–17.3).
Gong H et al. *J. Int. Med. Res.* 2021; 49: 300060521104707	19 observational studies were included for a total of 7,012,960 individuals with and without T2DM	NAFLD was associated with higher risks of AF (random-effects odds ratio 1.71, 95% confidence interval 1.14–2.57), prolonged QT interval (random-effects odds ratio 2.86, 95% confidence interval 1.64–4.99), premature atrial/ventricular contraction (random-effects odds ratio 2.53, 95% confidence interval 1.70–3.78) and heart block (random-effects odds ratio 2.65, 95% confidence interval 1.88–3.72)
	Chronic kidney disease (CKD)	
Mantovani A et al. *Metabolism* 2018; 79: 64–76	9 observational studies were included for a total of 96,595 individuals with and without T2DM	NAFLD was associated with a higher risk of incident CKD (random-effects hazard ratio 1.37, 95% confidence interval 1.20–1.53). Patients with severe forms of NAFLD were more likely to develop incident CKD (random-effects hazard ratio 1.50, 95% confidence interval 1.25–1.74)
Mantovani A et al. *Gut* 2022; 71: 156–162	13 observational studies were included for a total of 1,222,032 individuals with and without T2DM	NAFLD was associated with an increased risk of incident CKD (random-effects hazard ratio 1.43, 95% confidence interval 1.33–1.54)

Abbreviations: AF, atrial fibrillation; CKD chronic kidney disease; CVD, cardiovascular disease; NAFLD, non-alcoholic fatty liver disease; T2DM, type 2 diabetes.

Relating to heart valve calcifications, some cross-sectional studies have shown an independent association between NAFLD and risk of aortic valve sclerosis (AVS) and mitral annulus calcification (MAC) in patients with and without T2DM [22,62]. For instance, in a study involving nearly 250 consecutive outpatients with T2DM (~70% with NAFLD on ultrasonography), our research group documented that NAFLD was strongly associated with cardiac calcifications in both the aortic and mitral valves, even after adjustment for established CVD risk factors, diabetes-related covariates and other confounders [62]. These findings may be clinically relevant, as functional and structural myocardial abnormalities and AVS/MAC are strongly associated with all-cause and cardiovascular mortality in patients with and without T2DM [63].

Relating to cardiac arrhythmias, several observational studies and some meta-analyses [64–67] have documented that NAFLD (as detected by imaging techniques) is associated with prevalent and incident permanent atrial fibrillation (AF) in patients with and without T2DM (Table 1) [22]. Notably, AF is, at present, the most frequent cardiac arrhythmia observed day by day in clinical practice and, importantly, it is strongly linked to adverse cardiovascular outcomes [22]. In a recent meta-analysis of five observational studies for a total of roughly 240,000 adult individuals with and without T2DM, our research group documented that NAFLD (as detected by imaging techniques) was associated with higher prevalence and incidence of AF [66]. Interestingly, in a recent retrospective longitudinal study including 267 patients (33% with NAFLD as detected by ultrasonography and 17% with T2DM at baseline) undergoing AF ablation, Donnellan et al. reported that NAFLD was associated with increased arrhythmia recurrence rates following AF ablation, during a mean follow-up of nearly 2.5 years [68]. Other observational studies and meta-analyses, also enrolling T2DM patients, have reported that NAFLD (as detected by ultrasonography) was associated with an increased risk of prolonged QTc, ventricular arrhythmias or conduction defects, independent of established cardiovascular risk factors, diabetes-related covariates and other confounders [22,67,69–72]. Interestingly, in a 2021 meta-analysis of 19 observational studies, Gong et al. confirmed that NAFLD (as detected by indirect markers of steatosis or imaging techniques) was independently associated with higher risks of prolonged QT interval (random-effects odds ratio 2.86, 95% confidence interval 1.64–4.99), premature atrial/ventricular contraction (random-effects odds ratio 2.53, 95% confidence interval 1.70–3.78) and heart block (random-effects odds ratio 2.65, 95% confidence interval 1.88–3.72) [67]. These data are clinically relevant, because NAFLD-related cardiac arrhythmias complications might contribute to explaining, at least in part, the increased risk of fatal and non-fatal CVD events observed in NAFLD patients.

4.2. Fatal and Non-Fatal Cardiovascular Events

Over the last few decades, it has become increasingly evident that the leading cause of death in NAFLD patients is CVD [22,23,73–75]. In this regard, using data from the National Vital Statistics System multiple-cause mortality data (2007–2016), Paik et al. reported that CVD was the main cause of death among US patients with NAFLD, as detected by ICD codes [74]. In a meta-analysis of 45 observational studies for a total of approximately 8 million individuals followed up to 13 years, Younossi et al. also estimated that the pooled CVD-specific mortality rate among NAFLD patients with or without T2DM was nearly 5 per 1000 person-years [3]. Several longitudinal studies and some meta-analyses confirmed that patients with NAFLD (as detected by imaging techniques, ICD codes or liver biopsy) have an increased risk of developing fatal and non-fatal CVD events, even after adjustment for several traditional CVD risk factors, diabetes-related variables, specific medications and other potential confounders (Table 1) [22,23,54–56,76–79]. In a 2021 meta-analysis of 36 longitudinal studies for a total of 5,802,226 adults and 99,668 incident cases of fatal and non-fatal CVD events over a median follow-up of 6.5 years, our research group reported that NAFLD (as detected by imaging techniques, ICD codes or liver biopsy) was associated with a 45% increased risk of fatal or non-fatal CVD events, independent of age, sex, body mass index, waist circumference, presence of T2DM and other cardiovascular risk factors (random-effects hazard ratio 1.45, 95% confidence interval 1.31–1.61; $I^2 = 86.2\%$) [14]. Such risk further increased in patients with severe forms of NAFLD, especially those with advanced fibrosis [14]. Another 2021 meta-analysis confirmed that NAFLD (as detected by imaging techniques, ICD codes or liver biopsy) was independently associated with increased risk of myocardial infarction (random-effects odds ratio 1.66, 95% confidence interval 1.39–1.99), ischemic stroke (random-effects odds ratio 1.41, 95% confidence interval 1.29–1.55) and heart failure (random-effects odds ratio 1.62, 95% confidence interval 1.43–1.84) [26]. In this regard, it is important to underline that the magnitude of cardiovascular risk is strongly related to the severity of NAFLD [25,80–82]. For instance, in a nationwide, matched cohort study of 10,568 Swedish individuals with biopsy-confirmed NAFLD (11% with T2DM at baseline) who were followed for a median period of 14 years, Simon et al. reported that, when compared to 49,925 adults of the general population (3% with established T2DM at baseline), mortality rates from CVD were significantly elevated in patients with simple steatosis (adjusted-hazard ratio 1.25, 95% confidence interval 1.16–1.35), and that these risks progressively increased in patients with NASH without fibrosis (adjusted-hazard ratio 1.66, 95% confidence interval 1.38–2.01), in those with non-cirrhotic fibrosis (adjusted-hazard ratio 1.40, 95% confidence interval 1.17–1.69) and also in those with cirrhosis (adjusted-hazard ratio 2.11, 95% confidence interval 1.63–2.73) [80]. Similar findings were also documented in cohorts involving NAFLD patients with T2DM [22,23,53–56].

To date, data regarding whether the improvement of NAFLD may reduce the incidence of cardiovascular complications are scarce. Although some retrospective studies enrolling Asian adults without pre-existing CVD have reported that the improvement or resolution of NAFLD (on ultrasonography) could be associated with a reduced risk of (carotid) atherosclerotic development in patients with and without T2DM [56,83], we believe that additional information on this issue is needed. In addition, it is important to underline that current evidence also indicates that histologic resolution of NASH could be associated with beneficial changes in risk factors for CVD [56,83], thus suggesting a potential favorable effect on cardiac complications.

Lastly, novel evidence also suggests that MAFLD criteria might identify patients with CVD better than NAFLD criteria [84].

5. CVD Risk Assessment in Patients with NAFLD

Based on the aforementioned evidence, the EASL-EASO-EASD and American Association for the Study of Liver Diseases (AASLD) practice guidelines for diagnosing and managing NAFLD now recommend a CVD risk assessment in all patients with NAFLD [1,2]. In this context, as suggested by several experts in the field [13], a potential comprehensive CVD risk assessment may include (Table 2): (a) evaluation of coexisting risk factors (such as a prior history of CVD, family history of premature CVDs or T2DM, cigarette smoking, presence of T2DM, dyslipidemia, hypertension, obesity, metabolic syndrome, chronic kidney disease and erectile dysfunction), (b) physical examination (such as body weight, height, body mass index, waist circumference, blood pressure, arterial bruits and pulse examination), (c) laboratory tests (such as blood count, lipid profile, fasting plasma glucose, HbA1c, serum creatinine, transaminases, albumin, urinalysis, albuminuria) and (d) cardiovascular examination tests (such as resting electrocardiogram, carotid artery ultrasonography, and exercise stress test if coexisting CVD, CKD, T2DM or >2 CVD risk factors). In addition, the current evidence on this topic also calls attention to a holistic approach in managing and treating NAFLD patients [75,85].

Table 2. Essential comprehensive cardiovascular risk assessment in patients with NAFLD.

Cardiovascular risk factors	<ul><li>History of CVD,</li><li>family history of premature CVDs or T2DM,</li><li>cigarette smoking,</li><li>presence of T2DM, dyslipidemia, hypertension, obesity, CKD, erectile dysfunction (men),</li><li>alcohol use</li></ul>
Physical examination	<ul><li>Weight,</li><li>body mass index,</li><li>waist circumference,</li><li>blood pressure,</li><li>pulse examination</li></ul>
Laboratory tests	<ul><li>Blood count (including hemoglobin and platelets),</li><li>lipid profile,</li><li>fasting glucose,</li><li>HbA1c,</li><li>serum creatinine,</li><li>transaminases,</li><li>albumin,</li><li>albuminuria</li></ul>
Cardiovascular examination tests	<ul><li>Carotid artery ultrasonography,</li><li>resting electrocardiogram,</li><li>exercise stress test if coexisting CVD, CKD, T2DM or more than 2 CVD risk factors</li></ul>

This table is based on the review published by Byrne and Targher [13]. Abbreviations: CKD, chronic kidney disease; CVD, cardiovascular disease; T2DM type 2 diabetes.

6. Conclusions

The aforementioned data support the concept that NAFLD is a "multisystemic" disease [13]. Indeed, NAFLD is not only associated with serious hepatic complications, but it is also linked with macro- and microvascular complications. Importantly and notably, at present, the main cause of death among NAFLD patients is CVD [14]. For this reason, a comprehensive CVD risk assessment is essential in these patients [1,2,13]. That said, information regarding the impact of histological improvement of NAFLD on CVD risk is still scarce and needs further research [56,83]. In spite of our knowledge about epidemiology, pathogenesis and natural history of NAFLD, no specific pharmacological therapies have until now been approved for such a disease [86]. Lifestyle change promoting weight loss and the correction of modifiable cardio-metabolic risk factors are still the cornerstone of the treatment in NAFLD patients [86]. However, over the last few decades, several potential agents have been tested to treat NAFLD and its advanced forms [86,87]. They encompass some glucose-lowering drugs (especially pioglitazone, glucagon-like peptide-1 [GLP-1] receptor agonists and sodium-glucose co-transporter-2 [SGLT-2] inhibitors) [87], bile and non-bile acid farnesoid X activated receptor (FXR) agonists, anti-oxidants (i.e., vitamin E), statins and others [86,88]. In this regard, for instance, in a 2022 systematic review of randomised controlled trials testing the efficacy of peroxisome proliferator-activated receptor (PPAR) agonists, GLP-1 receptor agonists and SGLT-2 inhibitors for treating NAFLD in adults with or without type 2 diabetes, our research group found that pioglitazone (a PPAR-γ agonist), lanifibranor (a pan-PPAR agonist) and GLP1-R agonists (e.g., liraglutide and semaglutide) are able to obtain the resolution of NASH without worsening of fibrosis, whereas SGLT-2 inhibitors (e.g., empagliflozin and dapagliflozin) are able to reduce liver fat content, as detected by magnetic resonance-based techniques [87]. Given the strong relationship between NAFLD and macro- and microvascular complications, it is possible to speculate that these agents may exert a beneficial effect not only on the hepatic disease, but also in reducing the risk of developing cardiovascular and renal diseases [25,86–88]. However, herein it is important to note that pioglitazone is contraindicated in patients with symptomatic heart failure or in patients with a high risk of heart failure [25]. Seeing the multiple pathways implicated in the pathogenesis of NAFLD and its complications, as well as the single response from single-agent therapies across RCTs available so far, it is also reasonable to hypothesize that the combination of different therapies (e.g., GLP-1 receptor agonists *plus* SGLT-2 inhibitors) will be more appropriate for treating NAFLD patients [86,87,89]. In this context, as suggested by several experts in the field, a holistic approach in managing and treating NAFLD patients seems to be fundamental [75,85].

Author Contributions: Conceptualization, A.M. and F.G.-P.; methodology, A.M.; data curation, A.M.; writing—original draft preparation, A.M. and F.G.-P.; writing—review and editing, A.M., A.D., G.B., D.C. and F.G.-P.; supervision, A.M. and F.G.-P. All authors have read and agreed to the published version of the manuscript.

Funding: This research received no external funding.

Conflicts of Interest: The authors declare no conflict of interest.

References

1. European Association for the Study of the Liver; European Association for the Study of Diabetes; European Association for the Study of Obesity. EASL-EASD-EASO Clinical Practice Guidelines for the management of non-alcoholic fatty liver disease. *J. Hepatol.* **2016**, *64*, 1388–1402. [CrossRef] [PubMed]
2. Chalasani, N.; Younossi, Z.; LaVine, J.E.; Charlton, M.; Cusi, K.; Rinella, M.; Harrison, S.A.; Brunt, E.M.; Sanyal, A.J. The diagnosis and management of nonalcoholic fatty liver disease: Practice guidance from the American Association for the Study of Liver Diseases. *Hepatology* **2018**, *67*, 328–357. [CrossRef] [PubMed]
3. Younossi, Z.M.; Koenig, A.B.; Abdelatif, D.; Fazel, Y.; Henry, L.; Wymer, M. Global epidemiology of nonalcoholic fatty liver disease-Meta-analytic assessment of prevalence, incidence, and outcomes. *Hepatology* **2016**, *64*, 73–84. [CrossRef]
4. Younossi, Z.M.; Golabi, P.; de Avila, L.; Paik, J.M.; Srishord, M.; Fukui, N.; Qiu, Y.; Burns, L.; Afendy, A.; Nader, F. The global epidemiology of NAFLD and NASH in patients with type 2 diabetes: A systematic review and meta-analysis. *J. Hepatol.* **2019**, *71*, 793–801. [CrossRef]
5. Lonardo, A.; Mantovani, A.; Lugari, S.; Targher, G. Epidemiology and pathophysiology of the association between NAFLD and metabolically healthy or metabolically unhealthy obesity. *Ann Hepatol.* **2020**, *19*, 359–366. [CrossRef]
6. Sheka, A.C.; Adeyi, O.; Thompson, J.; Hameed, B.; Crawford, P.A.; Ikramuddin, S. Nonalcoholic Steatohepatitis: A Review. *JAMA* **2020**, *323*, 1175–1183. [CrossRef]
7. Byrne, C.D.; Patel, J.; Scorletti, E.; Targher, G. Tests for diagnosing and monitoring non-alcoholic fatty liver disease in adults. *BMJ* **2018**, *362*, k2734. [CrossRef]
8. Eslam, M.; Newsome, P.N.; Sarin, S.K.; Anstee, Q.M.; Targher, G.; Romero-Gomez, M.; Zelber-Sagi, S.; Wong, V.W.-S.; Dufour, J.-F.; Schattenberg, J.M.; et al. A new definition for metabolic dysfunction-associated fatty liver disease: An international expert consensus statement. *J. Hepatol.* **2020**, *73*, 202–209. [CrossRef]
9. Eslam, M.; Sanyal, A.J.; George, J.; International Consensus, P. MAFLD: A Consensus-Driven Proposed Nomenclature for Metabolic Associated Fatty Liver Disease. *Gastroenterology* **2020**, *158*, 1999–2014.e1. [CrossRef]
10. Ayada, I.; van Kleef, L.A.; Alferink, L.J.M.; Li, P.; de Knegt, R.J.; Pan, Q. Systematically comparing epidemiological and clinical features of MAFLD and NAFLD by meta-analysis: Focusing on the non-overlap groups. *Liver Int.* **2021**, *42*, 277–287. [CrossRef]
11. Mantovani, A. MAFLD vs NAFLD: Where are we? *Dig. Liver Dis.* **2021**, *53*, 1368–1372. [CrossRef]
12. Mantovani, A.; Dalbeni, A. NAFLD, MAFLD and DAFLD. *Dig. Liver Dis.* **2020**, *52*, 1519–1520. [CrossRef]
13. Byrne, C.D.; Targher, G. NAFLD: A multisystem disease. *J. Hepatol.* **2015**, *62* (Suppl. S1), S47–S64. [CrossRef]
14. Mantovani, A.; Csermely, A.; Petracca, G.; Beatrice, G.; Corey, K.E.; Simon, T.G.; Byrne, C.D.; Targher, G. Non-alcoholic fatty liver disease and risk of fatal and non-fatal cardiovascular events: An updated systematic review and meta-analysis. *Lancet Gastroenterol. Hepatol.* **2021**, *6*, 903–913. [CrossRef]
15. Mantovani, A.; Petracca, G.; Beatrice, G.; Tilg, H.; Byrne, C.D.; Targher, G. Non-alcoholic fatty liver disease and risk of incident diabetes mellitus: An updated meta-analysis of 501 022 adult individuals. *Gut* **2021**, *70*, 962–969. [CrossRef]
16. Mantovani, A.; Petracca, G.; Beatrice, G.; Csermely, A.; Lonardo, A.; Schattenberg, J.M.; Tilg, H.; Byrne, C.D.; Targher, G. Non-alcoholic fatty liver disease and risk of incident chronic kidney disease: An updated meta-analysis. *Gut* **2020**, *71*, 156–162. [CrossRef]
17. Mantovani, A.; Petracca, G.; Beatrice, G.; Csermely, A.; Tilg, H.; Byrne, C.D.; Targher, G. Non-alcoholic fatty liver disease and increased risk of incident extrahepatic cancers: A meta-analysis of observational cohort studies. *Gut* **2021**. [CrossRef]
18. Tilg, H.; Moschen, A.R. Insulin resistance, inflammation, and non-alcoholic fatty liver disease. *Trends Endocrinol. Metab.* **2008**, *19*, 371–379. [CrossRef]
19. Cantley, J.L.; Yoshimura, T.; Camporez, J.P.G.; Zhang, D.; Jornayvaz, F.; Kumashiro, N.; Guebre-Egziabher, F.; Jurczak, M.; Kahn, M.; Guigni, B.; et al. CGI-58 knockdown sequesters diacylglycerols in lipid droplets/ER-preventing diacylglycerol-mediated hepatic insulin resistance. *Proc. Natl. Acad. Sci. USA* **2013**, *110*, 1869–1874. [CrossRef] [PubMed]

20. Chen, Z.; Liu, J.; Zhou, F.; Li, H.; Zhang, X.-J.; She, Z.-G.; Lu, Z.; Cai, J.; Li, H. Nonalcoholic Fatty Liver Disease: An Emerging Driver of Cardiac Arrhythmia. *Circ. Res.* **2021**, *128*, 1747–1765. [CrossRef] [PubMed]
21. Zhou, J.; Bai, L.; Zhang, X.; Li, H.; Cai, J. Nonalcoholic Fatty Liver Disease and Cardiac Remodeling Risk: Pathophysiological Mechanisms and Clinical Implications. *Hepatology* **2021**, *74*, 2839–2847. [CrossRef]
22. Anstee, Q.M.; Mantovani, A.; Tilg, H.; Targher, G. Risk of cardiomyopathy and cardiac arrhythmias in patients with nonalcoholic fatty liver disease. *Nat. Rev. Gastroenterol. Hepatol.* **2018**, *15*, 425–439. [CrossRef] [PubMed]
23. Lonardo, A.; Nascimbeni, F.; Mantovani, A.; Targher, G. Hypertension, diabetes, atherosclerosis and NASH: Cause or consequence? *J. Hepatol.* **2017**, *68*, 335–352. [CrossRef]
24. Ciardullo, S.; Grassi, G.; Mancia, G.; Perseghin, G. Nonalcoholic fatty liver disease and risk of incident hypertension: A systematic review and meta-analysis. *Eur. J. Gastroenterol. Hepatol.* **2021**. [CrossRef] [PubMed]
25. Mantovani, A.; Byrne, C.D.; Benfari, G.; Bonapace, S.; Simon, T.G.; Targher, G. Risk of Heart Failure in Patients With Nonalcoholic Fatty Liver Disease: JACC Review Topic of the Week. *J. Am. Coll. Cardiol.* **2022**, *79*, 180–191. [CrossRef] [PubMed]
26. Alon, L.; Corica, B.; Raparelli, V.; Cangemi, R.; Basili, S.; Proietti, M.; Romiti, G.F. Risk of cardiovascular events in patients with non-alcoholic fatty liver disease: A systematic review and meta-analysis. *Eur. J. Prev. Cardiol.* **2021**. [CrossRef] [PubMed]
27. Manduteanu, I.; Simionescu, D.; Simionescu, A.; Simionescu, M. Aortic valve disease in diabetes: Molecular mechanisms and novel therapies. *J. Cell. Mol. Med.* **2021**, *25*, 9483–9495. [CrossRef]
28. Wang, T.-Y.; Wang, R.-F.; Bu, Z.-Y.; Targher, G.; Byrne, C.D.; Sun, D.-Q.; Zheng, M.-H. Association of metabolic dysfunction-associated fatty liver disease with kidney disease. *Nat. Rev. Nephrol.* **2022**. [CrossRef] [PubMed]
29. Eslam, M.; Valenti, L.; Romeo, S. Genetics and epigenetics of NAFLD and NASH: Clinical impact. *J. Hepatol.* **2017**, *68*, 268–279. [CrossRef] [PubMed]
30. Byrne, C.D.; Targher, G. NAFLD as a driver of chronic kidney disease. *J. Hepatol.* **2020**, *72*, 785–801. [CrossRef] [PubMed]
31. Mantovani, A.; Zaza, G.; Byrne, C.D.; Lonardo, A.; Zoppini, G.; Bonora, E.; Targher, G. Nonalcoholic fatty liver disease increases risk of incident chronic kidney disease: A systematic review and meta-analysis. *Metabolism* **2017**, *79*, 64–76. [CrossRef]
32. Ciardullo, S.; Ballabeni, C.; Trevisan, R.; Perseghin, G. Liver Stiffness, Albuminuria and Chronic Kidney Disease in Patients with NAFLD: A Systematic Review and Meta-Analysis. *Biomolecules* **2022**, *12*, 105. [CrossRef] [PubMed]
33. Mantovani, A.; Zusi, C.; Dalbeni, A.; Grani, G.; Buzzetti, E. Risk of Kidney Dysfunction IN Nafld. *Curr. Pharm. Des.* **2020**, *26*, 1045–1061. [CrossRef]
34. Jang, H.R.; Kang, D.; Sinn, D.H.; Gu, S.; Cho, S.J.; Lee, J.E.; Huh, W.; Paik, S.W.; Ryu, S.; Chang, Y.; et al. Nonalcoholic fatty liver disease accelerates kidney function decline in patients with chronic kidney disease: A cohort study. *Sci. Rep.* **2018**, *8*, 4718. [CrossRef] [PubMed]
35. Vilar-Gomez, E.; Bertot, L.C.; Friedman, S.L.; Gra-Oramas, B.; Gonzalez-Fabian, L.; Villa-Jimenez, O.; Vallin, S.L.-D.; Diago, M.; Adams, L.A.; Romero-Gómez, M.; et al. Improvement in liver histology due to lifestyle modification is independently associated with improved kidney function in patients with non-alcoholic steatohepatitis. *Aliment. Pharmacol. Ther.* **2016**, *45*, 332–344. [CrossRef] [PubMed]
36. Oniki, K.; Saruwatari, J.; Izuka, T.; Kajiwara, A.; Morita, K.; Sakata, M.; Otake, K.; Ogata, Y.; Nakagawa, K. Influence of the PNPLA3 rs738409 Polymorphism on Non-Alcoholic Fatty Liver Disease and Renal Function among Normal Weight Subjects. *PLoS ONE* **2015**, *10*, e0132640. [CrossRef]
37. Mantovani, A.; Taliento, A.; Zusi, C.; Baselli, G.A.; Prati, D.; Granata, S.; Zaza, G.; Colecchia, A.; Maffeis, C.; Byrne, C.D.; et al. PNPLA3 I148M gene variant and chronic kidney disease in type 2 diabetic patients with NAFLD: Clinical and experimental findings. *Liver Int.* **2020**, *40*, 1130–1141. [CrossRef]
38. Sun, D.Q.; Zheng, K.I.; Xu, G.; Ma, H.L.; Zhang, H.Y.; Pan, X.Y.; Zhu, P.W.; Wang, X.D.; Targher, G.; Byrne, C.D.; et al. PNPLA3 rs738409 is associated with renal glomerular and tubular injury in NAFLD patients with persistently normal ALT levels. *Liver Int.* **2020**, *40*, 107–119. [CrossRef] [PubMed]
39. Mantovani, A.; Zusi, C. PNPLA3 gene and kidney disease. *Explor. Med.* **2020**, *1*, 42–50. [CrossRef]
40. Targher, G.; Mantovani, A.; Alisi, A.; Mosca, A.; Panera, N.; Byrne, C.D.; Nobili, V. Relationship Between PNPLA3 rs738409 Polymorphism and Decreased Kidney Function in Children With NAFLD. *Hepatology* **2019**, *70*, 142–153. [CrossRef] [PubMed]
41. Marzuillo, P.; Di Sessa, A.; Guarino, S.; Capalbo, D.; Umano, G.R.; Pedullà, M.; La Manna, A.; Cirillo, G.; Del Giudice, E.M. Nonalcoholic fatty liver disease and eGFR levels could be linked by the PNPLA3 I148M polymorphism in children with obesity. *Pediatr. Obes.* **2019**, *14*, e12539. [CrossRef]
42. Di Costanzo, A.; Pacifico, L.; D'Erasmo, L.; Polito, L.; Di Martino, M.; Perla, F.M.; Iezzi, L.; Chiesa, C.; Arca, M.; Costanzo, D.; et al. Nonalcoholic Fatty Liver Disease (NAFLD), But not Its Susceptibility Gene Variants, Influences the Decrease of Kidney Function in Overweight/Obese Children. *Int. J. Mol. Sci.* **2019**, *20*, 4444. [CrossRef]
43. Sun, D.-Q.; Jin, Y.; Wang, T.-Y.; Zheng, K.I.; Rios, R.S.; Zhang, H.-Y.; Targher, G.; Byrne, C.D.; Yuan, W.-J.; Zheng, M.-H. MAFLD and risk of CKD. *Metabolism* **2021**, *115*, 154433. [CrossRef] [PubMed]
44. Yan, L.; Mu, B.; Guan, Y.; Liu, X.; Zhao, N.; Pan, D.; Wang, S. Assessment of the relationship between non-alcoholic fatty liver disease and diabetic complications. *J. Diabetes Investig.* **2016**, *7*, 889–894. [CrossRef]
45. Williams, K.H.; Burns, K.; Constantino, M.; Shackel, N.A.; Prakoso, E.; Wong, J.; Wu, T.; George, J.; McCaughan, G.W.; Twigg, S.M. An association of large-fibre peripheral nerve dysfunction with non-invasive measures of liver fibrosis secondary to non-alcoholic fatty liver disease in diabetes. *J. Diabetes Complicat.* **2015**, *29*, 1240–1247. [CrossRef] [PubMed]

46. Lombardi, R.; Airaghi, L.; Targher, G.; Serviddio, G.; Maffi, G.; Mantovani, A.; Maffeis, C.; Colecchia, A.; Villani, R.; Rinaldi, L.; et al. Liver fibrosis by FibroScan® independently of established cardiovascular risk parameters associates with macrovascular and microvascular complications in patients with type 2 diabetes. *Liver Int.* **2020**, *40*, 347–354. [CrossRef] [PubMed]
47. LLv, W.-S.; Sun, R.-X.; Gao, Y.-Y.; Wen, J.-P.; Pan, R.-F.; Li, L.; Wang, J.; Xian, Y.-X.; Cao, C.-X.; Zheng, M. Nonalcoholic fatty liver disease and microvascular complications in type 2 diabetes. *World J. Gastroenterol.* **2013**, *19*, 3134–3142. [CrossRef]
48. Kim, B.-Y.; Jung, C.-H.; Mok, J.-O.; Kang, S.K.; Kim, C.-H. Prevalences of diabetic retinopathy and nephropathy are lower in Korean type 2 diabetic patients with non-alcoholic fatty liver disease. *J. Diabetes Investig.* **2014**, *5*, 170–175. [CrossRef]
49. Houghton, D.; Zalewski, P.; Hallsworth, K.; Cassidy, S.; Thoma, C.; Avery, L.; Slomko, J.; Hardy, T.; Burt, A.D.; Tiniakos, D.; et al. The degree of hepatic steatosis associates with impaired cardiac and autonomic function. *J. Hepatol.* **2019**, *70*, 1203–1213. [CrossRef]
50. Targher, G.; Mantovani, A.; Grander, C.; Foco, L.; Motta, B.; Byrne, C.D.; Pramstaller, P.P.; Tilg, H. Association between non-alcoholic fatty liver disease and impaired cardiac sympathetic/parasympathetic balance in subjects with and without type 2 diabetes—The Cooperative Health Research in South Tyrol (CHRIS)-NAFLD sub-study. *Nutr. Metab. Cardiovasc. Dis.* **2021**, *31*, 3464–3473. [CrossRef]
51. Targher, G.; Bertolini, L.; Rodella, S.; Zoppini, G.; Lippi, G.; Day, C.; Muggeo, M. Non-alcoholic fatty liver disease is independently associated with an increased prevalence of chronic kidney disease and proliferative/laser-treated retinopathy in type 2 diabetic patients. *Diabetologia* **2008**, *51*, 444–450. [CrossRef]
52. Song, D.; Li, C.; Wang, Z.; Zhao, Y.; Shen, B.; Zhao, W. Association of non-alcoholic fatty liver disease with diabetic retinopathy in type 2 diabetic patients: A meta-analysis of observational studies. *J. Diabetes Investig.* **2021**, *12*, 1471–1479. [CrossRef]
53. Targher, G.; Bertolini, L.; Padovani, R.; Rodella, S.; Tessari, R.; Zenari, L.; Day, C.; Arcaro, G. Prevalence of Nonalcoholic Fatty Liver Disease and Its Association With Cardiovascular Disease Among Type 2 Diabetic Patients. *Diabetes Care* **2007**, *30*, 1212–1218. [CrossRef] [PubMed]
54. Anstee, Q.M.; Targher, G.; Day, C.P. Progression of NAFLD to diabetes mellitus, cardiovascular disease or cirrhosis. *Nat. Rev. Gastroenterol. Hepatol.* **2013**, *10*, 330–344. [CrossRef] [PubMed]
55. Targher, G.; Byrne, C.D. Clinical Review: Nonalcoholic fatty liver disease: A novel cardiometabolic risk factor for type 2 diabetes and its complications. *J. Clin. Endocrinol. Metab.* **2013**, *98*, 483–495. [CrossRef]
56. Targher, G.; Byrne, C.D.; Tilg, H. NAFLD and increased risk of cardiovascular disease: Clinical associations, pathophysiological mechanisms and pharmacological implications. *Gut* **2020**, *69*, 1691–1705. [CrossRef] [PubMed]
57. Mantovani, A.; Pernigo, M.; Bergamini, C.; Bonapace, S.; Lipari, P.; Pichiri, I.; Bertolini, L.; Valbusa, F.; Barbieri, E.; Zoppini, G.; et al. Nonalcoholic Fatty Liver Disease Is Independently Associated with Early Left Ventricular Diastolic Dysfunction in Patients with Type 2 Diabetes. *PLoS ONE* **2015**, *10*, e0135329. [CrossRef]
58. Borges-Canha, M.; Neves, J.S.; Libânio, D.; Von-Hafe, M.; Vale, C.; Araújo-Martins, M.; Leite, A.R.; Pimentel-Nunes, P.; Carvalho, D.; Leite-Moreira, A. Association between nonalcoholic fatty liver disease and cardiac function and structure—a meta-analysis. *Endocrine* **2019**, *66*, 467–476. [CrossRef]
59. VanWagner, L.B.; Wilcox, J.E.; Ning, H.; Lewis, C.E.; Carr, J.J.; Rinella, M.E.; Shah, S.J.; Lima, J.A.C.; Lloyd-Jones, D.M. Longitudinal Association of Non-Alcoholic Fatty Liver Disease With Changes in Myocardial Structure and Function: The CARDIA Study. *J. Am. Hear Assoc.* **2020**, *9*, e014279. [CrossRef]
60. Dong, Y.; Huang, D.; Sun, L.; Wang, Y.; Li, Y.; Chang, W.; Li, G.; Cui, H. Assessment of left ventricular function in type 2 diabetes mellitus patients with non-alcoholic fatty liver disease using three-dimensional speckle-tracking echocardiography. *Anatol. J. Cardiol.* **2020**, *23*, 41–48. [CrossRef]
61. Chang, W.; Wang, Y.; Sun, L.; Yu, N.; Li, Y.; Li, G. Evaluation of left atrial function in type 2 diabetes mellitus patients with nonalcoholic fatty liver disease by two-dimensional speckle tracking echocardiography. *Echocardiography* **2019**, *36*, 1290–1297. [CrossRef] [PubMed]
62. Mantovani, A.; Pernigo, M.; Bergamini, C.; Bonapace, S.; Lipari, P.; Valbusa, F.; Bertolini, L.; Zenari, L.; Pichiri, I.; Dauriz, M.; et al. Heart valve calcification in patients with type 2 diabetes and nonalcoholic fatty liver disease. *Metabolism* **2015**, *64*, 879–887. [CrossRef]
63. Rossi, A.; Targher, G.; Zoppini, G.; Cicoira, M.; Bonapace, S.; Negri, C.; Stoico, V.; Faggiano, P.; Vassanelli, C.; Bonora, E. Aortic and Mitral Annular Calcifications Are Predictive of All-Cause and Cardiovascular Mortality in Patients With Type 2 Diabetes. *Diabetes Care* **2012**, *35*, 1781–1786. [CrossRef]
64. Minhas, A.M.; Usman, M.S.; Khan, M.S.; Fatima, K.; Mangi, M.A.; Illovsky, M.A. Link Between Non-Alcoholic Fatty Liver Disease and Atrial Fibrillation: A Systematic Review and Meta-Analysis. *Cureus* **2017**, *9*, e1142. [CrossRef]
65. Wijarnpreecha, K.; Boonpheng, B.; Thongprayoon, C.; Jaruvongvanich, V.; Ungprasert, P. The association between non-alcoholic fatty liver disease and atrial fibrillation: A meta-analysis. *Clin. Res. Hepatol. Gastroenterol.* **2017**, *41*, 525–532. [CrossRef]
66. Mantovani, A.; Dauriz, M.; Sandri, D.; Bonapace, S.; Zoppini, G.; Tilg, H.; Byrne, C.D.; Targher, G. Association between non-alcoholic fatty liver disease and risk of atrial fibrillation in adult individuals: An updated meta-analysis. *Liver Int.* **2019**, *39*, 758–769. [CrossRef] [PubMed]
67. Gong, H.; Liu, X.; Cheng, F. Relationship between non-alcoholic fatty liver disease and cardiac arrhythmia: A systematic review and meta-analysis. *J. Int. Med. Res.* **2021**, *49*, 3000605211047074. [CrossRef]

68. Donnellan, E.; Cotter, T.G.; Wazni, O.M.; Elshazly, M.B.; Kochar, A.; Wilner, B.; Patel, D.; Kanj, M.; Hussein, A.; Baranowski, B.; et al. Impact of Nonalcoholic Fatty Liver Disease on Arrhythmia Recurrence Following Atrial Fibrillation Ablation. *JACC Clin. Electrophysiol.* **2020**, *6*, 1278–1287. [CrossRef] [PubMed]
69. Targher, G.; Valbusa, F.; Bonapace, S.; Bertolini, L.; Zenari, L.; Pichiri, I.; Mantovani, A.; Zoppini, G.; Bonora, E.; Barbieri, E.; et al. Association of nonalcoholic fatty liver disease with QTc interval in patients with type 2 diabetes. *Nutr. Metab. Cardiovasc. Dis.* **2014**, *24*, 663–669. [CrossRef] [PubMed]
70. Mantovani, A.; Rigolon, R.; Pichiri, I.; Bonapace, S.; Morani, G.; Zoppini, G.; Bonora, E.; Targher, G. Nonalcoholic fatty liver disease is associated with an increased risk of heart block in hospitalized patients with type 2 diabetes mellitus. *PLoS ONE* **2017**, *12*, e0185459. [CrossRef]
71. Mantovani, A. Nonalcoholic Fatty Liver Disease (NAFLD) and Risk of Cardiac Arrhythmias: A New Aspect of the Liver-heart Axis. *J. Clin. Transl. Hepatol.* **2017**, *5*, 134–141. [CrossRef]
72. Mantovani, A.; Rigamonti, A.; Bonapace, S.; Bolzan, B.; Pernigo, M.; Morani, G.; Franceschini, L.; Bergamini, C.; Bertolini, L.; Valbusa, F.; et al. Nonalcoholic Fatty Liver Disease Is Associated With Ventricular Arrhythmias in Patients With Type 2 Diabetes Referred for Clinically Indicated 24-Hour Holter Monitoring. *Diabetes Care* **2016**, *39*, 1416–1423. [CrossRef]
73. Mantovani, A.; Scorletti, E.; Mosca, A.; Alisi, A.; Byrne, C.D.; Targher, G. Complications, morbidity and mortality of nonalcoholic fatty liver disease. *Metabolism* **2020**, *111*, 154170. [CrossRef]
74. Paik, J.M.; Henry, L.; De Avila, L.; Younossi, E.; Racila, A.; Younossi, Z.M. Mortality Related to Nonalcoholic Fatty Liver Disease Is Increasing in the United States. *Hepatol. Commun.* **2019**, *3*, 1459–1471. [CrossRef]
75. Byrne, C.D.; Targher, G. Non-alcoholic fatty liver disease is a risk factor for cardiovascular and cardiac diseases: Further evidence that a holistic approach to treatment is needed. *Gut* **2021**. [CrossRef] [PubMed]
76. Targher, G.; Lonardo, A.; Byrne, C.D. Nonalcoholic fatty liver disease and chronic vascular complications of diabetes mellitus. *Nat. Rev. Endocrinol.* **2018**, *14*, 99–114. [CrossRef]
77. Targher, G.; Byrne, C.D.; Lonardo, A.; Zoppini, G.; Barbui, C. Non-alcoholic fatty liver disease and risk of incident cardiovascular disease: A meta-analysis. *J. Hepatol.* **2016**, *65*, 589–600. [CrossRef]
78. Morrison, A.E.; Zaccardi, F.; Khunti, K.; Davies, M.J. Causality between non-alcoholic fatty liver disease and risk of cardiovascular disease and type 2 diabetes: A meta-analysis with bias analysis. *Liver Int.* **2019**, *39*, 557–567. [CrossRef]
79. Liu, Y.; Zhong, G.-C.; Tan, H.-Y.; Hao, F.-B.; Hu, J.-J. Nonalcoholic fatty liver disease and mortality from all causes, cardiovascular disease, and cancer: A meta-analysis. *Sci. Rep.* **2019**, *9*, 11124. [CrossRef]
80. Simon, T.G.; Roelstraete, B.; Khalili, H.; Hagström, H.; Ludvigsson, J.F. Mortality in biopsy-confirmed nonalcoholic fatty liver disease: Results from a nationwide cohort. *Gut* **2021**, *70*, 1375–1382. [CrossRef]
81. Angulo, P.; Kleiner, D.E.; Dam-Larsen, S.; Adams, L.A.; Björnsson, E.S.; Charatcharoenwitthaya, P.; Mills, P.R.; Keach, J.C.; Lafferty, H.D.; Stahler, A.; et al. Liver Fibrosis, but No Other Histologic Features, Is Associated With Long-term Outcomes of Patients With Nonalcoholic Fatty Liver Disease. *Gastroenterology* **2015**, *149*, 389–397.e10. [CrossRef]
82. Ekstedt, M.; Hagström, H.; Nasr, P.; Fredrikson, M.; Stål, P.; Kechagias, S.; Hultcrantz, R. Fibrosis stage is the strongest predictor for disease-specific mortality in NAFLD after up to 33 years of follow-up. *Hepatology* **2015**, *61*, 1547–1554. [CrossRef] [PubMed]
83. Targher, G.; Corey, K.E.; Byrne, C.D. NAFLD, and cardiovascular and cardiac diseases: Factors influencing risk, prediction and treatment. *Diabetes Metab.* **2020**, *47*, 101215. [CrossRef]
84. Kim, D.; Konyn, P.; Sandhu, K.K.; Dennis, B.B.; Cheung, A.C.; Ahmed, A. Metabolic dysfunction-associated fatty liver disease is associated with increased all-cause mortality in the United States. *J. Hepatol.* **2021**, *75*, 1284–1291. [CrossRef]
85. Mantovani, A.; Valenti, L. A call to action for fatty liver disease. *Liver Int.* **2021**, *41*, 1182–1185. [CrossRef]
86. Mantovani, A.; Dalbeni, A. Treatments for NAFLD: State of Art. *Int. J. Mol. Sci.* **2021**, *22*, 2350. [CrossRef]
87. Mantovani, A.; Byrne, C.D.; Targher, G. Efficacy of peroxisome proliferator-activated receptor agonists, glucagon-like peptide-1 receptor agonists, or sodium-glucose cotransporter-2 inhibitors for treatment of non-alcoholic fatty liver disease: A systematic review. *Lancet Gastroenterol. Hepatol.* **2022**. [CrossRef]
88. Mantovani, A.; Byrne, C.D.; Scorletti, E.; Mantzoros, C.S.; Targher, G. Efficacy and safety of anti-hyperglycaemic drugs in patients with non-alcoholic fatty liver disease with or without diabetes: An updated systematic review of randomized controlled trials. *Diabetes Metab.* **2020**, *46*, 427–441. [CrossRef] [PubMed]
89. Dufour, J.-F.; Caussy, C.; Loomba, R. Combination therapy for non-alcoholic steatohepatitis: Rationale, opportunities and challenges. *Gut* **2020**, *69*, 1877–1884. [CrossRef] [PubMed]

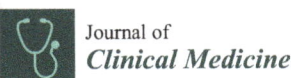 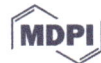

Communication

Low Screening Rates Despite a High Prevalence of Significant Liver Fibrosis in People with Diabetes from Primary and Secondary Care

Laurence J. Dobbie [1], Mohamed Kassab [2], Andrew S. Davison [3,4], Pete Grace [4], Daniel J. Cuthbertson [1] and Theresa J. Hydes [1,2,*]

1. Department of Cardiovascular and Metabolic Medicine, Institute of Life Course and Medical Sciences, University of Liverpool, Liverpool L9 7AL, UK; laurence.dobbie@liverpool.ac.uk (L.J.D.); dan.cuthbertson@liverpool.ac.uk (D.J.C.)
2. Department of Gastroenterology and Hepatology, Liverpool University Hospitals Foundation Trust, Liverpool L7 8XP, UK; mohamed.kassab@nhs.net
3. Department of Clinical Biochemistry and Metabolic Medicine, Liverpool Clinical Laboratories, Liverpool University Hospitals Foundation Trust, Liverpool L7 8XP, UK; andrew.davison@liverpoolft.nhs.uk
4. Liverpool Clinical Laboratories, Liverpool University Hospitals Foundation Trust, Liverpool L7 8XP, UK; pete.grace@liverpoolft.nhs.uk
* Correspondence: theresa.hydes@liverpool.ac.uk

Citation: Dobbie, L.J.; Kassab, M.; Davison, A.S.; Grace, P.; Cuthbertson, D.J.; Hydes, T.J. Low Screening Rates Despite a High Prevalence of Significant Liver Fibrosis in People with Diabetes from Primary and Secondary Care. *J. Clin. Med.* **2021**, *10*, 5755. https://doi.org/10.3390/jcm10245755

Academic Editor: Fernando Gómez-Peralta

Received: 16 November 2021
Accepted: 7 December 2021
Published: 9 December 2021

Publisher's Note: MDPI stays neutral with regard to jurisdictional claims in published maps and institutional affiliations.

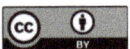

Copyright: © 2021 by the authors. Licensee MDPI, Basel, Switzerland. This article is an open access article distributed under the terms and conditions of the Creative Commons Attribution (CC BY) license (https:// creativecommons.org/licenses/by/ 4.0/).

Abstract: Diabetes is a driver of non-alcoholic fatty liver disease (NAFLD) and fibrosis. We determine current practices in examining liver fibrosis in people with diabetes and record prevalence levels in primary and secondary care. We extracted HbA_{1c} results ≥ 48 mmol/mol to identify people with diabetes, then examined the proportion who had AST, ALT, and platelets results, facilitating calculation of non-invasive fibrosis tests (NIT), or an enhanced liver fibrosis score. Fibrosis markers were requested in only 1.49% (390/26,090), of which 29.7% ($n = 106$) had evidence of significant fibrosis via NIT. All patients at risk of fibrosis had undergone transient elastography (TE), biopsy or imaging. TE and biopsy data showed that 80.6% of people with raised fibrosis markers had confirmed significant fibrosis. We also show that fibrosis levels as detected by NIT are marginally lower in patients treated with newer glucose lowering agents (sodium-glucose transporter protein 2 inhibitors, dipeptidyl peptidase-4 inhibitors and glucagon-like peptide-1 receptor agonists). In conclusion by utilising a large consecutively recruited dataset we demonstrate that liver fibrosis is infrequently screened for in patients with diabetes despite high prevalence rates of advanced fibrosis. This highlights the need for cost-effectiveness analyses to support the incorporation of widespread screening into national guidelines and the requirement for healthcare practitioners to incorporate NAFLD screening into routine diabetes care.

Keywords: fibrosis; NAFLD; diabetes; screening; primary care; secondary care

1. Introduction

Non-alcoholic fatty liver disease (NAFLD) is the most common cause of liver disease in the UK and Europe [1], soon to become the most common indication for liver transplantation in the next decade [2], as a result of the obesity and associated type 2 diabetes (T2D) epidemics. Expert consensus has suggested NAFLD be re-named metabolic-associated fatty liver disease (MAFLD) to reflect its strong association with insulin resistance and the metabolic syndrome [3]. Type 2 diabetes is a condition characterised by peripheral insulin resistance with inadequate compensatory pancreatic beta-cell insulin secretion. Insulin resistance and systemic inflammation lead to accumulation of free fatty acids and consequentially hepatocyte triglyceride accumulation characterising NAFLD [4,5]. NAFLD is generally benign in the majority of individuals, however in up to 40% of people it can progress to liver fibrosis [6,7]. Liver fibrosis describes the development of fibrous tissue due to the replacement of healthy tissue by extracellular matrix proteins, in NAFLD this is the result of hepatotoxic injury and initially leads to non-alcoholic steatohepatitis (NASH) and chronically to liver fibrosis [8]. Liver fibrosis, rather than simple steatosis or NASH, is associated with an increased risk of liver-related morbidity and mortality [6,9], overall mortality [10], and cardiovascular disease [11,12].

One of the most significant predictors of fibrosis progression and the development of advanced fibrosis is diabetes, particularly T2D [13–18]. NAFLD is reported to be present in 40–70% of individuals with T2D [19–21]. Furthermore, UK diabetes prevalence according to Quality Outcome Framework data is now 7.1% (2020/21), with an additional large number of undiagnosed cases [22]. While the European Association for the Study of the Liver (EASL) guidelines [23] and American Diabetes Association guidelines [24] suggest surveillance for NAFLD in people with T2D, the American [25], Asian [26], and UK [27,28] guidelines acknowledge that individuals with T2D are at greater risk of NAFLD, yet do not advocate widespread screening.

We aimed to perform a cross-sectional analysis of the burden of significant liver fibrosis in individuals with diabetes from both primary and secondary care to understand the prevalence of potentially clinically significant liver disease in these settings; and to provide a snapshot into current practice of examining fibrosis markers and ongoing risk stratification in people with diabetes.

2. Materials and Methods

Screening with HbA_{1c} We extracted glycated haemoglobin (HbA_{1c}) results over a 21-month period (31 December 2019 to 14 September 21) from the Liverpool (University Hospital Foundation Trust) Clinical Laboratories and identified a cohort of individuals with an $HbA_{1c} \geq 48$ mmol/mol indicative of a diagnosis of diabetes (Figure 1). Individuals under 35 years old were excluded as fibrosis scores are inaccurate in this age group. Results from blood requests from inpatient stays, the emergency department, cancer services, and dialysis units were excluded, leaving those taken from primary care and other outpatient departments.

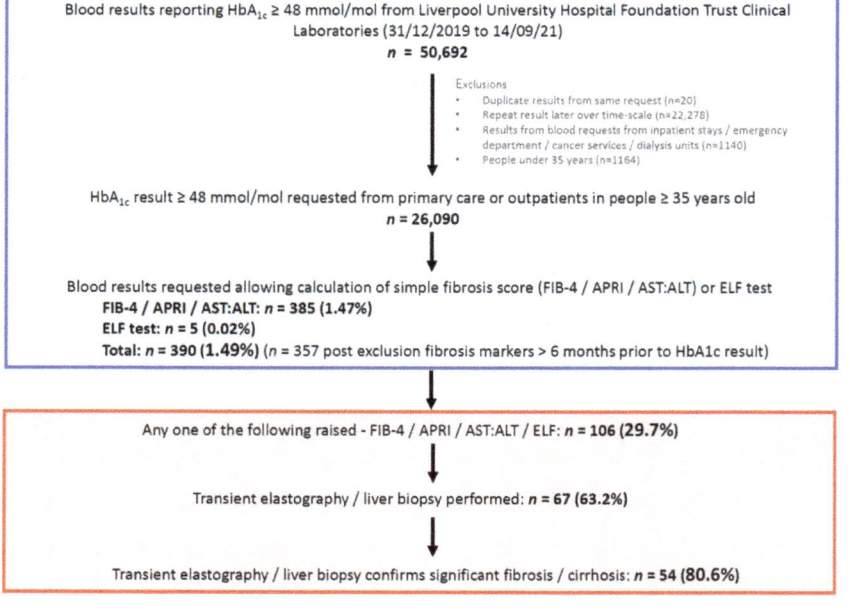

Figure 1. Study flow chart and summary of results. HbA_{1c}, glycated haemoglobin; FIB-4, fibrosis-4; APRI, aspartate transaminase to platelet ratio index; AST aspartate transaminase; ALT, alanine transaminase; ELF, enhanced liver fibrosis score.

2.1. Determination of Liver Biochemistry Results and Fibrosis Scores

We examined what proportion of these people had an aspartate transaminase (AST), alanine transaminase (ALT), and platelet levels taken within this time frame. From these results, we calculated three validated non-invasive scores of liver fibrosis, the fibrosis-4 (FIB-4) score [29], the AST to platelet ration index (APRI) [30], and the AST:ALT ratio (Supplementary Table S1) [31]. Significant fibrosis was defined as either a FIB-4 score > 2.67, APRI score $\geq$ 1.0, or AST:ALT ratio $\geq$ 1.0, where either the AST or ALT level was also >40 IU/L. We also included patients with an enhanced liver fibrosis score (ELF), based on tissue inhibitor metalloproteinases 1, amino-terminal pro-peptide of type III procollagen and hyaluronic acid [32]. Significant fibrosis was defined as an ELF score of >9.8. We then excluded results taken over 6 months prior to the HbA_{1c} to ensure that individuals were likely to have diabetes at the time the fibrosis tests were taken. We additionally compared prevalence rates of liver fibrosis detected by primary and secondary care.

2.2. Confirmation of Fibrosis Identified with Non-Invasive Testing Using Transient Elastography (TE) and/or Liver Biopsy

We further examined what proportion of individuals identified as being at risk of significant liver fibrosis according to non-invasive tests (NITs), had gone on to have confirmatory testing with either TE or liver biopsy. TE suggestive of fibrosis was defined according to a liver stiffness measurement > 8 kPa (Fibroscan, Echosens, Paris, France). Histological evidence of significant fibrosis or cirrhosis was confirmed by percutaneous liver biopsy and verified by an experienced liver histopathologist.

2.3. Association between Advanced Fibrosis According to FIB-4 Score and Glucose Lowering Agents

We examined prescription data for glucose lowering agents for patients who had data available to calculate a FIB-4 score. We additionally examined the proportion of people with a raised FIB-4 score > 2.67 according the number and classes of glucose lowering medications prescribed.

2.4. Statistical Analysis

Results are presented as the median and interquartile range. Data validity was ensured by examining ten random NHS numbers of both included and excluded patients and cross-checking them across databases. Data was analysed using R version 4.1.1 (R Foundation for Statistical Computing, Vienna, Austria) and Excel Kutools.

2.5. Ethics

As all patient data was anonymised this project did not require national ethical approval; clinical audit approval was obtained locally (number 10864).

3. Results

3.1. Description of Study Cohort

We identified 26,090 individuals who had an HbA_{1c} result $\geq$48 mmol/mol requested from primary care or secondary care (outpatients department). Data was available to calculate the APRI score, AST:ALT ratio and FIB-4 score in 385 (1.47%) of these individuals and a further 5 (0.02%) had an ELF score requested, meaning that overall 390 (1.49%) people with diabetes had undergone a non-invasive test for fibrosis. Following the exclusion of results taken >6 months prior to the HbA_{1c} result, the final study cohort consisted of 357 individuals with diabetes (Figure 1). In total 134 (37.5%) results were ordered from primary care and 223 from outpatients (62.5%). Baseline demographic data and laboratory results from this cohort are presented in Table 1.

Table 1. Baseline data from the cohort ($n = 357$).

Variable	Demographic Factor/Laboratory Finding
Sex (n (%))	204 (57.1) M, 153 (42.9) F
Age (years) (Median (IQR))	60 (53–67)
HbA$_{1c}$ (mmol/mol) (Median (IQR))	62 (53–76)
AST (IU/L) (Median (IQR))	30 (21–48)
ALT (IU/L) (Median (IQR))	35 (23–53)
Platelets ($\times 10^9$/L) (Median (IQR))	223 (170–284)
ELF score	10.1 (10–10.7)

M, male; F, Female; IQR, interquartile range; HbA$_{1c}$, glycated haemoglobin; AST aspartate transaminase; ALT, alanine transaminase; ELF, enhanced liver fibrosis.

3.2. Prevalence of Significant Fibrosis in Individuals with Diabetes According to Serum Fibrosis Scores

Between 13.7–19% individuals with diabetes were identified as having evidence of significant fibrosis using simple NITs (Table 2, Figure 2) and 80% (4/5) of people who had an ELF score requested had evidence of significant fibrosis. Using the previously described definitions of significant fibrosis (one or more of FIB-4 score > 2.67, APRI $\geq$ 1.0, AST:ALT $\geq$ 1.0, or ELF > 9.8), 106 (29.7%) people with diabetes were identified as being at risk. Of the 106 people at risk of significant fibrosis, 30 (28.3%) had fibrosis markers requested from primary care. Of the 76 outpatient blood requests, 66 (86.8%) came from the liver clinic. Overall fibrosis scores derived from blood requests sent from secondary care (34.1%) showed higher levels of significant fibrosis than primary care (22.4%) (Table 1, Figure 2). There was no positive correlation between HbA$_{1c}$ and fibrosis scores when examined on a continuous scale (Supplementary Figure S1).

Table 2. Percentage of people with diabetes found to have evidence of significant fibrosis determined by non-invasive markers.

Non-Invasive Serum Fibrosis Scores	Total, % (n)	Primary Care, % (n)	Secondary Care, % (n)
	n = 357	37.5 (134)	62.5 (223)
FIB-4 > 2.67	19.0 (68)	13.4 (18)	22.4 (50)
APRI $\geq$ 1.0	13.7 (49)	12.7 (17)	14.3 (32)
AST:ALT ratio $\geq$ 1.0 and AST or ALT > 40 IU/L	17.4 (62)	11.2 (15)	21.1 (47)
Any one of the above, or ELF > 9.8	29.7 (106)	22.4 (30)	34.1 (76)

FIB-4, fibrosis-4; APRI, aspartate transaminase to platelet ratio index; AST aspartate transaminase; ALT, alanine transaminase; ELF, enhanced liver fibrosis test; kPa kilopascal.

3.3. Prevalence of People with Diabetes and At-Risk Serum Fibrosis Scores with Confirmed Significant Fibrosis/Cirrhosis

Of the 106 individuals with diabetes identified to be at risk of significant fibrosis using non-invasive serum markers, 67/106 (63.2%) went on to have transient elastography (TE/Fibroscan) ($n = 50$, 47.2%), liver biopsy ($n = 24$, 22.6%), or both ($n = 7$, 6.6%). In total 54/67 (80.6%) of these individuals had a liver stiffness measurement >8 kPa or evidence of significant fibrosis or cirrhosis at biopsy. All 39 people with raised fibrosis markers who did not receive a fibroscan or liver biopsy, had prior liver imaging via ultrasound ($n = 30$, 76.9%) or CT ($n = 9$, 23.1%), and 21/39 (53.8%) had evidence of cirrhosis.

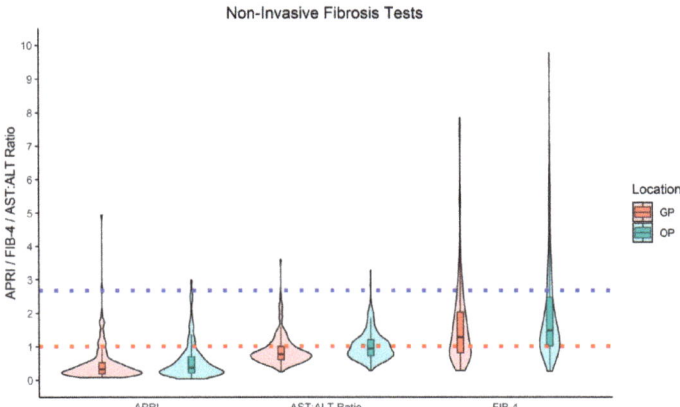

Figure 2. Summary Graphs of FIB-4, APRI, AST:ALT Ratio by Test Location. Red dotted line = cut-off for high-risk fibrosis via APRI and AST:ALT Ration. Blue dotted line = cut-off for high risk liver fibrosis via FIB-4, FIB-4 = Fibrosis 4, APRI = AST to Platelet Ratio Index, n = Number, GP = General Practice, OP = Outpatient.

3.4. Prevalence of a Raised FIB-4 Score According to the Number and Class of Glucose Lowering Agent

Medication data was available for 91.6% (327/357) patients. A further 4 patients were excluded who did not have data to calculate a FIB-4 score (final sample n = 323). A breakdown of the number of drugs and subclasses of glucose lowering agents prescribed are shown in Table 3. Patients who were not prescribed any glucose lowering therapies had lower levels of fibrosis according to the FIB-4 score (12.5%), compared to those on treatment (19.5%), however glycaemic control was also improved (Table 3, Supplementary Figure S2). Patients treated with SGLT2 inhibitors (16.4%), GLP-1 receptors agonists (16.0%) and DDP-4 inhibitors (15.1%) trended towards having non-significantly lower levels of NIT fibrosis (Table 3, Supplementary Figure S3), whilst having no noticeable differences in glycaemic control. Patients treated with metformin (18.6%) and sulphonylureas (18.4%) had similar levels of fibrosis to the overall cohort. Patients treated with insulin trended towards having non-significantly higher levels of fibrosis (23.8%) and higher HbA_{1c} levels (median 73 mmol/mol) (Table 3, Supplementary Figure S3).

Table 3. Results of Non-Invasive Serum Fibrosis Tests for People with Diabetes according to Number and Sub-class of Glucose-Lowering Agents Prescribed.

	People with Diabetes Who Had an NIT% (n)	Median HbA_{1c} [IQR] (mmol/mol)	FIB-4 > 2.67% (n)
	Number of Glucose Lowering Agents Prescribed		
None	12.4 (40)	51 (49–55)	12.5 (5)
1	40.6 (131)	58 (52–70)	22.1 (29)
2	29.1 (94)	67 (56–80)	17.0 (16)
≥3	19.2 (62)	73 (62–86)	17.7 (11)
	Subclasses of Glucose Lowering Agents Prescribed		
SGLT2 inhibitors	18.9 (61)	67 (59–79)	16.4 (10)
GLP-1 receptors agonists	7.7 (25)	69 (55–77)	16.0 (4)
DDP-4 inhibitors	26.6 (86)	67 (57–80)	15.1 (13)
Metformin	65.0 (210)	63 (53–77)	18.6 (39)
Insulin	24.8 (80)	73 (62–87)	23.8 (19)
Sulphonylurea	15.2 (49)	76 (63–86)	18.4 (9)
Thiazolidinediones	0.6 (2)	n/A	0.0 (0)

FIB-4, Fibrosis 4; SGLT-2 inhibitor, sodium-glucose cotransporter 2 inhibitor; GLP-1 receptor agonist, Glucagon-Like Peptide 1 Receptor Agonist; DDP-4 inhibitor, Dipeptidyl peptidase-4 inhibitor.

4. Discussion

4.1. Summary of Findings

In this brief report, we utilise real world UK regional data from local populations of people with diabetes and highlight two alarming findings. First, we demonstrate that <2% of people with diabetes are being screened for liver fibrosis, and that use of patented serum fibrosis biomarkers is minimal despite been advocated by the National Institute of Health and Clinical Excellence (NICE) as first line assessment for people with NAFLD [27]. Secondly, up to 29.7% of people with diabetes, in whom serum fibrosis markers were requested, were at risk of having significant liver fibrosis; subsequent confirmation of fibrosis was provided by second line tests, TE or liver biopsy, in a high proportion (80.6%) of cases. Thirdly, we report limited data showing a non-significant trend towards lower fibrosis scores in patients treated with DDP-4 inhibitors, SGLT-2 inhibitors, and GLP-1 receptor agonists. These findings reinforce the need for large prospective studies in this clinical population to develop cost-effective and easily implementable approaches to widespread screening for liver fibrosis in individuals with diabetes.

4.2. Comparison to the Existing Literature

While our estimates of fibrosis prevalence in people with diabetes are higher than comparable studies, there is consensus in the literature that clinically relevant liver fibrosis is highly prevalent in this group. Global meta-analysis data in 439 biopsied patient with NAFLD and T2D identified that 17% had advanced fibrosis [21]. Data from over 120,000 people with T2D from the Cleveland clinic suggests that 8.4% have a FIB-4 score >2.67; however, prevalence estimates varied widely depending on the non-invasive score used [33]. Among individuals with T2D and a reliable TE result in the NHANES study (n = 825), 15.4% had a liver stiffness measurement $\geq$9.7 kPa. In a recent cross-sectional study from the US, 561 individuals with T2D attending primary care or endocrinology clinics underwent non-invasive screening using serum markers and TE; liver biopsy was performed where there was a suggestion of fibrosis [34]. In total 9% of people with diabetes had advanced fibrosis (F3/F4) according to TE. Fibrosis prevalence levels with TE were similar to that estimated using the FIB-4 and APRI panels, and both modalities correlated well with biopsy findings. A similar analysis from the UK identified that 18.5% of people with T2D attending primary care clinics (n = 467) had a FIB-4 >1.3 for $\leq$65 years and >2.0 for >65 years, of which nearly two thirds had a TE >8 kPa [35].

4.3. Molecular Mechanisms Linking T2D and NAFLD

Pathogenic mechanisms linking T2D to NAFLD are complex; however, insulin resistance and inflammation are central [36]. High levels of circulating glucose and insulin increase rates of hepatic de novo lipogenesis leading to high levels of free fatty acids (FFA) in the liver; excess FFAs are stored as intrahepatic triglycerides [37]. Adiposity and the presence of insulin resistant adipose tissue leads to lipolysis; FFAs released from adipose tissue are taken up by peripheral tissues including the liver and muscle. NAFLD itself in turn leads to impairments in insulin signalling [38] and increased secretion of hepatokines. Adipokines are lipotoxic agents arising from chronically inflamed adipose tissue characterising T2D. These travel to the liver contributing to inflammation and NAFLD development [39]. Lipotoxicity, along with oxidative stress and a pro-inflammatory environment, result in steatohepatitis and eventually activation of hepatic stellate cells and extracellular matrix deposition. Clinical studies support this mechanism: stable isotope analyses show patients with increased hepatic adiposity have higher plasma FFA levels and ~3x greater de novo FFA synthesis [40].

4.4. Implications for Practice

We therefore propose that there is an urgent need for greater adoption of national and international guidelines to implement widespread screening for fibrosis in individuals with diabetes and undertake comprehensive cost-effectiveness analyses. Despite updated recommendations from the EASL advocating the use of NITs and that ALT, AST, and platelets should be part of the routine investigations in primary care in patients with suspected liver disease [41], a huge shift in practice towards more widespread screening is unlikely to be implemented in the UK without guidance from the NICE. Detection of liver cirrhosis, which develops insidiously and without abnormalities in liver biochemistry, allows entry of individuals into variceal and hepatocellular carcinoma surveillance programmes, the latter being particularly relevant for people with diabetes [42,43]. Liver fibrosis is a partially reversible state, achieved with weight loss (~7%) [44], while fibrosis progression may be retarded with optimisation of glycaemic control, so multi-component metabolic intervention programmes are likely to be highly effective. Detection of NAFLD, and associated fibrosis, will facilitate enrolment in relevant clinical trials, and may encourage prescription of glucose-lowering therapies that target steatosis, steatohepatitis, or even fibrosis (including DDP-4 inhibitors, GLP receptor agonists and SGLT2 inhibitors) [45]. The burden of NAFLD and liver fibrosis expands beyond the liver, with well-established associations with cardiovascular morbidity and mortality [11,12] and extrahepatic cancer [46], so the wider benefits of detection are considerable.

We additionally show that fewer patients treated with either GLP-1 receptor agonists, SGLT 2 inhibitors and DDP-4 inhibitors have elevated FIB-4 scores. Glucose lowering therapies are a potential therapy in NAFLD given the fact they reduce insulin resistance and thus potentially reduce liver fat. DDP-4 inhibitors have not shown therapeutic effect in NAFLD; however, data is limited so larger trials are required [45,47,48]. GLP-1 receptor agonists have shown more promising findings. One study reported GLP-1 agonists significantly reduce liver fat (relative reduction 42%) [49]. Similarly, in a larger randomised controlled trial (RCT) (n = 320), semaglutide therapy led to higher rate of NASH resolution than control. However, no clear dose–response relationship was reported between dosing regimens (0.1 mg vs 0.2 mg vs 0.4 mg) [50]. A meta-analysis (n = 4442) of patients treated with liraglutide demonstrated ALT reduction [51]. For SGLT-2 inhibitors, a large RCT, EMPA-REG OUTCOME, reported that empagliflozin reduced ALT with these findings independent of glycaemic control (HbA$_{1c}$) [52]. Similarly, in a moderately sized Swedish trial dapagliflozin reduced liver fat and ALT but did not improve glycaemic control. The conflicting findings between these two trials may or may delineate that SGLT-2 inhibitors have beneficial effects on NAFLD independent of glycaemic control [53]. Altogether, these trials show that GLP-1 agonists and SGLT 2 inhibitors have beneficial effects on liver biochemistry and liver fat levels in NAFLD. However, future trials need to assess the effects of these glucose lowering therapies on liver fibrosis. This could be via measuring non-invasive fibrosis scores (i.e., FIB-4, APRI, AST:ALT ratio), conducting fibroscans, liver multi-scan MRI testing, and liver biopsies.

4.5. Strengths and Limitations

This dataset benefits from a systematic approach to screening individuals with diabetes in both primary and secondary care. However, there are several limitations. The dataset is biased by the fact that we were only able to examine fibrosis markers in people in whom clinicians requested an AST level, i.e., influenced by clinical suspicion of liver disease. Most outpatient requests were made from hepatology clinics, with an inevitable bias towards higher rates of fibrosis or cirrhosis. These factors would lead to an over-estimation of fibrosis prevalence compared to the overall population with diabetes. The positive predictive values of NITs are only moderate, so the true prevalence of fibrosis confirmed by biopsy would also have been lower. Furthermore the performance of NITs is less well validated and less reliable in the diabetes population [54,55]. Individuals with exemplary glycaemic control, with HbA$_{1c}$ < 48 mmol/mol would also have been overlooked, leading to a selection bias towards a sub-population of lesser metabolic health at higher risk of diabetes-related end-organ damage. This study was reliant on electronic medical records and therefore we were unable to reliably determine the aetiology of diabetes (type 1 or type 2 diabetes), or liver disease (including alcohol excess or viral hepatitis). Approximately 95%

of people with diabetes in the UK are estimated to have T2D; however, and all individuals that we have assessed would have had either MAFLD or dual aetiology liver disease, given the fact that they had diabetes. We examined the current practice of examining fibrosis markers in individuals with diabetes over a 1 year window of an HbA_{1c}. Current guidelines advise screening every 1–3 years in people with confirmed NAFLD [41], so some individuals may have had bloods taken which could have been used to calculate a fibrosis score outside this time period. This study was limited by a significant proportion of the data being extracted over the COVID-19 pandemic. This may have negatively affected screening rates for fibrosis markers in both primary and secondary care and therefore may have affected the results. In addition, this study was limited by omission of the body mass index (BMI) data, which was not widely available from patient records. While we were able to access prescription records, unfortunately data on duration of diabetes, duration a glucose lowering agent had been prescribed and historic prescription data was no available to allow a comprehensive assessment of the role of newer glucose lowering therapies on fibrosis levels.

5. Conclusions

In summary, we found very limited evidence of systematic screening for liver fibrosis: only 1.5% of individuals with diabetes had a NIT for assessment of fibrosis, despite evidence of a high prevalence of significant fibrosis (29.8%) in those assessed. We also show that fibrosis levels as detected by NIT is lower in patients treated with SGLT2 inhibitors, DDP-4 inhibitors, and GLP-1 receptor agonists. There is an urgent and unmet need to assess, develop, and implement cost-effective methods to provide widespread screening of individuals with diabetes for liver fibrosis and for healthcare practitioners to incorporate NAFLD screening into routine diabetes care. This will undoubtedly reap longer-term clinical benefits in reducing the hepatic and extra-hepatic burden of NAFLD in patients with diabetes.

Supplementary Materials: The following are available online at https://www.mdpi.com/article/10.3390/jcm10245755/s1, Table S1: Algorithms used to calculate Hepatic Steatosis Index and Fibrosis scores, Figure S1: Correlation between HbA_{1c} and Fibrosis Marker scores; Figure S2: Percentage of people with a raised FIB-4 score according to Number of glucose lowering agents prescribed; Figure S3: Percentage of people with a raised FIB-4 score according to subclasses of glucose lowering agents prescribed.

Author Contributions: Conceptualization, all authors; methodology, all authors; formal analysis, L.J.D., M.K. and T.J.H.; data curation, A.S.D. and P.G.; writing—original draft preparation, T.J.H.; writing—review and editing, all authors; visualization, L.J.D.; supervision, D.J.C.; All authors have read and agreed to the published version of the manuscript.

Funding: This research received no external funding.

Institutional Review Board Statement: This project did not require ethical approval however was approved by Aintree University Hospital Local Audit Committee (number 10864).

Informed Consent Statement: Patient consent was not required for this study, however we obtained local approval from Aintree University Hospital Audit Committee (Number: 10864).

Data Availability Statement: Data is available upon reasonable request to the authors.

Conflicts of Interest: The authors declare no conflict of interest.

References

1. Younossi, Z.M.; Koenig, A.B.; Abdelatif, D.; Fazel, Y.; Henry, L.; Wymer, M. Global epidemiology of nonalcoholic fatty liver disease-Meta-analytic assessment of prevalence, incidence, and outcomes. *Hepatology* **2016**, *64*, 73–84. [CrossRef]
2. Estes, C.; Razavi, H.; Loomba, R.; Younossi, Z.; Sanyal, A.J. Modeling the epidemic of nonalcoholic fatty liver disease demonstrates an exponential increase in burden of disease. *Hepatology* **2018**, *67*, 123–133. [CrossRef] [PubMed]

3. Eslam, M.; Sanyal, A.J.; George, J.; Sanyal, A.; Neuschwander-Tetri, B.; Tiribelli, C.; Kleiner, D.E.; Brunt, E.; Bugianesi, E.; Yki-Järvinen, H.; et al. MAFLD: A Consensus-Driven Proposed Nomenclature for Metabolic Associated Fatty Liver Disease. *Gastroenterology* **2020**, *158*, 1999–2014.e1. [CrossRef] [PubMed]
4. DeFronzo, R.A.; Ferrannini, E.; Groop, L.; Henry, R.R.; Herman, W.H.; Holst, J.J.; Hu, F.B.; Kahn, C.R.; Raz, I.; Shulman, G.I.; et al. Type 2 diabetes mellitus. *Nat. Rev. Dis. Primers* **2015**, *1*, 15019. [CrossRef]
5. Tomah, S.; Alkhouri, N.; Hamdy, O. Non-alcoholic Fatty Liver Disease and Type 2 Diabetes: Where do Diabetologists stand? *Clin. Diabetes Endocrinol.* **2020**, *6*, 9. [CrossRef] [PubMed]
6. De, A.; Duseja, A. Natural History of Simple Steatosis or Nonalcoholic Fatty Liver. *J. Clin. Exp. Hepatol.* **2020**, *10*, 255–262. [CrossRef] [PubMed]
7. Singh, S.; Allen, A.M.; Wang, Z.; Prokop, L.J.; Murad, M.H.; Loomba, R. Fibrosis Progression in Nonalcoholic Fatty Liver vs Nonalcoholic Steatohepatitis: A Systematic Review and Meta-analysis of Paired-Biopsy Studies. *Clin. Gastroenterol. Hepatol.* **2015**, *13*, 643–654.e9. [CrossRef]
8. Kisseleva, T.; Brenner, D. Molecular and cellular mechanisms of liver fibrosis and its regression. *Nat. Rev. Gastroenterol. Hepatol.* **2021**, *18*, 151–166. [CrossRef] [PubMed]
9. Dulai, P.S.; Singh, S.; Patel, J.; Soni, M.; Prokop, L.J.; Younossi, Z.; Sebastiani, G.; Ekstedt, M.; Hagstrom, H.; Nasr, P.; et al. Increased risk of mortality by fibrosis stage in nonalcoholic fatty liver disease: Systematic review and meta-analysis. *Hepatology* **2017**, *65*, 1557–1565. [CrossRef]
10. Kim, D.; Kim, W.R.; Kim, H.J.; Therneau, T.M. Association between noninvasive fibrosis markers and mortality among adults with nonalcoholic fatty liver disease in the United States. *Hepatology* **2013**, *57*, 1357–1365. [CrossRef]
11. Simon, T.; Corey, K.; Cannon, C.; Blazing, M.; Park, J.; O'Donoghue, M.; Chung, R.; Giugliano, R. The nonalcoholic fatty liver disease (NAFLD) fibrosis score, cardiovascular risk stratification and a strategy for secondary prevention with ezetimibe. *Int. J. Cardiol.* **2018**, *270*, 245–252. [CrossRef] [PubMed]
12. Baratta, F.; Pastori, D.; Angelico, F.; Balla, A.; Paganini, A.M.; Cocomello, N.; Ferro, D.; Violi, F.; Sanyal, A.J.; del Ben, M. Nonalcoholic Fatty Liver Disease and Fibrosis Associated With Increased Risk of Cardiovascular Events in a Prospective Study. *Clin. Gastroenterol. Hepatol.* **2020**, *18*, 2324–2331.e4. [CrossRef]
13. Adams, L.A.; Sanderson, S.; Lindor, K.D.; Angulo, P. The histological course of nonalcoholic fatty liver disease: A longitudinal study of 103 patients with sequential liver biopsies. *J. Hepatol.* **2005**, *42*, 132–138. [CrossRef]
14. Koehler, E.M.; Plompen, E.P.C.; Schouten, J.N.L.; Hansen, B.E.; Darwish Murad, S.; Taimr, P.; Leebeek, F.W.G.; Hofman, A.; Stricker, B.H.; Castera, L.; et al. Presence of diabetes mellitus and steatosis is associated with liver stiffness in a general population: The Rotterdam study. *Hepatology* **2016**, *63*, 138–147. [CrossRef]
15. Bril, F.; Cusi, K. Management of Nonalcoholic Fatty Liver Disease in Patients with Type 2 Diabetes: A Call to Action. *Diabetes Care* **2017**, *40*, 419–430. [CrossRef] [PubMed]
16. Doycheva, I.; Cui, J.; Nguyen, P.; Costa, E.A.; Hooker, J.; Hofflich, H.; Bettencourt, R.; Brouha, S.; Sirlin, C.B.; Loomba, R. Non-invasive screening of diabetics in primary care for NAFLD and advanced fibrosis by MRI and MRE. *Aliment. Pharmacol. Ther.* **2016**, *43*, 83–95. [CrossRef]
17. McPherson, S.; Hardy, T.; Henderson, E.; Burt, A.D.; Day, C.P.; Anstee, Q.M. Evidence of NAFLD progression from steatosis to fibrosing-steatohepatitis using paired biopsies: Implications for prognosis and clinical management. *J. Hepatol.* **2015**, *62*, 1148–1155. [CrossRef] [PubMed]
18. Ekstedt, M.; Franzén, L.E.; Mathiesen, U.L.; Thorelius, L.; Holmqvist, M.; Bodemar, G.; Kechagias, S. Long-term follow-up of patients with NAFLD and elevated liver enzymes. *Hepatology* **2006**, *44*, 865–873. [CrossRef]
19. Liu, J.; Ayada, I.; Zhang, X.; Wang, L.; Li, Y.; Wen, T.; Ma, Z.; Bruno, M.J.; de Knegt, R.J.; Cao, W.; et al. Estimating global prevalence of metabolic dysfunction-associated fatty liver diseasein overweight or obese adults. *Clin. Gastroenterol. Hepatol.* **2021**, in press. [CrossRef]
20. Anstee, Q.M.; Targher, G.; Day, C.P. Progression of NAFLD to diabetes mellitus, cardiovascular disease or cirrhosis. *Nat. Rev. Gastroenterol. Hepatol.* **2013**, *10*, 330–344. [CrossRef] [PubMed]
21. Younossi, Z.M.; Golabi, P.; de Avila, L.; Paik, J.M.; Srishord, M.; Fukui, N.; Qiu, Y.; Burns, L.; Afendy, A.; Nader, F. The global epidemiology of NAFLD and NASH in patients with type 2 diabetes: A systematic review and meta-analysis. *J. Hepatol.* **2019**, *71*, 793–801. [CrossRef]
22. Public Health England. Public Health England Diabetes Statistics. Available online: https://fingertips.phe.org.uk/profile/diabetes-ft/data#page/0 (accessed on 1 November 2021).
23. European Association for the Study of the Liver (EASL); European Association for the Study of Diabetes (EASD); European Association for the Study of Obesity (EASO). EASL–EASD–EASO Clinical Practice Guidelines for the management of non-alcoholic fatty liver disease. *J. Hepatol.* **2016**, *64*, 1388–1402. [CrossRef] [PubMed]
24. Association, A.D. Comprehensive medical evaluation and assessment of comorbidities: Standards of Medical Care in Diabetes-2020. *Diabetes Care* **2020**, *43*, S37–S47. [CrossRef]
25. Chalasani, N.; Younossi, Z.; Lavine, J.E.; Charlton, M.; Cusi, K.; Rinella, M.; Harrison, S.A.; Brunt, E.M.; Sanyal, A.J. The diagnosis and management of nonalcoholic fatty liver disease: Practice guidance from the American Association for the Study of Liver Diseases. *Hepatology* **2018**, *67*, 328–357. [CrossRef]

26. Wong, V.W.S.; Chan, W.K.; Chitturi, S.; Chawla, Y.; Dan, Y.Y.; Duseja, A.; Fan, J.; Goh, K.L.; Hamaguchi, M.; Hashimoto, E.; et al. Asia–Pacific Working Party on Non-alcoholic Fatty Liver Disease guidelines 2017—Part 1: Definition, risk factors and assessment. *J. Gastroenterol. Hepatol.* **2018**, *33*, 70–85. [CrossRef] [PubMed]
27. National Guideline Centre (UK). *Non-Alcoholic Fatty Liver Disease (NAFLD): Assessment and Management*; National Institute for Health and Care Excellence: London, UK, 2016.
28. National Guideline Centre (UK). *Cirrhosis in over 16s: Assessment and Management*; National Institute for Health and Care Excellence: London, UK, 2016.
29. Sterling, R.K.; Lissen, E.; Clumeck, N.; Sola, R.; Correa, M.C.; Montaner, J.; Sulkowski, M.S.; Torriani, F.J.; Dieterich, D.T.; Thomas, D.L.; et al. Development of a simple noninvasive index to predict significant fibrosis in patients with HIV/HCV coinfection. *Hepatology* **2006**, *43*, 1317–1325. [CrossRef] [PubMed]
30. Wai, C.; Greenson, J.K.; Fontana, R.J.; Kalbfleisch, J.D.; Marrero, J.A.; Conjeevaram, H.S.; Lok, A.S.-F. A simple noninvasive index can predict both significant fibrosis and cirrhosis in patients with chronic hepatitis C. *Hepatology* **2003**, *38*, 518–526. [CrossRef]
31. Williams, A.L.; Hoofnagle, J.H. Ratio of serum aspartate to alanine aminotransferase in chronic hepatitis. Relationship to cirrhosis. *Gastroenterology* **1988**, *95*, 734–739. [CrossRef]
32. Lichtinghagen, R.; Pietsch, D.; Bantel, H.; Manns, M.P.; Brand, K.; Bahr, M.J. The Enhanced Liver Fibrosis (ELF) score: Normal values, influence factors and proposed cut-off values. *J. Hepatol.* **2013**, *59*, 236–242. [CrossRef] [PubMed]
33. Singh, A.; Le, P.; Peerzada, M.M.; Lopez, R.; Alkhouri, N. The Utility of Noninvasive Scores in Assessing the Prevalence of Nonalcoholic Fatty Liver Disease and Advanced Fibrosis in Type 2 Diabetic Patients. *J. Clin. Gastroenterol.* **2018**, *52*, 268–272. [CrossRef]
34. Lomonaco, R.; Leiva, E.G.; Bril, F.; Shrestha, S.; Mansour, L.; Budd, J.; Romero, J.P.; Schmidt, S.; Chang, K.-L.; Samraj, G.; et al. Advanced Liver Fibrosis Is Common in Patients With Type 2 Diabetes Followed in the Outpatient Setting: The Need for Systematic Screening. *Diabetes Care* **2021**, *44*, 399–406. [CrossRef]
35. Mansour, D.; Grapes, A.; Herscovitz, M.; Cassidy, P.; Vernazza, J.; Broad, A.; Anstee, Q.M.; McPherson, S. Embedding assessment of liver fibrosis into routine diabetic review in primary care. *JHEP Rep.* **2021**, *3*, 100293. [CrossRef] [PubMed]
36. Robertson, R.P.; Harmon, J.; Tran, P.O.T.; Poitout, V. β-cell glucose toxicity, lipotoxicity, and chronic oxidative stress in type 2 diabetes. *Diabetes* **2004**, *53* (Suppl. 1), S119–S124. [CrossRef] [PubMed]
37. Smith, G.I.; Shankaran, M.; Yoshino, M.; Schweitzer, G.G.; Chondronikola, M.; Beals, J.W.; Okunade, A.L.; Patterson, B.W.; Nyangau, E.; Field, T.; et al. Insulin resistance drives hepatic de novo lipogenesis in nonalcoholic fatty liver disease. *J. Clin. Investig.* **2020**, *130*, 1453–1460. [CrossRef] [PubMed]
38. Samuel, V.T.; Liu, Z.X.; Qu, X.; Elder, B.D.; Bilz, S.; Befroy, D.; Romanelli, A.J.; Shulman, G.I. Mechanism of hepatic insulin resistance in non-alcoholic fatty liver disease. *J. Biol. Chem.* **2004**, *279*, 32345–32353. [CrossRef] [PubMed]
39. Kantartzis, K.; MacHann, J.; Schick, F.; Fritsche, A.; Häring, H.U.; Stefan, N. The impact of liver fat vs visceral fat in determining categories of prediabetes. *Diabetologia* **2010**, *53*, 882–889. [CrossRef]
40. Lambert, J.E.; Ramos-Roman, M.A.; Browning, J.D.; Parks, E.J. Increased de novo lipogenesis is a distinct characteristic of individuals with nonalcoholic fatty liver disease. *Gastroenterology* **2014**, *146*, 726–735. [CrossRef]
41. Berzigotti, A.; Tsochatzis, E.; Boursier, J.; Castera, L.; Cazzagon, N.; Friedrich-Rust, M.; Petta, S.; Thiele, M. EASL Clinical Practice Guidelines on non-invasive tests for evaluation of liver disease severity and prognosis–2021 update. *J. Hepatol.* **2021**, *75*, 659–689. [CrossRef] [PubMed]
42. Rousseau, M.C.; Parent, M.É.; Pollak, M.N.; Siemiatycki, J. Diabetes mellitus and cancer risk in a population-based case-control study among men from Montreal, Canada. *Int. J. Cancer* **2006**, *118*, 2105–2109. [CrossRef]
43. Wang, P.; Kang, D.; Cao, W.; Wang, Y.; Liu, Z. Diabetes mellitus and risk of hepatocellular carcinoma: A systematic review and meta-analysis. *Diabetes. Metab. Res. Rev.* **2012**, *28*, 109–122. [CrossRef] [PubMed]
44. Vilar-Gomez, E.; Martinez-Perez, Y.; Calzadilla-Bertot, L.; Torres-Gonzalez, A.; Gra-Oramas, B.; Gonzalez-Fabian, L.; Friedman, S.L.; Diago, M.; Romero-Gomez, M. Weight Loss Through Lifestyle Modification Significantly Reduces Features of Nonalcoholic Steatohepatitis. *Gastroenterology* **2015**, *149*, 367–378.e5. [CrossRef]
45. Brown, E.; Hydes, T.; Hamid, A.; Cuthbertson, D. Emerging and Established Therapeutic Approaches for Nonalcoholic Fatty Liver Disease. *Clin. Ther.* **2021**, *43*, 1476–1504. [CrossRef] [PubMed]
46. Allen, A.M.; Hicks, S.B.; Mara, K.C.; Larson, J.J.; Therneau, T.M. The risk of incident extrahepatic cancers is higher in non-alcoholic fatty liver disease than obesity—A longitudinal cohort study. *J. Hepatol.* **2019**, *71*, 1229–1236. [CrossRef] [PubMed]
47. Cui, J.; Philo, L.; Nguyen, P.; Hofflich, H.; Hernandez, C.; Bettencourt, R.; Richards, L.; Salotti, J.; Bhatt, A.; Hooker, J.; et al. Sitagliptin vs. placebo for non-alcoholic fatty liver disease: A randomized controlled trial. *J. Hepatol.* **2016**, *65*, 369–376. [CrossRef] [PubMed]
48. Macauley, M.; Hollingsworth, K.G.; Smith, F.E.; Thelwall, P.E.; Al-Mrabeh, A.; Schweizer, A.; Foley, J.E.; Taylor, R. Effect of Vildagliptin on Hepatic Steatosis. *J. Clin. Endocrinol. Metab.* **2015**, *100*, 1578–1585. [CrossRef]
49. Cuthbertson, D.J.; Irwin, A.; Gardner, C.J.; Daousi, C.; Purewal, T.; Furlong, N.; Goenka, N.; Thomas, E.L.; Adams, V.L.; Pushpakom, S.P.; et al. Improved Glycaemia Correlates with Liver Fat Reduction in Obese, Type 2 Diabetes, Patients Given Glucagon-Like Peptide-1 (GLP-1) Receptor Agonists. *PLoS ONE* **2012**, *7*, e50117. [CrossRef] [PubMed]

50. Newsome, P.N.; Buchholtz, K.; Cusi, K.; Linder, M.; Okanoue, T.; Ratziu, V.; Sanyal, A.J.; Sejling, A.-S.; Harrison, S.A. A Placebo-Controlled Trial of Subcutaneous Semaglutide in Nonalcoholic Steatohepatitis. *N. Engl. J. Med.* **2021**, *384*, 1113–1124. [CrossRef]
51. Armstrong, M.J.; Houlihan, D.D.; Rowe, I.A.; Clausen, W.H.O.; Elbrønd, B.; Gough, S.C.L.; Tomlinson, J.W.; Newsome, P.N. Safety and efficacy of liraglutide in patients with type 2 diabetes and elevated liver enzymes: Individual patient data meta-analysis of the LEAD program. *Aliment. Pharmacol. Ther.* **2013**, *37*, 234–242. [CrossRef]
52. Sattar, N.; Fitchett, D.; Hantel, S.; George, J.T.; Zinman, B. Empagliflozin is associated with improvements in liver enzymes potentially consistent with reductions in liver fat: Results from randomised trials including the EMPA-REG OUTCOME® trial. *Diabetologia* **2018**, *61*, 2155–2163. [CrossRef]
53. Eriksson, J.W.; Lundkvist, P.; Jansson, P.-A.; Johansson, L.; Kvarnström, M.; Moris, L.; Miliotis, T.; Forsberg, G.-B.; Risérus, U.; Lind, L.; et al. Effects of dapagliflozin and n-3 carboxylic acids on non-alcoholic fatty liver disease in people with type 2 diabetes: A double-blind randomised placebo-controlled study. *Diabetologia* **2018**, *61*, 1923–1934. [CrossRef] [PubMed]
54. Grecian, S.M.; McLachlan, S.; Fallowfield, J.A.; Kearns, P.K.A.; Hayes, P.C.; Guha, N.I.; Morling, J.R.; Glancy, S.; Williamson, R.M.; Reynolds, R.M.; et al. Non-invasive risk scores do not reliably identify future cirrhosis or hepatocellular carcinoma in Type 2 diabetes: The Edinburgh type 2 diabetes study. *Liver Int.* **2020**, *40*, 2252–2262. [CrossRef] [PubMed]
55. Morling, J.R.; Fallowfield, J.A.; Guha, I.N.; Nee, L.D.; Glancy, S.; Williamson, R.M.; Robertson, C.M.; Strachan, M.W.J.; Price, J.F. Using non-invasive biomarkers to identify hepatic fibrosis in people with type 2 diabetes mellitus: The Edinburgh type 2 diabetes study. *J. Hepatol.* **2014**, *60*, 384–391. [CrossRef] [PubMed]

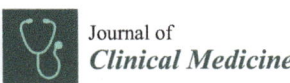

Article

Once-Weekly Semaglutide Use in Patients with Type 2 Diabetes: Results from the SURE Spain Multicentre, Prospective, Observational Study

Virginia Bellido [1,2,*], Cristina Abreu Padín [3], Andrei-Mircea Catarig [4], Alice Clark [4], Sofía Barreto Pittol [5] and Elias Delgado [6,7,8,9]

1. Unidad de Gestión Clínica de Endocrinología y Nutrición, Hospital Universitario Virgen del Rocío, 41013 Sevilla, Spain
2. Instituto de Biomedicina de Sevilla (IBiS), Hospital Universitario Virgen del Rocío, CSIC, Universidad de Sevilla, 41013 Sevilla, Spain
3. Hospital General de Segovia, 47002 Segovia, Spain
4. Novo Nordisk A/S, DK-2760 Søborg, Denmark
5. Novo Nordisk Pharma SA, 28033 Madrid, Spain
6. Department of Endocrinology and Nutrition, Hospital Universitario Central de Asturias (HUCA), 33011 Oviedo, Spain
7. Department of Medicine, University of Oviedo, 33006 Oviedo, Spain
8. Health Research Institute of the Principality of Asturias (ISPA), 33011 Oviedo, Spain
9. Spanish Biomedical Research Network in Rare Diseases (CIBERER), 28029 Madrid, Spain
* Correspondence: virginiabellido@gmail.com

Abstract: Type 2 diabetes (T2D) is a complex disease for which an individualised treatment approach is recommended. Once-weekly (OW) semaglutide is a glucagon-like peptide-1 receptor agonist approved for the treatment of insufficiently controlled T2D. The aim of this study was to investigate the use of OW semaglutide in adults with T2D in a real-world context. SURE Spain, from the 10-country SURE programme, was a prospective, multicentre, open-label, observational study, approximately 30 weeks in duration. Adults with T2D and ≥1 documented HbA_{1c} value ≤12 weeks before semaglutide initiation were enrolled. Change in HbA_{1c} from baseline to end of study (EOS) was the primary endpoint, with change in body weight (BW), waist circumference, and patient-reported outcomes as secondary endpoints. Of the 227 patients initiating semaglutide, 196 (86.3%) completed the study on-treatment with semaglutide. The estimated mean changes in HbA_{1c} and body weight between baseline and EOS were −1.3%-points (95% confidence interval (CI) −1.51;−1.18%-points) and −5.7 kg (95% CI −6.36;−4.98 kg). No new safety concerns were identified. Therefore, in routine clinical practice in Spain, OW semaglutide was shown to be associated with statistically significant and clinically relevant reductions in HbA_{1c} and BW in adults with T2D.

Keywords: body weight; glucagon-like peptide-1 receptor agonist; HbA_{1c}; real-world evidence; semaglutide; SURE study; type 2 diabetes

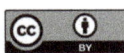

1. Introduction

Type 2 diabetes (T2D) places a heavy burden on individuals and healthcare systems across the world. In Spain, an estimated 13.8% of people have T2D, and this is expected to increase in the future [1,2].

The management of T2D is complex. The American Diabetes Association (ADA) Standards of Medical Care in Diabetes 2022 [3] and the 2020 joint consensus statement of the ADA and the European Association for the Study of Diabetes (EASD) [4] recommend that physicians should take an individualised treatment approach when prescribing medications for T2D, and that they consider drug efficacy, risk of hypoglycaemia, cardiorenal benefits, effect on body weight (BW), adverse effects, pricing, and convenience for the patient [4].

Glucagon-like peptide-1 receptor agonists (GLP-1RAs) are an established class of antihyperglycaemic drugs used for the treatment of T2D, which have demonstrated improvements in glycaemic control and reductions in BW in patients with T2D [5,6]. In addition to their glucose-dependent function resulting in a low risk for hypoglycaemia [7], some GLP-1RAs (dulaglutide, liraglutide, and semaglutide) have demonstrated cardiovascular (CV) benefits in patients with T2D at high risk of CV disease [8–10]. Despite these benefits, access to GLP-1RAs is limited in Spain, and GLP-1RAs are only reimbursed for patients with obesity (body mass index [BMI] $\geq$ 30 kg/m^2) and insufficient glycaemic control as a second-line therapy after metformin [11].

Semaglutide is a human GLP-1 analogue, approved as an add-on to diet and exercise for the treatment of adults with insufficiently controlled T2D, by the European Medicines Agency in February 2018 [12]. It has a long half-life, which makes it suitable for once-weekly (OW) dosing, [13] and is the only GLP-1RA that is available both in a OW subcutaneous (s.c.) injectable formulation and as an oral formulation administered once-daily [14].

The extensive SUSTAIN randomised clinical trial (RCT) programme, which investigated the efficacy and safety of OW s.c. semaglutide, demonstrated that 0.5 mg and 1.0 mg doses were associated with superior, clinically relevant improvements in glycaemic control and weight loss, compared with placebo or active comparators [8,15–23]. A safety profile similar to other GLP-1RAs was also observed.

SURE Spain is part of the SURE real-world study programme, which aimed to explore the use of OW semaglutide in a diverse population of adults with T2D in routine, real-world clinical practice across 10 countries (Canada, Denmark/Sweden, France, Germany, Italy, the Netherlands, Spain, Switzerland, and the United Kingdom) and to complement the results of the SUSTAIN RCTs. Unlike RCTs, the SURE studies are non-interventional and observational, allowing the assessment of patient outcomes, as well as product use and performance, in diverse patient populations in routine clinical practice [24].

The aim of this study was to evaluate the real-world use of OW semaglutide in a diverse T2D patient population in Spain.

2. Materials and Methods

2.1. Study Design

SURE Spain was a multicentre, prospective open-label, single-arm, non-interventional study assessing the use of OW semaglutide in adult patients with T2D in routine clinical practice in Spain. Informed consent and treatment initiation took place on the first visit (week 0), followed by an anticipated exposure period of ~30 weeks (range: 28–38 weeks). Intermediate visits scheduled according to local practice and data collection were performed throughout the entire study.

The decision to initiate semaglutide treatment was at the discretion of the treating physician, following requirements stated in the Summary of Product Characteristics (SmPC), therapeutic positioning report and local/regional guidelines, and clearly separated from the decision to include the patient in the SURE Spain study. All parameters collected in the study (except the patient-reported outcomes) were part of routine clinical practice. Patients were treated OW with commercially available s.c. semaglutide (Ozempic®; Novo Nordisk A/S, Bagsværd, Denmark), available in a pre-filled, multidose, pen injector. The treating physician determined the maintenance dose and any subsequent changes to it. Diet and physical activity counselling could be offered in line with routine clinical practice, with modifications to prescribed antihyperglycaemic treatment at the physician's discretion.

This study was conducted in accordance with the Declaration of Helsinki [25], the Guidelines for Pharmacovigilance Practices Module VI [26], and Good Pharmacoepidemiology Practices [27]. Prior to study initiation, the protocol, protocol amendment, patient information/informed consent form, together with any other written information to be provided to the patient and patient enrolment procedures, were reviewed and approved by the independent ethics committee/institutional review board at each study site (first approved in 2019 by the Ethics Committee of CEIm de EUSkadi, project identifier:

NN9535-4368). Written informed consent was obtained from all patients prior to any study-related activities. This study is registered on ClinicalTrials.gov (NCT04067999).

2.2. Study Population

Adult patients (age ≥ 18 years) diagnosed with T2D were included from 34 sites in Spain, with the first participant's first visit on 5 August 2019, and the last participant's last visit on 19 July 2021. Inclusion criteria included diagnosis of T2D and availability of one or more documented values of HbA_{1c} within 12 weeks prior to semaglutide treatment initiation. Exclusion criteria included previous participation in a SURE study, mental incapacity, unwillingness, or language barriers precluding adequate understanding or cooperation, prior treatment with any investigational drug (90 days before enrolment), and hypersensitivity to semaglutide or any of the excipients. The study duration of 30 weeks was considered sufficient to initiate and optimise the study treatment regimen and to obtain real-world data for the evaluation of the primary endpoint.

2.3. Endpoints

The primary endpoint was a change from baseline to end of study (EOS) in HbA_{1c} (%-point and mmol/mol). Supportive secondary endpoints included: change from baseline to EOS in BW (kg and %) and waist circumference (cm); proportion of patients achieving HbA_{1c} < 8.0% (64 mmol/mol), <7.5% (59 mmol/mol) and <7.0% (53 mmol/mol) [28]; reduction in HbA_{1c} from baseline to EOS of ≥1.0%-point; weight reduction from baseline to EOS of ≥3.0% [29] and ≥5.0%; HbA_{1c} reduction from baseline to EOS of ≥1.0% and weight reduction from baseline to EOS of ≥3.0% [29]; patient-reported severe or documented hypoglycaemia between baseline and EOS; and change from baseline to EOS in scores for patient-reported outcomes of: the Diabetes Treatment Satisfaction Questionnaire–status (DTSQs; absolute treatment satisfaction) comprising eight questions, of which six questions are combined into a total Treatment Satisfaction score (scale: 0 to 36); the Diabetes Treatment Satisfaction Questionnaire–change (DTSQc; relative treatment satisfaction), total treatment satisfaction (scale: −18.0 to 18.0); and the 36-item Short-Form Health Survey version 2 (SF-36®v2), physical and mental summary component. The proportion of patients who completed the study under treatment with semaglutide was also investigated.

Exploratory assessments included: weekly dose of semaglutide at EOS; proportion of patients who had not added new antihyperglycaemic drug(s) to semaglutide treatment at any time during the study, evaluated at EOS; proportion of patients who had achieved clinical success, in relation to the reason to initiate semaglutide treatment, as assessed by the physician at EOS; patient-reported 8-Item Morisky Medication Adherence Scale (MMAS-8) score at EOS (low, medium, high) [30–32]; and the number of severe or documented hypoglycaemic episodes. Post hoc assessments included change from baseline to EOS in BMI (kg/m^2). Permission for use of the MMAS-8 was granted prior to the study.

2.4. Safety

Only information on serious adverse drug reactions (SADRs), fatal events, pregnancies in female patients, and adverse events (AEs) in foetuses or newborns were systematically collected during the study. Voluntary reporting of other safety information by the physician followed the same process as for the systematic safety reporting. All episodes of patient-reported documented and/or severe hypoglycaemia were to be recorded.

2.5. Statistical Analyses

Power calculations showed that a sample size of 130 patients was required, based on the criterion of 90% probability of obtaining a 95% confidence interval (CI) for mean change from baseline in HbA_{1c} whose half-width was at most 0.30. The half-width of 0.30 was chosen as a reasonable uncertainty allowing for a robust evaluation of glycaemic efficacy, in line with diabetes guidelines [33]. To ensure sufficient statistical power to evaluate the efficacy of semaglutide on glycaemic control (on the basis of evidence from previous observational studies with GLP-1RA treatment), it was necessary to include at least 217 enrolled patients initiating semaglutide, to ensure that 130 patients completed the study on-treatment [34,35].

The Full Analysis Set (FAS), which included all patients in the study who initiated semaglutide treatment, was used for characterising baseline demographics, analysis of the secondary endpoint related to study completion on-treatment, the selected exploratory assessments, description of AEs, and the sensitivity analyses of the primary and secondary endpoints.

The Effectiveness Analysis Set (EAS) included all patients in the FAS who completed the study and were receiving semaglutide treatment at EOS. The EAS was used for characterising baseline demographics at EOS, the description of antihyperglycaemic medications at baseline and EOS, and the primary, secondary and exploratory endpoint analyses.

Baseline demographic data are summarised using descriptive statistics (mean ± standard deviation [SD] or median and interquartile range for continuous variables and number and proportion for categorical variables). Change in the continuous variables of the primary and secondary endpoints from baseline to EOS were analysed using the Analysis of Covariance (ANCOVA) model. Categorical endpoints were analysed using descriptive statistics.

Sensitivity analyses investigated the robustness of the conclusions from the main analyses and explored the impact of missing data in the primary analysis, for which patients were excluded if they did not complete the study or discontinued treatment, or if HbA_{1c} data were missing at EOS. The prespecified in-study sensitivity analysis of the primary endpoint included all patients in the FAS with at least one post-baseline HbA_{1c} measurement in the in-study period. For this analysis, the primary endpoint was analysed using a Mixed Model for Repeated Measures (MMRM) including all HbA_{1c} assessments in the in-study period. The on-treatment sensitivity analysis included patients in the FAS with at least one post-baseline HbA_{1c} assessment, but it only included HbA_{1c} assessments in the on-treatment period and used the same statistical approach as the in-study sensitivity analysis.

Because of the COVID-19 pandemic, the EOS visit (V6) window was extended beyond 38 weeks to allow participants to complete their EOS assessments. Consequently, an additional post hoc sensitivity analysis was performed to explore the impact of extending the EOS visit (V6) window on the primary endpoint. The sensitivity analysis of the primary endpoint was the same as the primary analysis of the primary endpoint but included only those patients who had an EOS visit between weeks 28 and 38 (the original visit window). An additional post hoc sensitivity analysis was performed to explore the impact of extending the EOS visit on the secondary endpoint of change from baseline to EOS in BW. This sensitivity analysis was the same as the main analysis of this endpoint but included only those patients who had an EOS visit between weeks 28 and 38.

3. Results

3.1. Patient Population and Baseline Characteristics

Of the 228 patients who signed the consent form, one did not meet the eligibility criteria. Therefore, the FAS comprised the 227 patients who were enrolled in the study and who had initiated semaglutide treatment (Figure 1). A total of 210 patients (92.5%) completed the study, and the mean treatment duration was 33.7 weeks. The reasons for non-completion were: death (n = 1; 0.4%), lost to follow-up (n = 3; 1.3%), withdrawal by patient (n = 3; 1.3%), and missed EOS visit within the visit window (n = 10; 4.4%) (Figure 1). The EAS comprised 196 patients (86.3%) who had completed the study on semaglutide treatment (Figure 1). Twelve patients (5.2% of the FAS) had an unknown treatment status at EOS. With regard to discontinuations, 16 patients (7.0%) discontinued treatment due to unacceptable gastrointestinal (GI) intolerability, and a further three patients (1.3%) had 'other' recorded as the reason (Figure 1).

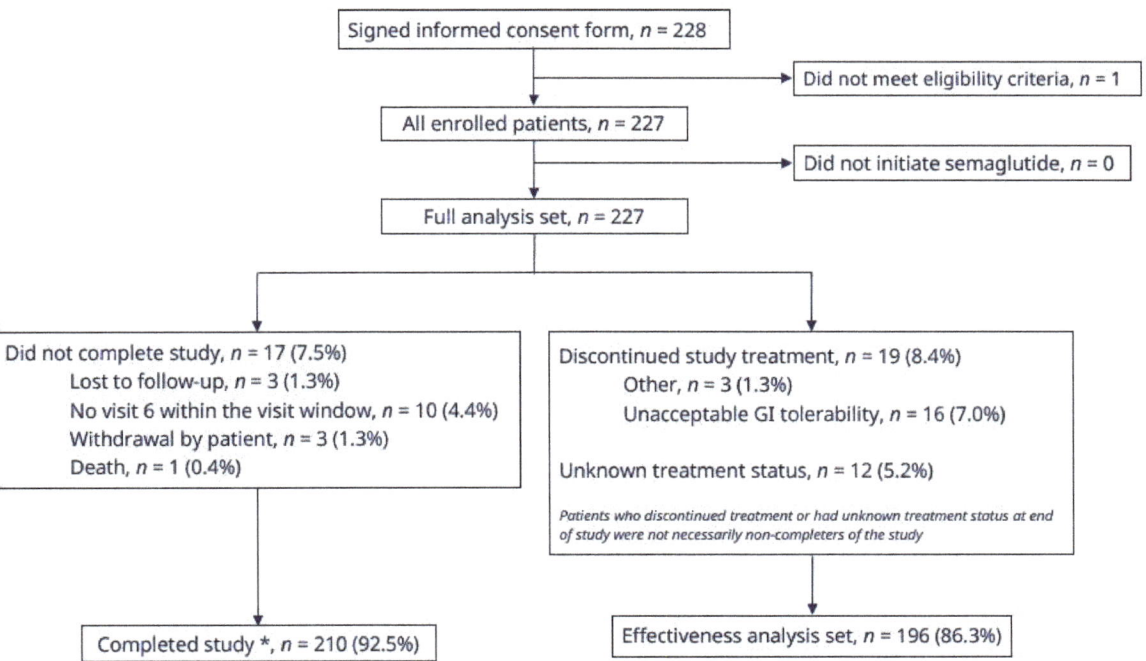

Figure 1. Patient disposition. * Patients who initiated semaglutide treatment and attended the end of study visit. GI, gastrointestinal.

Baseline characteristics of patients are summarised in Table 1. Hypertension and dyslipidaemia were the most frequent CV comorbidities at baseline, affecting 75.8% and 76.2% of patients, respectively.

Most patients initiated semaglutide at a dose of 0.25 mg (83.3%); 13.7% initiated at 0.5 mg and 3.1% at 1.0 mg. The most common reasons for initiating semaglutide as part of T2D treatment were weight reduction (94.3%) and to improve glycaemic control (88.5%).

The most frequent antihyperglycaemic drugs used by patients in the EAS at baseline were metformin (75.5% of patients), sodium–glucose cotransporter-2 inhibitors (SGLT-2is) (42.3%), basal insulin (32.7%), and dipeptidyl peptidase-4 inhibitors (DPP-4is) (20.4%) (Supplementary Table S1).

3.2. HbA_{1c}, BW, BMI, and Waist Circumference Outcomes

For patients in the EAS receiving semaglutide, statistically significant reductions were observed at EOS for mean HbA_{1c}, BW, waist circumference and BMI (Table 2). The mean HbA_{1c} at EOS was 7.1%, and the estimated mean change from baseline was -1.3%-points [95% CI $-1.51; -1.18$%-points; $p < 0.0001$] (Table 2, Supplementary Figure S1); mean BW at EOS was 93.2 kg, and the estimated mean change from baseline was -5.7 kg [95% CI $-6.36; -4.98$ kg; $p < 0.0001$] (Table 2, Supplementary Figure S1); mean BMI at EOS was 34.4 kg/m^2, and the estimated mean change from baseline was -2.1 kg/m^2 [95% CI $-2.37; -1.86$ kg/m^2; $p < 0.0001$]; and mean waist circumference at EOS was 113.4 cm, and the estimated mean change from baseline to EOS was -5.3 cm [95% CI $-6.29; -4.41$ cm; $p < 0.0001$] (Table 2, Supplementary Figure S1).

Table 1. Baseline characteristics of patients (FAS).

	N	227
	Age, years	59.1 (9.94)
	Female, n (%)	111 (48.9)
Race, n (%)		
	White	221 (97.4)
	American Indian or Alaska Native	2 (0.9)
	Other	4 (1.8)
	Body weight, kg	98.3 (17.89)
	Waist circumference, cm	118.8 (12.50)
	BMI, kg/m^2	36.4 (5.28)
BMI categories, n (%)		
	Normal (18.5–<25 kg/m^2)	0
	Overweight (25–<30 kg/m^2)	12 (5.3)
	Obese class I (30–<35 kg/m^2)	89 (39.6)
	Obese class II & III ($\geq$35 kg/m^2)	124 (55.1)
	Diabetes duration, years	11.8 (8.10)
	Baseline HbA$_{1c}$, %	8.5 (1.58)
HbA$_{1c}$ level, n (%)		
	<8.0%	93 (41.0)
	<7.5%	62 (27.3)
	<7.0%	34 (15.0)
	Baseline HbA$_{1c}$, mmol/L	69.1 (17.3)
	FPG, mmol/L	9.9 (3.46)
	eGFR, mL/min/1.73 m^2	82.4 (22.58)
Lipid composition, mg/dL		
	HDL cholesterol	44.8 (13.31)
	LDL cholesterol	92.5 (30.76)
	Total cholesterol	175.7 (45.41)
	Triglycerides	243.9 (298.8)
Lipid composition, mmol/L		
	HDL cholesterol	1.2 (0.34)
	LDL cholesterol	2.4 (0.80)
	Total cholesterol	4.6 (1.18)
	Triglycerides	2.8 (3.37)
Comorbid conditions at baseline, n (%)		
	Diabetic retinopathy	29 (12.9)
	Diabetic neuropathy	18 (7.9)
	Diabetic nephropathy	38 (16.7)
	Dyslipidaemia	173 (76.2)
	Hypertension	172 (75.8)

Values based on FAS (n = 227). Data for continuous variables are mean (SD) unless otherwise specified. BMI, body mass index; eGFR, estimated glomerular filtration rate; FAS, Full Analysis Set; FPG, fasting plasma glucose; HDL, high-density lipoprotein; LDL, low-density lipoprotein; SD, standard deviation.

At EOS, 81.0%, 67.7% and 54.0% of patients in the EAS had an HbA$_{1c}$ of < 8.0%, <7.5% and <7.0%, respectively (Figure 2). The proportion of patients achieving an HbA$_{1c}$ reduction $\geq$1%-point was 56.6% and the proportions achieving weight reduction of $\geq$ 3.0% and $\geq$5.0% were, respectively, 69.2% and 49.7% (Figure 2). The proportion of patients in the EAS achieving the composite endpoint of an HbA$_{1c}$ reduction of $\geq$ 1.0% and weight reduction $\geq$3.0% at EOS was 44.3% (Figure 2). In the FAS, 86.3% of patients completed the study on-treatment with semaglutide (Figure 1).

3.3. Sensitivity Analyses

Prespecified sensitivity analyses were used to explore the impact of missing data in the main analysis. The on-treatment sensitivity analysis of the FAS showed that the mean HbA$_{1c}$ decreased over time from initiation of semaglutide to week 30, with an estimated change of −1.4%-points [95% CI −1.59; −1.27%-points] (Supplementary Figure S2). The estimated mean changes from baseline to EOS and associated 95% CIs were similar across sensitivity analyses and showed that the mean changes in HbA_{1c} were statistically significantly different from having no mean change in HbA_{1c} (Supplementary Table S2, Supplementary Figure S2). Moreover, the estimated mean HbA_{1c} and estimated change in HbA_{1c} were similar over the course of the study for both the in-study and on-treatment period.

Table 2. Change from baseline to EOS in HbA_{1c}, body weight, waist circumference, and BMI (EAS).

	N	n	Estimate	95% CI	p-Value
HbA_{1c}, %	196	187	-	-	-
Observed mean at baseline	-	-	8.4	-	-
Estimated mean at EOS	-	-	7.1	-	-
Change from baseline to EOS	-	-	−1.3	[−1.51; −1.18]	<0.0001
HbA_{1c}, mmol/mol	196	187	-	-	-
Observed mean at baseline	-	-	68.5	-	-
Estimated mean at EOS	-	-	53.8	-	-
Change from baseline to EOS	-	-	−14.7	[−16.48; −12.86]	<0.0001
Body weight, kg	196	194	-	-	-
Observed mean at baseline	-	-	98.9	-	-
Estimated mean at EOS	-	-	93.2	-	-
Change from baseline to EOS	-	-	−5.7	[−6.36; −4.98]	<0.0001
Percent change from baseline to EOS	-	-	−5.7	[−6.41; −5.03]	<0.0001
Waist circumference, cm	196	165	-	-	-
Observed mean at baseline	-	-	118.8	-	-
Estimated mean at EOS	-	-	113.4	-	-
Change from baseline to EOS	-	-	−5.3	[−6.29; −4.41]	<0.0001
BMI, kg/m^2	196	194	-	-	-
Observed mean at baseline	-	-	36.5	-	-
Estimated mean at EOS	-	-	34.4	-	-
Change from baseline to EOS	-	-	−2.1	[−2.37; −1.86]	<0.0001

Data are based on the EAS, which included patients who attended the EOS visit and were still receiving semaglutide. Change in response from baseline to EOS is analysed using baseline, T2D duration, age, BMI, pre-initiation use of GLP-1RA, pre-initiation use of DPP-4i, pre-initiation use of insulin, number of OADs used pre-initiation (0–1/2+) and sex as covariates. p-value is reported for no average change in response from baseline to EOS. The assessment of BMI was performed as a post hoc analysis. BMI, body mass index; CI, confidence interval; DPP-4i, dipeptidyl peptidase-4 inhibitor; EAS, Effectiveness Analysis Set; EOS, end of study; GLP-1RA, glucagon-like peptide-1 receptor agonist; N, total number of patients in EAS; n, total number of patients included in analyses; OAD, oral antihyperglycaemic drug; T2D, type 2 diabetes.

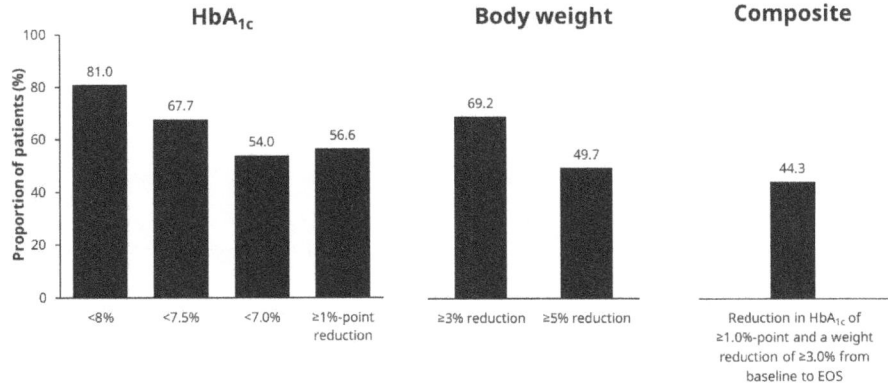

Figure 2. Proportion of patients achieving HbA_{1c} targets and weight-loss goals (EAS). EAS, Effectiveness Analysis Set; EOS, end of study.

Additional post hoc sensitivity analyses were performed in patients who had their EOS visit within the original visit window (week 28–38). The post hoc analyses of the mean changes from baseline to EOS for HbA_{1c} and for BW showed similar results to those seen in the primary analysis (Supplementary Table S3).

Collectively, the sensitivity analyses supported the conclusions from the primary analysis, which included assessments for patients who were on-treatment at the EOS visit (V6), also including those completing the study after week 38.

3.4. Semaglutide Dose

The mean ± SD weekly dose of semaglutide at EOS was 0.85 ± 0.24 mg. At EOS, five (2.6%) patients were receiving 0.25 mg OW semaglutide, 50 (25.5%) were receiving 0.5 mg, two (1.0%) were receiving between >0.5 mg and <1.0 mg, and 139 (70.9%) were receiving 1.0 mg.

3.5. Patient-Reported Outcomes

In patients receiving semaglutide at EOS, DTSQs score increased by 4.4 [95% CI 3.66; 5.07; $p < 0.0001$] from baseline to EOS, representing a significant increase in absolute treatment satisfaction (Figure 3). Patients receiving semaglutide also reported a DTSQc score at EOS of 13.1 (95% CI 12.36; 13.85) out of a maximum score of 18, indicating a significant relative improvement in treatment satisfaction ($p < 0.0001$) (Figure 3).

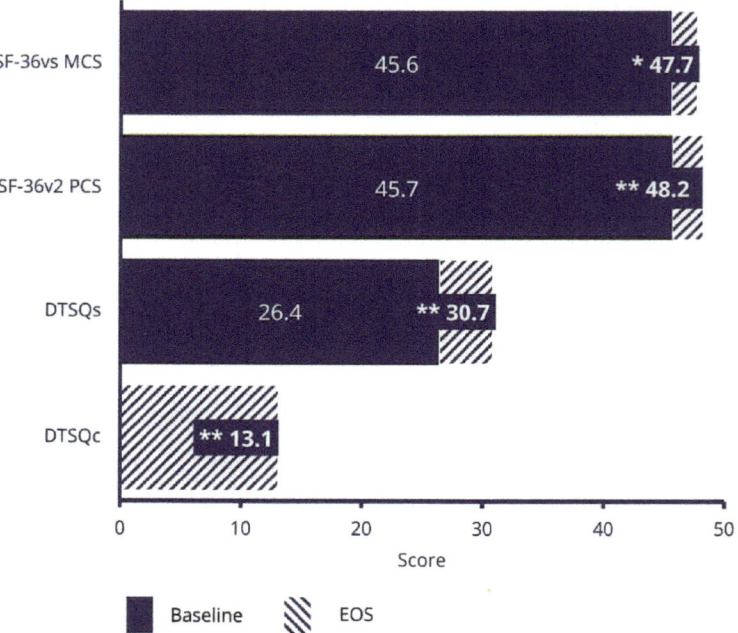

Figure 3. Treatment satisfaction and HRQoL (EAS). * $p = 0.0013$; ** $p < 0.0001$. Data are based on EAS. DTSQ status version (DTSQs) was measured at the informed consent and initiation visit, and the EOS visit; with responses ranging from 0 (very dissatisfied) to 6 (very satisfied) for each item of the questionnaire. The maximum total score is 36. The SF-36®v2 questionnaire has 36 questions grouped into eight domains, which can be combined into two summary component scores (overall mental and physical health); a higher SF-36®v2 score indicates lower disability. DTSQ, Diabetes Treatment Satisfaction Questionnaire; DTSQc, DTSQ change version; DTSQs, DTSQ status version; EAS, Effectiveness Analysis Set; EOS, end of study; HRQoL, health-related quality of life; MCS, mental component summary; PCS, physical component summary; SF-36®v2, 36-Item Short-Form Health Survey version 2.

At EOS, significant increases were observed in both the SF-36®v2 health-related quality-of life (HRQoL) questionnaire physical component score ($p < 0.0001$) and the mental component score ($p = 0.0013$), indicating an improvement in quality of life from baseline to EOS (Figure 3).

Mean MMAS-8 score was 7.0 at baseline and 7.4 at EOS, indicating a medium level of treatment adherence. The proportion of participants with medium and high adherence was, respectively, 49.5% and 36.6% at baseline and 34.1% and 57.3% at EOS.

3.6. Adverse Events and Hypoglycaemia

AEs and severe or documented hypoglycaemic episodes in patients receiving semaglutide are summarised in Table 3. In the FAS, 15 patients (6.6%) reported 26 treatment-emergent AEs: 88.5% of AEs were non-serious (13 [5.7%] patients; 23 events) and 46.2% were moderate in intensity (7 [3.1%] patients; 12 events). A total of 13 patients reported 22 GI AEs, which accounted for the highest number of AEs by system organ class. Three serious AEs (SAEs) were reported (Medical Dictionary for Regulatory Activities preferred terms: atrial fibrillation, left ventricular failure, and myocardial infarction) by two patients (0.9%), which were all judged as unlikely to be related to semaglutide treatment by the investigators. One severe SAE (preferred term: myocardial infarction) was reported, which had a fatal outcome.

Table 3. AEs and severe or documented hypoglycaemic episodes in patients receiving semaglutide (FAS).

	Serious			Non-Serious			Total		
	N	(%)	E	N	(%)	E	N	(%)	E
AE	2	0.9	3	13	5.7	23	15	6.6	26
Severity									
Mild	0	0	0	6	2.6	12	6	2.6	12
Moderate	1	0.4	2	6	2.6	10	7	3.1	12
Severe	1	0.4	1	1	0.4	1	2	0.9	2
GI disorders	0	0	0	13	5.7	22	13	5.7	22
Nausea	0	0	0	7	3.1	7	7	3.1	7
Vomiting	0	0	0	5	2.2	5	5	2.2	5
Diarrhoea	0	0	0	3	1.3	3	3	1.3	3
AEs leading to treatment discontinuation	0	0	0	5	2.2	6	5	2.2	6
SADRs	0	0	0	0	0	0	0	0	0
							N	(%)	
Patients with severe or documented hypoglycaemic episodes							8	4.1	

All other events were reported on a voluntary basis (FAS). AE, adverse event; E, event; FAS, Full Analysis Set; GI, gastrointestinal; N, total number of patients in FAS; SADR, serious adverse drug reaction.

Eight patients (4.1%) in the EAS reported severe or documented hypoglycaemia episodes between baseline and EOS, with similar results in the FAS (12 patients; 5.3%). At EOS, 20 severe or documented hypoglycaemic episodes were reported in the EAS, and 26 were reported in the FAS. Of these 26 events, 22 were reported by patients while using insulin and 3 occurred while using sulphonylureas. The date of one hypoglycaemic episode was unrecorded, which prevented an assessment of concurrent medication use. No severe hypoglycaemic episodes were reported during the study.

4. Discussion

The SURE Spain study is part of the SURE study programme, which consists of nine observational studies in ten countries and was conducted to assess the real-world use of OW semaglutide.

The data reported indicate that when OW s.c. semaglutide was taken according to local clinical practice by adult patients with T2D in Spain, a clinically relevant and statistically significant reduction, compared with baseline, was observed for HbA_{1c} at EOS ($p < 0.0001$) [36]. This was observed despite 14.5% of the study population switching from another GLP-1RA to semaglutide at baseline. While previous treatment may be expected to influence outcomes, improvements have been reported in patients treated with semaglutide who were not naïve to GLP-1RAs [36].

At EOS, patients also experienced statistically significant decreases from baseline in BW and waist circumference. A total of 97 (49.7%) patients achieved a weight reduction from baseline of ≥5%. This weight reduction is a key consideration in terms of reducing CV risk, in view of the beneficial reductions in triglycerides, total cholesterol, and low-density lipoprotein cholesterol that are associated with a weight loss of 5–10% [37].

Furthermore, patients reported substantial improvements in treatment satisfaction and HRQoL, as measured by the DTSQ and the SF-36®v2, respectively. In addition, patients' adherence to OW semaglutide treatment was good, with 91.4% of patients reporting either high (57.3%) or medium (34.1%) adherence at EOS. Adherence to OW semaglutide in the SURE Spain study compares favourably to the adherence rates of 39.1–64.5% at 1 year reported for GLP-1RAs (including semaglutide) in retrospective, real-world cohort studies [37,38].

Additionally, the patient population in this study had advanced T2D, as indicated by the mean disease duration of 11.8 years from diagnosis and the complex pharmacological treatment at baseline, with 41.9% of patients taking more than two antihyperglycaemic medications and 47.5% taking insulin. These factors are associated with poorer treatment outcomes and make it more difficult to achieve treatment goals.

Drawing comparisons between GLP-1RA RCTs and real-world evidence studies from different countries can be challenging. Local T2D clinical guidelines vary and can restrict clinical access to GLP-1RAs, while local reimbursement policies may impose further barriers to patient access. In Spain, outside of private practice, GLP-1RAs are only reimbursed for patients with a BMI ≥ 30 kg/m². This is in contrast with Denmark, where the recommendation is independent of BMI, and the UK, where use is recommended in those with a BMI ≥ 35 kg/m² who show an adequate metabolic response.

Overall, the results of this study support previously reported data on the real-world use of OW semaglutide in Spain [39–41]. The reduction in HbA_{1c} and BW observed in Spain align with those observed in the countries that have published results from the SURE programme to date—Canada, Denmark/Sweden, Switzerland, and the UK—for which the mean change in HbA_{1c} from baseline to EOS was between −0.8 and −1.5%-points and the mean change in BW from baseline to EOS was between −4.3 and −5.8 kg [42–45]. The results are also aligned with real-world evidence from other countries, for example, a study by Marzullo et al., that showed reductions in HbA1c and body weight after 6 and 12 months of OW semaglutide treatment in people with T2D in Italy [46].

Metabolic control in patients with T2D is assessed using multiple factors (e.g., BW, waist circumference), and not only HbA_{1c}. In SURE Spain, the majority (70.9%) of patients were receiving the recommended dose of 1.0 mg OW of semaglutide by EOS, and the significant improvements in primary and secondary endpoints in the study may indicate that this dose is appropriate for the goal of achieving global metabolic control. The safety findings of the real-world T2D population in Spain were also consistent with the safety profile of semaglutide established in the SUSTAIN programme and with that of the GLP-1RA class, with no unexpected safety issues reported.

Study Limitations

The SURE Spain study was non-interventional and single-armed, so the potential impact of other predictive factors cannot be excluded. The fundamental limitation of such a study design is the absence of a randomised comparator, which would otherwise have enabled differentiation of the changes caused by treatment, and the impact of other factors. Data in this study were collected during routine clinical practice, rather than through mandated examinations at predetermined time points, which may have impacted the robustness and completeness of the dataset.

The primary analysis was based on data from patients who completed the study on semaglutide treatment and with their HbA_{1c} levels recorded at EOS. This could have resulted in selection bias, because patients who benefit from the study treatment are more likely to continue than those who do not. To account for this, sensitivity analyses of the primary endpoint included all post-baseline HbA_{1c} assessments as well as evaluations from intermediate visits also including patients who did not complete the study or discontinued semaglutide during the study. In addition, secondary supportive analyses assessed the percentage of patients who had started semaglutide treatment and were receiving it at the EOS.

The inclusion criteria were purposely designed to be broad and reflect a real-world T2D population, which is rarely the case in a standard RCT. However, it is likely that physicians who were highly motivated would have been overrepresented among the participating centres, and that the centres included either highly motivated patients or patients who were difficult to treat with the other therapies available. As a result, the enrolled group may only represent subsets of individuals who are eligible for semaglutide therapy. Nevertheless, study participants were profiled in terms of demographics and clinical data, which allowed for the assessment of the representativeness of the recruited population. Details of medical history (including T2D diagnosis) and concurrent diseases were obtained without further confirmation as provided by the investigators.

A potential limitation of SURE Spain is the study's geographical location and time of initiation. The study was conducted soon after the launch of OW semaglutide, in a real-world setting, in a diverse T2D population recruited by investigators at 34 sites in Spain. However, the 34 sites that enrolled patients account for approximately half of the communities/regions within Spain, so may not be representative of the entire population. Furthermore, in Spain, GLP-1RAs are only reimbursed for patients who have a $BMI \geq 30$ kg/m^2, and only approximately 8% of Spanish patients with T2D are prescribed GLP-1RAs [11,47]. Therefore, none of the patients enrolled in the study had a 'normal' BMI (≥ 18.5–<25 kg/m^2). These country-specific factors may have influenced the study results; in the future, however, semaglutide will likely be prescribed to a broader range of patients with T2D, including those with less severe disease progression.

The COVID-19 pandemic impacted intermediate and EOS visits in SURE Spain. Because of accessibility issues, several of these visits were instead conducted by telephone, rather than in-person. To further mitigate the challenges raised by the pandemic, changes were made to the study design that allowed patients to postpone their last visit (after the 38-week timepoint). An additional post hoc sensitivity analysis was performed to assess how the primary and secondary endpoints were affected by extending the EOS visit window. Extending the EOS visit window had no impact on the study outcomes.

Evidence has been reported that patients with T2D in Spain may have gained weight during the COVID-19 lockdown, due to their substantial lifestyle changes [48]. Sánchez et al. noted that if another lockdown were to be imposed, there should be greater emphasis on avoiding weight gain, in which case GLP-1RAs might be an effective therapy for these patients. Despite the influence of COVID-19, the data from this study are regarded as robust, and are suitable for further interpretation.

5. Conclusions

In SURE Spain, patients treated with OW semaglutide experienced statistically significant and clinically relevant reductions from baseline to EOS in HbA_{1c}, BW, and waist circumference, and improvements in other clinical parameters such as treatment satisfaction and HRQoL in a real-world setting. These findings were significant, despite the nature of the population (advanced T2D) included in the SURE Spain study and the local limitations on prescribing GLP-1RAs. The reported AEs were consistent with the known safety profile of semaglutide, with no new safety concerns reported. These results support the use of OW semaglutide in routine clinical practice in adults with T2D in Spain.

Supplementary Materials: The following supporting information can be downloaded at: https://www.mdpi.com/article/10.3390/jcm11174938/s1.

Author Contributions: Conceptualisation, V.B., C.A.P., A.-M.C., A.C., S.B.P. and E.D.; investigation, V.B., C.A.P., A.-M.C., A.C., S.B.P. and E.D.; writing—review and editing, V.B., C.A.P., A.-M.C., A.C., S.B.P. and E.D. All authors have read and agreed to the published version of the manuscript.

Funding: This work was supported by Novo Nordisk A/S.

Institutional Review Board Statement: The study was conducted in accordance with the Declaration of Helsinki, and first approved in 2019 by the Ethics Committee of CEIm de EUSkadi, project identifier: NN9535-4368.

Informed Consent Statement: Informed consent was obtained from all subjects involved in the study.

Data Availability Statement: The datasets analysed during the current study are available from the corresponding author on reasonable request.

Acknowledgments: This study was funded by Novo Nordisk A/S. We thank all the participants, investigators, and study-site staff, as well as Kamal Kant Mangla and Sanskruti Jayesh Patel from Novo Nordisk for their review and input to the manuscript, and Julia Peics (AXON Communications) for medical writing and editorial assistance (funded by Novo Nordisk A/S). Use of the ©MMAS is protected by US Copyright laws. Permission for use is required. A license agreement is available from Donald E. Morisky, MMAS Research LLC 14725 NE 20th St. Bellevue WA 98007 or from dmorisky@gmail.com.

Conflicts of Interest: V.B. has received unrestricted research support from Abbot, Novo Nordisk, and Sanofi, and has received speaker/advisory honoraria from Abbott, AstraZeneca, Boehringer Ingelheim, Eli Lilly, Esteve, Janssen, Merck, Mundipharma, Novartis, Novo Nordisk, Roche, and Sanofi. E.D. has received unrestricted research support from AstraZeneca, Novo Nordisk, Pfizer, Roche, and Sanofi, and has received consulting fees and/or honoraria for membership on advisory boards and speaker's bureau from Abbott Laboratories, Almirall, AstraZeneca, Esteve, GlaxoSmithKline, Lilly, Merck Sharp & Dohme, Novartis, Novo Nordisk, Pfizer, and Sanofi.

References

1. Soriguer, F.; Goday, A.; Bosch-Comas, A.; Bordiú, E.; Calle-Pascual, A.; Carmena, R.; Casamitjana, R.; Castaño, L.; Castell, C.; Catalá, M.; et al. Prevalence of diabetes mellitus and impaired glucose regulation in Spain: The Di@bet.es Study. *Diabetologia* **2012**, *55*, 88–93. [CrossRef] [PubMed]
2. International Diabetes Federation Diabetes Atlas 2021, Tenth Edition. Available online: https://diabetesatlas.org/atlas/tenth-edition/ (accessed on 3 March 2022).
3. American Diabetes Association. 8. Obesity Management for the Treatment of Type 2 Diabetes: Standards of Medical Care in Diabetes–2020. *Diabetes Care* **2020**, *43* (Suppl. 1), S89–S97. [CrossRef]
4. Chung, W.K.; Erion, K.; Florez, J.C.; Hattersley, A.T.; Hivert, M.F.; Lee, C.G.; McCarthy, M.I.; Nolan, J.J.; Norris, J.M.; Pearson, E.R.; et al. Precision Medicine in Diabetes: A consensus report from the American Diabetes Association (ADA) and the European Association for the Study of Diabetes (EASD). *Diabetes Care* **2020**, *43*, 1617–1635. [CrossRef] [PubMed]
5. Meier, J.J. GLP-1 receptor agonists for individualized treatment of type 2 diabetes mellitus. *Nat. Rev. Endocrinol.* **2012**, *8*, 728–742. [CrossRef] [PubMed]
6. Inzucchi, S.E.; Bergenstal, R.M.; Buse, J.B.; Diamant, M.; Ferrannini, E.; Nauck, M.; Peters, A.L.; Tsapas, A.; Wender, R.; Matthews, D.R. Management of hyperglycemia in type 2 diabetes, 2015: A patient-centered approach: Update to a position statement of the American Diabetes Association and the European Association for the Study of Diabetes. *Diabetes Care* **2015**, *38*, 140–149. [CrossRef] [PubMed]
7. Prasad-Reddy, L.; Isaacs, D. A clinical review of GLP-1 receptor agonists: Efficacy and safety in diabetes and beyond. *Drugs Context* **2015**, *4*, 212283. [CrossRef]
8. Marso, S.P.; Bain, S.C.; Consoli, A.; Eliaschewitz, F.G.; Jódar, E.; Leiter, L.A.; Lingvay, I.; Rosenstock, J.; Seufert, J.; Warren, M.L.; et al. Semaglutide and cardiovascular outcomes in patients with type 2 diabetes. *N. Engl. J. Med.* **2016**, *375*, 1834–1844. [CrossRef]
9. Marso, S.P.; Daniels, G.H.; Brown-Fransen, K.; Kristensen, P.; Mann, J.F.E.; Nauck, M.A.; Nissen, S.E.; Pocock, S.; Poulter, N.R.; Ravn, L.S.; et al. Liraglutide and cardiovascular outcomes in type 2 diabetes. *N. Engl. J. Med.* **2016**, *375*, 311–322. [CrossRef]
10. Gerstein, H.C.; Colhoun, H.M.; Dagenais, G.R.; Diaz, R.; Lakshamanan, M.; Pais, P.; Probstfield, J.; Riesmeyer, J.S.; Riddle, M.C.; Rydén, L.; et al. Dulaglutide and cardiovascular outcomes in type 2 diabetes (REWIND): A double-blind, randomised placebo-controlled trial. *Lancet* **2019**, *394*, 121–130. [CrossRef]

11. Reyes-García, R.; Moreno-Pérez, Ó.; Tejera-Pérez, C.; Fernández-García, D.; Bellido-Castañeda, V.; de la Torre Casares, M.L.; Rozas-Moreno, P.; Fernández-García, J.C.; Martínez, A.M.; Escalada-San Martín, J.; et al. Document on a comprehensive approach to type 2 diabetes mellitus. *Endocrinol. Diabetes Nutr. (Engl. Ed.)* **2019**, *66*, 443–458. [CrossRef]
12. Novo Nordisk. Ozempic® (Semaglutide) Summary of Product Characteristics. 2018. Available online: http://www.ema.europa.eu/docs/en_GB/document_library/EPAR_-_Product_Information/human/004174/WC500244163.pdf (accessed on 23 March 2022).
13. Lau, J.; Bloch, P.; Schäffer, L.; Pettersson, I.; Spetzler, J.; Kofoed, J.; Madsen, K.; Knudsen, L.B.; McGuire, J.; Steensgaard, D.B.; et al. Discovery of the once-weekly glucagon-like peptide-1 (GLP-1) analogue semaglutide. *J. Med. Chem.* **2015**, *58*, 7370–7380. [CrossRef] [PubMed]
14. Nauck, M.A.; Meier, J.J. Pioneering oral peptide therapy for patients with type 2 diabetes. *Lancet Diabetes Endocrinol.* **2019**, *7*, 500–502. [CrossRef]
15. Ahmann, A.J.; Capehorn, M.; Charpentier, G.; Dotta, F.; Henkel, E.; Lingvay, I.; Holst, A.G.; Annett, M.P.; Aroda, V.R. Efficacy and safety of once-weekly semaglutide versus exenatide ER in subjects with type 2 diabetes (SUSTAIN 3): A 56-week, open-label, randomized clinical trial. *Diabetes Care* **2018**, *41*, 258–266. [CrossRef] [PubMed]
16. Ahrén, B.; Masmiquel, L.; Kumar, H.; Sargin, M.; Karsbøl, J.D.; Jacobsen, S.H.; Chow, F. Efficacy and safety of once-weekly semaglutide versus once-daily sitagliptin as an add-on to metformin, thiazolidinediones, or both, in patients with type 2 diabetes (SUSTAIN 2): A 56-week, double-blind, phase 3a, randomised trial. *Lancet Diabetes Endocrinol.* **2017**, *5*, 341–354. [CrossRef]
17. Capehorn, M.S.; Catarig, A.-M.; Furberg, J.K.; Janez, A.; Price, H.C.; Tadayon, S.; Vergès, B.; Marre, M. Efficacy and safety of once-weekly semaglutide 1.0 mg vs once-daily liraglutide 1.2 mg as add-on to 1–3 oral antidiabetic drugs in subjects with type 2 diabetes (SUSTAIN 10). *Diabetes Metab.* **2020**, *46*, 100–109. [CrossRef] [PubMed]
18. Aroda, V.R.; Bain, S.C.; Cariou, B.; Piletič, M.; Rose, L.; Axelsen, M.; Rowe, E.; DeVries, J.H. Efficacy and safety of once-weekly semaglutide versus once-daily insulin glargine as add-on to metformin (with or without sulfonylureas) in insulin-naive patients with type 2 diabetes (SUSTAIN 4): A randomised, open-label, parallel-group, multicentre, multinational, phase 3a trial. *Lancet Diabetes Endocrinol.* **2017**, *5*, 355–366. [PubMed]
19. Lingvay, I.; Catarig, A.-M.; Frias, J.P.; Kumar, H.; Lausvig, N.L.; le Roux, C.W.; Thielke, D.; Viljoen, A.; McCrimmon, R.J. Efficacy and safety of once-weekly semaglutide versus daily canagliflozin as add-on to metformin in patients with type 2 diabetes (SUSTAIN 8): A double-blind, phase 3b, randomised controlled trial. *Lancet Diabetes Endocrinol.* **2019**, *7*, 834–844. [CrossRef]
20. Pratley, R.E.; Aroda, V.R.; Lingvay, I.; Lüdemann, J.; Andreassen, C.; Navarria, A.; Viljoen, A. SUSTAIN 7 investigators; Semaglutide versus dulaglutide once weekly in patients with type 2 diabetes (SUSTAIN 7): A randomised, open-label, phase 3b trial. *Lancet Diabetes Endocrinol.* **2018**, *6*, 275–286. [CrossRef]
21. Rodbard, H.W.; Lingvay, I.; Reed, J.; de la Rosa, R.; Rose, L.; Sugimoto, D.; Araki, E.; Chu, P.-L.; Wijayasinghe, N.; Norwood, P. Semaglutide added to basal insulin in type 2 diabetes (SUSTAIN 5): A randomized, controlled trial. *J. Clin. Endocrinol. Metab.* **2018**, *103*, 2291–2301. [CrossRef]
22. Sorli, C.; Harashima, S.; Tsoukas, G.M.; Unger, J.; Karsbøl, J.D.; Hansen, T.; Bain, S.C. Efficacy and safety of once-weekly semaglutide monotherapy versus placebo in subjects with type 2 diabetes (SUSTAIN 1): A double-blind, randomised, placebo-controlled, parallel-group, multinational, multicentre phase 3a trial. *Lancet Diabetes Endocrinol.* **2017**, *5*, 251–260. [CrossRef]
23. Zinman, B.; Bhosekar, V.; Bush, R.; Holst, I.; Ludvik, B.; Thielke, D.; Thrasher, J.; Woo, V.; Philis-Tsimikas, A. Semaglutide once weekly as add-on to SGLT-2 inhibitor therapy in type 2 diabetes (SUSTAIN 9): A randomized, placebo-controlled trial. 2019. *Lancet Diabetes Endocrinol.* **2019**, *7*, 356–367. [CrossRef]
24. Blonde, L.; Khunti, K.; Harris, S.B.; Meizinger, C.; Skolnik, N.S. Interpretation and impact of real-world clinical data for the practicing clinician. *Adv. Ther.* **2018**, *35*, 1763–1774. [CrossRef] [PubMed]
25. World Medical Association. World Medical Association Declaration of Helsinki: Ethical principles for medical research involving human subjects. *JAMA* **2013**, *310*, 2191–2194. [CrossRef] [PubMed]
26. European Medicines Agency, Guideline on Good Pharmacovigilance Practices (GVP)-Module VI. 2017. Available online: https://www.ema.europa.eu/en/documents/regulatory-procedural-guideline/guideline-good-pharmacovigilance-practices-gvp-module-vi-collection-management-submission-reports_en.pdf (accessed on 8 March 2022).
27. International Society of Pharmacoepidemiology. Guidelines for good pharmacoepidemiology practice (GPP). *Pharmacoepidemiol. Drug Saf.* **2016**, *25*, 2–10. [CrossRef]
28. American Diabetes Association. 6. Glycemic Targets: Standards of Medical Care in Diabetes-2018. *Diabetes Care* **2018**, *41* (Suppl. 1), S55–S64. [CrossRef]
29. National Institute for Clinical Excellence. Type 2 Diabetes in Adults: Management [NG28]. 2015. Available online: http://www.nice.org.uk/guidance/ng28 (accessed on 8 March 2022).
30. Morisky, D.E.; Ang, A.; Krousel-Wood, M.; Ward, H.J. Predictive validity of a medication adherence measure in an outpatient setting. *J. Clin. Hypertens.* **2008**, *10*, 348–354. [CrossRef]
31. Krousel-Wood, M.; Islam, T.; Webber, L.S.; Re, R.N.; Morisky, D.E.; Muntner, P. New medication adherence scale versus pharmacy fill rates in seniors with hypertension. *Am. J. Manag. Care* **2009**, *15*, 59–66.
32. Morisky, D.E.; DiMatteo, M.R. Improving the measurement of self-reported medication nonadherence: Response to authors. *J. Clin. Epidemiol.* **2011**, *64*, 255–257. [CrossRef]

33. Mody, R.; Grabner, M.; Yu, M.; Turner, R.; Kwan, A.Y.M.; York, W.; Landó, L.F. Real-world effectiveness, adherence and persistence among patients with type 2 diabetes mellitus initiating dulaglutide treatment. *Curr. Med. Res. Opin.* **2018**, *34*, 995–1003. [CrossRef]
34. Wilke, T.; Mueller, S.; Groth, A.; Berg, B.; Fuchs, A.; Sikirica, M.; Logie, J.; Martin, A.; Maywald, U. Non-persistence and non-adherence of patients with type 2 diabetes mellitus in therapy with GLP-1 receptor agonists: A retrospective analysis. *Diabetes Ther.* **2016**, *7*, 105–124. [CrossRef]
35. Divino, V.; DeKoven, M.; Hallinan, S.; Varo, N.; Wirta, S.B.; Lee, W.C.; Reaney, M. Glucagon-like peptide-1 receptor agonist treatment patterns among type 2 diabetes patients in six European countries. *Diabetes Ther.* **2014**, *5*, 499–520. [CrossRef] [PubMed]
36. Di Loreto, C.; Minarelli, V.; Nasini, G.; Norgiolini, R.; Del Sindaco, P. Effectiveness in real world of once weekly semaglutide in people with type 2 diabetes: Glucagon-like peptide receptor agonist naïve or switchers from other glucagon-like peptide receptor agonists: Results from a retrospective observational study in Umbria. *Diabetes Ther.* **2022**, *13*, 551–567. [CrossRef] [PubMed]
37. Weiss, T.; Yang, L.; Carr, R.D.; Pal, S.; Sawhney, B.; Boggs, R.; Rajpathak, S.; Iglay, K. Real-world weight change, adherence, and discontinuation among patients with type 2 diabetes initiating glucagon-like peptide-1 receptor agonists in the UK. *BMJ Open Diabetes Res. Care* **2022**, *10*, e002517. [CrossRef] [PubMed]
38. Uzoigwe, C.; Liang, Y.; Whitmire, S.; Paprocki, Y. Semaglutide once-weekly persistence and adherence versus other GLP-1RAs in patients with type 2 diabetes in a US real-world setting. *Diabetes Ther.* **2021**, *12*, 1475–1489. [CrossRef]
39. Ferrer-García, J.C.; Galera, R.A.; Arribas Sr., L.; Torrens, M.T.; Lorente, A.S.; Portilla, A.J.; Artero, A.; Sánchez-Juan, C. Receptor agonist in type 2 diabetes: A study to evaluate real-world effectiveness. In Proceedings of the American Diabetes Association 80th Scientific Sessions, Chicago, IL, USA, 12–16 June 2020. Poster number 947-P.
40. Cárdenas-Salas, J.J.; Sierra, R.; Luca, B.L.; Sánchez, B.; Modroño, N.; Casado, C.; Sánchez, N.M.; Cruces, E.; Vázquez, C. Semaglutide in patients with type 2 diabetes: Real-world data from Spain. In Proceedings of the American Diabetes Association 81st Scientific Sessions, Washington, DC, USA, 25–29 June 2021. Poster number 690-P.
41. Garcia De Lucas, M.D.; Avilés Bueno, B.; Pérez Belmonte, L.M.; Jiménez Millán, A.B.; Rivas Ruiz, F. Semaglutide Achieves Better Metabolic and Weight Control than Other GLP-1 RA in Real Life after 12 Months of Follow-up. In Proceedings of the American Diabetes Association 81st Scientific Sessions, Washington, DC, USA, 25–29 June 2021. Poster number 676-P.
42. Holmes, P.; Bell, H.E.; Bozkurt, K.; Catarig, A.-M.; Clark, A.; Machell, A.; Sathyapalan, T. Real-world use of once-weekly semaglutide in type 2 diabetes: Results from the SURE UK multicentre, prospective, observational study. *Diabetes Ther.* **2021**, *12*, 2891–2905. [CrossRef]
43. Ekberg, N.R.; Bodholt, U.; Catarig, A.-M.; Catrina, S.-B.; Grau, K.; Holmberg, C.N.; Klanger, B.; Knudsen, S.T. Real-world use of once-weekly semaglutide in patients with type 2 diabetes: Results from the SURE Denmark/Sweden multicentre, prospective, observational study. *Prim. Care Diabetes* **2021**, *15*, 871–878. [CrossRef]
44. Yale, J.F.; Catarig, A.-M.; Grau, K.; Harris, S.; Klimek-Abercrombie, A.; Rabasa-Lhoret, R.; Reardon, L.; Woo, V.; Liutkus, J. Use of once-weekly semaglutide in patients with type 2 diabetes in routine clinical practice: Results from the SURE Canada multicentre, prospective, observational study. *Diabetes Obes. Metab.* **2021**, *23*, 2269–2278. [CrossRef]
45. Rudofsky, G.; Catarig, A.-M.; Favre, L.; Grau, K.; Häfliger, S.; Thomann, R.; Schultes, B. Real-world use of once-weekly semaglutide in patients with type 2 diabetes: Results from the SURE Switzerland multicentre, prospective, observational study. *Diabetes Res. Clin. Pract.* **2021**, *178*, 108931. [CrossRef]
46. Instituto Aragonés de Ciencias de la Salud. Un Nuevo Atlas Muestra la Prescripción Recibida Por la Población Diabética de Aragón en 2020. Available online: https://www.iacs.es/un-nuevo-atlas-muestra-la-prescripcion-recibida-por-la-poblacion-diabetica-de-aragon-en-2020/ (accessed on 8 March 2022).
47. Marzullo, P.; Daffara, T.; Mele, C.; Zavattaro, M.; Ferrero, A.; Caputo, M.; Prodam, F.; Aimaretti, G. Real-world evaluation of weekly subcutaneous treatment with semaglutide in a cohort of Italian diabetic patients. *J. Endocrinol. Invest.* **2022**, *45*, 1587–1598.
48. Sánchez, E.; Lecube, A.; Bellido, D.; Monereo, S.; Malagón, M.M.; Tinahones, F.J.; on behalf of the Spanish Society for the Study of Obesity. Leading factors for weight gain during COVID-19 lockdown in a Spanish population: A cross-sectional study. *Nutrients* **2021**, *13*, 894. [CrossRef]

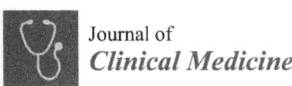

Systematic Review

Efficacy of Liraglutide in Non-Diabetic Obese Adults: A Systematic Review and Meta-Analysis of Randomized Controlled Trials

Joshuan J. Barboza [1,2,*], Mariella R. Huamán [3], Beatriz Melgar [1,4], Carlos Diaz-Arocutipa [1], German Valenzuela-Rodriguez [1] and Adrian V. Hernandez [1,5]

1. Unidad de Revisiones Sistemáticas y Meta-Análisis (URSIGET), Vicerrectorado de Investigación, Universidad San Ignacio de Loyola (USIL), Lima 15024, Peru; beamelgar@gmail.com (B.M.); carlosdiaz013@gmail.com (C.D.-A.); german.v.valenzuela@gmail.com (G.V.-R.); adrian.hernandez-diaz@uconn.edu (A.V.H.)
2. Tau Relaped Group, Trujillo 13007, Peru
3. Facultad de Medicina Humana, Universidad Nacional Mayor de San Marcos, Lima 15001, Peru; mariella.huaman@unmsm.edu.pe
4. Programa de Atencion Domiciliaria (PADOMI)—EsSalud, Lima, Peru
5. Health Outcomes, Policy, and Evidence Synthesis (HOPES) Group, University of Connecticut School of Pharmacy, Storrs, CT 06269, USA
* Correspondence: jbarbozameca@relaped.com; Tel.: +51-992108520

Abstract: Objective: We systematically assessed the efficacy of liraglutide in non-diabetic obese adults. Methods: Six databases were searched up to July 2021 for randomized controlled trials (RCTs) assessing liraglutide versus placebo in obese adults. Primary outcomes were body weight and body mass index (BMI). Secondary outcomes were treatment-emergent adverse events (TEAEs), hypoglycemic episodes, HbA1c, and blood pressure. Effect measures were risk ratio (RR) or mean difference (MD) with their confidence interval (95%CI). Random-effects models and inverse variance meta-analyses were used. Quality of evidence was assessed using GRADE. Results: Twelve RCTs (n = 8249) were included. In comparison to placebo, liraglutide reduced body weight (MD −3.35 kg; 95%CI −4.65 to −2.05; p < 0.0001), and BMI (MD −1.45 kg/m^2; 95%CI −1.98 to −0.91; p < 0.0001). Liraglutide did not reduce TEAEs (RR 1.08; 95%CI 0.92 to 1.27; p = 0.25), and Hb1Ac (MD −0.76%; 95%CI −2.24 to 0.72; p = 0.31). Furthermore, it did not increase hypoglycemic episodes (RR 2.01; 95%CI 0.37 to 11.02; p = 0.28). Finally, liraglutide reduced systolic blood pressure (MD −3.07 mmHg; 95%CI −3.66 to −2.48; p < 0.0001) and diastolic blood pressure (MD −1.01 mmHg; 95%CI −1.55 to −0.47; p = 0.0003). Seven RCTs had a high risk of bias. Subgroup analyses by length of treatment and doses had effects similar to the overall analyses. Quality of evidence was low or very low for most outcomes. Conclusions: In non-diabetic obese adults, liraglutide reduced body weight, BMI and blood pressure in comparison to placebo. Adverse events, Hb1Ac levels and hypoglycemic episodes were not different than placebo.

Keywords: liraglutide; body weight; obesity; hypoglycemia; meta-analysis

1. Introduction

Obesity is a major public health problem, affecting more than 603 million adults across the globe [1]. It may also increase the risk of several diseases, including hypertension, dyslipidemia, type 2 diabetes (T2D), and coronary artery disease. Initial management of obese patients includes a combination of dietary changes, exercise, and behavior modification. Nevertheless, in some cases, this strategy is insufficient and pharmacological treatment is required to achieve and maintain therapeutic goals in terms of weight loss.

Liraglutide is a glucagon-like peptide-1 (GLP-1) agonist and potential weight loss drug [2]. It increases insulin concentrations after eating, prior to the elevation of blood glucose levels [3,4]. Liraglutide is a drug used in obese diabetic patients, which justified the investigation of liraglutide as a treatment for non-diabetic obese people. A study evaluated the efficacy at 12 weeks of low-dose liraglutide on the weight of Taiwanese patients without T2D. Compared to baseline, 5.6% of patients in the liraglutide 1.2 mg group reached weight reduction ($p < 0.001$), whereas in the 0.6 mg group 6.4% reached weight reduction ($p < 0.001$) [5]. However, there was no difference in weight reduction between liraglutide doses (absolute difference 1.2 mg vs. 0.6 mg −0.8%, 95%CI −0.12 to 0.11).

We conducted a systematic review and meta-analysis to evaluate the efficacy and safety of liraglutide in non-diabetic obese adults.

2. Materials and Methods

We report the systematic review considering the guidelines of the PRISMA-2020 statement [6]. The protocol of this systematic review has been previously published in PROSPERO (CRD42020172654).

2.1. Search of Studies

We searched in different search engines such as Web of Science, Pubmed, Embase, Cochrane Central and Scopus, from inception to 7 October 2021. We performed Mesh terms, Emtree terms and TIAB terms, and we designed different strategies for the selected databases (Search strategy, Supplement). We did not limit our searches by language or year of publication.

2.2. Eligibility Criteria

We included studies based on: (i) randomized controlled trials (RCTs), (ii) assessed adults with obesity without diabetes type 1 or 2, (iii) evaluated liraglutide compared with placebo or other drugs. Observational studies (case-control studies or cohort), systematic reviews, case series/reports, abstract of conferences and editorials were excluded.

2.3. Selection of Studies

One author (JJB) downloaded all registers, and these were added to Rayyan (https://rayyan.qcri.org/, accessed on 23 March 2022), and duplicate records were removed. Two authors (JBM, MHR) independently reviewed the title and abstract regarding eligibility criteria. Following this step, the full-texts were screened for further evaluation. Differences in selections were addressed with a third author (AVH). Endnote 20 software (Philadelphia, PA, USA) was used for saved registers.

2.4. Outcomes

Primary outcomes a were decrease in body mass index (BMI) and body weight loss. Secondary outcomes were treatment-emergent adverse events (TEAEs), hypoglycemic episodes, decrease of HbA1c, and blood pressure. The concepts and definitions of outcomes described by the authors in each of the eligible studies were applied. TEAEs are defined as undesirable or unexpected events, which are not present before medical treatment. It can also be considered as an already present event that worsens in intensity or frequency after the treatment provided [7]. TEAEs included gastro-intestinal disorders (nausea, abdominal pain, vomiting, or diarrhea), nervous system disorders, infections and infestations, and vascular disorders. Types of hypoglycemic events in non-diabetic child and adult were: (a) reactive hypoglycemia (glycemia level <70 mg/dL at the time of symptoms and relief after eating); and (b) fasting hypoglycemia (glycemia <50 mg/dL after an overnight fast, between meals, or after physical activity) [8] Specific types of hypoglycemic events for any hypoglycemia were extracted. Also, author-reported definitions were used.

2.5. Data Extraction and Management

Two authors (JBM, MRH) independently extracted the data using a pre-developed standard data extraction form. Disagreements were resolved by consensus, and a third author (AVH) was consulted if needed. Data extracted per study were: name of author, year, type of research, country, number of participants, mean age, initial and maximum dosage of liraglutide, duration of treatment, and primary and secondary outcomes per trial arm with baseline values of continuous outcomes.

2.6. Risk of Bias Assessment

The RoB 2.0 tool (Bristol, UK) of the Cochrane Collaboration was used for risk of bias assessment [9]. The risk of bias judged the results as low risk, some concerns, or high risk. RoB 2.0 assessment was performed independently by two authors (JBM and MRH), and discrepancies resolved by discussion or with consultation with a third author (AVH).

2.7. Statistical Analyses

For meta-analysis, we performed random effects models and followed the inverse variance method. The Paule-Mandel estimator was used for the assessment of the between-study variance [10]. For continuous outcomes, effects of liraglutide on outcomes were expressed as mean difference (MD) with 95% confidence intervals (95% CIs). For dichotomous outcomes, relative risk (RR) with 95% CIs were assessed. Baseline values of continuous outcomes were adjusted for per trial arm. Statistical heterogeneity of effects among RCTs were evaluated using the I^2 statistic, with values corresponding to low (<30%), medium (30–60%), and high (>60%) levels of heterogeneity. Subgroup analyses by length of treatment ($\leq$16 versus >16 weeks) and maximum dosage (1.8 versus 3.0 mg/day) for all outcomes were performed. For sensitivity analysis, we changed the model and method of meta-analysis. With regard to the model, we applied fixed-effects, and regarding the methods, the Mantel-Haenzel method for sensitivity analyses for the primary outcomes were performed. We used the *metabin* and *metacont* functions of the meta library of R 3.5.1 (www.r-project.org, 23 March 2022). For publication bias analysis, a funnel plot was used to assess asymmetry that may indicate publication bias.

A summary of findings by GRADE methodology was used to rate the quality of evidence (QoE) per outcome [11]. Risk of bias, indirectness, imprecision, inconsistency, and publication bias were assessed, and QoE were rated as high, moderate, low, and very low. QoE was described in the summary of findings (SoF) tables; GRADEpro GDT was used to create SoF tables (GRADEpro).

3. Results

3.1. Selection of Studies

After the search, 2171 registers were found in all databases (Figure 1); 702 duplicate registers were deleted. Of 1469 registers, 1447 were excluded by title and abstract. Thus, 22 full-text studies were assessed for eligibility and 10 studies were excluded. Finally, 12 RCTs were included for qualitative and quantitative analyses [4,12–22].

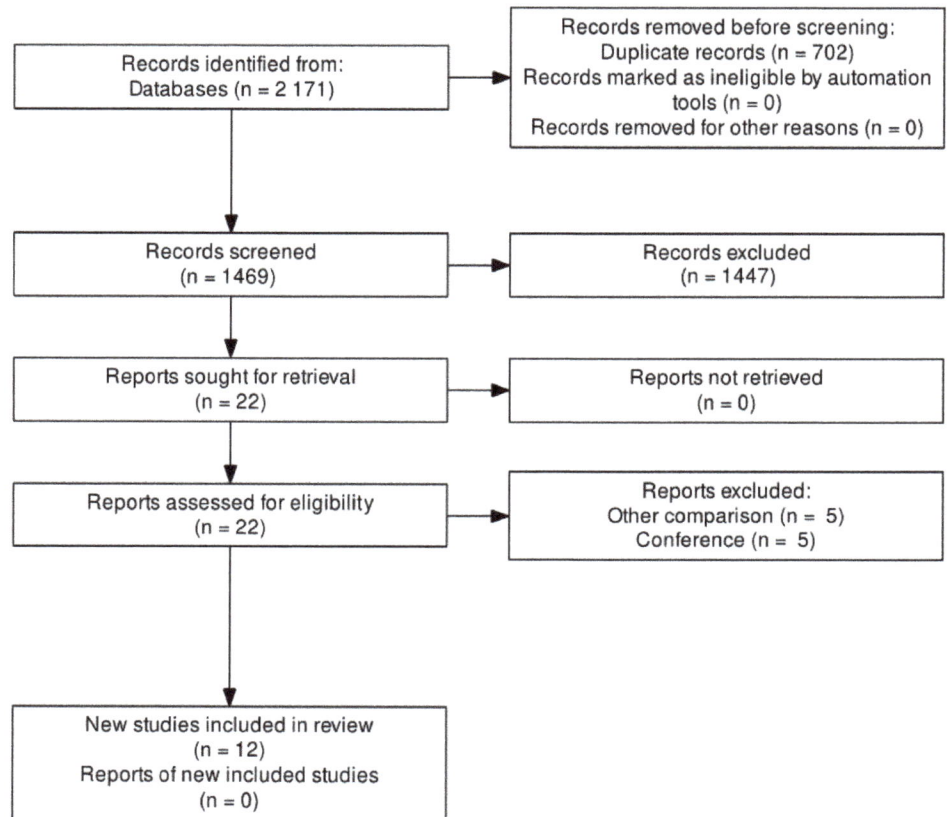

Figure 1. PRISMA flow chart of the study selection process.

3.2. Characteristics of Included Studies

The main characteristics of the included RCTs are summarized in Table 1. A total of 8249 adults treated with liraglutide were evaluated. The mean age was 45.9 ± 5.5 years and 24% of patients were men. Liraglutide was started at 0.6 mg/day with a progressive increase of 0.6 weekly up to a maximum of 1.8 mg/day [13,19,21] and 3.0 mg/day [4,12,14–18,20,22]. The mean duration of treatment was 35.1 ± 19.1 weeks. All studies included body weight loss as primary outcome, and other studies added inflammatory markers [13], glucose tolerance [19], proportion of individuals with T2D [4], and adverse events only [15]. At baseline, the mean Hb1Ac was 5.6% ± 0.09% in the liraglutide arm and 5.6% ± 0.07% in the control arm. Also, the mean BMI was 36.6 ± 2.6 kg/m^2 in the liraglutide arm and 36.8 ± 2.9 in the control arm.

Table 1. Baseline characteristics of included randomized controlled trials.

Author	Country	Number of Participants	Age (Mean, SD)	Male (n, %)	HbA1c at Baseline (Mean, SD)	BMI kg/m² at Baseline (Mean, SD)	Liraglutide Starting and Maximum Doses	Type of Control	Length of Treatment or Following	Primary Outcomes
Astrup, 2012	Denmark	191	45.9 (10.7)	48 (25%)	LG: 5.6 (0.4); Control: 5.6 (0.4)	NR	Liraglutide 3.0 mg once-daily (increased by 0.6 mg/week)	Placebo	52 weeks	Body weight loss and glycemic parameters
Blackman, 2016	USA	359	48.6 (9.9)	258 (73%)	LG: 5.7 (0.4); Control: 5.6 (0.4)	LG: 38.9 (6.4); Control: 39.4 (7.4)	Liraglutide 3.0 mg once-daily (increased by 0.6 mg/week)	Placebo	32 weeks	Apnea–hypopnea index and Body weight loss
Halawi, 2017	USA	40	37 (29.2)	NR	NR	LG: 37.2 (8.2); Control: 34.6 (6.4)	Liraglutide was administered as recommended by the FDA: initiated at 0.6 mg daily for 1 week, with instructions to increase by 0.6 mg weekly until 3.0 mg was reached (over 4 weeks).	Placebo	16 weeks	Body weight loss
Kim, 2013	USA	51	58 (7)	18 (35%)	NR	LG: 31.9 (2.7); Control: 31.9 (3.5)	The starting dose of medication was 0.6 mg; the dose was titrated by 0.6 mg weekly to a maximum dose of 1.8 mg.	Placebo	14 weeks	Body weight loss and inflammatory markers
Larsen, 2017	Denmark	103	42.1 (10.7)	60 (58%)	LG: 5.6 (0.4); Control: 5.5 (0.4)	LG: 33.7 (5.1); Control: 33.9 (6.6)	The participants followed a fixed uptitration schedule of 0.6 mg per week to a daily dose of 1.8 mg.	Placebo	16 weeks	Glucose tolerance, Body weight loss
Lean, 2014	UK	188	45.9 (10.7)	48 (26%)	NR	LG: 34.8 (2.8); Control: 34.9 (2.8)	Liraglutide doses of 3.0 mg were administered once daily by evening subcutaneous injection, starting with doses of 0.6 mg per day and increasing by weekly increments of 0.6 mg (dose escalation).	Placebo	20 weeks	Adverse events
Le Roux, 2017	USA	2254	NR	540 (24%)	LG: 5.8 (0.3); Control: 5.7 (0.3)	LG: 38.8 (6.4); Control: 39 (6.3)	Start Liraglutide at 0.6 mg with weekly 0.6 mg incremental increases to 3.0 mg.	Placebo	56 weeks	Proportion of individuals with type 2 diabetes, Body weight loss

Table 1. Cont.

Author	Country	Number of Participants	Age (Mean, SD)	Male (n, %)	HbA1c at Baseline (Mean, SD)	BMI kg/m² at Baseline (Mean, SD)	Liraglutide Starting and Maximum Doses	Type of Control	Length of Treatment or Following	Primary Outcomes
O'Neil	USA	957	47 (12)	338 (35%)	LG: 5.5 (0.4); Control: 5.5 (0.4)	LG: 38.6 (6.6); Control: 40.1 (7.2)	Liraglutide (3.0 mg) as once-daily subcutaneous injections	Placebo	52 weeks	Body weight loss
Pi-sunyer, 2015	USA	3731	45.2 (12.1)	803 (22%)	LG: 5.6 (0.4); Control: 5.6 (0.4)	LG: 38.3 (6.4); Control: 39.3 (6.3)	Starting at a dose of 0.6 mg with weekly 0.6 mg increments to 3.0 mg	Placebo	56 weeks	Body weight loss
Saxena	USA	56	46 (10.9)	18 (32%)	NR	NR	Liraglutide initiated at a dose of 0.6 mg/day and escalated by 0.6 mg/week up to a maximum of 3.0 mg/day)	Placebo	6 weeks	Change from baseline (CFB) in mean EI (in kcal) during ad libitum lunch meals.
Svensson, 2019	Denmark	97	42.1 (10.7)	60 (62%)	NR	LG: 38.9 (6.4); Control: 39.4 (7.4)	Starting at a dose of 0.6 mg with weekly 0.6-mg increments to 1.8 mg	Placebo	16 weeks	Body weight loss
Wadden, 2013	USA	222	45.9 (11.9)	37 (17%)	LG: 5.6 (0.4); Control: 5.6 (0.4)	LG: 36(5.9); Control: 35.2 (5.9)	Liraglutide 3.0 mg once-daily	Placebo	56 weeks	Body weight loss

SD: Standard deviation; BMI: Body mass index; LG: Liraglutide group; NR: No registered.

3.3. Risk of Bias

Overall, seven RCTs were scored as high risk of bias [12–15,20–22]. One RCT showed high risk in the randomization process [13]. Three RCTs showed high risk of deviations from intended interventions [13,15,16], and five RCTs showed high risk of missing outcome data [12–14,20,22]. The other RCTs showed low or unclear risk of bias (Supplementary Figure S1).

3.4. Effect on Primary Outcomes

In comparison to placebo, liraglutide significantly reduced body weight (MD −3.35 kg; 95% CI −4.65 to −2.05; $p < 0.0001$; $I^2 = 100\%$; Figure 2A), and reduced BMI (MD −1.45 kg/m^2; 95% CI −1.98 to −0.91; $p < 0.0001$; $I^2 = 99.5\%$; Figure 2B).

A

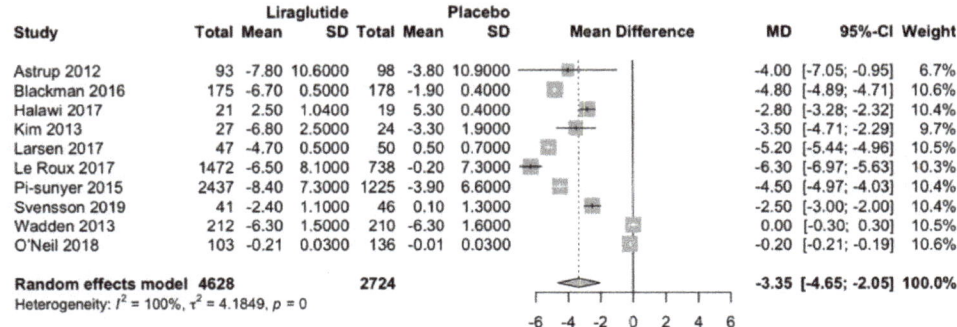

B

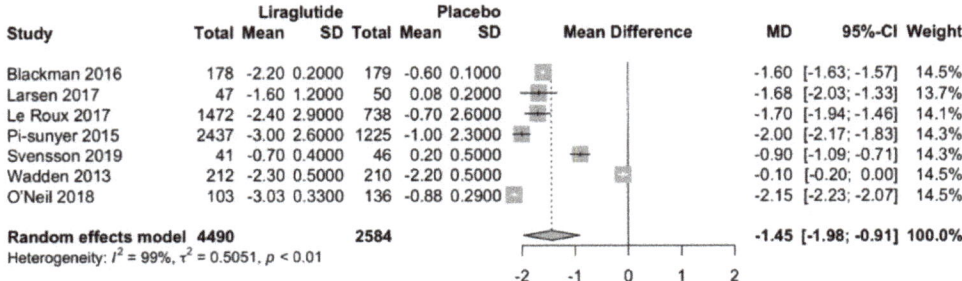

Figure 2. Forest plot of primary outcomes. (**A**): body weight, (**B**): BMI.

3.5. Effect on Secondary Outcomes

Liraglutide did not significantly reduce TEAEs (RR 1.08; 95% CI 0.92 to 1.27; $p = 0.25$; $I^2 = 90.2\%$; Figure 3a), and did not significantly increase hypoglycemic episodes (RR 2.01; 95% CI 0.37 to 11.02; $p = 0.28$; $I^2 = 54\%$; Figure 3b) in comparison to placebo. Liraglutide did not reduce Hb1Ac in comparison to placebo (MD −0.76; 95% CI −2.24 to 0.72; $p = 0.31$; $I^2 = 99.7\%$; Figure 3c). Finally, liraglutide significantly reduced systolic blood pressure (MD −3.07 mmHg; 95% CI −3.66 to −2.48; $p = <0.0001$; $I^2 = 71\%$; Figure 3d), and diastolic blood pressure (MD −1.01 mmHg; 95% CI −1.55 to −0.47; $p = 0.0003$; $I^2 = 92.2\%$; Figure 3e).

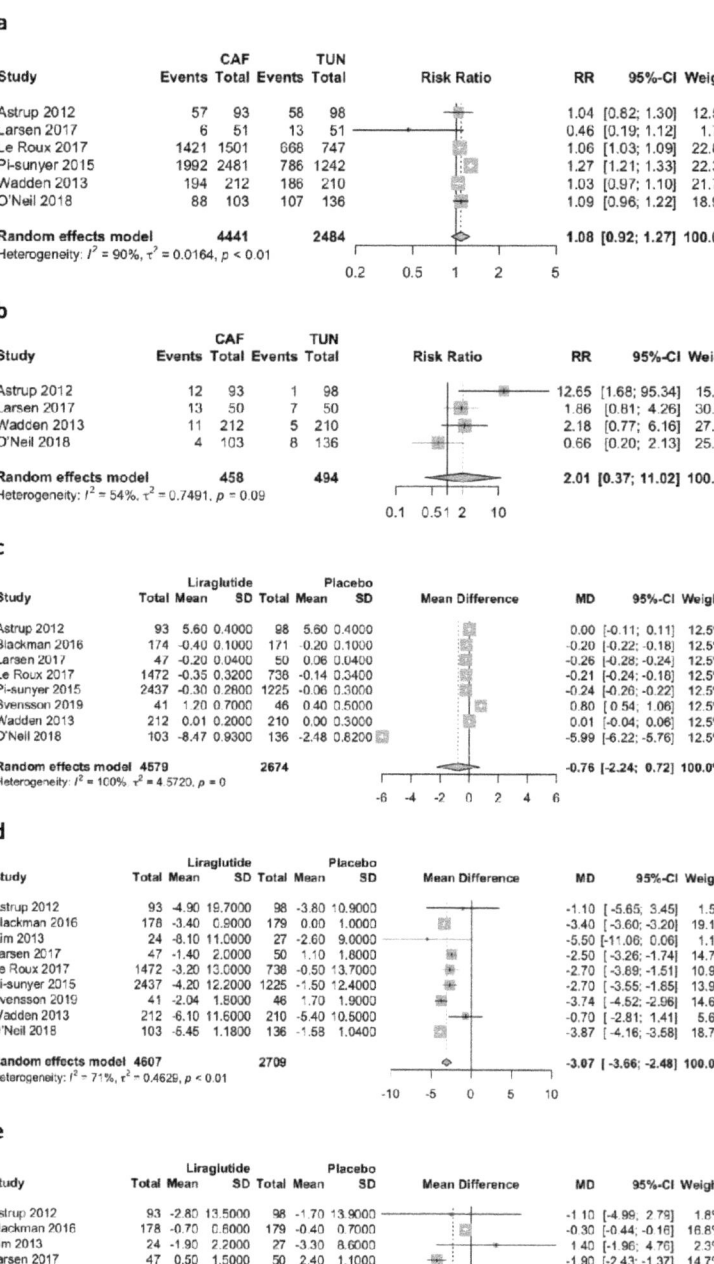

Figure 3. Forest plot of secondary outcomes. (**a**): TEAEs, (**b**): hypoglycemic episodes, (**c**): Hb1Ac, (**d**): Systolic blood pressure, (**e**): Diastolic blood pressure.

3.6. Subgroup Analyses

Subgroup analyses by length of treatment and maximum dosage were like the overall analyses for all outcomes (Supplementary Figures S2–S15).

3.7. Sensitivity Analyses

Effects on primary outcomes were the same, except for the effects of liraglutide vs. placebo on TEAEs, where liraglutide was associated with higher TEAEs compared to placebo (RR 1.15; 95% CI 1.12 to 1.18; $p < 0.01$) (Supplementary Figures S16 and S17).

3.8. Quality of Evidence

QoE was low or very low for most of the primary and secondary outcomes (Supplementary Table S1). In body weight, body mass index, TEAEs, hypoglycemic episodes, Hb1Ac, systolic blood pressure, and diastolic blood pressure, the QoE was very low due to high risk of bias; the heterogeneity among the studies and the imprecision of the effect. In systolic blood pressure, the QoE was low with regard to moderate heterogeneity among the studies.

3.9. Publication Bias

In the graphical test for publication bias, no significant asymmetry indicating high publication bias was observed (Supplementary Figure S18).

4. Discussion

Main Findings

In our systematic review in non-diabetic obese adults, liraglutide reduced body weight, BMI and blood pressure. However, it did not reduce TEAEs episodes or HbA1c, or the risk of hypoglycemic episodes compared with placebo. We also found that liraglutide reduced body weight, BMI, systolic blood pressure, and diastolic blood pressure in comparison to placebo. Subgroup analyses by duration of treatment and maximum dosage were like the main analyses. The risk of bias was high in 30% of the trials. The QoE was low or very low for most of the outcomes.

Liraglutide is a GLP-1 receptor agonist [23]. GLP-1 is known to be a hormone secreted in the intestine, which is activated after food ingestion by enteroendocrine L cells located in the distal jejunum and ileum [24]. It has been found that GLP-1 receptor agonists reduce cardiovascular events in people with T2D and are also a recommended treatment for weight reduction in these patients [25].

GLP-1 receptors are associated with weight loss by attenuating the fall in the anorexigenic hormone leptin that conditions this decrease [3,26]. Based on this, it has been reported that although GLP-1 can increase energy expenditure, its influence on weight is related to decreased energy intake through factors involved with the appetite reward centers of the brain and through local gastrointestinal effects [27].

Some studies have evaluated the efficacy of liraglutide for weight reduction in non-diabetic obese people. For example, a retrospective cohort study [5] evaluated the efficacy of low-dose liraglutide (0.6 vs. 1.2 mg/day) for 12 weeks on body weight among Taiwanese non-diabetic patients. The authors found that among patients in the liraglutide 1.2 mg group, 5.6% reached weight reduction compared to baseline ($p < 0.001$), whereas in the 0.6 mg group 6.4% reached weight reduction ($p < 0.001$); however, no significant differences in weight reduction were found between the two dose groups (absolute difference 1.2 mg vs. 0.6 mg -0.8%, 95%CI -0.12 to 0.11).

In a similar population, a prospective cohort study [28] evaluated the effect of liraglutide on body weight and microvascular function in non-diabetic overweight women with coronary microvascular dysfunction. The authors evaluated the intervention with Liraglutide 3 mg daily for 11 to 13 weeks of treatment, compared to a previous control stage, without treatment, for four to six weeks, and the baseline features. The authors found that a period of 12 weeks of liraglutide 3 mg daily led to a significant weight loss vs. baseline (absolute difference −6.03 kg; 95%CI: −5.22 to −6.84; $p < 0.001$).

A systematic review and Bayesian meta-analysis of RCTs by Khera et al. [29] assessed the effects of different drugs on weight loss and adverse effects in 29,018 patients. The authors included studies that assessed obese (BMI $\geq$ 30) or overweight (BMI $\geq$ 27) adults (aged $\geq$18 years), with or without weight-associated comorbidities. The authors found higher odds of >5% weight loss with the liraglutide group compared to placebo (three studies, 3301 patients, OR 5.09, 95%CI 4.07 to 6.37). A network meta-analysis suggested that phentermine-topiramate, 15 mg/92 mg once daily, was associated with the highest probability of achieving at least 5% weight loss (surface under the cumulative ranking [SUCRA], 0.95), followed by liraglutide (SUCRA, 0.83) and other drugs.

In the 2016 systematic review by Khera et al. [29], the authors did not evaluate the adverse effects or hypoglycemic events. For the liraglutide versus placebo comparison, Khera et al. included 4424 patients, whereas our study included 7236 patients. The Khera et al. study included studies published before 2016. The primary and secondary outcomes were also different, as we included TEAEs, hypoglycemic episodes, body weight, BMI, systolic and diastolic blood pressure and Hb1Ac levels; and they included proportion of patients achieving at least 5% weight loss from baseline, weight loss and adverse events. We used the Cochrane Collaboration RoB 2.0 tool, whereas the study by Khera et al. did not specify the tool used. The study by Khera et al. did not perform subgroup analyses due to a small number of included studies. The inclusion and exclusion criteria between Khera et al. and our study were similar and searched the same databases, but with a different search strategy. In addition, the search and selection of abstracts and full texts was performed independently by two people in the same way as our selection has been carried out. Something in common with the Khera et al. study was the use of the GRADE methodology to evaluate QoE per outcome.

Another systematic review published by Zhang et al. [30], assessed the efficacy and safety of liraglutide in obese, non-diabetic individuals. The authors reported five RCTs involving a total of 4754 patients, and found that mean weight loss (MD = −5.52, 95% CI = −5.93 to −5.11, $p < 0.00001$); loss of more than 5% of body weight (OR = 5.46, 95% CI = 3.57 to 8.34, $p < 0.00001$), and key secondary efficacy end points: SBP decreased (the MD = −2.56, 95% CI = −3.28 to −1.84, $p < 0.00001$). These results are similar to those of our study. However, it is noteworthy that the authors reported a low risk of bias in the trials included in the meta-analysis, whereas our study reported a comprehensive risk of bias analysis, where the majority of trials were found to be at high risk of bias. Another observation is that the authors refer to having used two different models for the meta-analysis, and did not consider the implicit heterogeneity among the studies, and there is no exact distinction about the model applied. Our study, on the other hand, used the random effects model for all meta-analyses under the assumption of heterogeneity and differences between studies.

5. Limitations

We have identified several limitations. First, there were differences in the starting and maintenance dose of liraglutide. However, we did not find differences in the weight loss effects between lower or higher liraglutide doses. Second, there was a difference in follow-up time among studies. Most of the included studies had a follow-up time longer than 17 weeks, and our subgroup analyses showed no difference between shorter and longer follow up times. Third, the risk of bias in most studies was high, which may compromise the true effect of most of the outcomes described, as in other studies that applied meta-analysis with included studies and high risk of bias [31–34]. Finally, in the evaluation of the QoE using GRADE methodology, we found low and very low quality of evidence for most outcomes, which should be considered when interpreting the significant effects that may favor the treatment.

6. Conclusions

In non-diabetic obese adults, liraglutide reduced body weight, BMI, and blood pressure in comparison to placebo. TEAEs rates, Hb1Ac and hypoglycemic episodes were not different than placebo. However, the effects in the outcomes may have been compromised due to the true effect related to the high risk of bias in the most studies, and the low or very low level of recommendation in GRADE.

Supplementary Materials: The following supporting information can be downloaded at: https://www.mdpi.com/article/10.3390/jcm11112998/s1. Figure S1: Risk of bias assessment of included trials. Figure S2: Subgroup analyses by length of treatment of the effects of Liraglutide vs placebo on TEAEs. Figure S3: Subgroup analyses by doses of the effects of Liraglutide vs placebo on hypoglycemia TEAES. Figure S4: Subgroup analyses by length of treatment of the effects of Liraglutide vs placebo on hypoglycemia episodes. Figure S5: Subgroup analyses by doses of the effects of Liraglutide vs placebo on hypoglycemia episodes. Figure S6: Subgroup analyses by length of treatment of the effects of Liraglutide vs placebo on body weight loss. Figure S7: Subgroup analyses by doses of the effects of Liraglutide vs placebo on body weight loss. Figure S8: Subgroup analyses by length of treatment of the effects of Liraglutide vs placebo on BMI. Figure S9: Subgroup analyses by doses of the effects of Liraglutide vs placebo on BMI. Figure S10: Subgroup analyses by length of treatment of the effects of Liraglutide vs placebo on SBP. Figure S11: Subgroup analyses by doses of the effects of Liraglutide vs placebo on SBP. Figure S12: Subgroup analyses by length of treatment of the effects of Liraglutide vs placebo on DBP. Figure S13: Subgroup analyses by doses of the effects of Liraglutide vs placebo on DBP. Figure S14: Subgroup analyses by length of treatment of the effects of Liraglutide vs placebo on Hb1Ac. Figure S15: Subgroup analyses by doses of the effects of Liraglutide vs placebo on Hb1Ac. Figure S16: Sensitivity analyses of the effects of Liraglutide vs placebo on body weight loss. Figure S17: Sensitivity analyses of the effects of Liraglutide vs placebo on BMI. Figure S18: Publication bias. Table S1: GRADE summary of findings table.

Author Contributions: J.J.B., M.R.H., B.M., C.D.-A., G.V.-R. and A.V.H.: conceptualization, methodology, software, validation, formal analysis, investigation, resources, data curation, writing—original draft preparation, writing—review and editing, visualization, supervision. All authors have read and agreed to the published version of the manuscript.

Funding: This research received no external funding.

Institutional Review Board Statement: Not applicable.

Informed Consent Statement: Not applicable.

Data Availability Statement: Not applicable.

Conflicts of Interest: The authors declare that they have no conflict of interest.

References

1. GBD 2015 Obesity Collaborators; Afshin, A.; Forouzanfar, M.H.; Reitsma, M.B.; Sur, P.; Estep, K.; Lee, A.; Marczak, L.; Mokdad, A.H.; Moradi-Lakeh, M.; et al. Health Effects of Overweight and Obesity in 195 Countries over 25 Years. *N. Engl. J. Med.* **2017**, *377*, 13–27. [CrossRef]
2. Ahrén, B. Glucagon-like peptide-1 receptor agonists for type 2 diabetes: A rational drug development. *J. Diabetes Investig.* **2019**, *10*, 196–201. [CrossRef] [PubMed]
3. Ladenheim, E. Liraglutide and obesity: A review of the data so far. *Drug Des. Dev. Ther.* **2015**, *9*, 1867–1875. [CrossRef] [PubMed]
4. le Roux, C.W.; Astrup, A.; Fujioka, K.; Greenway, F.; Lau, D.C.W.; Van Gaal, L.; Ortiz, R.V.; Wilding, J.P.H.; Skjøth, T.V.; Manning, L.S.; et al. 3 years of liraglutide versus placebo for type 2 diabetes risk reduction and weight management in individuals with prediabetes: A randomised, double-blind trial. *Lancet* **2017**, *389*, 1399–1409. [CrossRef]
5. Chou, C.; Chuang, S. Evaluation of the efficacy of low-dose liraglutide in weight control among Taiwanese non-diabetes patients. *J. Diabetes Investig.* **2020**, *11*, 1524–1531. [CrossRef] [PubMed]
6. Page, M.; McKenzie, J.; Bossuyt, P.; Boutron, I.; Hoffmann, T.; Mulrow, C.D.; Shamseer, L.; Tetzlaff, J.M.; Akl, E.A.; Brennan, S.E.; et al. The PRISMA 2020 statement: An up-dated guideline for reporting systematic reviews. *Int. J. Surg.* **2020**, *88*, 105906. [CrossRef]
7. Nilsson, M.E.; Koke, S.C. Defining Treatment-Emergent Adverse Events with the Medical Dictionary for Regulatory Activities (MedDRA). *Drug Inf. J.* **2001**, *35*, 1289–1299. [CrossRef]
8. Santiago, J.V.; Pereira, M.B.; Avioli, L.V. Fasting hypoglycemia in adults. *Arch. Intern. Med.* **1982**, *142*, 465–468. [CrossRef]

9. Sterne, J.A.C.; Savović, J.; Page, M.J.; Elbers, R.G.; Blencowe, N.S.; Boutron, I.; Cates, C.J.; Cheng, H.Y.; Corbett, M.S.; Eldridge, S.M.; et al. RoB 2: A revised tool for assessing risk of bias in randomised trials. *BMJ* **2019**, *366*, l4898. [CrossRef]
10. Van Aert, R.C.M.; Jackson, D. Multistep estimators of the between-study variance: The relationship with the Paule-Mandel estimator. *Stat. Med.* **2018**, *37*, 2616–2629. [CrossRef]
11. Guyatt, G.H.; Oxman, A.D.; Schuenemann, H.J.; Tugwell, P.; Knottnerus, A. GRADE guidelines: A new series of articles in the Journal of Clinical Epidemiology. *J. Clin. Epidemiol.* **2011**, *64*, 380–382. [CrossRef] [PubMed]
12. Astrup, A.; Carraro, R.; Finer, N.; Harper, A.; Kunesova, M.; Lean, M.E.J.; Niskanen, L.; Rasmussen, M.F.; Rissanen, A.; Rössner, S.; et al. Safety, tolerability and sustained weight loss over 2 years with the once-daily human GLP-1 analog, liraglutide. *Int. J. Obes.* **2012**, *36*, 843–854. [CrossRef] [PubMed]
13. Kim, S.H.; Abbasi, F.; Lamendola, C.; Liu, A.; Ariel, D.; Schaaf, P.; Grove, K.; Tomasso, V.; Ochoa, H.; Liu, Y.V.; et al. Benefits of Liraglutide Treatment in Overweight and Obese Older Individuals with Prediabetes. *Diabetes Care* **2013**, *36*, 3276–3282. [CrossRef] [PubMed]
14. Wadden, T.A.; Hollander, P.; Klein, S.; Niswender, K.; Woo, V.; Hale, P.M.; Aronne, L. Weight maintenance and additional weight loss with liraglutide after low-calorie-diet-induced weight loss: The SCALE Maintenance randomized study. *Int. J. Obes.* **2013**, *37*, 1443–1451. [CrossRef]
15. Lean, M.E.J.; Carraro, R.; Finer, N.; Hartvig, H.; Lindegaard, M.L.; Rössner, S.; van Gaal, L.; Astrup, A.; on behalf of the NN8022-1807 Investigators. Tolerability of nausea and vomiting and associations with weight loss in a randomized trial of liraglutide in obese, non-diabetic adults. *Int. J. Obes.* **2014**, *38*, 689–697. [CrossRef]
16. Pi-Sunyer, X.; Astrup, A.; Fujioka, K.; Greenway, F.; Halpern, A.; Krempf, M.; Lau, D.C.W.; Le Roux, C.W.; Ortiz, R.V.; Jensen, C.B.; et al. A Randomized, Controlled Trial of 3.0 mg of Liraglutide in Weight Management. *N. Engl. J. Med.* **2015**, *373*, 11–22. [CrossRef]
17. Blackman, A.; Foster, G.D.; Zammit, G.; Rosenberg, R.; Aronne, L.; Wadden, T.; Claudius, B.; Jensen, C.B.; Mignot, E.; on behalf of the SCALE study group. Effect of liraglutide 3.0 mg in individuals with obesity and moderate or severe obstructive sleep apnea: The SCALE Sleep Apnea randomized clinical trial. *Int. J. Obes.* **2016**, *40*, 1310–1319. [CrossRef]
18. Halawi, H.; Khemani, D.; Eckert, D.; O'Neill, J.; Kadouh, H.; Grothe, K.; Clark, M.M.; Burton, D.D.; Vella, A.; Acosta, A.; et al. Effects of liraglutide on weight, satiation, and gastric functions in obesity: A randomised, placebo-controlled pilot trial. *Lancet Gastroenterol. Hepatol.* **2017**, *2*, 890–899. [CrossRef]
19. Larsen, J.R.; Vedtofte, L.; Jakobsen, M.S.L.; Jespersen, H.R.; Jakobsen, M.I.; Svensson, C.K.; Koyuncu, K.; Schjerning, O.; Oturai, P.S.; Kjaer, A.; et al. Effect of Liraglutide Treatment on Prediabetes and Overweight or Obesity in Clozapine- or Olanzapine-Treated Patients with Schizophrenia Spectrum Disorder: A Randomized Clinical Trial. *JAMA Psychiatry* **2017**, *74*, 719–728. [CrossRef]
20. O'Neil, P.; Birkenfeld, A.L.; McGowan, B.; Mosenzon, O.; Pedersen, S.D.; Wharton, S.; Carson, C.G.; Jepsen, C.H.; Kabisch, M.; Wilding, J.P.H. Efficacy and safety of semaglutide compared with liraglutide and placebo for weight loss in patients with obesity: A randomised, double-blind, placebo and active controlled, dose-ranging, phase 2 trial. *Lancet* **2018**, *392*, 637–649. [CrossRef]
21. Svensson, C.K.; Larsen, J.R.; Vedtofte, L.; Jakobsen, M.S.L.; Jespersen, H.R.; Jakobsen, M.I.; Koyuncu, K.; Schjerning, O.; Nielsen, J.; Ekstrøm, C.T.; et al. One-year follow-up on liraglutide treatment for prediabetes and overweight/obesity in clozapine- or olanzapine-treated patients. *Acta Psychiatr. Scand.* **2019**, *139*, 26–36. [CrossRef] [PubMed]
22. Saxena, A.R.; Banerjee, A.; Corbin, K.D.; Parsons, S.A.; Smith, S.R. Energy intake as a short-term biomarker for weight loss in adults with obesity receiving liraglutide: A randomized trial. *Obes. Sci. Pract.* **2021**, *7*, 281–290. [CrossRef] [PubMed]
23. Tronieri, J.S.; Fabricatore, A.N.; Wadden, T.A.; Auerbach, P.; Endahl, L.; Sugimoto, D.; Rubino, D. Effects of Dietary Self-Monitoring, Physical Activity, Liraglutide 3.0 mg, and Placebo on Weight Loss in the SCALE IBT Trial. *Obes. Facts* **2020**, *13*, 572–583. [CrossRef]
24. Thakur, U.; Bhansali, A.; Gupta, R.; Rastogi, A. Liraglutide Augments Weight Loss After Laparoscopic Sleeve Gastrectomy: A Randomised, Double-Blind, Placebo-Control Study. *Obes. Surg.* **2020**, *31*, 84–92. [CrossRef] [PubMed]
25. Verma, S.; McGuire, D.K.; Bain, S.C.; Bhatt, D.L.; Leiter, L.A.; Mazer, C.D.; Fries, T.M.; Pratley, R.E.; Rasmussen, S.; Vrazic, H.; et al. Effects of glucagon-like peptide-1 receptor agonists liraglutide and semaglutide on cardiovascular and renal outcomes across body mass index categories in type 2 diabetes: Results of the LEADER and SUSTAIN 6 trials. *Diabetes Obes. Metab.* **2020**, *22*, 2487–2492. [CrossRef]
26. Kaji, N.; Takagi, Y.; Matsuda, S.; Takahashi, A.; Fujio, S.; Asai, F. Effects of liraglutide on metabolic syndrome in WBN/Kob diabetic fatty rats supplemented with a high-fat diet. *Anim. Model. Exp. Med.* **2020**, *3*, 62–68. [CrossRef]
27. Li, Z.; Yang, P.; Liang, Y.; Xia, N.; Li, Y.; Su, H.; Pan, H. Effects of liraglutide on lipolysis and the AC3/PKA/HSL pathway. *Diabetes Metab. Syndr. Obes. Targets Ther.* **2019**, *12*, 1697–1703. [CrossRef]
28. Suhrs, H.E.; Raft, K.F.; Bové, K.; Madsbad, S.; Holst, J.J.; Zander, M.; Prescott, E. Effect of liraglutide on body weight and microvascular function in non-diabetic overweight women with coronary microvascular dysfunction. *Int. J. Cardiol.* **2019**, *283*, 28–34. [CrossRef]
29. Khera, R.; Murad, M.H.; Chandar, A.K.; Dulai, P.S.; Wang, Z.; Prokop, L.J.; Loomba, R.; Camilleri, M.; Singh, S. Association of Pharmacological Treatments for Obesity with Weight Loss and Adverse Events: A Systematic Review and Meta-analysis. *JAMA* **2016**, *315*, 2424–2434. [CrossRef]
30. Zhang, P.; Liu, Y.; Ren, Y.; Bai, J.; Zhang, G.; Cui, Y. The efficacy and safety of liraglutide in the obese, non-diabetic individuals: A systematic review and meta-analysis. *Afr. Health Sci.* **2019**, *19*, 2591–2599. [CrossRef]

31. Diaz-Arocutipa, C.; Benites-Meza, J.K.; Chambergo-Michilot, D.; Barboza, J.J.; Pasupuleti, V.; Bueno, H.; Sambola, A.; Hernandez, A.V. Efficacy and Safety of Colchicine in Post-acute Myocardial Infarction Patients: A Systematic Review and Meta-Analysis of Randomized Controlled Trials. *Front. Cardiovasc. Med.* **2021**, *8*, 676771. [CrossRef] [PubMed]
32. Barboza, J.J.; Albitres-Flores, L.; Rivera-Meza, M.; Rodriguez-Huapaya, J.; Caballero-Alvarado, J.; Pasupuleti, V.; Hernandez, A.V. Short-term efficacy of umbilical cord milking in preterm infants: Systematic review and meta-analysis. *Pediatr. Res.* **2021**, *89*, 22–30. [CrossRef] [PubMed]
33. Barboza, J.J.; Chambergo-Michilot, D.; Velasquez-Sotomayor, M.; Silva-Rengifo, C.; Diaz-Arocutipa, C.; Caballero-Alvarado, J.; Garcia-Solorzano, F.O.; Alarcon-Ruiz, C.A.; Albitres-Flores, L.; Rodriguez-Morales, A.J.; et al. Assessment and management of asymptomatic COVID-19 infection: A systematic review. *Travel Med. Infect. Dis.* **2021**, *41*, 102058. [CrossRef] [PubMed]
34. Hernandez, A.V.; Ingemi, J., III; Sherman, M.; Pasupuleti, V.; Barboza, J.J.; Piscoya, A.; Roman, Y.M.; White, C.M. Impact of Prophylactic Hydroxychloroquine on People at High Risk of COVID-19: A Systematic Review and Meta-Analysis. *J. Clin. Med.* **2021**, *10*, 2609. [CrossRef] [PubMed]

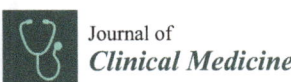 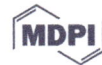

Article

Association between Add-On Dipeptidyl Peptidase-4 Inhibitor Therapy and Diabetic Retinopathy Progression

Eugene Yu-Chuan Kang [1,2], Chunya Kang [3], Wei-Chi Wu [1,2], Chi-Chin Sun [2,4,5], Kuan-Jen Chen [1,2], Chi-Chun Lai [1,2,4], Tien-Hsing Chen [2,5,6,*] and Yih-Shiou Hwang [1,2,*]

1. Department of Ophthalmology, Chang Gung Memorial Hospital, Linkou Medical Center, Taoyuan 333, Taiwan; yckang0321@gmail.com (E.Y.-C.K.); weichi666@gmail.com (W.-C.W.); cgr999@gmail.com (K.-J.C.); chichun.lai@gmail.com (C.-C.L.)
2. College of Medicine, Chang Gung University, Taoyuan 333, Taiwan; arvinsun@cgmh.org.tw
3. School of Medicine, Medical University of Lublin, 20529 Lublin, Poland; miranda52879@gmail.com
4. Department of Ophthalmology, Chang Gung Memorial Hospital, Keelung 204, Taiwan
5. Biostatistical Consultation Center, Chang Gung Memorial Hospital, Keelung 204, Taiwan
6. Department of Internal Medicine, Division of Cardiology, Chang Gung Memorial Hospital, Keelung 204, Taiwan
* Correspondence: skyheart0826@gmail.com (T.-H.C.); yihshiou.hwang@gmail.com (Y.-S.H.); Tel.: +886-2-2431-3131 (ext. 6314) (T.-H.C.); +886-3-328-1200 (ext. 8666) (Y.-S.H.)

Abstract: This study aimed to investigate the association of add-on dipeptidyl peptidase-4 inhibitor (DPP4i) therapy and the progression of diabetic retinopathy (DR). In this retrospective population-based cohort study, we examined Taiwanese patients with type 2 diabetes, preexisting DR, and aged ≥40 years from 2009 to 2013. Prescription of DPP4i was defined as a medication possession ratio of ≥80% during the first 6 months. The outcomes included vitreous hemorrhage (VH), tractional retinal detachment, macular edema, and interventions including retinal laser therapy, intravitreal injection (IVI), and vitrectomy. Of 1,767,640 patients, 62,824 were eligible for analysis. After matching, the DPP4i and non-DPP4i groups each contained 20,444 patients. The risks of VH (p = 0.013) and macular edema (p = 0.035) were higher in the DPP4i group. The DPP4i group also had higher risks of receiving surgical interventions (retinal laser therapy (p < 0.001), IVI (p = 0.049), vitrectomy (p < 0.001), and any surgical intervention (p < 0.001)). More patients in the DPP4i group received retinal laser therapy (p < 0.001) and IVI (p = 0.001) than in the non-DPP4i group. No between-group differences in cardiovascular outcomes were noted. In the real-world database study, add-on DPP4i therapy may be associated with the progression of DR in patients with type 2 diabetes. No additional cardiovascular risks were found. The early progression of DR in rapid glycemic control was inconclusive in our study. The possible effect of add-on DPP4i therapy in the progression of DR in patients with type 2 diabetes requires further research.

Keywords: dipeptidyl peptidase-4 inhibitor; diabetes mellitus; diabetic retinopathy; progression

Citation: Kang, E.Y.-C.; Kang, C.; Wu, W.-C.; Sun, C.-C.; Chen, K.-J.; Lai, C.-C.; Chen, T.-H.; Hwang, Y.-S. Association between Add-On Dipeptidyl Peptidase-4 Inhibitor Therapy and Diabetic Retinopathy Progression. *J. Clin. Med.* **2021**, *10*, 2871. https://doi.org/10.3390/jcm10132871

Academic Editor: Fernando Gómez-Peralta

Received: 3 June 2021
Accepted: 28 June 2021
Published: 28 June 2021

Publisher's Note: MDPI stays neutral with regard to jurisdictional claims in published maps and institutional affiliations.

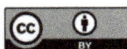

Copyright: © 2021 by the authors. Licensee MDPI, Basel, Switzerland. This article is an open access article distributed under the terms and conditions of the Creative Commons Attribution (CC BY) license (https://creativecommons.org/licenses/by/4.0/).

1. Introduction

Diabetic retinopathy (DR), a common microvascular complication in patients with diabetes, is also a major cause of blindness in working-age adults [1]. The global number of patients with diabetes is estimated to reach 600 million by 2040, one-third of whom are expected to have DR [2]. Severe DR can lead to complications such as vitreous hemorrhage (VH), tractional retinal detachment (RD), and macular edema [3,4]. DR and its complications may require surgical intervention such as retinal laser therapy, intravitreal injection (IVI) of anti-vascular endothelial growth factor, and in some cases vitrectomy [3,4]. This imposes a substantial economic burden on patients with such conditions and their families [5].

Numerous studies have been conducted on preventing or slowing the progression of diabetic complications. A randomized controlled trial reported that appropriate glucose-lowering reduced the risk of cardiovascular diseases, microvascular complications, and all-cause mortality in patients with diabetes [6]. Another randomized controlled trial indicated that intensive glucose control effectively slowed DR progression in patients with type 2 diabetes [7]. Treatment for systemic conditions, such as hypertension and dyslipidemia, has been demonstrated to be associated with a low risk of DR development or progression [7,8].

Dipeptidyl peptidase-4 (DPP4) inhibitors (DPP4i) are a class of oral hypoglycemics, of which the first agent sitagliptin was approved in 2006 by the US Food and Drug Administration [9]. DPP4i suppress the function of DPP4 and indirectly prolong the serum level of glucagon-like peptide-1 (GLP-1), increasing insulin secretion and reducing glucagon secretion from the pancreas [10]. Although a meta-analysis reported that DPP4i exerted a better hypoglycemic effect than α-glucosidase inhibitors [11], other studies have observed associations between its use and an increased risk of heart failure [12,13]. Moreover, another meta-analysis indicated no beneficial association between DPP4i use and all-cause mortality [14]. Regarding DPP4i use in DR, sitagliptin prevented the effect of diabetes on the blood-retinal barrier in male Zucker diabetic fatty rats. Specifically, it improved endothelial function and prevented inflammation, nitrative stress, and apoptosis in animals [15]. However, the association between DPP4i and DR has not been fully characterized [16,17]. The first clinical study of the possible protective effects of DPP4i on DR progression, published in 2016, included 28 patients with type 2 diabetes [18]. A 2018 population-based study by Kim et al. that used data from the South Korean National Health Insurance Service reported a possible association of DPP4i use with an increased risk of DR events early in the treatment phase [19]. Using the same database, Chung et al. found a neutral association between DPP4i use and sulfonylurea added to metformin therapy and the risk of DR progression. The aggravation of DR by DPP4i remains a concern and requires more clinical investigation [20]. In this study, we investigated the association between add-on DPP4i therapy and DR progression in patients with type 2 diabetes and preexisting DR in a real-world setting.

2. Materials and Methods

2.1. Data Source

This retrospective population-based cohort study was conducted using the Taiwan National Health Insurance (NHI) Research Database (NHIRD) (Center for Biomedical Resources of National Health Research Institutes, Miaoli, Taiwan). More than 99.8% of the population in Taiwan (approximately 23.7 million people as of 2020) is covered by the NHI program, a single-payer system established in March 1995. The NHIRD contains de-identified information including medical claims data. Information on the NHI program and its databases has been described in detail in previous publications [21,22]. The present study was approved by the Chang Gung Memorial Hospital Ethics Institutional Review Board (IRB No. 201800199B1) and adheres to the principles of the Declaration of Helsinki.

2.2. Inclusion and Exclusion Criteria

From 2009 to 2013, we identified patients with diabetes in the NHIRD by using the diagnostic codes of the International Classification of Diseases, Ninth Revision, Clinical Modification (ICD-9-CM). These codes were validated in a study on the accuracy of diabetes diagnosis in NHI claims data. Specifically, at least four outpatient visits for diabetes corresponded to a 95.7% accuracy [23]. Another study observed that a prescription of any oral hypoglycemic agent corresponded to an accuracy of 99% [24]. Therefore, in the present study, we included patients with at least five outpatient diagnoses of type 2 diabetes who were also taking any oral hypoglycemics. Patients with type 2 diabetes and preexisting DR were included in the analysis. We excluded patients who were aged under 40 years as well as those with missing demographic data, type 1 diabetes, retinal disorders (including retinal vascular occlusion, separation of retinal layers, retina degeneration, and chorioretinal inflammation), a history of receiving vitreoretinal interventions (including

IVI, retinal laser therapy, scleral buckling, and vitrectomy), or were followed up for less than 6 months (Figure 1).

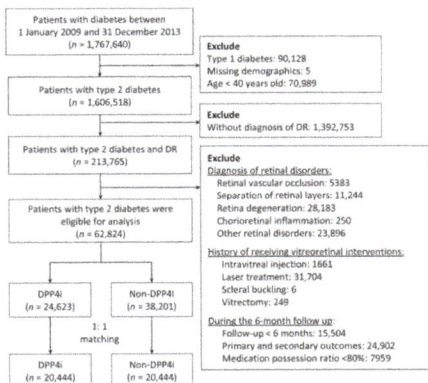

Figure 1. Flowchart of the inclusion and exclusion criteria of the patients. DR, diabetes retinopathy; DPP4i, dipeptidyl peptidase 4 inhibitors.

2.3. Group Definition

The index date of the DPP4i group was defined as the date of the first DPP4i prescription between 2009 and 2013. To prevent the immortal time bias, the index date of the non-DPP4i group was assigned as the index date of the DPP4i group through an approach known as prescription time-distribution matching [25]. To ascertain the compliance of DPP4i use, patients in the DPP4i group with a medication possession ratio (MPR) of less than 80% during the first 6 months of follow-up [26], specifically 144 days (180 days × 0.8), were excluded from further analysis (Figure 1).

2.4. Outcomes

In this study, the primary ocular outcome was the composite DR outcome, which consisted of any one of the following: VH, tractional RD, and macular edema. The secondary ocular outcome was the composite outcome of any surgical intervention, namely retinal laser therapy, IVI, and vitrectomy. The cardiovascular outcomes, including myocardial infarction, hospitalization for heart failure, ischemic stroke, and hemorrhagic stroke, were defined as safety outcomes. The primary DR outcome and its components were defined as diagnosis after at least three outpatient diagnoses or one inpatient diagnosis. The surgical interventions and other ocular outcomes were examined using the Taiwan NHI reimbursement codes from the claims data for outpatient and inpatient visits. The occurrence of safety outcomes was determined using the principal discharge diagnosis. Mortality and cardiovascular events selected for analysis have been validated previously [27,28].

2.5. Covariates

Covariates were sex, age, proxy variables for compliance (i.e., the number of outpatient visits for diabetes management), proxy variables for DR severity (previous proliferative DR and previous DR duration), comorbidities as well as scores on the Charlson Comorbidity Index, indicators for diabetic severity (diabetes duration, diabetic neuropathy, and diabetic foot ulcer), and concomitant medications. Comorbidities, namely dyslipidemia, hypertension, ischemic heart disease, chronic kidney disease, peripheral arterial disease, ischemic stroke, heart failure, and atrial fibrillation, were confirmed after at least three outpatient diagnoses or one inpatient diagnosis in the previous year. Medications during the first 6 months of follow-up were classified into three categories: antidiabetics, antihypertensives, and other medications. Details of the ICD-9-CM diagnostic codes used in this study are provided in Supplementary Materials (Table S1). The Charlson Comorbidity Index scores were calculated as described previously [29].

2.6. Statistics

To reduce confounding effects, the analysis of differences in outcomes between the DPP4i and non-DPP4i groups was performed after propensity score matching (PSM). The propensity score was the predicted probability given the value of the covariates, which was calculated using a multivariable logistic regression model in which the study groups (1: DPP4i and 0: non-DPP4i) were regressed on the selected covariates. The matching was processed using a greedy nearest-neighbor algorithm with a caliper of 0.2 times the standard deviation of the logit of the propensity score. The matching order was random, and replacement was not allowed. Each patient in the DPP4i group was matched with a non-DPP4i control. The matching quality was assessed after PSM by using the absolute value of the standardized difference between the groups, where a value of less than 0.1 was considered negligible.

The Fine–Gray subdistribution hazard model, which considers all-cause mortality a competing risk, was used to compare the occurrence of time-to-event outcomes between the groups. The average number of surgical interventions per decade was also analyzed and compared using the Poisson model, in which the natural logarithm of the follow-up duration was an offset variable. The study groups (DPP4i vs. non-DPP4i) were the only explanatory variable in the regression analysis. The within-pair clustering of outcomes after PSM was accounted for by using robust standard errors through the generalized estimating equation approach [30]. Further subgroup analyses were conducted to evaluate the consistency of the observed treatment effect on the specified outcomes across different levels of subgroup variables. The outcomes of interest comprised the primary and secondary endpoints, namely the composite DR outcome and the composite outcome of any surgical intervention, respectively. The selected subgroups were sex, age (dichotomized at 65 years), previous proliferative DR, hypertension, dyslipidemia, ischemic heart disease, ischemic stroke, chronic kidney disease, peripheral arterial disease, diabetes duration (dichotomized at 10 years), diabetic neuropathy, diabetic foot ulcer, and the use of concomitant antidiabetics (e.g., metformin, sulfonylurea, thiazolidinediones, alpha-glucosidase inhibitors, meglitinides, and insulin). A two-sided p-value of <0.05 was considered to be significant. All analyses were performed using SAS software, Version 9.4 of the SAS System (SAS Institute Inc., Cary, NC, USA), including the % cif macro for generating cumulative incidence functions under the Fine–Gray sub-distribution hazard method.

3. Results

3.1. Participants

Between 2009 and 2013, a total of 1,767,640 patients with diabetes were identified. After the exclusion of patients aged under 40 years as well as those with type 1 diabetes, missing demographic data, and no DR diagnosis, 213,765 patients remained. We further excluded patients who were followed up for less than 6 months or developed any of the primary or secondary ocular outcomes within 6 months after the index date, as well as those with retinal disorders, a history of receiving vitreoretinal interventions or who had an MPR of less than 80%. After these procedures, 62,824 patients remained. After 1:1 PSM, the non-DPP4i and DPP4i groups comprised 20,444 patients each (Figure 1).

3.2. Demographic Characteristics

Table 1 presents the demographic characteristics of the study groups before and after matching. Before matching, the patients in the DPP4i group were younger; had more outpatient visits for diabetes management in the previous year; were more likely to have undergone a dilated fundus examination in the previous year; had a higher prevalence of dyslipidemia; had a longer diabetes duration; had more prescriptions of sulfonylurea, alpha-glucosidase inhibitors, meglitinides, beta-blockers, angiotensin-converting enzyme inhibitors/angiotensin II receptor blockers, antiplatelets, statins, and fenofibrates, and fewer prescriptions of insulin. After matching, the two groups were well balanced in terms of sex, age, comorbidities, indicators for diabetic severity, underlying ocular diseases, medications, and follow-up duration.

Table 1. Characteristics of patients with type 2 diabetes and diabetic retinopathy before and after matching. Balance achieved between the DPP4i and non-DPP4i groups after matching.

Variable	before Matching			after Matching		
	DDP4i (n = 24,623)	Non-DDP4i (n = 38,201)	STD	DDP4i (n = 20,444)	Non-DDP4i (n = 20,444)	STD
Sex (male)	10,745 (43.6)	17,084 (44.7)	−0.02	8936 (43.7)	9013 (44.1)	−0.01
Age (years)	66.5 ± 10.5	68.0 ± 11.0	−0.14	66.7 ± 10.5	66.7 ± 10.8	<0.01
Age ≥ 65 years	13,606 (55.3)	22,849 (59.8)	−0.09	11,416 (55.8)	11,448 (56.0)	<0.01
No. of outpatient visit in the prior year	16.8 ± 8.9	14.1 ± 9.0	0.31	16.1 ± 8.3	16.1 ± 9.7	<0.01
Previous proliferative DR	2195 (8.9)	3605 (9.4)	−0.02	1862 (9.1)	1879 (9.2)	<0.01
Duration of DR (years)	6.1 ± 3.5	6.0 ± 3.5	0.03	6.0 ± 3.4	6.0 ± 3.5	<0.01
Comorbidity						
Dyslipidemia	20,277 (82.3)	29,405 (77.0)	0.13	16,560 (81.0)	16,673 (81.6)	−0.01
Hypertension	17,202 (69.9)	25,236 (66.1)	0.08	14,038 (68.7)	14,140 (69.2)	−0.01
Ischemic heart disease	11,746 (47.7)	17,433 (45.6)	0.04	9626 (47.1)	9608 (47.0)	<0.01
Chronic kidney disease	6126 (24.9)	8035 (21.0)	0.09	4724 (23.1)	4745 (23.2)	<0.01
Peripheral arterial disease	3350 (13.6)	5480 (14.3)	−0.02	2804 (13.7)	2739 (13.4)	0.01
Ischemic stroke	3015 (12.2)	4989 (13.1)	−0.02	2526 (12.4)	2512 (12.3)	<0.01
Heart failure	1470 (6.0)	2464 (6.5)	−0.02	1186 (5.8)	1171 (5.7)	<0.01
Atrial fibrillation	882 (3.6)	1459 (3.8)	−0.01	716 (3.5)	699 (3.4)	<0.01
Charlson Comorbidity Index score	2.5 ± 1.7	2.3 ± 1.8	0.07	2.4 ± 1.7	2.4 ± 1.8	<0.01
Indicator for diabetic severity						
Diabetes duration, years	11.3 ± 2.7	11.0 ± 3.0	0.11	11.2 ± 2.8	11.2 ± 2.9	−0.01
Diabetic neuropathy	9887 (40.2)	14,112 (36.9)	0.07	7980 (39.0)	8065 (39.4)	−0.01
Diabetic foot ulcer	3366 (13.7)	5152 (13.5)	0.01	2762 (13.5)	2751 (13.5)	<0.01
Antidiabetics						
Sulfonylurea	14,543 (59.1)	19,954 (52.2)	0.14	11,921 (58.3)	12,065 (59.0)	−0.01
Metformin	13,162 (53.5)	22,197 (58.1)	−0.09	11,396 (55.7)	11,537 (56.4)	−0.01
Alpha-glucosidase inhibitors	4636 (18.8)	4,779 (12.5)	0.17	3514 (17.2)	3490 (17.1)	<0.01
Thiazolidinediones	3076 (12.5)	210 (13.6)	−0.03	2683 (13.1)	2812 (13.8)	−0.02
Meglitinides	2574 (10.5)	2918 (7.6)	0.10	1996 (9.8)	2024 (9.9)	<0.01
Insulin	3873 (15.7)	8299 (21.7)	−0.15	3488 (17.1)	3633 (17.8)	−0.02
Antihypertensives						
Angiotensin-converting enzyme inhibitors/angiotensin II receptor blockers	15,630 (63.5)	20,002 (52.4)	0.23	12,445 (60.9)	12,577 (61.5)	−0.01
Calcium channel blockers	8509 (34.6)	14,036 (36.7)	−0.05	7174 (35.1)	7213 (35.3)	<0.01
Beta blockers	7654 (31.1)	9780 (25.6)	0.12	6048 (29.6)	6023 (29.5)	<0.01
Alpha blockers	1403 (5.7)	2154 (5.6)	<0.01	1163 (5.7)	1176 (5.8)	<0.01
Thiazide	1075 (4.4)	1545 (4.0)	0.02	886 (4.3)	866 (4.2)	<0.01
Other medications						
Antiplatelets	8767 (35.6)	11,115 (29.1)	0.14	6970 (34.1)	7074 (34.6)	−0.01
Anticoagulants	380 (1.5)	473 (1.2)	0.03	304 (1.5)	284 (1.4)	0.01
Statins	10,788 (43.8)	12,319 (32.2)	0.24	8381 (41.0)	8346 (40.8)	<0.01
Fenofibrates	2552 (10.4)	2894 (7.6)	0.10	1975 (9.7)	1972 (9.6)	<0.01
Follow-up (years)	2.5 ± 1.3	2.4 ± 1.1	0.06	2.6 ± 1.2	2.5 ± 1.2	0.08

DDP4i, dipeptidyl peptidase 4 inhibitor; STD, standardized difference; DR, diabetic retinopathy. Data are presented as frequency (percentage) or mean ± standard deviation.

3.3. Primary Ocular Outcomes

Table 2 presents the primary ocular outcomes of the patients, including any surgical intervention taken. Over a mean follow-up duration of 2.5 years, 366 and 294 patients (1.8% and 1.4%, respectively) in the DPP4i and non-DPP4i groups developed the primary ocular outcome, namely the composite DR outcome. The risk of developing the composite DR outcome was significantly higher in the DPP4i group (sub-distribution hazard ratio [SHR] 1.23, 95% confidence interval [CI] 1.06–1.44; Figure 2A). Among the individual components of the composite DR outcome, the risks of VH (SHR 1.24, 95% CI 1.05–1.48) and macular edema (SHR 1.48, 95% CI 1.03–2.13) were significantly higher in the DPP4i group.

Table 2. Primary ocular outcomes, including any surgical intervention taken, of patients with type 2 diabetes and diabetic retinopathy demonstrating significantly higher risks of composite diabetic retinopathy and surgical interventions in the DPP4i group.

Outcome	DDP4i (n = 20,444)	Non-DDP4i (n = 20,444)	DPP4i vs. Non-DPP4i SHR (95% CI)	p-Value
Primary ocular outcome (composite DR outcome)	366 (1.8)	294 (1.4)	1.23 (1.06–1.44)	0.008
Individual component of composite DR outcome				
VH	292 (1.4)	232 (1.1)	1.24 (1.05–1.48)	0.013
Tractional RD	50 (0.24)	35 (0.17)	1.41 (0.91–2.17)	0.122
Macular edema	72 (0.35)	48 (0.23)	1.48 (1.03–2.13)	0.035
Surgical intervention				
Retinal laser therapy	824 (4.0)	582 (2.8)	1.75 (1.33–2.30)	<0.001
IVI	140 (0.68)	79 (0.39)	1.32 (1.001–1.74)	0.049
Vitrectomy	118 (0.58)	88 (0.43)	1.32 (1.24–1.40)	<0.001
Composite outcome of any surgical intervention	891 (4.4)	636 (3.1)	1.40 (1.26–1.55)	<0.001
Number of interventions per 10 years			RR (95% CI) *	p-value
Retinal laser therapy	0.6 ± 3.4	0.4 ± 2.9	1.39 (1.23–1.58)	<0.001
IVI	0.06 ± 0.94	0.03 ± 0.67	1.84 (1.28–2.63)	0.001
Vitrectomy	0.03 ± 0.42	0.02 ± 0.38	1.29 (0.94–1.79)	0.117

DDP4i, dipeptidyl peptidase 4 inhibitor; SHR, sub-distribution hazard ratio; CI, confidence interval; RD, retinal detachment; DR, diabetic retinopathy; RR, rate ratio; VH, vitreous hemorrhage; IVI, intravitreal injection. * Estimated using a Poisson model in which the logarithm of follow-up duration was treated as an offset variable.

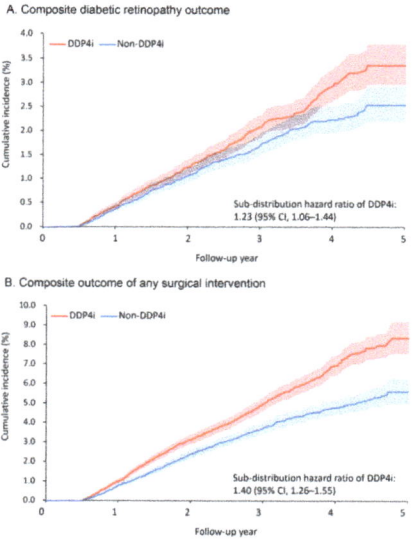

Figure 2. Cumulative incidence function of (**A**) composite diabetic retinopathy outcome and (**B**) composite outcome of any surgical intervention between the DPP4i and non-DPP4i group after propensity score matching. DPP4i, dipeptidyl peptidase 4 inhibitor; CI, confidence interval.

The DPP4i group also had a higher risk of receiving surgical intervention for severe DR or its complications (retinal laser therapy: SHR 1.75, 95% CI 1.33–2.30; IVI: SHR 1.32, 95% CI 1.001–1.74; vitrectomy: SHR 1.32, 95% CI 1.24–1.40; any surgical intervention: SHR 1.40, 95% CI 1.26–1.55; Figure 2B). As for the number of interventions, more patients in the DPP4i group received retinal laser therapy (rate ratio (RR) 1.39, 95% CI 1.23–1.58) and IVI (RR 1.84, 95% CI 1.28–2.63) than in the non-DPP4i group.

3.4. Safety Outcomes

The results of the safety outcomes are shown in Table 3. No between-group differences were observed in any of the safety outcomes, namely myocardial infarction, hospitalization for heart failure, ischemic stroke, hemorrhagic stroke, and the composite outcome of major adverse cardiovascular events.

Table 3. Safety outcomes of patients with type 2 diabetes and diabetic retinopathy showing no significant risk in both groups.

Outcome	DDP4i (n = 20,444)	Non-DDP4i (n = 20,444)	DPP4i vs. Non-DPP4i SHR (95% CI)	p-Value
Myocardial infarction	252 (1.2)	268 (1.3)	0.93 (0.78–1.10)	0.396
Hospitalization for heart failure	495 (2.4)	441 (2.2)	1.11 (0.98–1.26)	0.115
Ischemic stroke	872 (4.3)	839 (4.1)	1.02 (0.93–1.13)	0.621
Hemorrhagic stroke	131 (0.64)	151 (0.74)	0.85 (0.68–1.08)	0.183
Major adverse cardiovascular events *	1600 (7.8)	1529 (7.5)	1.05 (0.98–1.12)	0.198

DDP4i, dipeptidyl peptidase 4 inhibitor; SHR, sub-distribution hazard ratio; CI, confidence interval. * Any one of myocardial infarction, heart failure, or stroke.

3.5. Subgroup Analysis

We further conducted subgroup analysis on the primary composite DR outcome and the composite outcome of any surgical interventions. The results showed that the observed hazardous effect of DPP4i on the risk of primary composite DR outcome was particularly obvious in the following population: females, younger patients, patients with relatively shorter diabetes duration, and those without taking insulin (All p-values for interaction <0.05; Figure 3A). Similarly, the observed increased risk of the composite outcome of any surgical interventions due to DPP4i was more apparent in patients with relatively shorter diabetes duration, and those who took sulfonylurea, and those without insulin therapy (All p-values for interaction <0.05; Figure 3B).

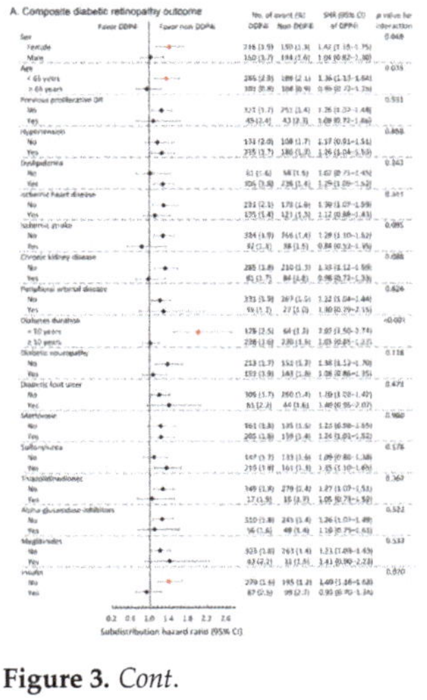

Figure 3. Cont.

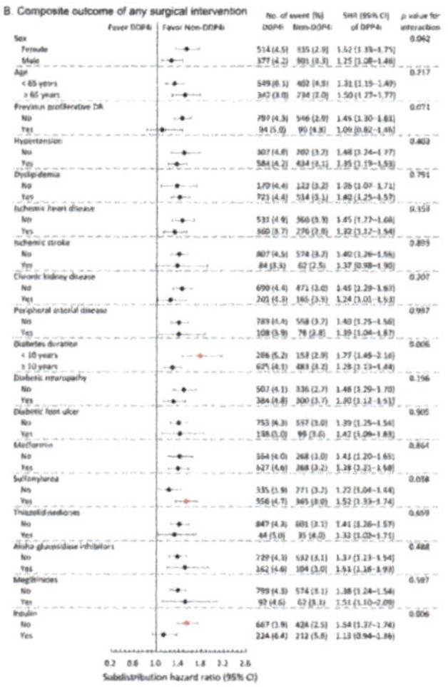

Figure 3. Subgroup analysis of (**A**) composite diabetic retinopathy outcomes and (**B**) composite outcome of any surgical interventions of the diabetic patients with DR between the DPP4i users and non-DPP4i controls in the propensity score-matched cohort. The red color indicates a statistical significance.

4. Discussion

The use of DPP4i in glucose-lowering for diabetes has increased considerably over the past decade after being introduced in 2006 [31]. To reduce mortality and morbidity, measuring drugs' protective effects and related diabetes complications are essential. As mentioned, DR, a major microvascular complication in diabetes, can cause severe visual impairment. Thus, in this population-based study, we evaluated the association between the add-on DPP4i therapy and the progression of preexisting DR in patients with type 2 diabetes aged ≥ 40 years. During the 2.5-year follow-up, the add-on DPP4i therapy was associated with increased risks of composite DR outcome and needs of surgical interventions. However, it did not increase the risk of cardiovascular events.

The association between DPP4i and DR remains a matter of contention in the literature. A study including 82 patients with type 2 diabetes reported that DPP4i use had protective effects on DR progression [18]. A study using a cohort representative of individuals in the US population aged ≥ 65 years observed that DPP4i use had a neutral effect on DR [32]. Some other studies have found that DPP4i cause adverse retinal outcomes. In the Trial Evaluating Cardiovascular Outcomes With Sitagliptin (TECOS), DR occurred more frequently in patients under add-on sitagliptin therapy than in those who were not (2.8% vs. 2.2%) [33]. Another study, using a sample representative of the South Korean population, also indicated an increased risk of DR in early DPP4i treatment (<12 months) [19]. These findings indicate that the pharmacodynamic or effects of DPP4i may vary with population or patient characteristics.

The non-DPP4i and DPP4i groups in the present study comprised 20,444 patients (after matching) with type 2 diabetes (mean duration of 11 years since onset) and preexisting DR, respectively. VH and macular edema occurred significantly more frequently in the DPP4i group than in the non-DPP4i group. Furthermore, patients in the DPP4i group under add-on DPP4i therapy for diabetes control were more likely to receive surgical intervention for advanced DR. In short, add-on DPP4i therapy increased the risk of DR progression. However, no significant between-group differences in safety outcomes were noted. In addition, DPP4i was not associated with an increased risk of cardiovascular events.

Although the exact mechanism remains uncertain, biochemical changes in retinal cells after DPP4i administration in experimental studies have been inconsistent. Numerous laboratory studies have reported the protective effects of DPP4i on retinal health. For example, Gonçalves et al. found that sitagliptin had an antioxidative effect on rat retinas [34]. In another of their studies, sitagliptin ameliorated bovine retinal endothelial dysfunction caused by inflammation [15]. Another study noted that linagliptin had anti-angiogenic effects on mice with oxygen-induced retinopathy [35]. However, Lee et al. indicated that DPP4i caused disruptions in endothelial cell-to-cell junctions by accumulating stromal cell-derived factor 1α and phosphorylating vascular endothelial cadherin, as well as further increasing retinal vascular permeability [36]. In a 2020 experimental study, the results revealed that prolonged DPP4 inhibition destabilized the blood-retina barrier, potentially inducing retinal edema [37]. Early deterioration of DR was also reported in a GLP-1 analog, semaglutide, although the pharmacodynamic may be different with the DPP4i [38]. Retinal changes under DPP4i therapy may depend on the duration of DPP4i treatment and the severity of diabetes and its complications. Long-term administration of DPP4i in patients with preexisting DR might induce the development of excess vasculature as well as vascular permeability, potentially contributing to exudate production and further exacerbating DR. Thus, more awareness of DR progression may be necessary for patients under long-term DPP4i treatment.

Cardiovascular complications of DPP4i remain the topic of an ongoing debate. Some studies have reported a decreased risk of cardiovascular events after DPP4i therapy [39,40]. By contrast, other studies have indicated that DPP4i use increased the risk of cardiovascular disorders [17,41]. In our study, the safety outcomes (including myocardial infarction, heart failure, ischemic stroke, hemorrhagic stroke, and composite cardiovascular outcomes) did not differ significantly between the groups. This is consistent with the assessment from the TECOS [33], the Examination of Cardiovascular Outcomes with Alogliptin versus Standard of Care, and the Saxagliptin Assessment of Vascular Outcomes Recorded in Patients with Diabetes Mellitus (SAVOR)—Thrombolysis in Myocardial Infarction (TIMI) [12]. Thus, our additional finding also supported a neutral association between DPP4i use and the occurrence of major adverse cardiovascular events.

A limited number of large-scale clinical studies have evaluated the association of DPP4i and the progression of retinopathy in patients with diabetes. The strength of the present study is that, to the best of our knowledge, it is the first observational investigation of the association of an add-on DPP4i in DR progression in a population-based cohort. By systemically assessing the possible confounding factors and making adjustments through PSM, we minimized detection bias and balanced the clinical characteristics between the groups. The approximately 2.5-year follow-up also means that the present findings demonstrate the long-term impacts—as opposed to the short-term effects—of DPP4i use. The potential harm that may accompany DPP4i use indicated in the present study raises substantial concerns regarding its safe use as an antidiabetic.

This study has some limitations. First, because only patients older than 40 years were included, the present findings cannot be extrapolated to other age groups. Moreover, because the patients were all Taiwanese, it remains unclear whether our findings are generalizable to other populations. Second, we could not completely prevent confounding effects. Nevertheless, we performed matching by systematically considering various variables, minimizing any imbalance between the groups. Third, we could not obtain information on the patients' diabetes control, as well as the hypoglycemic events, which are important factors of diabetes management. Nevertheless, we have matched the patients in the two groups based on their hypoglycemic agent use. Fourth, data on laboratory tests, such as the serum glucose level or hemoglobin A1c, are not available in the NHIRD. Rapid reduction of hemoglobin A1c may affect early worsening of DR [8]. However, this phenomenon should be counterbalanced in a long-term observation in the patients with better glucose control, which has been reported in the Semaglutide Unabated Sustainability in Treatment of Type 2 Diabetes (SUSTAIN) study [38]. In our study, the follow-up period of 2.5 years is comparable with the previous study, and our case number (n = 20,444 in both study and control groups) is higher than the SUSTAIN study (n = 8105 across the SUSTAIN 1 to 6 studies) [38]. Whether the DR progression in the add-on DPP4i use is related to rapid hypoglycemic response needs further study. Fifth, the between-patient variation in diabetes severity (with some patients in severe condition) means that the alleviation of systemic disorders with medications remains challenging. The blood pressure change in our study was also not available. Nevertheless, we have matched the groups according to their disease duration, complications, medications, and underlying conditions. Therefore, the clinical characteristics of patients in the two groups were comparable at least in theory. Last, the database did not contain the results of ocular exams including optical coherence tomography, which is essential to differentiate the involvement of diabetic macular edema. The association of DPP4i and the involvement of diabetic macular edema may need further investigations. A prospective randomized trial may be required for understanding the possible effect of add-on DPP4i therapy in the progression of DR in patients with type 2 diabetes.

5. Conclusions

In conclusion, add-on DPP4i therapy may be associated with the progression of preexisting DR in patients with type 2 diabetes aged ≥40 years, but the cause and effect need further research DPP4i therapy did not increase the risk of cardiovascular events. Therefore, when choosing hypoglycemic treatments for patients with diabetes and preexisting DR, the possible promoting effect of DPP4i on DR progression should be considered. A close retinal evaluation may be necessary for long-term DPP4i administration.

Supplementary Materials: The following are available online at https://www.mdpi.com/article/10.3390/jcm10132871/s1, Table S1: ICD-9 CM diagnostic codes used in the study.

Author Contributions: Y.-S.H. and T.-H.C. have full access to the data and takes overall responsibility. Conception and design: E.Y.-C.K., T.-H.C. and Y.-S.H.; Data collection and collation: C.K., W.-C.W. and C.-C.S.; Data analysis and interpretation: K.-J.C. and C.-C.L.; Writing: E.Y.-C.K. and C.K. All authors have read and agreed to the published version of the manuscript.

Funding: The study was supported by the Ministry of Science and Technology, Taiwan (MOST 106-2314-B-182A-045 -MY3), and Chang Gung Memorial Hospital, Taiwan (BMRPF29). The sponsor had no role in the design or conduct of this research.

Institutional Review Board Statement: The study was conducted according to the guidelines of the Declaration of Helsinki and approved by the Institutional Review Board of Chang Gung Memorial Hospital, Taiwan (No. 201800199B1).

Informed Consent Statement: Patient consent was waived due to the de-identified database.

Data Availability Statement: The data used for the current study cannot be made publicly available according to the NHIRD regulations of personal data protection, allowing only the person responsible for the data management to approach the data after approval from Taiwan NHI bureau.

Acknowledgments: We thank two biostatisticians, Alfred Hsing-Fen Lin and Ben Yu-Lin Chou, for their valuable assistance with the statistical analysis in the present study.

Conflicts of Interest: The authors declare no conflict of interest.

References

1. Klein, B.E. Overview of epidemiologic studies of diabetic retinopathy. *Ophthalmic Epidemiol.* **2007**, *14*, 179–183. [CrossRef] [PubMed]
2. Yau, J.W.; Rogers, S.L.; Kawasaki, R.; Lamoureux, E.L.; Kowalski, J.W.; Bek, T.; Chen, S.J.; Dekker, J.M.; Fletcher, A.; Grauslund, J.; et al. Global prevalence and major risk factors of diabetic retinopathy. *Diabetes Care* **2012**, *35*, 556–564. [CrossRef] [PubMed]
3. Cheung, N.; Mitchell, P.; Wong, T.Y. Diabetic retinopathy. *Lancet* **2010**, *376*, 124–136. [CrossRef]
4. Antonetti, D.A.; Klein, R.; Gardner, T.W. Diabetic retinopathy. *N. Engl. J. Med.* **2012**, *366*, 1227–1239. [CrossRef]
5. International Diabetes Federation. *IDF Diabetes Atlas*, 8th ed.; International Diabetes Federation: Brussels, Belgium, 2019; Available online: http://www.diabetesatlas.org/ (accessed on 13 January 2021).
6. Gerstein, H.C.; Miller, M.E.; Genuth, S.; Ismail-Beigi, F.; Buse, J.B.; Goff, D.C., Jr.; Probstfield, J.L.; Cushman, W.C.; Ginsberg, H.N.; Bigger, J.T.; et al. Long-term effects of intensive glucose lowering on cardiovascular outcomes. *N. Engl. J. Med.* **2011**, *364*, 818–828. [CrossRef]

7. Chew, E.Y.; Ambrosius, W.T.; Davis, M.D.; Danis, R.P.; Gangaputra, S.; Greven, C.M.; Hubbard, L.; Esser, B.A.; Lovato, J.F.; Perdue, L.H.; et al. Effects of medical therapies on retinopathy progression in type 2 diabetes. *N. Engl. J. Med.* **2010**, *363*, 233–244. [CrossRef]
8. UK Prospective Diabetes Study (UKPDS) Group. Intensive blood-glucose control with sulphonylureas or insulin compared with conventional treatment and risk of complications in patients with type 2 diabetes (UKPDS 33). UK Prospective Diabetes Study (UKPDS) Group. *Lancet* **1998**, *352*, 837–853. [CrossRef]
9. The, U.S. *Food and Drug Administration. Drug Approval Package*; U.S. Food and Drug Administration: Silver Spring, MD, USA, 2006. Available online: https://www.accessdata.fda.gov/drugsatfda_docs/nda/2006/021995s000TOC.cfm (accessed on 13 January 2021).
10. Baetta, R.; Corsini, A. Pharmacology of dipeptidyl peptidase-4 inhibitors: Similarities and differences. *Drugs* **2011**, *71*, 1441–1467. [CrossRef]
11. Li, Z.; Zhao, L.; Yu, L.; Yang, J. Head-to-Head Comparison of the Hypoglycemic Efficacy and Safety Between Dipeptidyl Peptidase-4 Inhibitors and alpha-Glucosidase Inhibitors in Patients With Type 2 Diabetes Mellitus: A Meta-Analysis of Randomized Controlled Trials. *Front. Pharmacol.* **2019**, *10*, 777. [CrossRef]
12. Scirica, B.M.; Bhatt, D.L.; Braunwald, E.; Steg, P.G.; Davidson, J.; Hirshberg, B.; Ohman, P.; Frederich, R.; Wiviott, S.D.; Hoffman, E.B.; et al. Saxagliptin and cardiovascular outcomes in patients with type 2 diabetes mellitus. *N. Engl. J. Med.* **2013**, *369*, 1317–1326. [CrossRef]
13. Zannad, F.; Cannon, C.P.; Cushman, W.C.; Bakris, G.L.; Menon, V.; Perez, A.T.; Fleck, P.R.; Mehta, C.R.; Kupfer, S.; Wilson, C.; et al. Heart failure and mortality outcomes in patients with type 2 diabetes taking alogliptin versus placebo in EXAMINE: A multicentre, randomised, double-blind trial. *Lancet* **2015**, *385*, 2067–2076. [CrossRef]
14. Zheng, S.L.; Roddick, A.J.; Aghar-Jaffar, R.; Shun-Shin, M.J.; Francis, D.; Oliver, N.; Meeran, K. Association Between Use of Sodium-Glucose Cotransporter 2 Inhibitors, Glucagon-like Peptide 1 Agonists, and Dipeptidyl Peptidase 4 Inhibitors With All-Cause Mortality in Patients With Type 2 Diabetes: A Systematic Review and Meta-analysis. *JAMA* **2018**, *319*, 1580–1591. [CrossRef]
15. Gonçalves, A.; Leal, E.; Paiva, A.; Teixeira Lemos, E.; Teixeira, F.; Ribeiro, C.F.; Reis, F.; Ambrosio, A.F.; Fernandes, R. Protective effects of the dipeptidyl peptidase IV inhibitor sitagliptin in the blood-retinal barrier in a type 2 diabetes animal model. *Diabetes Obes. Metab.* **2012**, *14*, 454–463. [CrossRef]
16. Avogaro, A.; Fadini, G.P. The effects of dipeptidyl peptidase-4 inhibition on microvascular diabetes complications. *Diabetes Care* **2014**, *37*, 2884–2894. [CrossRef]
17. Rehman, M.B.; Tudrej, B.V.; Soustre, J.; Buisson, M.; Archambault, P.; Pouchain, D.; Vaillant-Roussel, H.; Gueyffier, F.; Faillie, J.L.; Perault-Pochat, M.C.; et al. Efficacy and safety of DPP-4 inhibitors in patients with type 2 diabetes: Meta-analysis of placebo-controlled randomized clinical trials. *Diabetes Obes. Metab.* **2017**, *43*, 48–58. [CrossRef]
18. Chung, Y.R.; Park, S.W.; Kim, J.W.; Kim, J.H.; Lee, K. Protective Effects of Dipeptidyl peptidase-4 inhibitors on Progression of Diabetic Retinopathy in Patient with Type 2 Diabetes. *Retina* **2016**, *36*, 2357–2363. [CrossRef]
19. Kim, N.H.; Choi, J.; Kim, N.H.; Choi, K.M.; Baik, S.H.; Lee, J.; Kim, S.G. Dipeptidyl peptidase-4 inhibitor use and risk of diabetic retinopathy: A population-based study. *Diabetes Obes. Metab.* **2018**, *44*, 361–367. [CrossRef]
20. Chung, Y.R.; Ha, K.H.; Kim, H.C.; Park, S.J.; Lee, K.; Kim, D.J. Dipeptidyl Peptidase-4 Inhibitors versus Other Antidiabetic Drugs Added to Metformin Monotherapy in Diabetic Retinopathy Progression: A Real World-Based Cohort Study. *Diabetes Metab. J.* **2019**. [CrossRef]
21. Hsieh, C.Y.; Su, C.C.; Shao, S.C.; Sung, S.F.; Lin, S.J.; Kao Yang, Y.H.; Lai, E.C. Taiwan's National Health Insurance Research Database: Past and future. *Clin. Epidemiol.* **2019**, *11*, 349–358. [CrossRef]
22. Hsing, A.W.; Ioannidis, J.P. Nationwide Population Science: Lessons From the Taiwan National Health Insurance Research Database. *JAMA Intern. Med.* **2015**, *175*, 1527–1529. [CrossRef]
23. Lin, C.C.; Lai, M.S.; Syu, C.Y.; Chang, S.C.; Tseng, F.Y. Accuracy of diabetes diagnosis in health insurance claims data in Taiwan. *J. Med. Assoc.* **2005**, *104*, 157–163.
24. Wu, C.S.; Lai, M.S.; Gau, S.S.; Wang, S.C.; Tsai, H.J. Concordance between patient self-reports and claims data on clinical diagnoses, medication use, and health system utilization in Taiwan. *PLoS ONE* **2014**, *9*, e112257. [CrossRef]
25. Zhou, Z.; Rahme, E.; Abrahamowicz, M.; Pilote, L. Survival bias associated with time-to-treatment initiation in drug effectiveness evaluation: A comparison of methods. *Am. J. Epidemiol.* **2005**, *162*, 1016–1023. [CrossRef]
26. Kang, E.Y.; Chen, T.H.; Garg, S.J.; Sun, C.C.; Kang, J.H.; Wu, W.C.; Hung, M.J.; Lai, C.C.; Cherng, W.J.; Hwang, Y.S. Association of Statin Therapy With Prevention of Vision-Threatening Diabetic Retinopathy. *JAMA Ophthal.* **2019**, *137*, 363–371. [CrossRef]
27. Cheng, C.L.; Chien, H.C.; Lee, C.H.; Lin, S.J.; Yang, Y.H. Validity of in-hospital mortality data among patients with acute myocardial infarction or stroke in National Health Insurance Research Database in Taiwan. *Int. J. Cardiol.* **2015**, *201*, 96–101. [CrossRef] [PubMed]
28. Cheng, C.-L.; Lee, C.-H.; Chen, P.-S.; Li, Y.-H.; Lin, S.-J.; Yang, Y.-H.K. Validation of Acute Myocardial Infarction Cases in the National Health Insurance Research Database in Taiwan. *J. Epidemiol.* **2014**, *24*, 500–507. [CrossRef]
29. Charlson, M.E.; Pompei, P.; Ales, K.L.; MacKenzie, C.R. A new method of classifying prognostic comorbidity in longitudinal studies: Development and validation. *J. Chronic Dis.* **1987**, *40*, 373–383. [CrossRef]

30. Austin, P.C.; Fine, J.P. Propensity-score matching with competing risks in survival analysis. *Stat. Med.* **2019**, *38*, 751–777. [CrossRef]
31. Gallwitz, B. Clinical Use of DPP-4 Inhibitors. *Front. Endocrinol.* **2019**, *10*, 389. [CrossRef]
32. Wang, T.; Hong, J.L.; Gower, E.W.; Pate, V.; Garg, S.; Buse, J.B.; Stürmer, T. Incretin-Based Therapies and Diabetic Retinopathy: Real-World Evidence in Older U.S. Adults. *Diabetes Care* **2018**, *41*, 1998–2009. [CrossRef]
33. Green, J.B.; Bethel, M.A.; Armstrong, P.W.; Buse, J.B.; Engel, S.S.; Garg, J.; Josse, R.; Kaufman, K.D.; Koglin, J.; Korn, S.; et al. Effect of Sitagliptin on Cardiovascular Outcomes in Type 2 Diabetes. *N. Engl. J. Med.* **2015**, *373* (Suppl. 235S), 232–242. [CrossRef]
34. Gonçalves, A.; Almeida, L.; Silva, A.P.; Fontes-Ribeiro, C.; Ambrósio, A.F.; Cristóvão, A.; Fernandes, R. The dipeptidyl peptidase-4 (DPP-4) inhibitor sitagliptin ameliorates retinal endothelial cell dysfunction triggered by inflammation. *Biomed. Pharmacother.* **2018**, *102*, 833–838. [CrossRef] [PubMed]
35. Kolibabka, M.; Dietrich, N.; Klein, T.; Hammes, H.P. Anti-angiogenic effects of the DPP-4 inhibitor linagliptin via inhibition of VEGFR signalling in the mouse model of oxygen-induced retinopathy. *Diabetologia* **2018**, *61*, 2412–2421. [CrossRef] [PubMed]
36. Lee, C.S.; Kim, Y.G.; Cho, H.J.; Park, J.; Jeong, H.; Lee, S.E.; Lee, S.P.; Kang, H.J.; Kim, H.S. Dipeptidyl Peptidase-4 Inhibitor Increases Vascular Leakage in Retina through VE-cadherin Phosphorylation. *Sci. Rep.* **2016**, *6*, 29393. [CrossRef] [PubMed]
37. Jäckle, A.; Ziemssen, F.; Kuhn, E.M.; Kampmeier, J.; Lang, G.K.; Lang, G.E.; Deissler, H.; Deissler, H.L. Sitagliptin and the Blood-Retina Barrier: Effects on Retinal Endothelial Cells Manifested Only after Prolonged Exposure. *J. Diabetes Res.* **2020**, *2020*, 2450781. [CrossRef] [PubMed]
38. Vilsbøll, T.; Bain, S.C.; Leiter, L.A.; Lingvay, I.; Matthews, D.; Simó, R.; Helmark, I.C.; Wijayasinghe, N.; Larsen, M. Semaglutide, reduction in glycated haemoglobin and the risk of diabetic retinopathy. *Diabetes Obes. Metab.* **2018**, *20*, 889–897. [CrossRef] [PubMed]
39. Ussher, J.R.; Drucker, D.J. Cardiovascular actions of incretin-based therapies. *Circ. Res.* **2014**, *114*, 1788–1803. [CrossRef]
40. Bae, E.J. DPP-4 inhibitors in diabetic complications: Role of DPP-4 beyond glucose control. *Arch. Pharmacal. Res.* **2016**, *39*, 1114–1128. [CrossRef]
41. Li, L.; Li, S.; Deng, K.; Liu, J.; Vandvik, P.O.; Zhao, P.; Zhang, L.; Shen, J.; Bala, M.M.; Sohani, Z.N.; et al. Dipeptidyl peptidase-4 inhibitors and risk of heart failure in type 2 diabetes: Systematic review and meta-analysis of randomised and observational studies. *BMJ* **2016**, *352*, i610. [CrossRef]

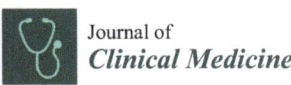

Review

Pneumatosis Intestinalis Induced by Alpha-Glucosidase Inhibitors in Patients with Diabetes Mellitus

Blake J. McKinley [1], Mariangela Santiago [2], Christi Pak [2], Nataly Nguyen [2] and Qing Zhong [2,*]

1. Department of Internal Medicine, Mayo Clinic, Jacksonville, FL 32224, USA
2. Department of Biomedical Science, Rocky Vista University College of Osteopathic Medicine, Ivins, UT 84738, USA
* Correspondence: qzhong@rvu.edu; Tel.: +43-52-221-285

Abstract: Alpha-glucosidase inhibitor (αGIs)-induced pneumatosis intestinalis (PI) has been narrated in case reports but never systematically investigated. This study aimed to investigate the concurrency of PI and αGIs. A literature search was performed in PubMed, Google Scholar, WorldCat, and the Directory of Open-Access Journals (DOAJ) by using the keywords "pneumatosis intestinalis", "alpha-glucosidase inhibitors", and "diabetes". In total, 29 cases of αGIs-induced PI in 28 articles were included. There were 11 men, 17 women, and one undefined sex, with a median age of 67. The most used αGI was voglibose (44.8%), followed by acarbose (41.4%) and miglitol (6.8%). Nine (31%) patients reported concomitant use of prednisone/prednisolone with or without immunosuppressants. The main symptoms were abdominal pain (54.5%) and distention (50%). The ascending colon (55.2%) and the ileum (34.5%) were the most affected. Nineteen (65.5%) patients had comorbidities. Patients with comorbidities had higher rates of air in body cavities, the portal vein, extraintestinal tissues, and the wall of the small intestine. Only one patient was found to have non-occlusive mesenteric ischemia. Twenty-five patients were treated with conservative therapy alone, and two patients received surgical intervention. All patients recovered. In conclusion, comorbidities, glucocorticoids, and immunosuppressants aggravate αGIs-induced PI. Conservative therapy is recommended when treating αGIs-induced PI.

Keywords: pneumatosis intestinalis; diabetes; alpha-glucosidase inhibitors; acarbose; voglibose; miglitol; comorbidities; concomitant drugs; prednisone; immunosuppressants

1. Introduction

Pneumatosis intestinalis (PI) is a condition in which gas is present within the walls of the intestines [1]. It is characterized by gas and free air in the mucosa, submucosa, and subserosa, and it can present in linear and/or cystic forms [2]. It is also called pneumatosis cystoides intestinalis. The incidence of PI is 2/6553 (0.03%) in autopsies [3]. There are two subtypes of PI: primary/idiopathic and secondary; secondary PI consists of up to 85% of all PI cases in adults [1,2].

PI is diagnosed via imaging techniques that include X-ray, computed tomography (CT), and endoscopy [4]. CT is the most sensitive medium for diagnosing PI.

PI can cause a wide range of symptoms with varying levels of severity. Some patients are asymptomatic, while others have life-threatening symptoms [5]. When patients with PI are asymptomatic, they may go undiagnosed [6]. On the other hand, the rupture of the subserosal cysts of PI could result in pneumoperitoneum without clinical peritonitis, and portal venous gas is often associated with pathological lesions [3]. Some PI cases may be secondary to transmural ischemia or necrosis of the gastrointestinal wall [7]. The mortality rates of PI increase in patients with bowel obstruction, toxic megacolon, cecal ileus, bone marrow transplants, and collagen vascular diseases [8].

Given that PI is a rare finding, its etiology is not well understood. However, PI has been reported in association with different disorders, including inflammatory bowel diseases,

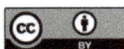

cytomegalovirus (CMV) colitis, acquired immunodeficiency syndrome (AIDS), emphysema, chronic obstructive pulmonary disease (COPD), cystic fibrosis, asthma, diabetes, cancer, organ transplants, fecal impaction, and mesenteric ischemia and necrosis [6,8,9].

While uncommon, some drugs are suspected of causing PI [8]. In particular, PI has been described in patients receiving corticosteroids, immunosuppressants, anticancer drugs, alpha-glucosidase inhibitors (αGIs), lactulose, and sorbitol [2,8,10]. In a multicenter study in Japan, out of 167 PI patients, 31 (19%) cases were related to diabetes. Among those 31 patients, 74.2% of them (23/31) had used αGIs [11].

αGIs competitively inhibit the intestinal α-glucosidase, thus delaying carbohydrate absorption in the small intestine. αGIs are commonly used to treat diabetes, especially type II diabetes. It has been thought that αGIs increase gastrointestinal luminal gas, contributing to the development of PI [12]. This raises a question: why does PI occur in some patients but not in others? So far, there have not yet been any systematic investigations on αGIs and PI. This study investigated the concurrency of PI and αGIs in patients with diabetes and sought to identify what other factors precipitate αGIs-induced PI.

2. Methods
2.1. Literature Search

A literature search was performed up to 7 June 2022, in PubMed/MEDLINE, World-Cat, Google Scholar, and the Directory of Open-Access Journals (DOAJ). We searched for articles using the following keywords: "pneumatosis intestinalis" AND "diabetes", or "pneumatosis intestinalis" AND "alpha-glucosidase inhibitors", or "acarbose" OR "voglibose" OR "miglitol" AND "pneumatosis intestinalis". Inclusion criteria were the following: clinical trials/observational studies/case series or case reports that identified patients with intramural intestinal air, the usage of alpha-glucosidase inhibitors, and studies written in English. Exclusion criteria were the following: congress abstracts, and no alpha-glucosidase inhibitors involved.

All authors participated in the initial screening. Data extraction was performed by all authors and confirmed independently by two authors (B.M. and Q.Z.) to assess for correctness and bias. Data syntheses and analyses were performed by one author (Q.Z.) and confirmed by another (M.S.). Interpretations of the results were agreed upon by all authors.

2.2. Statistical Analysis

The characteristics of αGIs-induced PI cases were compared in patients with or without comorbidities, and between patients treated with voglibose and patients treated with acarbose, using the Student's t-test or X^2 test with a $p < 0.05$ as statistically significant.

3. Results
3.1. Articles Included

Our search resulted in 151 unique titles. All titles were screened, after which 30 full-text articles were assessed for eligibility. Ultimately, 28 articles with a total of 29 cases met our inclusion criteria, as shown in Figure 1. No clinical trials and observational studies were found. Details regarding patients' information and characters are provided in Supplemental Tables S1 and S2 [4,12–38].

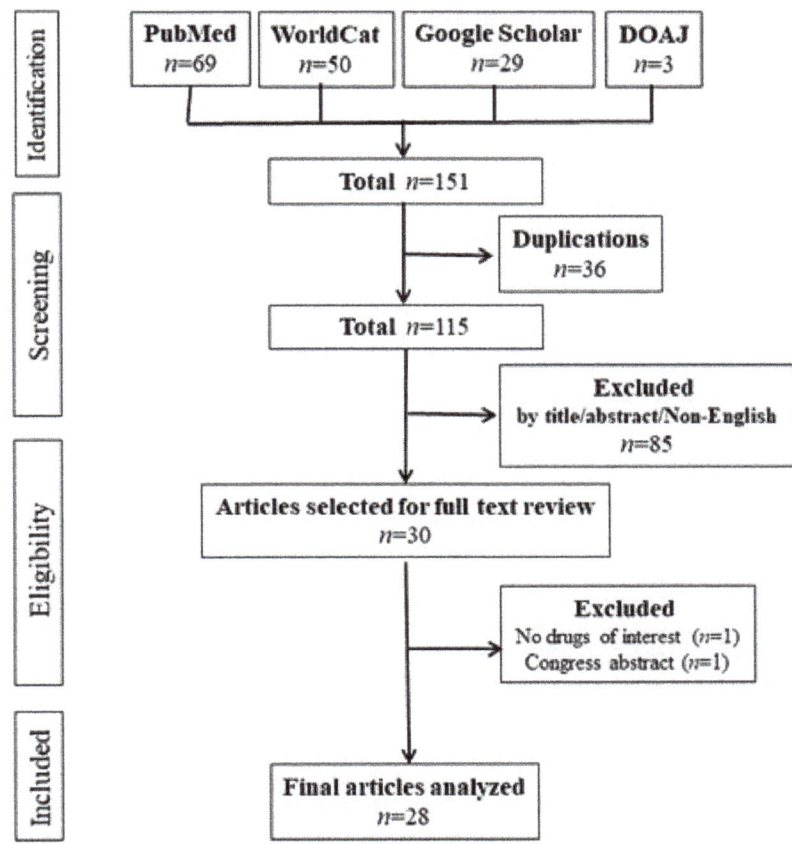

Figure 1. Literature search flow. Legend: A total of 151 abstracts were found from four databases of Pubmed, WorldCat, Google Scholar, and DOAJ. Twenty-eight articles met the inclusion criteria.

3.2. Clinical Characteristics of PI

A total of 29 patients' general information, comorbidities, past medical histories, and medication uses (Sections 3.2–3.4) are shown in Table 1. Twenty-three patients were diagnosed with type II diabetes, and six patients were diagnosed with steroid-induced diabetes as their diabetes occurred after prednisone use [23,25,26,28,34].

Eleven patients were men, 17 were women, and the sex of one patient was not defined. Ages ranged from 48 to 87, with a median of 67. The duration of time with diabetes varied from 2 days to 20 years.

Nineteen (65.5%) patients had comorbidities. Seven cases had connective tissue disorders/autoimmune diseases, including dermatomyositis [25], neuropsychiatric systemic lupus erythematosus [28], polymyalgia rheumatica [32], rheumatoid arthritis [34], granulomatosis with polyangiitis [34], hypothyroidism [22], and myasthenia gravis [26]. Three cases had immunocompromising conditions, including post-lung transplantation [38], minimal change disease-nephrotic syndrome [24], and non-specific interstitial pneumonitis (NSIP) [23]. Three patients had concomitant infections: one with acute cholecystitis [31], one with *E.coli* sepsis [24], and another with *Pseudomonas putida* detected in peritoneal dialysate effluent [37]. Five patients had hypertension, three of them with ischemic disease (post-cerebral infarction, vascular ischemia, heart ischemia, and/or nonocclusive mesenteric ischemia (NOMI)) and/or kidney failure [27,29,30,33,37].

Only 10 (34.5%) patients had no comorbidities. The number of patients with comorbidities was 1.9 times the number of patients without comorbidities.

Table 1. Clinical characteristics of patients with pneumatosis intestinalis.

Characteristics	n	(% of Cases)
Number of patients	29	
Men/women/undefined sex	11/17/1	
Age in years (mean ± SD) (median)	68.1 ± 10.3 (67)	
Age range	48–87	
Diabetes' duration (mean ± SD) (median)	6.0 ± 6.1 (4)	
Range	2 days to 20 years	
Comorbidities and/or past medical history		
Number of patients	19	(65.5)
Connective tissue disorders/autoimmune diseases	7	(24.1)
Hypertension	2	(6.9)
Hypertension + post cerebral infarction	1	(3.4)
Hypertension + diabetic nephropathy + ischemic heart disease	1	(3.4)
Hypertension + diabetic nephropathy + peritonitis + nonocclusive mesenteric ischemia (NOMI) + ischemic disease + post cerebral infarction	1	(3.4)
Minimal change disease—nephrotic syndrome + E. coli sepsis	1	(3.4)
Chronic inflammatory colitis	2	(6.9)
Post lung transplantation + pneumonia 1 month prior	1	(3.4)
Sigmoid volvulus/dolichocolon	1	(3.4)
Non-specific interstitial pneumonitis (NSIP)	1	(3.4)
Acute cholecystitis	1	(3.4)
Medications		
Alpha-glucosidase inhibitors		
Acarbose	12	(41.4)
Median of duration (year) (Range)	5 (1–12)	
Voglibose	13	(44.8)
Median of duration (year) (Range)	0.6 (0.005–10)	
Miglitol	2	(6.9)
Median of duration (year) (Range)	3.8 (0.7–7)	
Undefined	2	(6.9)
Concomitant drugs/supplements		
Prednisone/prednisolone	6	(20.7)
Prednisolone + tacrolimus	1	(3.4)
Prednisolone + mizoribine	1	(3.4)
Prednisolone + methotrexate	1	(3.4)
Insulin	7	(24.1)
Sulfonylurea	4	(13.8)
Dipeptidyl peptidase-4 inhibitors	2	(6.9)
Metformin	1	(3.4)
Maltitol	1	(3.4)

3.3. Type of αGIs

All three available αGIs—acarbose, voglibose, and miglitol—were related to PI. The most common one was voglibose (44.8%), followed by acarbose (41.4%). There were only two cases of miglitol (6.9%). Two cases did not define a specific alpha-glucosidase inhibitor [17,30].

3.4. Concomitant Use of Other Drugs

As shown in Table 1, nine (31%) patients used prednisone or prednisolone ± other immunosuppressants or cytotoxic drugs [23–26,28,32,34,38]. Among those cases, one was combined with mizoribine (inhibiting guanosine synthesis), one with methotrexate, and one with tacrolimus [24,25,38]. Other antidiabetic drugs that were used consisted of insulin (seven cases), sulfonylurea (four cases), dipeptidyl peptidase-4 inhibitors (two cases), and metformin (one case). One patient used the carbohydrate supplement maltitol [22].

3.5. Symptoms

Characteristics of PI, including symptoms; diagnostic imaging; complications; the segments involved; the presence of free gas in cavities or other tissues; treatment; and outcomes (Sections 3.5–3.11) are shown in Table 2.

Table 2. Characteristics of PI.

Characteristics	n	(%)
Symptoms		
Asymptomatic	7	(24.1)
Symptomatic	22	(75.9)
Imaging		
Abdominal X-ray	29	(100)
Abdominal CT	29	(100)
Colonoscopy	11	(37.9)
Segments involved		
Large bowel only		
Ascending colon only	5	(17.2)
Sigmoid only	5	(17.2)
Ascending + sigmoid	1	(3.4)
Ascending + transverse colon	2	(6.9)
Ascending + descending colon	2	(6.9)
Cecum + splenic flexure colon	1	(3.4)
Cecum + ascending + transverse + sigmoid colon	1	(3.4)
All colon	2	(6.9)
Small intestine only		
Ileum only	1	(3.4)
Whole small intestine	6	(20.7)
Combined		
Ileum + ascending colon	2	(6.9)
Ileum + ascending + transverse colon	1	(3.4)
Free gas in cavities or other tissue		

Table 2. Cont.

Characteristics	n	(%)
Pneumoperitoneum	7	(24.1)
Pneumoretroperitoneum	2	(6.9)
Portal venous gas	2	(6.9)
Portal venous gas + pneumoperitoneum	1	(3.4)
Subcutaneous air in the cervical region + pneumomediastinum + pneumoretroperitoneum + pneumoperitoneum	1	(3.4)
Pneumomediastinum + pneumopericardium + pneumoretroperitoneum	1	(3.4)
Treatment		
Termination of alpha-glucosidase inhibitors	29	(100)
Conservative	25	(86.2)
Fasting	12	(41.4)
Fluid supplementation	8	(27.6)
Antibiotics	7	(24.1)
Oxygen therapy		
Conventional	5	(17.2)
Mechanical	1	(3.4)
Endoscopy (colonoscopy) therapy		
Needle puncture + electro-resection of gas cysts	1	(3.4)
Hemofiltration	2	(6.9)
Exploratory laparotomy but with conservative therapy	2	(6.9)
Laparoscopic sigmoidectomy	1	(3.4)
Laparotomy and hemicolectomy	1	(3.4)
Outcome		
Survival	29	(100)
Free air disappearance was confirmed radiologically	22	(75.9)
Median of duration in days (range)	18 (2-180)	

Abbreviations: CT: computed tomography; PI: pneumatosis intestinalis.

Patients presented with symptoms in 22/29 (75.9%) of the cases. As shown in Figure 2, the most common symptoms were abdominal pain (54.5%) and abdominal distention (50%), followed by diarrhea (22.7%), bloody stool (22.7%), and constipation (13.6%).

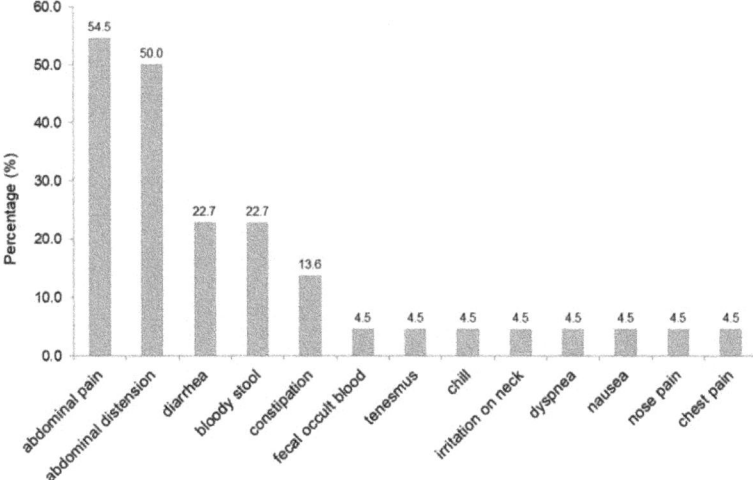

Figure 2. Overview of the symptoms of αGIs-induced PI. Legend: abdominal pain and distention were the most common symptoms, followed by diarrhea and bloody stool.

3.6. Segment of Bowel Involved

The location of PI had a wide distribution throughout the intestines. Nineteen (65.5%) cases had only large intestine involvement, seven (24.1%) had only small intestine involvement, and three (10.3%) had combinations of small and large intestine involvement. The ascending colon was the most involved (16/29, 55.2%), followed by the ileum (10/29, 34.5%).

3.7. Free Air in the Portal Vein and Intraabdominal Cavities and Extraintestinal Involvement

As shown in Table 3, patients with comorbidities had significantly higher rates of free air in the peritoneum or retroperitoneum (9/19 (47.4%) vs. 1/10 (10%), $p < 0.05$), and with small intestine involvement (8/19 (42.1%) vs. 2/10 (20%), $p < 0.05$), compared to patients without comorbidities. Only in patients with comorbidities was free air found in the mediastinum, pericardium, or subcutaneous space (2/19 (10.5%) vs. 0/10 (0%)) or the portal vein (3/19 (15.8%) vs. 0/10 (0%)).

Table 3. Comparison between patients with and without comorbidities.

	Patient without Comorbidities ($n = 10$)	Patients with Comorbidities ($n = 19$)
Age (years) (mean±SD) (median)	65.5 ± 8.4 (64.5)	69.6 ± 11.0 (70)
Pneumoperitoneum or pneumoretroperitoneum	1	9 *
Pneumomediastinum or pneumopericardium or subcutaneous air	0	2
Portal venous gas	0	3
Small intestine involvement	2	8 *
Combination of small and large intestines	1	2
Exploratory laparotomy	1	2
Surgery	1	1
PI disappearance (days) (median) (range)	21.5 (4–180)	21 (4–90)

* $p < 0.05$ compared to patients without comorbidities.

3.8. Comparison between Patients Treated with Acarbose and Patients Treated with Voglibose

As shown in Table 1, the duration range for voglibose usage was 2 days to 10 years, with 6/13 (46.2%) having a duration shorter than 2 months. The duration range for acarbose usage was 1 year to 12 years, with 5/12 (41.7%) having a duration of less than five years. The median time of voglibose usage was relatively shorter than that of acarbose usage (0.6 years vs. 5 years).

As shown in Table 4, 7/12 (58.3%) patients who used acarbose and 10/13 (76.9%) patients who used voglibose had comorbidities. The durations of voglibose usage were shorter than those of acarbose regardless of the presence of comorbidities (without comorbidities: median 0.17 years vs. 3 years; with comorbidities: median 1.7 years vs. 8 years).

Table 4. Comparison between patients who used acarbose and patients who used voglibose.

	Acarbose		Voglibose	
	Without Comorbidities	With Comorbidities	Without Comorbidities	With Comorbidities
Number of patients	5	7	3	10
Age (years) (mean±SD) (median)	63.6 ± 8.2 (65)	72.6 ± 9.3 (72)	67.7 ± 9.1 (64)	64.8 ± 10.1 (69.5)
Diabetes' duration (years) (mean ± SD) (median)	Unknown	9.8 ± 3.5 (10)	11.5 ± 12 (11.5)	1.1 ± 1.6 (0.08)
αGIs duration range (years) (median)	1–10 (3)	2–12 (8)	0.05–5 (0.17)	0.005–10 (1.7)
Concomitant prednisone/prednisolone ± immunosuppressants (case) (%)		1 (14.3%)		8 (80%) **
Portal venous gas		1 (14.3%)		2 (20%)
Pneumoperitoneum +/− Pneumoretroperitoneum		3 (42.9%)		5 (50%)
Pneumomediastinum, Pneumopericardium, Pneumoretroperitoneum				1(10%)
Subcutaneous air in the cervical region, pneumomediastinum, pneumoperitoneum, pneumoretroperitoneum				1(10%)
Exploratory laparotomy		1 (14.3%)		1(10%)
Laparoscopic sigmoidectomy		1 (14.3%)		

** $p < 0.01$ compared to the acarbose group with comorbidities.

The voglibose group with comorbidities had a significantly higher ratio of concomitant usage of glucocorticoids compared to the acarbose group with comorbidities (80% vs. 14.3%, $p < 0.01$). The three cases of glucocorticoids + immunosuppressants were all in the voglibose group. Free air in the mediastinum, pericardium, or subcutaneous space only developed in the voglibose group with comorbidities (two cases, 20%).

3.9. Diagnosis

All cases of PI were confirmed by X-ray and computed tomography. Eleven (37.9%) patients were also checked with colonoscopy, and two patients were examined with endoscopic ultrasonography [26,35].

3.10. Treatment and Complications

The αGIs were recognized as potential causal drugs in all cases and were terminated. Twenty-five (86.2%) patients were only treated with conservative therapy: fasting was initiated at the onset of the disease in 12 (41.4%) patients, fluid supplementation in eight

(27.5%) patients, antibiotic therapy in seven (24.1%) patients, and O_2 therapy in six (20.6%) patients. One case delayed terminating the αGIs treatment until three months later, when the PI disappeared [35]. This same patient also received unique endoscopic needle puncture and high-frequency electro-scission of submucosal air cysts [35].

An exploratory laparotomy ruled out ischemia and necrosis in two (6.9%) patients with portal venous gas; therefore, no surgical intervention was needed, and the patients were treated with conservative therapy [31,33]. One case of portal venous gas was confirmed to have non-occlusive mesenteric ischemia by CT and endoscopic ultrasound examination, and the patient developed peritonitis and hypotension [37]. This case was treated with antibiotics, vasopressors, and continuous hemodiafiltration [37]. One patient developed E. coli sepsis that resulted in disseminated intravascular coagulation (DIC), acute renal failure, and acute respiratory distress syndrome [24]. This patient was treated with antibiotics, continuous hemofiltration, and mechanical ventilation [24].

Surgical intervention was performed in two cases. Laparotomy and hemicolectomy were performed on one patient [17], and a sigmoidectomy was performed on another to release a sigmoid volvulus [36].

3.11. Outcome or Duration of PI

All patients completely recovered. Symptom resolution ranged from 4 to 90 days, with a median of 7 days recorded in 16 (55.2%) patients. Resolution of PI was confirmed via images (CT and/or X-ray) or colonoscopy in 4 to 180 days, with a median of 18 days in 22 (75.9%) patients.

Although patients with comorbidities had increased rates of free air in cavities or extraintestinal tissues compared to patients without comorbidities, the median time of disappearance of PI was similar between those two groups, with a median of 21 to 21.5 days, as shown in Table 3.

4. Discussion

4.1. Mechanisms of αGIs-Induced PI

We summarized 29 cases of αGIs-induced PI. The number of patients with other comorbidities was 1.9 times the number of patients without comorbidities. The exact pathophysiological mechanism of PI is unclear, but there are three theories: "mechanical theory" (the air penetrates the bowel wall), "bacterial theory" (gas-forming bacteria penetrate the submucosa), and "biochemical theory" (luminal carbohydrates are fermented, increasing intraluminal pressure) [2,36]. Based on those theories, the authors propose that multiple factors contribute to the development of αGIs-induced PI: increased production of intestinal gas, the hypomotility of the gastrointestinal tract, weakened intestinal mucosa and wall, and/or air carried from the lungs. These mechanisms are depicted in Figure 3.

Increased production of intestinal gas could be due to αGIs, supplemental carbohydrates, and bacterial infection. αGIs lead to an increase in intestinal gas by suppressing carbohydrate absorption, resulting in the retention of carbohydrates in the lumen of the intestine. The unabsorbed carbohydrates are subsequently fermented by normal flora to produce carbon dioxide, methane, and hydrogen [22,35]. An additional carbohydrate supplement maltitol, a natural sweetener that is considered a sugar alcohol, or polyol may have played a concomitant role in one case of αGIs-induced PI as it is not readily absorbed in the small intestine and thus is fermented in the large intestine [22]. Three cases had bacterial infections [21,31,37]. Bacterial infection, especially gas-producing bacteria, not only increases gas production in the lumen of the intestine but also can invade and produce gas within the intestinal wall [39].

Hypomotility of the gastrointestinal (GI) tract will prolong the fermentation of carbohydrates and increase luminal pressure. In our series of cases, the hypomotility of the GI tract could be caused by diabetic autonomic nerve damage, hypothyroidism [22], dolichocolon (an abnormally long large intestine) [36], and atrophy and fibrosis of smooth-muscle cells of GI in dermatomyositis [25]. Increased intraluminal pressure could cause mechanical damage to the intestinal mucosa, resulting in gas migration into the intestinal wall [36].

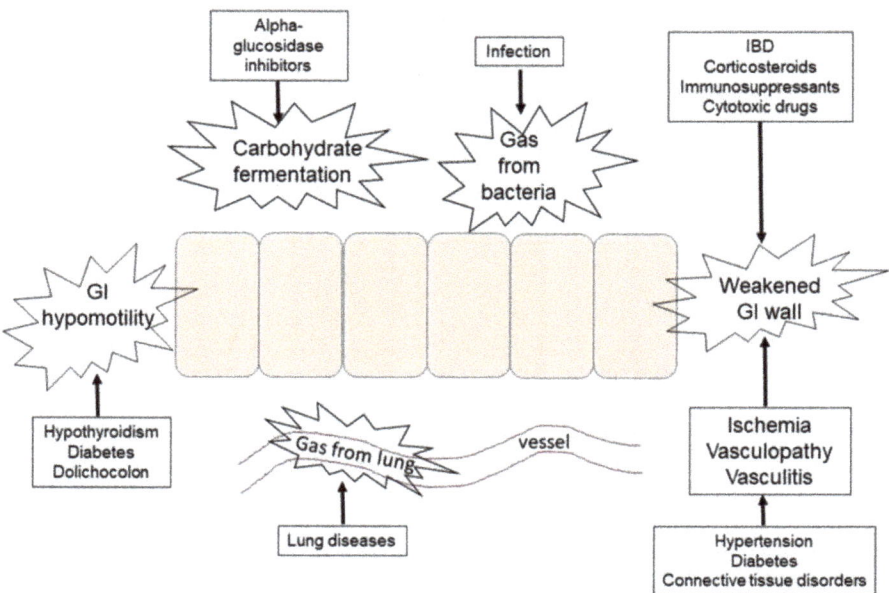

Figure 3. Possible mechanisms of αGIs-induced PI. Legend: There are multiple contributors to the development of αGIs-induced PI: increased production of intestinal gas, hypomotility of the gastrointestinal tract, weakened intestinal mucosa and wall, and/or air carried from the lungs. Abbreviations: IBD: inflammatory bowel disease; GI: the gastrointestinal tract.

The intestinal mucosa and wall could be weakened or damaged by inflammation, infection, or low blood perfusion. In our case series, there were two cases of colitis [4,35], three cases of infection [24,31,37], five cases of hypertension with or without vasculopathy (one of them with non-occlusive mesenteric ischemia), five cases of connective tissue disorders [25,28,32,34], and three cases of autoimmune diseases [22,23,26]. Bowel inflammatory diseases, including ulcerative colitis and Crohn's disease, have been reported to be related to PI [9]. Hypertension and vasculopathy are important contributors to mesenteric ischemia in the elderly [16]. Connective tissue disorders could cause vasculitis or atrophy and fibrosis of smooth muscles of the GI tract, resulting in hypomotility [40].

Some drugs could also weaken or damage the intestinal mucosa and wall as well. In our series of cases, nine patients used prednisone/prednisolone, with three of them adding immunosuppressants or cytotoxic drugs [23–26,28,32,34,38]. Prednisone and immunosuppressants could deplete lymphocytes and shrink Peyer's patches, facilitating gas entry into the intestinal wall [41]. Mizoribine and methotrexate are cytotoxic and may cause mucosa and epithelial cell damage directly [2]. In our case series, the patient with dermatomyositis treated with prednisolone and methotrexate was the only one developing subcutaneous air in the cervical area, along with pneumomediastinum, pneumoperitoneum, pneumoretroperitoneum, and PI [25].

Furthermore, a pulmonary cause needs consideration. Pulmonary diseases, such as chronic obstructive pulmonary disease, asthma, cystic fibrosis, and chronic cough, may force gas to enter the blood vessels and be carried from the lungs to the intestines [8]. In Hisamoto et al.'s study, the patient had non-specific interstitial pneumonitis; after using prednisone and voglibose, the patient presented with pneumomediastinum, pneumopericardium, pneumoretroperitoneum, and PI [23]. In Otsuka et al.'s study, the patient was a lung transplantation recipient for 1031 days and had pneumonia 47 days before finding

PI [38]. In these two cases, chronic cough-induced alveolar rupture and PI could not be completely ruled out.

Patients with comorbidities not only have a higher risk of developing αGIs-induced PI but also have more severe imaging findings. Patients with comorbidities had a higher incidence of free air in cavities or extraintestinal tissues and a higher rate of small intestine involvement. Portal venous gas was only found in three patients, all of whom had comorbidities [31,33,37]. Only one of the three cases was confirmed to have non-occlusive mesenteric ischemia [37]. Although portal venous gas may suggest intestinal ischemia [42], it has been reported that 30% of patients with portal venous gas and PI were due to benign idiopathic causes [43].

4.2. Comparison of Three αGIs

αGIs are especially effective in reducing postprandial hyperglycemia and are frequently used to treat patients with type II diabetes in combination with other antidiabetic drugs. The αGIs' effect on lowering blood glucose is modest, but αGIs have the advantage of a very low risk of hypoglycemia compared to sulfonylurea drugs. αGIs often cause side effects of abdominal distention, flatulence, diarrhea, and abdominal pain. Because of the side effects, αGIs should not be used in patients who have gastrointestinal disorders [44–46].

PI is a rare side effect of αGIs. Voglibose and acarbose were more commonly reported than miglitol in causing PI. This may be due to different pharmacokinetics. Acarbose and voglibose are poorly absorbed in the intestine and primarily excreted in the feces, with approximately 30% that undergo fermentation by colonic microbiota [44]. In contrast, miglitol is absorbed by the gut and excreted unchanged in the kidneys [45]. Fermentation of voglibose and acarbose may increase luminal gas.

We found that PI developed more rapidly in patients treated with voglibose than in patients treated with acarbose. In our case series, patients with comorbidities on voglibose treatment had a higher ratio of simultaneous usage of glucocorticoids/immunosuppressants than those on acarbose treatment. As we discussed in Section 4.1, concomitant glucocorticoids/immunosuppressants may precipitate the development of PI. In addition, voglibose is 190 to 270 times more potent than acarbose [46]. Therefore, the authors hypothesize that a higher ratio of concomitant usage of glucocorticoids/immunosuppressants and a higher potency of voglibose contribute to a short duration of time that is needed to trigger PI compared to that with acarbose. Clinicians should be alerted that voglibose may cause PI in the first few months of its usage, whereas acarbose has the propensity to cause PI at any time during its usage, even a decade after its initiation.

4.3. Symptoms and Treatments

The most common symptoms are abdominal distension and pain, followed by diarrhea and bloody stool in the cases we analyzed. As these are non-specific symptoms, physicians should have a high level of suspicion for possible PI in patients that present with gastrointestinal complaints while taking αGIs. Additionally, physicians should be aware that PI may be identified incidentally on radiological imaging, endoscopy, or laparotomy in patients taking αGIs because several of the reviewed cases were asymptomatic.

The majority of patients fully recovered after conservative therapy, which includes the termination of alpha-glucosidases, fasting, fluid supplementation, antibiotics, and inhalation of oxygen. The authors recommend conservative treatment to be the mainstay of treatment in αGIs-induced PI.

We recommend sustaining from surgery, including exploratory laparotomies, if patients are stable without guarding or rebound tenderness. Taking into context the clinical presentation of the patients, PI and pneumoperitoneum or portal venous gas should not be used as an indication by themselves for an exploratory laparotomy. Additional criteria, including higher C-reactive protein concentrations, higher white blood cell counts, higher lactate levels, and ascites, may be required to indicate inflammatory syndrome and the likelihood of intestinal necrosis from mesenteric ischemia [7,47,48].

It is worth mentioning that although our case series had mild clinical features in most cases with patients recovering, severe complications from PI such as perforation and death have been reported in PI patients of other etiologies [2,7,47]. It is important to combine detailed history, laboratory, and image examinations to make differential diagnoses. While it is beneficial to avoid unnecessary laparotomy in patients with non-inflammatory signs, it is also important to keep patients whose clinical features worsen under careful observation.

4.4. Strength and Limitations

The strength of this study is its analysis of the contributions to PI from three alpha-glucosidase inhibitors, comorbidities, and other offending drugs. To our knowledge, this is the first thorough review of αGIs-induced PI.

This review, however, also has some limitations. Due to the low incidence rate, we cannot calculate the actual prevalence of αGIs-induced PI. Moreover, this study is only a description and observation, and no correlation or causative assessment has been generated. Furthermore, the possibilities of PI induced by other types of antidiabetic drugs have not been analyzed.

5. Conclusions

Alpha-glucosidase inhibitors are related to the development of PI. The most common ones are voglibose and acarbose. Voglibose usage may cause a much more rapid development of PI than acarbose. Patients with comorbidities and concurrent usage of glucocorticoids and/or immunosuppressants have a relatively higher risk of developing αGIs-induced PI with complications of free gas in cavities, portal veins, and extraintestinal tissues. The authors propose that multiple factors contribute to the development of PI when using αGIs. Intestinal ischemia or necrosis in αGIs-induced PI is uncommon, with only 1/29 (3.4%) patients having non-occlusive mesenteric ischemia in our study. The majority of patients recovered after conservative therapy. Therefore, the authors advocate for conservative therapy and the avoidance of any unnecessary surgery.

Supplementary Materials: The following supporting information can be downloaded at https://www.mdpi.com/article/10.3390/jcm11195918/s1, Table S1: Clinical features of patients without comorbidities (n = 10) [12–21], and Table S2: Clinical features of patients with comorbidities (n = 19) [4,22–38] can be found in the supplementary materials.

Author Contributions: B.J.M. and Q.Z. contributed to the conception and design of the study; all authors contributed to screening and sorting the literature; Q.Z. and M.S. analyzed the data; all authors contributed to the first draft of the manuscript; M.S., C.P. and N.N. edited the manuscript; B.J.M. critically revised the manuscript; and Q.Z. finalized the manuscript. All authors have read and agreed to the published version of the manuscript.

Funding: This research received no external funding.

Informed Consent Statement: Not applicable.

Conflicts of Interest: All authors declare no conflict of interest.

References

1. Im, J.; Anjum, F. *Pneumatosis Intestinalis*; StatPearls Publishing: Treasure Island, FL, USA, 2022. Available online: https://www.ncbi.nlm.nih.gov/books/NBK564381/ (accessed on 1 August 2022).
2. Gazzaniga, G.; Villa, F.; Tosi, F.; Pizzutilo, E.G.; Colla, S.; D'Onghia, S.; Sanza, G.D.; Fornasier, G.; Gringeri, M.; Lucatelli, M.V.; et al. Pneumatosis Intestinalis Induced by Anticancer Treatment: A Systematic Review. *Cancers* **2022**, *14*, 1666. [CrossRef]
3. Heng, Y.; Schuffler, M.D.; Haggitt, R.C.; Rohrmann, C.A. Pneumatosis intestinalis: A review. *Am. J. Gastroenterol.* **1995**, *90*, 1747–1758.
4. Ksiadzyna, D.; Peña, A.S. Segmental pneumatosis cystoides coli: Computed tomography-facilitated diagnosis. *Rev. Esp. Enferm. Dig.* **2016**, *108*, 510–513. [CrossRef]

5. Alpuim Costa, D.; Modas Daniel, P.; Vieira Branco, J. The Role of Hyperbaric Oxygen Therapy in Pneumatosis Cystoides Intestinalis-A Scoping Review. *Front. Med.* **2021**, *8*, 601872. [CrossRef]
6. Lee, A.H.H.; Tellambura, S. Pneumatosis intestinalis: Not always bowel ischemia. *Radiol. Case Rep.* **2022**, *17*, 1305–1308. [CrossRef]
7. Sato, T.; Ohbe, H.; Fujita, M.; Kushimoto, S. Clinical characteristics and prediction of the asymptomatic phenotype of pneumatosis intestinalis in critically ill patients: A retrospective observational study. *Acute Med. Surg.* **2020**, *7*, e556. [CrossRef]
8. Ho, L.M.; Paulson, E.K.; Thompson, W.M. Pneumatosis intestinalis in the adult: Benign to life-threatening causes. *AJR Am. J. Roentgenol.* **2007**, *188*, 1604–1613. [CrossRef]
9. Gao, Y.; Uffenheimer, M.; Ashamallah, M.; Grimaldi, G.; Swaminath, A.; Sultan, K. Presentation and outcomes among inflammatory bowel disease patients with concurrent pneumatosis intestinalis: A case series and systematic review. *Intest. Res.* **2020**, *18*, 289–296. [CrossRef]
10. McGettigan, M.J.; Menias, C.O.; Gao, Z.J.; Mellnick, V.M.; Hara, A.K. Imaging of Drug-induced Complications in the Gastrointestinal System. *RadioGraphics* **2016**, *36*, 71–87. [CrossRef]
11. Ohmiya, N.; Hirata, I.; Sakamoto, H.; Morishita, T.; Saito, E.; Matsuoka, K.; Nagaya, T.; Nagata, S.; Mukae, M.; Sano, K.; et al. Multicenter epidemiological survey of pneumatosis intestinalis in Japan. *BMC Gastroenterol.* **2022**, *22*, 272. [CrossRef]
12. Kojima, K.; Tsujimoto, T.; Fujii, H.; Morimoto, T.; Yoshioka, S.; Kato, S.; Yasuhara, Y.; Aizawa, S.; Sawai, M.; Makutani, S.; et al. Pneumatosis cystoides intestinalis induced by the α-glucosidase inhibitor miglitol. *Intern. Med.* **2010**, *49*, 1545–1548. [CrossRef]
13. Hayakawa, T.; Yoneshima, M.; Abe, T.; Nomura, G. Pneumatosis cystoides intestinalis after treatment with an alpha-glucosidase inhibitor. *Diabetes Care* **1999**, *22*, 366–367. [CrossRef]
14. Yanaru, R.; Hizawa, K.; Nakamura, S.; Yoshimura, R.; Watanabe, K.; Nakamura, U.; Yoshinari, M.; Matsumoto, T. Regression of pneumatosis cystoides intestinalis after discontinuing of alpha-glucosidase inhibitor administration. *J. Clin. Gastroenterol.* **2002**, *35*, 204–205. [CrossRef]
15. Furio, L.; Vergura, M.; Russo, A.; Bisceglia, N.; Talarico, S.; Gatta, R.; Tomaiuolo, M.; Tomaiuolo, P. Pneumatosis coli induced by acarbose administration for diabetes mellitus. Case report and literature review. *Minerva Gastroenterol. Dietol.* **2006**, *52*, 339–346.
16. Wu, X.; Bao, Z. Population-Based Study of the Clinical Characteristics and Risk Factors of Ischemic Colitis. *Turk. J. Gastroenterol.* **2021**, *32*, 393–400. [CrossRef]
17. Tseng, C.J.; Yen, C.S.; Ming-Jenn Chen, M.J. Pneumatosis cystoides intestinalis. *Formos. J. Surg.* **2011**, *44*, 192–195. [CrossRef]
18. Takase, A.; Akuzawa, N.; Naitoh, H.; Aoki, J. Pneumatosis intestinalis with a benign clinical course: A report of two cases. *BMC Res. Notes* **2017**, *10*, 319. [CrossRef]
19. Liao, Y.H.; Lo, Y.P.; Liao, Y.K.; Lin, C.H. Pneumatosis Cystoides Coli Related to Acarbose Treatment. *Am. J. Gastroenterol.* **2017**, *112*, 984. [CrossRef]
20. Wang, Y.J.; Wang, Y.M.; Zheng, Y.M.; Jiang, H.Q.; Zhang, J. Pneumatosis cystoides intestinalis: Six case reports and a review of the literature. *BMC Gastroenterol.* **2018**, *18*, 100. [CrossRef]
21. Lin, W.C.; Wang, K.C. Pneumatosis Cystoides Intestinalis Secondary to Use of an α-Glucosidase Inhibitor. *Radiology* **2019**, *290*, 619. [CrossRef]
22. Azami, Y. Paralytic ileus accompanied by pneumatosis cystoides intestinalis after acarbose treatment in an elderly diabetic patient with a history of heavy intake of maltitol. *Intern. Med.* **2000**, *39*, 826–829. [CrossRef] [PubMed]
23. Hisamoto, A.; Mizushima, T.; Sato, K.; Haruta, Y.; Tanimoto, Y.; Tanimoto, M.; Matsuo, K. Pneumatosis cystoides intestinalis after alpha-glucosidase inhibitor treatment in a patient with interstitial pneumonitis. *Intern. Med.* **2006**, *45*, 73–76. [CrossRef] [PubMed]
24. Maeda, Y.; Inaba, N.; Aoyagi, M.; Kanda, E.; Shiigai, T. Fulminant pneumatosis intestinalis in a patient with diabetes mellitus and minimal change nephrotic syndrome. *Intern. Med.* **2007**, *46*, 41–44. [CrossRef] [PubMed]
25. Saito, M.; Tanikawa, A.; Nakasute, K.; Tanaka, M.; Nishikawa, T. Additive contribution of multiple factors in the development of pneumatosis intestinalis: A case report and review of the literature. *Clin. Rheumatol.* **2007**, *26*, 601–603. [CrossRef] [PubMed]
26. Tsujimoto, T.; Shioyama, E.; Moriya, K.; Kawaratani, H.; Shirai, Y.; Toyohara, M.; Mitoro, A.; Yamao, J.; Fujii, H.; Fukui, H. Pneumatosis cystoides intestinalis following alpha-glucosidase inhibitor treatment: A case report and review of the literature. *World J. Gastroenterol.* **2008**, *14*, 6087–6092. [CrossRef] [PubMed]
27. Vogel, Y.; Buchner, N.J.; Szpakowski, M.; Tannapfel, A.; Henning, B.F. Pneumatosis cystoides intestinalis of the ascending colon related to acarbose treatment: A case report. *J. Med. Case Rep.* **2009**, *3*, 9216. [CrossRef] [PubMed]
28. Shimojima, Y.; Ishii, W.; Matsuda, M.; Tojo, K.; Watanabe, R.; Ikeda, S. Pneumatosis cystoides intestinalis in neuropsychiatric systemic lupus erythematosus with diabetes mellitus: Case report and literature review. *Mod. Rheumatol.* **2011**, *21*, 415–419. [CrossRef] [PubMed]
29. Imai, K.; Doi, Y.; Takata, N.; Yoshinaka, I.; Harada, K. Successful conservative treatment of pneumatosis intestinalis associated with intraperitoneal free air: Report of a case. *Surg. Today* **2012**, *42*, 992–996. [CrossRef]
30. Tanabe, S.; Shirakawa, Y.; Takehara, Y.; Maeda, N.; Katsube, R.; Ohara, T.; Sakurama, K.; Noma, K.; Fujiwara, T. Successfully treated pneumatosis cystoides intestinalis with pneumoperitoneum onset in a patient administered α-glucosidase inhibitor. *Acta Med. Okayama* **2013**, *67*, 123–128. [CrossRef]
31. Makiyama, H.; Kataoka, R.; Tauchi, M.; Sumitomo, Y.; Fuita, R. Do alpha-glucosidase inhibitors have the potential to induce portal venous gas? -Two clinical case reports. *Intern. Med.* **2014**, *53*, 691–694. [CrossRef] [PubMed]
32. Ogo, A.; Hasuzawa, N.; Sakaki, Y.; Sakamoto, R.; Matoba, Y. Pneumatosis cystoides intestinalis related to α-glucosidase inhibitor treatment in a polymyalgia rheumatica patient with diabetes mellitus. *Diabetol. Int.* **2014**, *5*, 244–248. [CrossRef]

33. Rottenstreich, A.; Agmon, Y.; Elazary, R. A Rare Case of Benign Pneumatosis Intestinalis with Portal Venous Gas and Pneumoperitoneum Induced by Acarbose. *Intern. Med.* **2015**, *54*, 1733–1736. [CrossRef] [PubMed]
34. Suzuki, E.; Kanno, T.; Hazama, M.; Kobayashi, H.; Watanabe, H.; Ohira, H. Four Cases of Pneumatosis Cystoides Intestinalis Complicated by Connective Tissue Diseases. *Intern. Med.* **2017**, *56*, 1101–1106. [CrossRef]
35. Ling, F.; Guo, D.; Zhu, L. Pneumatosis cystoides intestinalis: A case report and literature review. *BMC Gastroenterol.* **2019**, *19*, 176. [CrossRef] [PubMed]
36. Police, A.; Charre, L.; Volpin, E.; Antonopulos, C.; Braham, H.; El Arbi, N. Pneumatosis cystoides intestinalis induced by the alpha-glucosidase inhibitor complicated from sigmoid volvulus in a diabetic patient. *Int. J. Colorectal. Dis.* **2020**, *35*, 943–946. [CrossRef]
37. Oda, Y.; Ishioka, K.; Moriya, H.; Taguchi, S.; Oki, R.; Matsui, K.; Mochida, Y.; Hidaka, S.; Ohtake, T.; Kobayashi, S. Peritoneal dialysis-related peritonitis complicated with nonocclusive mesenteric ischemia. *CEN Case Rep.* **2021**, *10*, 74–77. [CrossRef] [PubMed]
38. Otsuka, S.; Ujiie, H.; Kato, T.; Shiiya, H.; Fujiwara-Kuroda, A.; Hida, Y.; Kaga, K.; Wakasa, S.; Inoue, R.; Iimura, Y. Pneumatosis Intestinalis After Living Donor Lung Transplantation Associated With Alpha-Glucosidase Inhibitor Treatment: A Case Report. *Transplant. Proc.* **2021**, *53*, 1379–1381. [CrossRef] [PubMed]
39. Gillon, J.; Tadesse, K.; Logan, R.F.; Holt, S.; Sircus, W. Breath hydrogen in pneumatosis cystoides intestinalis. *Gut* **1979**, *20*, 1008–1011. [CrossRef]
40. Sagara, A.; Kitagawa, K.; Furuichi, K.; Kitajima, S.; Toyama, T.; Okumura, T.; Hara, A.; Sakai, Y.; Kaneko, S.; Wada, T. Three cases of pneumatosis intestinalis presenting in autoimmune diseases. *Mod. Rheumatol.* **2012**, *22*, 610–615. [CrossRef] [PubMed]
41. Mannes, G.P.; de Boer, W.J.; van der Jagt, E.J.; Meinesz, A.F.; Meuzelaar, J.J.; van der Bij, W. Pneumatosis intestinalis and active cytomegaloviral infection after lung transplantation. Groningen Lung Transplant Group. *Chest* **1994**, *105*, 929–930. [CrossRef]
42. Kernagis, L.Y.; Levine, M.S.; Jacobs, J.E. Pneumatosis intestinalis in patients with ischemia: Correlation of CT findings with viability of the bowel. *AJR Am. J. Roentgenol.* **2003**, *180*, 733–736. [CrossRef]
43. Wayne, E.; Ough, M.; Wu, A.; Liao, J.; Andresen, K.J.; Kuehn, D.; Wilkinson, N. Management algorithm for pneumatosis intestinalis and portal venous gas: Treatment and outcome of 88 consecutive cases. *J. Gastrointest. Surg.* **2010**, *14*, 437–448. [CrossRef]
44. Bischoff, H. *Pharmacology of α-Glycosidase Inhibitors Drugs in Development α-Glycosidase Inhibition Potential Use in Diabetes*; Neva: Branford, CT, USA, 1995; Volume 1, pp. 1–13.
45. Standl, E.; Schernthaner, G.; Rybka, J.; Hanefeld, M.; Raptis, S.A.; Naditch, L. Improved glycaemic control with miglitol in inadequately-controlled type 2 diabetics. *Diabetes Res. Clin. Pract.* **2001**, *51*, 205–213. [CrossRef]
46. Dabhi, A.S.; Bhatt, N.R.; Shah, M.J. Voglibose: An alpha glucosidase inhibitor. *J. Clin. Diagn. Res.* **2013**, *7*, 3023–3027. [CrossRef] [PubMed]
47. Fujii, M.; Yamashita, S.; Tashiro, J.; Tanaka, M.; Takenaka, Y.; Yamasaki, K.; Masaki, Y. Clinical characteristics of patients with pneumatosis intestinalis. *ANZ J. Surg.* **2021**, *91*, 1826–1831. [CrossRef] [PubMed]
48. Zhao, H.; Meng, Y.; Zhang, P.; Zhang, Q.; Wang, F.; Li, Y. Predictors and risk factors for intestinal necrosis in patients with mesenteric ischemia. *Ann. Transl. Med.* **2021**, *9*, 337. [CrossRef]

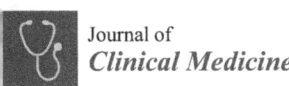

Article

The Sodium-Glucose Co-Transporter 2 (SGLT2) Inhibitor Empagliflozin Reverses Hyperglycemia-Induced Monocyte and Endothelial Dysfunction Primarily through Glucose Transport-Independent but Redox-Dependent Mechanisms

Dilvin Semo [1], Julius Obergassel [1], Marc Dorenkamp [1], Pia Hemling [1], Jasmin Strutz [2], Ursula Hiden [2], Nicolle Müller [3], Ulrich Alfons Müller [3], Sajan Ahmad Zulfikar [4], Rinesh Godfrey [1,5,*,†] and Johannes Waltenberger [5,6,7,*,†]

1. Vascular Signalling, Molecular Cardiology, Department of Cardiology I—Coronary and Peripheral Vascular Disease, Heart Failure, University Hospital Münster, 48149 Münster, Germany
2. Department of Obstetrics and Gynecology, Medical University of Graz, 8036 Graz, Austria
3. Department of Internal Medicine III, University Hospital Jena, 07743 Jena, Germany
4. Department of Cardiology, St. Gregorios Hospital, Parumala, Kerala 689626, India
5. Department of Physiology, Cardiovascular Research Institute Maastricht (CARIM), 6229 ER Maastricht, The Netherlands
6. Department of Cardiovascular Medicine, Medical Faculty, University of Münster, 48149 Münster, Germany
7. Hirslanden Klinik Im Park, Cardiovascular Medicine, Diagnostic and Therapeutic Heart Center AG, 8002 Zürich, Switzerland
* Correspondence: rine.godfrey@gmail.com (R.G.); waltenberger@email.de (J.W.); Tel.: +49-251-8357089 (R.G.); +49-157-331-991-61 (J.W.)
† R.G. and J.W. are joint senior authors.

Abstract: Purpose: Hyperglycaemia-induced oxidative stress and inflammation contribute to vascular cell dysfunction and subsequent cardiovascular events in T2DM. Selective sodium-glucose co-transporter-2 (SGL-2) inhibitor empagliflozin significantly improves cardiovascular mortality in T2DM patients (EMPA-REG trial). Since SGL-2 is known to be expressed on cells other than the kidney cells, we investigated the potential ability of empagliflozin to regulate glucose transport and alleviate hyperglycaemia-induced dysfunction of these cells. Methods: Primary human monocytes were isolated from the peripheral blood of T2DM patients and healthy individuals. Primary human umbilical vein endothelial cells (HUVECs) and primary human coronary artery endothelial cells (HCAECs), and fetoplacental endothelial cells (HPECs) were used as the EC model cells. Cells were exposed to hyperglycaemic conditions in vitro in 40 ng/mL or 100 ng/mL empagliflozin. The expression levels of the relevant molecules were analysed by RT-qPCR and confirmed by FACS. Glucose uptake assays were carried out with a fluorescent derivative of glucose, 2-NBDG. Reactive oxygen species (ROS) accumulation was measured using the H_2DFFDA method. Monocyte and endothelial cell chemotaxis were measured using modified Boyden chamber assays. Results: Both primary human monocytes and endothelial cells express SGL-2. Hyperglycaemic conditions did not significantly alter the SGL-2 levels in monocytes and ECs in vitro or in T2DM conditions. Glucose uptake assays carried out in the presence of GLUT inhibitors revealed that SGL-2 inhibition very mildly, but not significantly, suppressed glucose uptake by monocytes and endothelial cells. However, we detected the significant suppression of hyperglycaemia-induced ROS accumulation in monocytes and ECs when empagliflozin was used to inhibit SGL-2 function. Hyperglycaemic monocytes and endothelial cells readily exhibited impaired chemotaxis behaviour. The co-treatment with empagliflozin reversed the PlGF-1 resistance phenotype of hyperglycaemic monocytes. Similarly, the blunted VEGF-A responses of hyperglycaemic ECs were also restored by empagliflozin, which could be attributed to the restoration of the VEGFR-2 receptor levels on the EC surface. The induction of oxidative stress completely recapitulated most of the aberrant phenotypes exhibited by hyperglycaemic monocytes and endothelial cells, and a general antioxidant N-acetyl-L-cysteine (NAC) was able to mimic the effects of empagliflozin. Conclusions: This study provides data indicating

Citation: Semo, D.; Obergassel, J.; Dorenkamp, M.; Hemling, P.; Strutz, J.; Hiden, U.; Müller, N.; Müller, U.A.; Zulfikar, S.A.; Godfrey, R.; et al. The Sodium-Glucose Co-Transporter 2 (SGLT2) Inhibitor Empagliflozin Reverses Hyperglycemia-Induced Monocyte and Endothelial Dysfunction Primarily through Glucose Transport-Independent but Redox-Dependent Mechanisms. *J. Clin. Med.* **2023**, *12*, 1356. https://doi.org/10.3390/jcm12041356

Academic Editor: Fernando Gómez-Peralta

Received: 19 January 2023
Accepted: 2 February 2023
Published: 8 February 2023

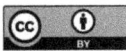

Copyright: © 2023 by the authors. Licensee MDPI, Basel, Switzerland. This article is an open access article distributed under the terms and conditions of the Creative Commons Attribution (CC BY) license (https://creativecommons.org/licenses/by/4.0/).

the beneficial role of empagliflozin in reversing hyperglycaemia-induced vascular cell dysfunction. Even though both monocytes and endothelial cells express functional SGLT-2, SGLT-2 is not the primary glucose transporter in these cells. Therefore, it seems likely that empagliflozin does not directly prevent hyperglycaemia-mediated enhanced glucotoxicity in these cells by inhibiting glucose uptake. We identified the reduction of oxidative stress by empagliflozin as a primary reason for the improved function of monocytes and endothelial cells in hyperglycaemic conditions. In conclusion, empagliflozin reverses vascular cell dysfunction independent of glucose transport but could partially contribute to its beneficial cardiovascular effects.

Keywords: diabetes mellitus; empagliflozin; SGLT-2; monocytes; endothelial cells; vascular dysfunction; chemotaxis; reactive oxygen species (ROS); glucose transport; VEGFR-2; VEGFR-1

1. Introduction

Diabetes mellitus-associated hyperglycaemia is a significant risk factor for developing cardiovascular disease (CVD) and associated cardiovascular mortality [1]. Diabetic vascular disease is responsible for a 2–4-fold rise in the development of coronary artery disease (CAD) [2,3]. Oxidative stress plays a vital role in developing complications associated with diabetes by inducing vascular cell dysfunction [4]. There are a variety of pathways through which hyperglycaemia transduces its deleterious effects downstream. The induction of inflammation through the activation of NF-κB pathway is one of the major determinants contributing to vascular complications in diabetes [5]. Prolonged hyperglycaemia-induced advanced glycation end products (AGEs) through the Receptor for Advanced Glycation End-products (RAGE)–NF-κB pathway contribute heavily to inflammation induction in T2DM [6]. RAGE has also been implicated in mediating the dysfunction of both monocytes [7] and endothelial cells [8]. There is significant cross-talk between oxidative stress induction and AGE-RAGE signalling [9,10].

The sodium-glucose co-transporter 2 (SGLT2) is a major glucose transporter accountable for the renal reabsorption of almost 90% of the glucose from the urine [11]. SGLT-2 inhibitor empagliflozin, is used to treat T2DM and heart failure. It is considered a new therapy for cardiovascular diseases as numerous clinical trials have shown favourable outcomes. These include the EMPA-REG OUTCOME (NCT01131676) [1,12], DAPA-HF (NCT03036124) [13] and the EMPORER-Reduced (NCT03057977) [14]. The EMPA-REG OUTCOME trial demonstrated the ability of empagliflozin to reduce cardiovascular events and overall mortality in T2DM patients with higher cardiovascular risk [1,12,15], and this by far outweighs the benefits of other glucose-lowering T2DM medications such as dipeptidyl peptidase 4 inhibitors or glucagon-like peptide-1 analogues.

Several animal studies have reported the pleiotropic effects of empagliflozin, and this drug is known to give protection against high glucose level-independent diseases such as atherosclerosis [16], heart failure [17,18] and myocardial infarction [19]. Therefore, it is highly likely that the cardiovascular benefits of empagliflozin are not solely through the reduction of blood glucose levels. The favourable pleiotropic effects of empagliflozin have already been described and discussed in several studies [20,21]. Empagliflozin is known to interfere with cellular redox status by attenuating ROS generation [22,23]. Previous studies from our laboratory have shown that in the T2DM environment, monocytes [7] and endothelial cells [24] are dysfunctional due to the accumulation of reactive oxygen species (ROS). Both monocytes and endothelial cells carry out vital functions in cardiovascular physiology, and their function is compromised during T2DM conditions [7,24–26]. Indeed, the reversal of endothelial dysfunction and imparting vascular protective effects by empagliflozin has been described in both T1DM [27] and T2DM [28]. However, Empagliflozin's beneficial effects on monocyte function have not been reported so far.

The increased incidence of CAD in T2DM patients has been linked to the impaired arteriogenesis and angiogenesis found in these patient groups [29–31]. Lack of proper

VEGF responses contributes to endothelial and monocyte dysfunction in T2DM [24,31–33]. The inability of T2DM endothelial cells to respond to VEGF-2 activating growth factors leads to impaired VEGFR-2-dependent processes such as proliferation, migration and angiogenesis [24,31]. Abnormalities of angiogenesis induced by T2DM directly contribute in the pathogenesis of diabetes complications [34]. Furthermore, T2DM individuals have reduced coronary collateral formation compared to non-diabetics [35]. The defective arteriogenesis is hypothesised to be due to the dysfunction of "arteriogenic" cells, leading to the disability of these cells to home to the sites of vessel growth. Monocytes from T2DM patients were found to be defective in their migratory potential towards VEGFA and PlGF-1, previously described as "VEGF resistance" [7,26,33]. VEGF resistance is based on the non-specific activation of downstream signalling pathways in vascular cells. Pre-activation results in these cells' resistance to respond to more specific signals. As the VEGFA or PlGF-1 responses are very specific for endothelial cells and monocytes, resistance to these growth factors results in monocyte and endothelial dysfunction [36,37].

Considering the importance of oxidative stress in contributing to both monocyte and endothelial dysfunction, the proposed role of empagliflozin as a redox modulator and the ability of empagliflozin to improve cardiovascular outcomes, we hypothesised that empagliflozin could circumvent both monocyte and endothelial dysfunction through a glucose transport-dependent or independent mechanism, thereby improving vascular health. Such a possibility was investigated in this study.

2. Results

2.1. Primary Human Monocytes and Primary Endothelial Cells Express SGLT-2

SGLT-2 is the glucose transporter is primarily expressed in the kidneys on the epithelial cells lining the first segment of the proximal tubule. Since the reports about the expression of SGLT-2 in monocytes and endothelial cells were not robust, we decided to analyse the expression pattern of SGLT-2 in these two cell types. First, we used Immortalised Human Kidney Epithelial cells (IHKE1) as a positive control to detect a positive signal for SGLT-2. We used $CD14^{++}CD16^{-}$ primary monocytes and THP-1 monocytic cell line and detected the mRNA levels of SGLT-2 using RT-qCR. We used two sets of primers, one designed to span the boundaries of exons 6 and 7 and another located at exon 13 of SGLT-2, as reported previously [38]. The exon 13 primers were reported robust in amplifying the SGLT-2 gene. Figure 1A,B shows that both primary monocytes and THP-1 monocytic cells express SGLT-2 mRNA. Both set of primers amplified the SGLT-2 gene. Even though only at a 50% expression level compared to the positive control, IHKE-1 cells, both monocytic cells expressed SGLT-2 transcripts. As reported, the exon 13 primer was more efficient in amplifying the SGLT-2 gene. In order to confirm the gene product, we sequenced the product, and it was confirmed to be the SGLT-2 gene (results not shown).

Furthermore, using FACS, we reliably detected the surface levels of the SGLT-2 protein. Similar to the situation in monocytic cells, three different types of endothelial cells, the Human Umbilical Vein Endothelial Cells (HUVEC), Human Coronary Artery Endothelial Cells (HCAEC) and Human fetoplacental Endothelial Cells (HPEC), showed varying degrees of SGLT-2 gene expression, with HPEC expressing the lowest levels (Figure 1C). Interestingly, we detected the SGLT-2 transcript amplification only when we used the exon 13 primers. We could not detect any SGLT-2 transcripts reliably when the exon 6/7 was used (Figure 1D). Nevertheless, using FACS, we detected SGLT-2 protein levels on the surfaces of these three endothelial cell types and the protein expression pattern matched with the transcript levels, with HPEC showing the lowest SGLT-2 expression. (Figure 1E). Taken together, these data confirm that both monocytes and endothelial cells express SGLT-2.

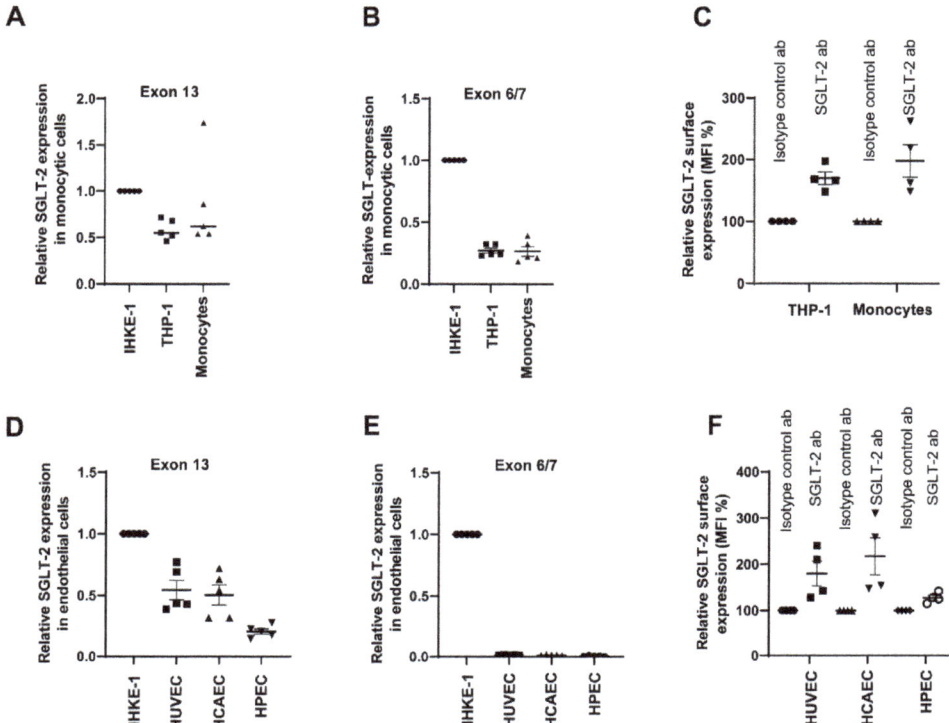

Figure 1. Monocytic and endothelial cells express SGLT-2. (**A**,**B**) CD14++CD16 monocytes isolated from healthy individuals ($n = 5$) and THP-1 monocytic cells ($n = 5$) were analysed for the transcript levels of SGLT-2 using two different primer pairs targeting the exon 13 and exon 6/7 using RT-qPCR. Immortalised Human Kidney Epithelial cells (IHKE1) were used as a positive control. rPLO was used as the house/keeping gene to normalise the gene expression. All data are means ± SEM. (**C**) CD14++CD16 monocytes isolated from healthy individuals ($n = 4$), and THP-1 monocytic cells were analysed by flow cytometry for the surface expression of SGLT-2 compared to the signal from the isotype-specific antibody. The mean fluorescence intensity (MFI) was then quantified. All data are means ± SEM. (**D**,**E**) Human Umbilical Vein Endothelial Cells (HUVEC), Human Coronary Artery Endothelial Cells (HCAEC) and Human fetoplacental Endothelial Cells (HPEC) ($n = 5$ each) were analysed for the transcript levels of SGLT-2 using two different primer pairs targeting the exon 13 and exon 6/7 using RT-qPCR. Immortalised Human Kidney Epithelial cells (IHKE1) were used as a positive control. rPLO was used as the house/keeping gene to normalise the gene expression. All data are means ± SEM. (**F**) Human Umbilical Vein Endothelial Cells (HUVEC), Human Coronary Artery Endothelial Cells (HCAEC) and Human fetoplacental Endothelial Cells (HPEC) ($n = 5$ each) were analysed by flow cytometry for the surface expression of SGLT-2 compared to the signal from the isotype-specific antibody. The mean fluorescence intensity (MFI) was then quantified. All data are means ± SEM.

2.2. $CD14^{++}CD16^{-}$ Monocytes Exposed to Hyperglycemic Conditions Do Not Exhibit an Enhanced Transmigration Phenotype

Since there are reports that diabetic conditions upregulate the expression of SGLT-2 [39], we wondered whether hyperglycaemic conditions or diabetes could modulate the expression of SGLT-2 in monocytes and endothelial cells. For that, we used monocytic cells and endothelial cells cultured under hyperglycaemic conditions in vitro. In addition, we also used $CD14^{++}CD16^{-}$ monocytes isolated from T2DM patients and human fetoplacental endothelial cells (HPEC) isolated from gestational diabetes patients. As shown in Figure 2A, hyperglycaemic conditions did not alter the expression of SGLT-2 transcripts in both THP-1 monocytic cells and primary monocytes. Furthermore, T2DM monocytes did not reveal any significant modulation of SGLT-2 expression (Figure 2B).

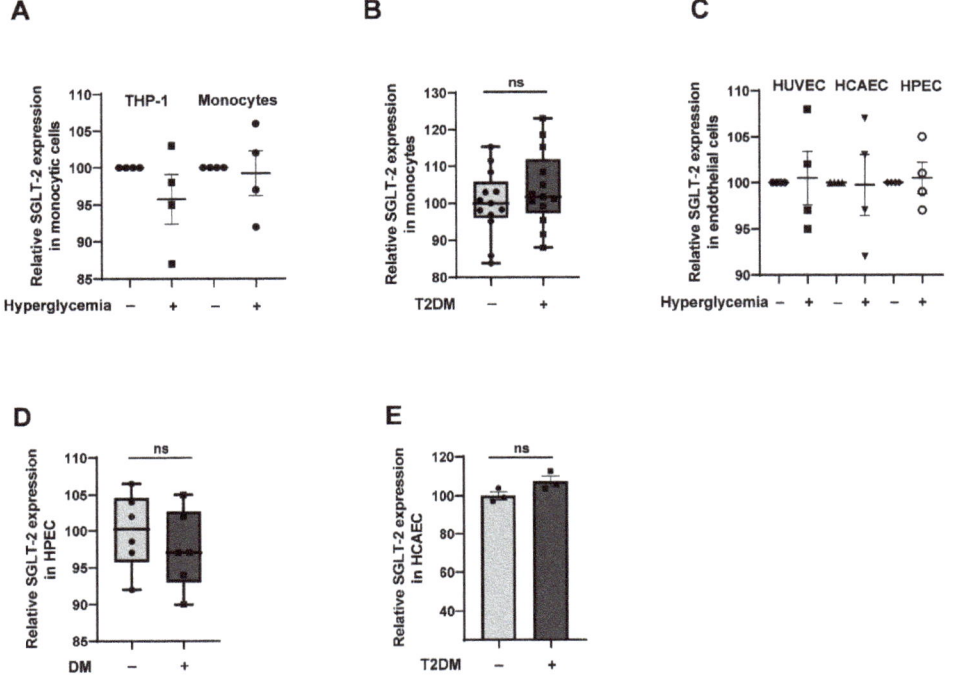

Figure 2. Diabetic conditions do not alter the expression of SGLT-2 in monocytes and endothelial cells. (**A**) CD14^{++}CD16^{-} monocytes isolated from healthy individuals ($n = 4$) and THP-1 monocytic cells ($n = 4$) were exposed to either normoglycemic or hyperglycaemic conditions for 48 h. The cells were then analysed for the transcript levels of SGLT-2 using primer pairs targeting the exon 13 using RT-qPCR. rPLO was used as the house/keeping gene to normalise the gene expression. All data are means ± SEM. (**B**) CD14++CD16 monocytes isolated from T2DM patients ($n = 12$) and non-T2DM individuals ($n = 12$) were analysed for the transcript levels of SGLT-2 using primer pairs targeting the exon 13 using RT-qPCR. rPLO was used as the house/keeping gene to normalise the gene expression. (**C**) Human Umbilical Vein Endothelial Cells (HUVEC), Human Coronary Artery Endothelial Cells (HCAEC) and Human fetoplacental Endothelial Cells (HPEC) ($n = 4$ each) were exposed to either normoglycemic or hyperglycaemic conditions for 48 h. The cells were then analysed for the transcript levels of SGLT-2 using primer pairs targeting the exon 13 using RT-qPCR. rPLO was used as the house/keeping gene to normalise the gene expression. All data are means ± SEM. (**D**) HPECs (Human fetoplacental Endothelial Cells) isolated from gestational diabetes patients ($n = 6$) and non-diabetic individuals ($n = 6$) were analysed for the transcript levels of SGLT-2 using primer pairs targeting the exon 13 using RT-qPCR. rPLO was used as the house/keeping gene to normalise the gene expression. (**E**) HCAECs (Human Coronary Artery Endothelial Cells) isolated from T2DM patients ($n = 3$) and non-T2DM individuals ($n = 3$) were analysed for the transcript levels of SGLT-2 using primer pairs targeting the exon 13 using RT-qPCR. rPLO was used as the house/keeping gene to normalise the gene expression. All data are means ± SEM. ns = non-significant.

Similarly, the in vitro hyperglycaemia treatment of HUVEC, HCAEC and HPEC did not alter the levels of SGLT-2 (Figure 2C). Again, neither gestational DM nor T2DM conditions were found to alter the expression levels of SGLT-2 (Figure 2D,E). These data indicate that diabetic conditions do not alter the SGLT-2 expression levels in monocytes and endothelial cells.

2.3. SGLT-2 Is Weakly Involved in the Glucose Transport in Both Monocytes and Endothelial Cells

Since we detected the transcripts and surface expression of SGLT-2 in monocytes and endothelial cells, we wondered about the potential function of these transporters in these cells. In order to understand the role of SGLT-2 as a glucose transporter, we used fluorescent-tagged glucose derivative (2-NBDG) and carried out glucose transport assays. Since GLUT-dependent transport has been reported in monocytes [40] and endothelial cells [41], we employed a GLUT1 inhibitor to understand GLUT-dependent glucose transport. As shown in Figure 3A, inhibition of GLUT resulted in the significant reduction of 2-NBDG accumulation in primary monocytes. However, the inhibition of SGLT-2 using empagliflozin resulted in a steady but not significant reduction in the 2-NBDG uptake. Both GLUT and SGLT-2 inhibitors did not synergistically influence the glucose uptake (Figure 3A). A similar trend was observed for GLUT inhibition in HUVEC, but the inhibition of SGLT-2 resulted in a meagre but significant difference in the 2-NBDG accumulation (Figure 3B). For HCAEC, SGLT-2 inhibition did not result in a significant difference in the glucose transport but showed a clear tendency in that direction (Figure 3C).

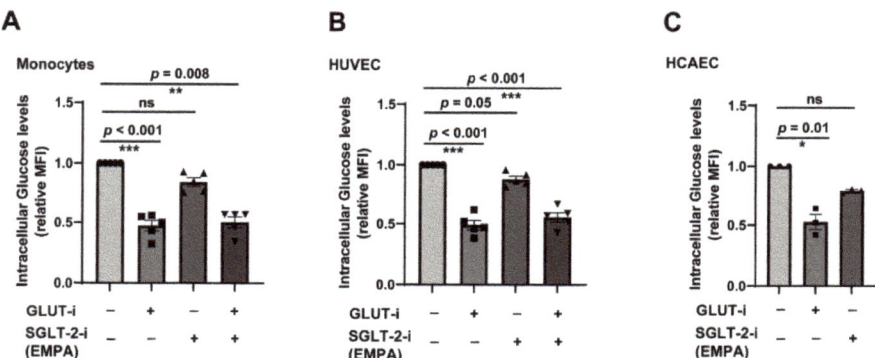

Figure 3. SGLT-2-dependent glucose transport in monocytes and endothelial cells. (**A**) CD14^{++}CD16^{-} monocytes were starved without glucose and serum for 2 h, along with either GLUT inhibitor or SGLT-2 inhibitor. Afterwards, the cells were exposed to the fluorescent-tagged derivative of glucose (2-NBDG) for 2–4 h in the presence of GLUT or SGLT-2 inhibitor or both in combination. Cells were then washed and analysed for intracellular fluorescence using FACS or fluorescence plate reader. $n = 5$. All data are means ± SEM. (**B**) HUVECs were starved without glucose and serum for 2 h, along with either GLUT inhibitor or SGLT-2 inhibitor. After that, the cells were exposed to the fluorescent-tagged derivative of glucose (2-NBDG) for 2–4 h in the presence of a GLUT or SGLT-2 inhibitor or both in combination. Cells were then washed and analysed for intracellular fluorescence using FACS or fluorescence plate reader. $n = 5$. All data are means ± SEM. (**C**) HCAECs were starved without glucose and serum for 2 h, along with either GLUT inhibitor or SGLT-2 inhibitor. Afterwards, the cells were exposed to the fluorescent-tagged derivative of glucose (2-NBDG) for 2–4 h in the presence of GLUT or SGLT-2 inhibitor or both in combination. Cells were then washed and analysed for intracellular fluorescence using FACS or fluorescence spectroscopy. $n = 5$. All data are means ± SEM. ns = non-significant. * $p < 0.05$, ** $p < 0.01$ and *** $p < 0.001$.

2.4. Hyperglycemia-Induced Monocyte Dysfunction Is Oxidative Stress-Dependent, and Empagliflozin Alleviates ROS Accumulation and Reverses Monocyte Dysfunction

Monocytes are rendered dysfunctional in T2DM conditions. As shown in Figure 4A, hyperglycaemic monocytes cannot migrate toward a strong arteriogenic stimulus, the placental growth factor-1 (PlGF-1), which is a direct readout indicating monocyte dysfunction. This inability is partly attributed to the ligand-independent activation monocytes resulting in random motility. The random motile monocytes (termed chemokinesis) cannot sense and specifically respond to growth factor stimulation. As expected, the hyperglycaemic monocytes readily undergo chemokinesis (Figure 4B). Oxidative stress was found to be a primary driver of monocyte dysfunction. The exogenous addition of hydrogen peroxide (H_2O_2) was found to be sufficient to induce monocytes' refractoriness to respond to PlGF-1 (Figure 4C). Exactly as in hyperglycaemic conditions, H_2O_2 treatment alone was sufficient to induce monocyte chemokinesis (Figure 4D). Since empagliflozin has several pleiotropic effects and is considered to be a redox modulator [28], we hypothesised that empagliflozin could interfere with hyperglycaemia-induced ROS accumulation. As shown in Figure 4E, empagliflozin significantly attenuated hyperglycaemia-induced ROS accumulation. Similarly, hyperglycaemia-induced monocyte dysfunction (Figure 4F) and the induction of monocyte chemokinesis (Figure 4G) were significantly reinstated by empagliflozin. Since empagliflozin does not significantly modulate glucose transport in monocytes, these beneficial effects are independent of the intracellular glucose levels.

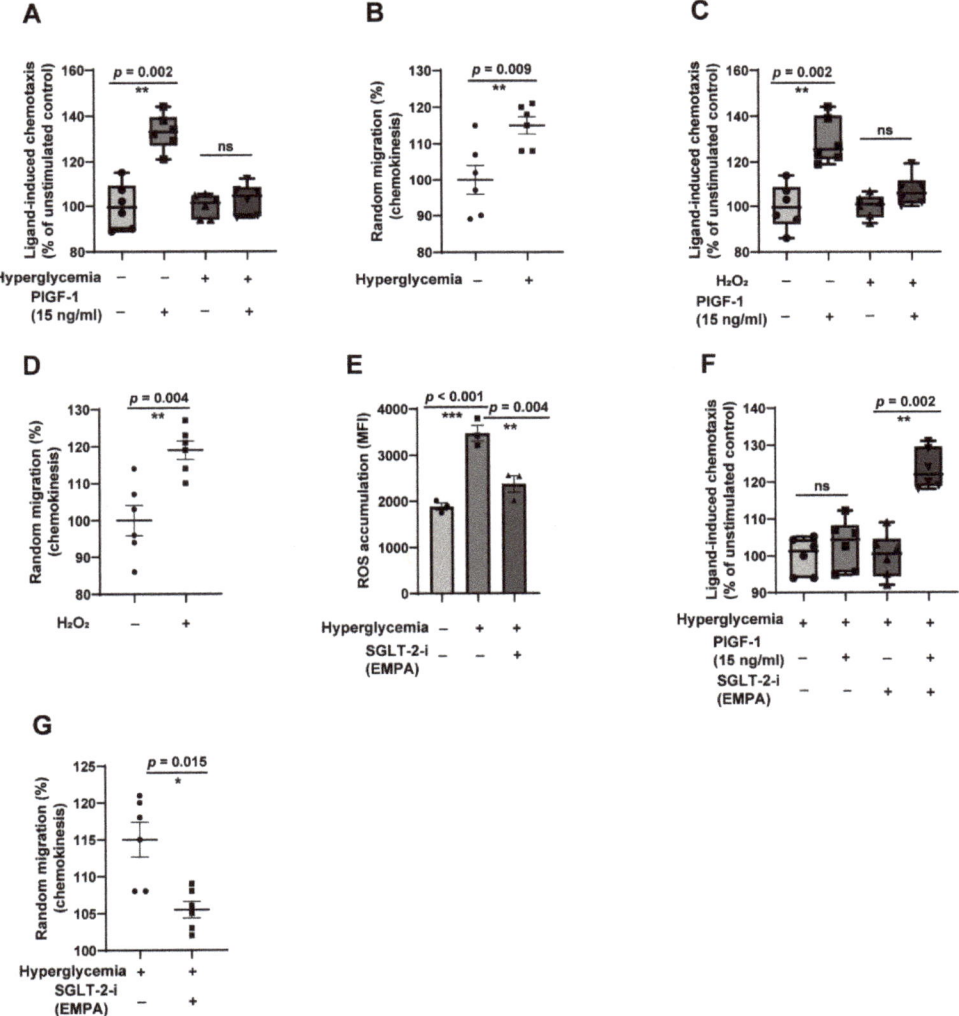

Figure 4. Hyperglycaemia-induced monocyte dysfunction is reversed by empagliflozin through the modulation of oxidative stress. (**A**) CD14^{++}CD16$^-$ monocytes were cultured in vitro in normoglycemic (5 mM glucose) or hyperglycaemic (30 mM glucose + 100 µM methylglyoxal) for 48 h and were analysed for their ability to undergo chemotaxis (directional migration) towards arteriogenic

stimuli PlGF-1. Boyden chamber assays were performed. $n = 6$. (**B**) CD14^{++}CD16^{-} monocytes were cultured in vitro in normoglycemic (5 mM glucose) or hyperglycaemic (30 mM glucose + 100 µM methylglyoxal) for 48 h and were analysed for their ability to undergo chemokinesis (random migration). Checkerboard analyses were performed for this. $n = 6$. All data are means ± SEM. (**C,D**) CD14^{++}CD16^{-} monocytes were cultured in vitro in normoglycemic (5 mM glucose) conditions in the presence of 200 µM H_2O_2 for 24 h. After that, the cells were analysed for their ability to undergo chemotaxis towards PlGF-1 and chemokinesis using Boyden chamber assays. $n = 6$. All data are means ± SEM. (**E**) CD14^{++}CD16^{-} monocytes were cultured in vitro in normoglycemic (5 mM glucose) or hyperglycaemic (30 mM glucose + 100 µM methylglyoxal) for 48 h. The reactive oxygen species (ROS) accumulated was detected by fluorescence spectroscopy using 5-(and-6)-carboxy-2′,7′-difluorodihydrofluorescein diacetate (H2-DFFDA) reagent. $n = 3$. All data are means ± SEM. (**F,G**) CD14^{++}CD16^{-} monocytes were cultured in vitro under hyperglycaemic (30 mM glucose + 100 µM methylglyoxal) conditions for 48 h in the presence or absence of 100 ng/mL SGLT-2 inhibitor empagliflozin. After that, the cells were analysed for their ability to undergo chemotaxis towards PlGF-1 and chemokinesis using Boyden chamber assays. $n = 6$. All data are means ± SEM. ns = non-significant. * $p < 0.05$, ** $p < 0.01$ and *** $p < 0.001$.

2.5. Oxidative Stress-Dependent Impairment of VEGFR-2 Contributes to Endothelial Dysfunction in Hyperglycemia, and Empagliflozin Restores VEGFR-2 to Alleviate Endothelial Dysfunction

Similar to dysfunctional monocytes, diabetes conditions render endothelial cells unable to carry out their primary physiological functions. Most of the signals from the physiological functions of the endothelial cells are transduced through the Vascular Endothelial Growth Factor Receptor-2 (VEGFR-2), and defective VEGFR-2 signalling characterises endothelial dysfunction. We tested this. The ability to respond to VEGFR-2 ligand VEGF-A was significantly reduced in hyperglycaemic endothelial cells (Figure 5A). This defect was found to be due to the reduction of VEGFR-2 surface expression (Figure 5B). Indeed, oxidative stress is vital in mediating the refractoriness of endothelial cells to VEGF-A. The treatment of endothelial cells with exogenous H_2O_2 readily recapitulated the impaired ability to respond to VEGF-A stimulation (Figure 5C), and the induction of oxidative stress was sufficient to impair the surface expression of VEGFR-2 levels (Figure 5D). Confirming the role of empagliflozin as a redox modulator, hyperglycaemia-induced ROS accumulated was reduced in empagliflozin-treated endothelial cells (Figure 5E). Furthermore, empagliflozin restored the ability of hyperglycaemic endothelial cells to respond to VEGF-A (Figure 5F), and this was due to the improved surface expression of the VEGFR-2 receptor (Figure 5G). Taken together, these data indicate that empagliflozin modulates redox homeostasis in endothelial cells.

2.6. A General Antioxidant Improves Cell Function, Whereas Induction of Oxidative Stress Reverses the Beneficial Effects of Empagliflozin

From the results described so far, it seems likely that the modulation of oxidative stress by empagliflozin contributes to improving cell function in hyperglycaemic conditions. We used a very commonly used antioxidant, N-acetyl cysteine (NAC), in our system. In fact, NAC is known to impart a protective effect against diabetes-associated cardiovascular complications [42]. As hypothesised, the application of NAC reversed hyperglycaemia-induced monocyte and endothelial dysfunction (Figure 6A,B). NAC, such as empagliflozin, significantly restored both the impairment of PlGF-1 and VEGF-A responses. This indicated that oxidative alleviation is central to improving vascular cell function. Next, we asked if we were able to suppress the beneficial effects of empagliflozin by the induction of oxidative stress. For that, we used H_2O_2. Oxidative stress significantly attenuated the improvement of monocyte and endothelial cell function induced by empagliflozin in hyperglycaemic conditions (Figure 6C,D). These data further confirmed the role of empagliflozin as a redox regulator in monocytes and endothelial cells.

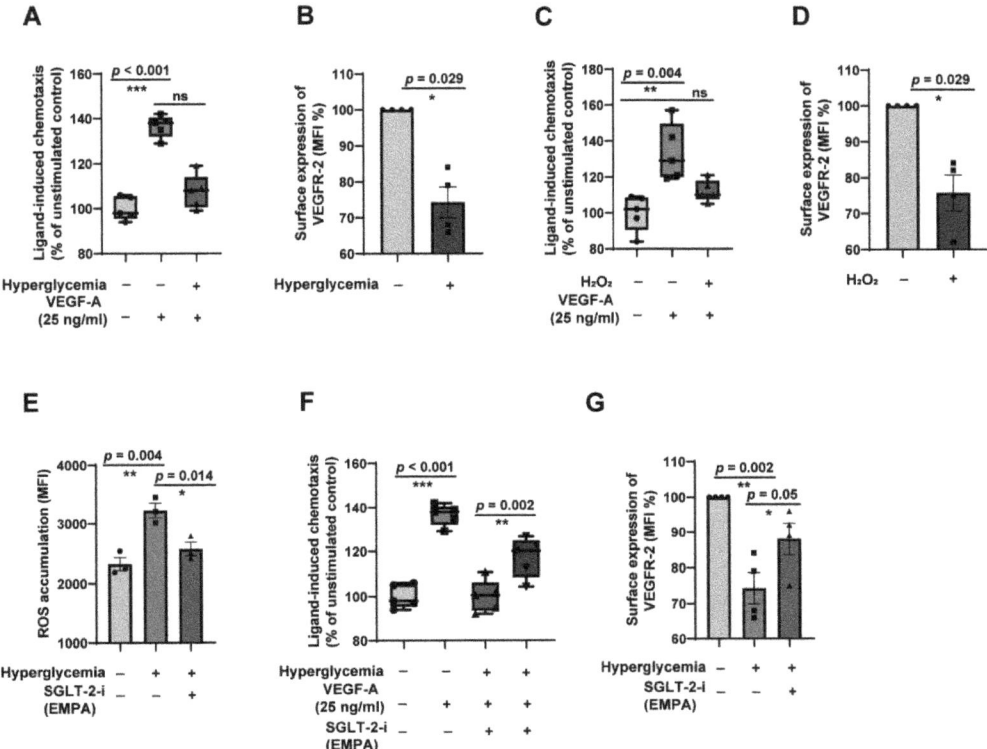

Figure 5. Empagliflozin reverses hyperglycaemia-induced endothelial dysfunction by reducing oxidative stress. (**A**) HUVECs were exposed to in vitro normoglycemic conditions (5 mM glucose) or hyperglycaemic conditions mimicking a diabetic milieu (30 mM glucose + 100 µM methylglyoxal) for 24 h. The cells were then analysed for their ability to undergo chemotaxis (directional migration) towards angiogenic stimuli VEGF-A. Boyden chamber assays were performed. n = 5. (**B**) HUVECs were exposed to in vitro normoglycemic conditions (5 mM glucose) or hyperglycaemic conditions mimicking a diabetic milieu (30 mM Glucose + 100 µM methylglyoxal) for 24 h. Thereafter, FACS analysis of the surface expression of VEGFR-2 on hyperglycaemic HUVECs was done. (n = 5). All data are means ± SEM. (**C**) HUVECs were exposed to in vitro normoglycemic conditions (5 mM glucose) in the presence of 200 µM H_2O_2 for 24 h. After that, the cells were analysed for their ability to undergo chemotaxis towards VEGF-A using Boyden chamber assays. n = 5. (**D**) HUVECs were exposed to in vitro normoglycemic conditions (5 mM glucose) in the presence of 200 µM H_2O_2 for 24 h. After that, the cells were analysed for the surface expression of VEGFR-2 using FACS. n = 4. Data are means ± SEM. (**E**) HUVECs were exposed to in vitro normoglycemic conditions (5 mM glucose) or hyperglycaemic conditions mimicking a diabetic milieu (30 mM Glucose + 100 µM methylglyoxal) for 24 h. The reactive oxygen species (ROS) accumulated was detected by fluorescence spectroscopy using 5-(and-6)-carboxy-2′,7′-difluorodihydrofluorescein diacetate (H2-DFFDA) reagent. n = 3. All data are means ± SEM. (**F**) HUVECs were exposed to in vitro normoglycemic conditions (5 mM glucose) or hyperglycaemic conditions mimicking a diabetic milieu (30 mM Glucose + 100 µM methylglyoxal) for 24 h in the presence or absence of 100 ng/mL SGLT-2 inhibitor empagliflozin. After that, the cells were analysed for their ability to undergo chemotaxis towards VEGF-A using Boyden chamber assays. n = 5 (**G**) FACS analysis of the surface expression of VEGFR-2 of the cells grown under conditions as described for F. n = 4. All data are means ± SEM. ns = non-significant. * $p < 0.05$, ** $p < 0.01$ and *** $p < 0.001$.

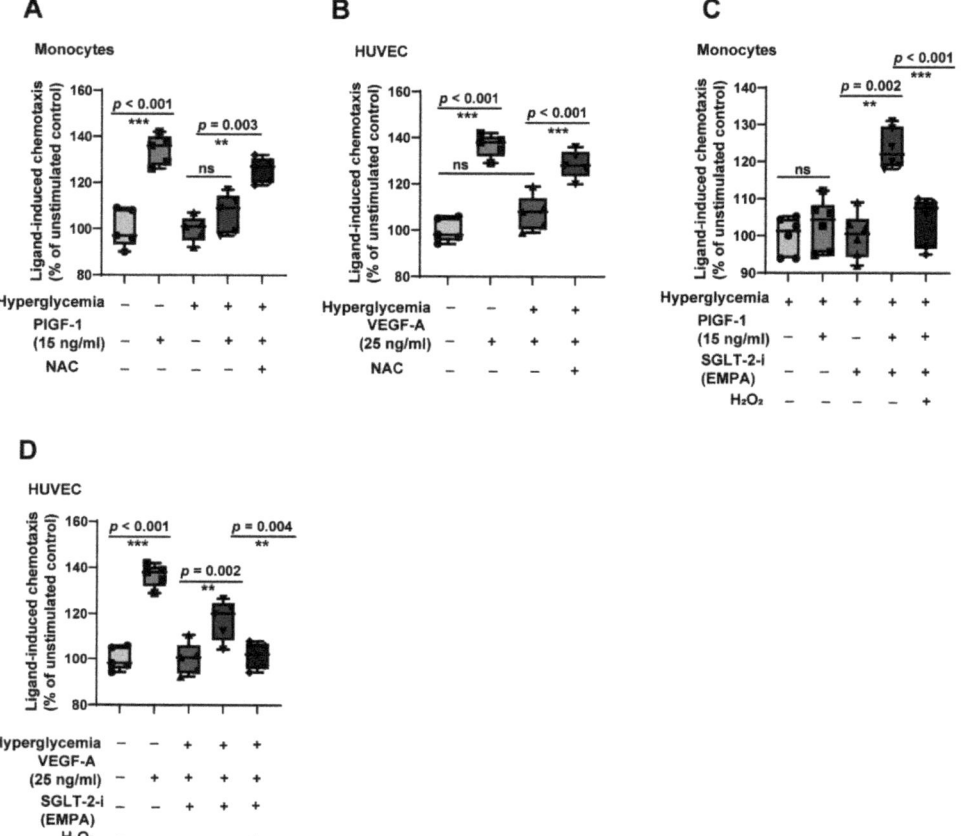

Figure 6. Manipulating the redox status of the cells recapitulates the dysfunction phenotype. (**A**) CD14^{++}CD16$^-$ monocytes were cultured in vitro in normoglycemic (5 mM glucose) or hyperglycaemic (30 mM glucose + 100 µM methylglyoxal) for 48 h in the presence or absence of 5 mM N-acetylcysteine (NAC) and were analysed for their ability to undergo chemotaxis (directional migration) towards arteriogenic stimuli PlGF-1. Boyden chamber assays were performed. n = 5. (**B**) HUVECs were exposed to in vitro normoglycemic conditions (5 mM glucose) or hyperglycaemic conditions mimicking a diabetic milieu (30 mM Glucose + 100 µM methylglyoxal) for 24 h in the presence or absence of 5 mM N-acetylcysteine (NAC). The cells were then analysed for their ability to undergo chemotaxis (directional migration) towards angiogenic stimuli VEGF-A. Boyden chamber assays were performed. n = 5. (**C**) CD14^{++}CD16$^-$ monocytes were cultured in vitro under hyperglycaemic (30 mM glucose + 100 µM methylglyoxal) conditions for 48 h in the presence or absence of 100 ng/mL SGLT-2 inhibitor empagliflozin. In addition, cells were treated with or without 200 µM H$_2$O$_2$. After that, the cells were analysed for their ability to undergo chemotaxis towards PlGF-1 in the presence of 200 µM H$_2$O$_2$. n = 5. (**D**) HUVECs were exposed to in vitro normoglycemic conditions (5 mM glucose) or hyperglycaemic conditions mimicking a diabetic milieu (30 mM Glucose + 100 µM methylglyoxal) for 24 h in the presence or absence of 100 ng/mL SGLT-2 inhibitor empagliflozin. In addition, cells were treated with or without 200 µM H$_2$O$_2$. After that, the cells were analysed for their ability to undergo chemotaxis towards VEGF-A using Boyden chamber assays in the presence of 200 µM H$_2$O$_2$. n = 5. ns = non-significant. ** $p < 0.01$ and *** $p < 0.001$.

3. Discussion

The present study demonstrates that the two important cell types, the monocytes and endothelial cells, are dysfunctional in hyperglycaemic conditions. These cells are required for vascular repair processes and contribute to atherosclerosis development in diabetic patients when dysfunctional. Empagliflozin, the SGLT-2 inhibitor—developed to attenuate the glucose reabsorption by the kidneys as a strategy to reduce blood glucose levels in diabetes patients—improves both hyperglycaemia-induced monocyte and endothelial cell dysfunction by glucose transport-independent mechanisms. Even though monocytes and endothelial cells express functional SGLT-2, glucose transport is not primarily mediated through SGLT-2 but via GLUT. Empagliflozin interferes with the hyperglycaemia-induced oxidative stress induction and attenuates ROS accumulation. Empagliflozin-treated hyperglycaemic monocytes displayed attenuated chemokinesis and were readily responding to arteriogenic stimuli.

Similarly, empagliflozin-treated endothelial cells displayed improved VEGFR-2 receptor levels on the cell surface and responded robustly to angiogenic stimuli. The attenuation of arteriogenesis and angiogenesis is a hallmark of diabetes mellitus contributing to micro- and macrovascular complications [30,34]. Other than interfering with the glucose transport in the proximal kidney tubules and contributing positively to the reduction of glucotoxicity-dependent alterations in cell function, the results described here highlight the pleiotropic effects of empagliflozin and can be a contributing pathway through which this drug offers protection in diabetic and heart failure patients.

Even though SGLT-2 expression is primarily confined to the kidneys, its expression has been reported in various other cell types, including endothelial cells [23,43] and smooth muscle cells [44]. However, the expression of SGLT-2 on monocytes and monocytic cell lines was not reported. Here, we detected the mRNA and protein expression of SGLT-2 in both primary monocytes and several primary endothelial cell types. These data confirm that SGLT-2 is expressed in vascular cells. SGLT-2 expression is regulated dynamically, and several biochemical stimuli such as TNFα and Ang-II have been reported to increase its expression [23,45]. Furthermore, there are reports about the upregulation of SGLT-2 in diabetes [46,47] and heart failure patients [48]. However, our investigations using in vitro hyperglycaemic conditions and monocytes and endothelial cells from T2DM patients did not reveal any differences in the expression pattern of SGLT-2, indicating that diabetes conditions do not stimulate SGLT-2 expression in these cells. The signalling pathways responsible for the induction of SGLT2 in monocytes and endothelial cells have not been delineated.

We identified that the SGLT-2 expressed on monocytes and endothelial cells are also functionally active. Even though to a very low level, the inhibition of SGLT-2 using empagliflozin resulted in slightly altered glucose transport in both these cell types. Although the differences were minimal, there was always a tendency to downgrade glucose transport. This indicates that SGLT-2 is able to transport glucose in these cells, albeit to a lower level. These also validate our data that the positive effect of empagliflozin on monocyte and endothelial function is not secondary to the reduction of glucose transport. As expected, GLUT inhibition significantly blocked glucose transport in both monocytes and endothelial cells. This is in line with the published data on the vital role of GLUT in transporting glucose [49,50].

This study's most exciting and novel finding is the influence of empagliflozin in improving monocyte function in hyperglycaemic conditions. Even though several animal studies have shown that empagliflozin is able to improve endothelial function [27,28,51], its positive effects on monocyte function have not yet been reported. Furthermore, most of the positive effects of empagliflozin on endothelial function in vivo are also secondary to its role in reducing glucotoxicity. However, we report that empagliflozin imparts positive effects on endothelial cells and monocytes through a pleiotropic mechanism. Indeed, this ambiguous role of empagliflozin has been reported in several studies [20]. Our data refer to the specific contribution of empagliflozin in alleviating the oxidative stress-dependent induction of monocyte and endothelial cell function. Further studies are required to evaluate the improvement of endothelial function in vivo using the flow-mediated dilation (FMD) method [52].

Translational data suggest that SGLT2 inhibitors may positively affect plaque composition and burden through the reduction of inflammatory and cell adhesion pathways. Still, human data are not available to make solid conclusions. However, endothelial dysfunction represents an important mechanism underlying heart failure with preserved ejection fraction (HFpEF) [53]. Impaired coronary microvascular function is strongly associated with the severity of heart failure [54]. Even though published data do not completely support a causative role for monocytes and heart failure, their role in atrial fibrillation (AF) has been postulated [55]. Therefore, the improvement of both endothelial and monocyte function by empagliflozin could improve heart failure outcomes.

The modulation of oxidative stress by empagliflozin is a pleiotropic mechanism on which several positive effects of this drug could be based. Such a possibility is currently being tested in patients with type 2 diabetes (EMPOX study) in a clinical trial. (ClinicalTrials.gov Identifier: NCT02890745). Our data confirm the notion that empagliflozin can reduce the ROS accumulation induced by hyperglycaemia. This could be secondary to reducing oxidative stress-inducing machinery such as NADPH oxidases (NOXs) or improving the antioxidant system [56]. The dysfunction of monocytes and endothelial cells induced by hyperglycaemia is oxidative stress-dependent [24,33], and the complete alleviation of this dysfunction phenotype of empagliflozin demonstrates its function as a redox regulator. The alleviation of the beneficial effects of empagliflozin by the induction of oxidative stress demonstrates that the beneficial effects of empagliflozin are redox-dependent. Since functionally active monocytes and endothelial cells could carry out a wide array of repair and regeneration processes in diabetes, empagliflozin-mediated improvement of these two cell types would contribute to the beneficial aspects of empagliflozin. Further investigations are necessary to understand how empagliflozin is able to impart its effects as a redox modulator.

4. Materials and Methods

4.1. Monocyte Isolation from Clinical Cohorts and Healthy Individuals

$CD14^{++}CD16^-$ human monocytes were isolated from healthy donors and from non-T2DM individuals or T2DM patients according to a published protocol [33] using Magnet-assisted cell sorting (MACS) using negative selection with the human Monocyte Isolation Kit II from Miltenyi Biotec (Bergisch Gladbach, Germany). The study was approved by the scientific and ethics committee of the University of Münster and the University of Jena and conformed to the principles of the Declaration of Helsinki. Written informed consent was obtained from all donors by the blood bank, and thrombocyte reduction filters were provided anonymously without sharing personal and detailed information. The purity of isolated cells was confirmed by FACS, and they were around 98% pure. The clinical characteristics are described in detail in Supplementary Table S1.

4.2. Human Umbilical Vein Endothelial Cells Isolation and Ethics

Human umbilical vein endothelial cells (HUVEC) were isolated from anonymously acquired umbilical cords according to the Declaration of Helsinki, "Ethical Principles for Medical Research Involving Human Subjects" (1964), as described previously [57]. The study was approved by the Jena University Hospital Ethics Committee (no. 3130-05/11), and donors were informed and gave written consent. For cell preparation, umbilical cord veins were cleaned with 0.9% NaCl solution, and cells were detached with 0.01% collagenase dissolved in M199 for 3 min at 37 °C. Veins were then rinsed with M199/10% FCS, and the cell suspension was centrifuged ($500\times g$, 6 min). The pellet was resuspended in M199/10% FCS and seeded on a cell culture flask coated with 0.2% gelatine. After 24 h, cells were washed and cultured in full growth medium (M199, 20% FCS, 7.5 U/mL heparin, 100 U/mL penicillin and 100 μg/mL streptomycin).

4.3. Human Fetoplacental Endothelial Cell Isolation from Clinical Cohorts and Healthy Individuals

Primary HPEC were isolated from arterial vessels of human term placentas obtained from healthy and GDM pregnancies, as described previously [58]. In brief, arterial vessels from the apical surface of the chorionic plate were dissected and cells were isolated by perfusion of the arteries with Hank's balanced salt solution (HBSS, Invitrogen, Waltham, MA, USA) containing 0.1 U/mL collagenase, 0.8 U/mL dispase II (Roche, Basel, Switzerland) and 10 mg/mL penicillin/streptomycin for 8 min. Digested suspension was centrifuged ($200 \times g$, 5 min), the cell pellet resuspended in EBM-2 Media supplemented with the EGM-2 MV Bullet Kit (Lonza, Basel, Switzerland), containing 5% human heat-inactivated serum of pregnant women instead of FCS and plated on 1% gelatine-coated wells of a 12-well plate. Cells were split into a 12 cm^2 flask, 25 cm^2 flask and, finally, 75 cm^2 flask accordingly when cells were confluent. The identity and purity of HPEC were confirmed by immunocytochemistry staining of specific endothelial markers for von Willebrand factor and CD31 (PECAM1), fibroblast markers (CD90 and TE-7) and smooth muscle cell markers (SMA and Desmin). For maintaining a culture, primary cells were grown in EBM-2 Media supplemented with the EGM-2 MV Bullet Kit containing 5% FCS, and cells split for less than 10 passages were used for experiments. The ethics committee of the Medical University of Graz approved this study (27-265 ex 14/15). All individuals gave voluntary informed consent and underwent an oral glucose tolerance test (OGTT) at 24 weeks of gestation. Control subjects were selected based on negative OGGT. Women with GDM diagnosed according to the WHO/IADPSG criteria, but without other pregnancy complications, were recruited before delivery. All subjects included in the GDM group were managed by diet and lifestyle modifications during the remaining time of pregnancy. The study conforms to the Declaration of Helsinki. Clinical characteristics are listed in Supplementary Table S2.

4.4. Monocyte, HUVEC, HCAEC and HPEC Culture

Primary human monocytes were maintained in RPMI-1640 medium (+L-glutamine, D(+)-glucose; Thermo Scientific, Waltham, MA, USA) supplemented with 5 mM glucose, 10% foetal bovine serum (FBS) and 1% penicillin/streptomycin (P/S). For migration experiments, cells were starved for 2–4 h in FBS-free RPMI-1640 medium. Monocytes were kept in an incubator at 37 °C and 5% CO$_2$. Normoglycemic medium contained 5 mM glucose and 25 mM mannitol. In hyperglycaemic medium, 30 mM glucose and 100 µM methylglyoxal were used, and the cells were treated for 48 h. HUVECs were cultured in full growth medium (M199, 20% FCS, 7.5 U/mL heparin and 1% penicillin/streptomycin). In general, HUVEC from 2–5 passages were used for the experiments. For migration experiments, cells were starved for 2–4 h in FBS-free M199 medium. Monocytes were kept in an incubator at 37 °C and 10% CO$_2$. Normoglycemic medium contained 5 mM glucose and 25 mM mannitol. In hyperglycaemic medium, 30 mM glucose and 100 µM methylglyoxal were used, and the cells were treated for 24 h. HCAECs were obtained from Lonza and were maintained in EBM™-2 Basal Medium (CC-3156) and EGM™-2 MV Microvascular Endothelial Cell Growth Medium SingleQuots™ supplements (CC-4147), as per the recommendations of the manufacturer. Cells up to a passage of 6 were used for the experiments. HPECs were grown in EBM-2 media supplemented with the EGM-2 MV Bullet Kit containing 5% FCS, and cells split for less than 10 passages were used for experiments.

4.5. Reagents

Cell culture media RPMI 1640 Medium GlutaMAX™ was obtained from Life Technologies. Human VEGF-A and PlGF-1 were from Peprotech. H$_2$DFFDA and CellROX were from Life Technologies. Hydrogen peroxide, methylglyoxal, NAC and 2-NBDG were from Sigma Aldrich. All the primers for qPCR were custom synthesised from Sigma Aldrich. Primer sequences are described in Supplementary Table S3.

4.6. RNA Isolation and qPCR

For the extraction of RNA, roughly $5\text{--}8 \times 10^6$ monocytes were used. For in vitro experiments, the RNA was extracted between 8 and 12 h post-cell treatment. Total RNA purification was performed using a NucleoSpin RNA isolation kit (Macherey-Nagel, Dueren, Germany), and cDNA was synthesised using a RevertAid First Strand cDNA Synthesis Kit (Thermo Scientific, Waltham, MA, USA). qPCR was carried out using iTaq™ Universal SYBR®® Green supermix (Bio-Rad, Hercules, CA, USA) in the Connect Real-Time PCR Detection System (Bio-Rad, Hercules, CA, USA). The threshold cycle (Cq) value of each sample was calculated, and the expression of the target gene mRNA relative to rpl0 was determined by the $2^{-\Delta\Delta Ct}$ method. The sequences of the primers used can be found in Supplementary Table S3.

4.7. Glucose Uptake Assay

Cells were equilibrated in glucose-free medium with 1% serum for three hours prior to being treated with 10 µM of 2-NBDG for 30 min at 37 °C, together with GLUT inhibitor or empagliflozin. Cells were washed two times, and the flow cytometry analysis was carried out using Guava easyCyte (Millipore, Burlington, MA, USA).

4.8. Monocyte Chemotaxis and Chemokinesis Assay

Chemotaxis assays were performed as described previously [7,59] using a 48-well Boyden chamber (Neuroprobe, Gaithersburg, MD, USA) and Nucleopore PET membrane (Whatman, Maidstone, UK) with 5 µm diameter pores. Cells in a concentration from 0.5×10^6 cells/mL were allowed to migrate for 90 min at 37 °C and 5% CO_2. The cells that migrated through the pores were counted. For quantification, migrated cells were counted by 20 high-power fields in four wells using the Axioskop 2 Plus microscope (Carl Zeiss, Jena, Germany).

4.9. Chemotaxis Assay of Endothelial Cells

For the detection of endothelial cell chemotaxis, a modified 48-well Boyden chamber (Nucleopore) and a polycarbonate membrane with a pore diameter of 8 mm (Nucleopore) were used as described earlier [24,33]. Endothelial cells were cultured for 24 h under normal and high glucose conditions with or without empagliflozin. For the assay, cells were starved in a serum-free M199 medium for 1 h, trypsinised, washed and resuspended in serum-free medium. Cells were seeded in a concentration of 0.35×10^6 cells/mL and allowed to migrate for 1.5 h at 37 °C and 5% CO_2 with and without 25 ng/mL VEGF-A stimulation. Migrated cells were fixed with 99% ethanol for 10 min and stained with Giemsa staining solution. Cells at the upper side of the filter membrane were scraped off. Migrated cells were counted using ZEISS Axioskop 2 Plus at 10X magnification from 3 different wells.

4.10. Intracellular Reactive Oxygen Species Detection

HUVECs were seeded in a 12-well plate in different glucose conditions with or without 100 ng/mL empagliflozin for 24–48 h. The method was based on the modification of the published protocol [60]. After that, cells were washed twice with Krebs-Ringer phosphate glucose buffer (KRPG; 145 mM NaCl, 5.7 mM KH_2PO_4, 4.86 mM KCl, 0.54 mM $CaCl_2$, 1.22 mM $MgSO4$ and 5.5 mM glucose) and then resuspended in 1 mL KRPG. Carboxy-H_2DFFDA (20 µM) or CellROX (5 µM) was added; the suspension mixed well and then incubated in dark for 20 to 30 min at room temperature. The subsequent steps were strictly carried out in the dark. The cells were washed twice with KRPG. The fluorescence intensity was quantified with a fluorescence multimode microplate reader (Vector, Perkin Elmer) with excitation at 485 nm and emission at 530 nm or by Guava easyCyte FACS using the FITC-channel (Millipore, Burlington, MA, USA).

4.11. Detection of the Surface Expression of VEGFR-2

HUVECs were cultured in normoglycemic or hyperglycaemic conditions with or without 100 ng/mL empagliflozin for 24 h in a 12-well plate. For the assay, the cells were trysinised, washed once with 1X PBS and resuspended in 500 µL of PBS/BSA (0.5% BSA) solution. Fc-R blocking reagent was added for 10 min at room temperature, and 2 µL of PE-VEGFR2 antibody (Miltenyi Biotec, Bergisch Gladbach, Germany) were added and incubated for 15 min at room temperature in the dark, and the FACS analysis was done using Guava easyCyte (Millipore, Burlington, MA, USA).

4.12. Statistical Analysis

To analyse the significance of differences in experiments with monocytes isolated from diabetic or healthy individuals/mice, the Mann–Whitney Rank Sum Test (for intergroup comparisons) or Kruskal–Wallis One-Way Analysis of Variance on Ranks with Tukey's or Dunn's post hoc correction was used. For all the other experiments, two-sample independent t-tests or when multiple comparisons were made, Kruskal–Wallis One-Way Analysis of Variance on Ranks with Tukey's or Dunn's post hoc correction was performed. SigmaPlot 12 software was used for the statistical analysis. The level of significance was defined as $p < 0.05$. All other statistics and graphs were generated using GraphPad Prism 8 software.

5. Conclusions

In conclusion, using the cell culture model of in vitro hyperglycaemia and T2DM monocytes and T2DM endothelial cells and endothelial cells from gestational diabetes patients, we identified that both monocytes and endothelial cells express SGLT-2 transcripts and harbour functionally active SGLT-2 on their surface. SGLT-2 was not responsible for the glucose transport in these cells. However, the empagliflozin treatment significantly reversed the monocyte and endothelial cell dysfunction induced by hyperglycaemia. This was completely independent of glucose transport but through the reduction of oxidative stress. Mechanistically, empagliflozin attenuated the oxidative stress-dependent chemokinesis of monocytes and restored the surface levels of VEGFR-2 on endothelial cells. Furthermore, our results highlight the pleiotropic role of empagliflozin as a redox modulator.

Supplementary Materials: The following supporting information can be downloaded at: https://www.mdpi.com/article/10.3390/jcm12041356/s1: Table S1. Clinical characteristics of the non-T2DM and T2DM individuals used in the study. Table S2. Clinical characteristics of non-diabetic and diabetic individuals used for the HPEC isolation. Table S3. RT-qPCR primer sequences used in the study.

Author Contributions: R.G. and J.W. conceived and developed the concept; R.G., D.S., J.O., M.D. and J.W. designed the experiments and interpreted the data; D.S., J.O., M.D., P.H. and R.G. did the experiments; J.S. and U.H. isolated, characterized, provided, and supported the experiments using HPECs. N.M., U.A.M. and R.G. were involved with patient characterization, recruitment, and isolation of diabetic and non-diabetic monocytes; R.G. drafted the manuscript; S.A.Z. and J.W. contributed to the redrafting of the manuscript; R.G. and J.W. finalised the manuscript with input from all the authors and R.G. and J.W. supervised the study. All authors have read and agreed to the published version of the manuscript.

Funding: This study was supported, in part, by the Innovative Medizinische Forschung (IMF) grant GO121222 (to Godfrey), Interdisziplinäre Zentrum für Klinische Forschung (IZKF) grant IZKF-SEED 014/20 (to Dorenkamp), grants from the Deutsche Forschungsgemeinschaft (DFG), Collaborative Research Centre 656 Münster (project C12) and grants from the Deanery of the Medical Faculty of the Westfälische Wilhelms-Universität Münster (all to Waltenberger).

Institutional Review Board Statement: Human blood leukocyte reduction filters from healthy subjects were received from the blood bank of the University Hospital Münster. Written informed consent was obtained from all donors by the blood bank, and leukocyte reduction filters were provided anonymously without sharing personal and detailed information. This study was approved by the local ethics committee of Münster University Hospital, Germany, and Jena University Hospital, Germany. All the DM patients and non-DM individuals provided written informed consent to participate in the study. The ethical permission number is 2011-612-f-S (Münster) and 4125-06/14 (Jena). The study was conducted according to the principles of the Declaration of Helsinki.

Informed Consent Statement: Informed consent was obtained from all subjects involved in the study.

Data Availability Statement: Not applicable.

Acknowledgments: We thank Merle Leffers and Sybille Koch for their technical support.

Conflicts of Interest: The authors declare no conflict of interest.

References

1. Zinman, B.; Lachin, J.M.; Inzucchi, S.E. Empagliflozin, Cardiovascular Outcomes, and Mortality in Type 2 Diabetes. *N. Engl. J. Med.* **2016**, *374*, 1094. [CrossRef] [PubMed]
2. Prevalence of small vessel and large vessel disease in diabetic patients from 14 centres. The World Health Organisation Multinational Study of Vascular Disease in Diabetics. Diabetes Drafting Group. *Diabetologia* **1985**, *28*, 615–640. [CrossRef] [PubMed]
3. Aronson, D.; Edelman, E.R. Coronary artery disease and diabetes mellitus. *Cardiol. Clin.* **2014**, *32*, 439–455. [CrossRef]
4. Giacco, F.; Brownlee, M. Oxidative stress and diabetic complications. *Circ. Res.* **2010**, *107*, 1058–1070. [CrossRef] [PubMed]
5. Suryavanshi, S.V.; Kulkarni, Y.A. NF-kappabeta: A Potential Target in the Management of Vascular Complications of Diabetes. *Front. Pharmacol.* **2017**, *8*, 798. [CrossRef]
6. Yamamoto, Y.; Yamamoto, H. RAGE-Mediated Inflammation, Type 2 Diabetes, and Diabetic Vascular Complication. *Front. Endocrinol.* **2013**, *4*, 105. [CrossRef]
7. Tchaikovski, V.; Olieslagers, S.; Bohmer, F.D.; Waltenberger, J. Diabetes mellitus activates signal transduction pathways resulting in vascular endothelial growth factor resistance of human monocytes. *Circulation* **2009**, *120*, 150–159. [CrossRef]
8. Gao, X.; Zhang, H.; Schmidt, A.M.; Zhang, C. AGE/RAGE produces endothelial dysfunction in coronary arterioles in type 2 diabetic mice. *Am. J. Physiol. Heart Circ. Physiol.* **2008**, *295*, H491–H498. [CrossRef]
9. Coughlan, M.T.; Thorburn, D.R.; Penfold, S.A.; Laskowski, A.; Harcourt, B.E.; Sourris, K.C.; Tan, A.L.; Fukami, K.; Thallas-Bonke, V.; Nawroth, P.P.; et al. RAGE-induced cytosolic ROS promote mitochondrial superoxide generation in diabetes. *J. Am. Soc. Nephrol.* **2009**, *20*, 742–752. [CrossRef]
10. Wautier, M.P.; Chappey, O.; Corda, S.; Stern, D.M.; Schmidt, A.M.; Wautier, J.L. Activation of NADPH oxidase by AGE links oxidant stress to altered gene expression via RAGE. *Am. J. Physiol. Endocrinol. Metab.* **2001**, *280*, E685–E694. [CrossRef]
11. Rieg, T.; Masuda, T.; Gerasimova, M.; Mayoux, E.; Platt, K.; Powell, D.R.; Thomson, S.C.; Koepsell, H.; Vallon, V. Increase in SGLT1-mediated transport explains renal glucose reabsorption during genetic and pharmacological SGLT2 inhibition in euglycemia. *Am. J. Physiol. Ren. Physiol.* **2014**, *306*, F188–F193. [CrossRef]
12. Zinman, B.; Wanner, C.; Lachin, J.M.; Fitchett, D.; Bluhmki, E.; Hantel, S.; Mattheus, M.; Devins, T.; Johansen, O.E.; Woerle, H.J.; et al. Empagliflozin, Cardiovascular Outcomes, and Mortality in Type 2 Diabetes. *N. Engl. J. Med.* **2015**, *373*, 2117–2128. [CrossRef]
13. Packer, M.; Anker, S.D.; Butler, J.; Filippatos, G.; Pocock, S.J.; Carson, P.; Januzzi, J.; Verma, S.; Tsutsui, H.; Brueckmann, M.; et al. Cardiovascular and Renal Outcomes with Empagliflozin in Heart Failure. *N. Engl. J. Med.* **2020**, *383*, 1413–1424. [CrossRef]
14. Zannad, F.; Ferreira, J.P.; Pocock, S.J.; Anker, S.D.; Butler, J.; Filippatos, G.; Brueckmann, M.; Ofstad, A.P.; Pfarr, E.; Jamal, W.; et al. SGLT2 inhibitors in patients with heart failure with reduced ejection fraction: A meta-analysis of the EMPEROR-Reduced and DAPA-HF trials. *Lancet* **2020**, *396*, 819–829. [CrossRef]
15. Fitchett, D.; Zinman, B.; Wanner, C.; Lachin, J.M.; Hantel, S.; Salsali, A.; Johansen, O.E.; Woerle, H.J.; Broedl, U.C.; Inzucchi, S.E.; et al. Heart failure outcomes with empagliflozin in patients with type 2 diabetes at high cardiovascular risk: Results of the EMPA-REG OUTCOME(R) trial. *Eur. Heart J.* **2016**, *37*, 1526–1534. [CrossRef]
16. Han, J.H.; Oh, T.J.; Lee, G.; Maeng, H.J.; Lee, D.H.; Kim, K.M.; Choi, S.H.; Jang, H.C.; Lee, H.S.; Park, K.S.; et al. The beneficial effects of empagliflozin, an SGLT2 inhibitor, on atherosclerosis in ApoE (-/-) mice fed a western diet. *Diabetologia* **2017**, *60*, 364–376. [CrossRef]
17. Byrne, N.J.; Parajuli, N.; Levasseur, J.L.; Boisvenue, J.; Beker, D.L.; Masson, G.; Fedak, P.W.M.; Verma, S.; Dyck, J.R.B. Empagliflozin Prevents Worsening of Cardiac Function in an Experimental Model of Pressure Overload-Induced Heart Failure. *JACC Basic Transl. Sci.* **2017**, *2*, 347–354. [CrossRef]
18. Park, S.H.; Farooq, M.A.; Gaertner, S.; Bruckert, C.; Qureshi, A.W.; Lee, H.H.; Benrahla, D.; Pollet, B.; Stephan, D.; Ohlmann, P.; et al. Empagliflozin improved systolic blood pressure, endothelial dysfunction and heart remodeling in the metabolic syndrome ZSF1 rat. *Cardiovasc. Diabetol.* **2020**, *19*, 19. [CrossRef]
19. Andreadou, I.; Efentakis, P.; Balafas, E.; Togliatto, G.; Davos, C.H.; Varela, A.; Dimitriou, C.A.; Nikolaou, P.E.; Maratou, E.; Lambadiari, V.; et al. Empagliflozin Limits Myocardial Infarction in Vivo and Cell Death in Vitro: Role of STAT3, Mitochondria, and Redox Aspects. *Front. Physiol.* **2017**, *8*, 1077. [CrossRef]

20. Patel, D.K.; Strong, J. The Pleiotropic Effects of Sodium-Glucose Cotransporter-2 Inhibitors: Beyond the Glycemic Benefit. *Diabetes Ther.* **2019**, *10*, 1771–1792. [CrossRef]
21. Satoh, H. Pleiotropic effects of SGLT2 inhibitors beyond the effect on glycemic control. *Diabetol. Int.* **2018**, *9*, 212–214. [CrossRef] [PubMed]
22. Mone, P.; Varzideh, F.; Jankauskas, S.S.; Pansini, A.; Lombardi, A.; Frullone, S.; Santulli, G. SGLT2 Inhibition via Empagliflozin Improves Endothelial Function and Reduces Mitochondrial Oxidative Stress: Insights From Frail Hypertensive and Diabetic Patients. *Hypertension* **2022**, *79*, 1633–1643. [CrossRef] [PubMed]
23. Uthman, L.; Homayr, A.; Juni, R.P.; Spin, E.L.; Kerindongo, R.; Boomsma, M.; Hollmann, M.W.; Preckel, B.; Koolwijk, P.; van Hinsbergh, V.W.M.; et al. Empagliflozin and Dapagliflozin Reduce ROS Generation and Restore NO Bioavailability in Tumor Necrosis Factor alpha-Stimulated Human Coronary Arterial Endothelial Cells. *Cell Physiol. Biochem.* **2019**, *53*, 865–886. [CrossRef]
24. Hemling, P.; Zibrova, D.; Strutz, J.; Sohrabi, Y.; Desoye, G.; Schulten, H.; Findeisen, H.; Heller, R.; Godfrey, R.; Waltenberger, J. Hyperglycemia-induced endothelial dysfunction is alleviated by thioredoxin mimetic peptides through the restoration of VEGFR-2-induced responses and improved cell survival. *Int. J. Cardiol.* **2020**, *308*, 73–81. [CrossRef] [PubMed]
25. Avogaro, A.; Fadini, G.P.; Gallo, A.; Pagnin, E.; de Kreutzenberg, S. Endothelial dysfunction in type 2 diabetes mellitus. *Nutr. Metab. Cardiovasc. Dis.* **2006**, *16* (Suppl. S1), S39–S45. [CrossRef]
26. Waltenberger, J.; Lange, J.; Kranz, A. Vascular endothelial growth factor-A-induced chemotaxis of monocytes is attenuated in patients with diabetes mellitus: A potential predictor for the individual capacity to develop collaterals. *Circulation* **2000**, *102*, 185–190. [CrossRef]
27. Oelze, M.; Kroller-Schon, S.; Welschof, P.; Jansen, T.; Hausding, M.; Mikhed, Y.; Stamm, P.; Mader, M.; Zinssius, E.; Agdauletova, S.; et al. The sodium-glucose co-transporter 2 inhibitor empagliflozin improves diabetes-induced vascular dysfunction in the streptozotocin diabetes rat model by interfering with oxidative stress and glucotoxicity. *PLoS ONE* **2014**, *9*, e112394. [CrossRef]
28. Steven, S.; Oelze, M.; Hanf, A.; Kroller-Schon, S.; Kashani, F.; Roohani, S.; Welschof, P.; Kopp, M.; Godtel-Armbrust, U.; Xia, N.; et al. The SGLT2 inhibitor empagliflozin improves the primary diabetic complications in ZDF rats. *Redox Biol.* **2017**, *13*, 370–385. [CrossRef]
29. Werner, G.S.; Richartz, B.M.; Heinke, S.; Ferrari, M.; Figulla, H.R. Impaired acute collateral recruitment as a possible mechanism for increased cardiac adverse events in patients with diabetes mellitus. *Eur. Heart J.* **2003**, *24*, 1134–1142. [CrossRef]
30. Waltenberger, J. Impaired collateral vessel development in diabetes: Potential cellular mechanisms and therapeutic implications. *Cardiovasc. Res.* **2001**, *49*, 554–560. [CrossRef]
31. Warren, C.M.; Ziyad, S.; Briot, A.; Der, A.; Iruela-Arispe, M.L. A ligand-independent VEGFR2 signaling pathway limits angiogenic responses in diabetes. *Sci. Signal.* **2014**, *7*, ra1. [CrossRef]
32. Sasso, F.C.; Torella, D.; Carbonara, O.; Ellison, G.M.; Torella, M.; Scardone, M.; Marra, C.; Nasti, R.; Marfella, R.; Cozzolino, D.; et al. Increased vascular endothelial growth factor expression but impaired vascular endothelial growth factor receptor signaling in the myocardium of type 2 diabetic patients with chronic coronary heart disease. *J. Am. Coll. Cardiol.* **2005**, *46*, 827–834. [CrossRef]
33. Dorenkamp, M.; Muller, J.P.; Shanmuganathan, K.S.; Schulten, H.; Muller, N.; Loffler, I.; Muller, U.A.; Wolf, G.; Bohmer, F.D.; Godfrey, R.; et al. Hyperglycaemia-induced methylglyoxal accumulation potentiates VEGF resistance of diabetic monocytes through the aberrant activation of tyrosine phosphatase SHP-2/SRC kinase signalling axis. *Sci. Rep.* **2018**, *8*, 14684. [CrossRef]
34. Fadini, G.P.; Albiero, M.; Bonora, B.M.; Avogaro, A. Angiogenic Abnormalities in Diabetes Mellitus: Mechanistic and Clinical Aspects. *J. Clin. Endocrinol. Metab.* **2019**, *104*, 5431–5444. [CrossRef]
35. Ruiter, M.S.; van Golde, J.M.; Schaper, N.C.; Stehouwer, C.D.; Huijberts, M.S. Diabetes impairs arteriogenesis in the peripheral circulation: Review of molecular mechanisms. *Clin. Sci.* **2010**, *119*, 225–238. [CrossRef]
36. Waltenberger, J. VEGF resistance as a molecular basis to explain the angiogenesis paradox in diabetes mellitus. *Biochem. Soc. Trans.* **2009**, *37*, 1167–1170. [CrossRef]
37. Waltenberger, J. Stress testing at the cellular and molecular level to unravel cellular dysfunction and growth factor signal transduction defects: What Molecular Cell Biology can learn from Cardiology. *Thromb. Haemost.* **2007**, *98*, 975–979. [CrossRef]
38. Chen, J.; Williams, S.; Ho, S.; Loraine, H.; Hagan, D.; Whaley, J.M.; Feder, J.N. Quantitative PCR tissue expression profiling of the human SGLT2 gene and related family members. *Diabetes Ther.* **2010**, *1*, 57–92. [CrossRef]
39. Rahmoune, H.; Thompson, P.W.; Ward, J.M.; Smith, C.D.; Hong, G.; Brown, J. Glucose transporters in human renal proximal tubular cells isolated from the urine of patients with non-insulin-dependent diabetes. *Diabetes* **2005**, *54*, 3427–3434. [CrossRef]
40. Dimitriadis, G.; Maratou, E.; Boutati, E.; Psarra, K.; Papasteriades, C.; Raptis, S.A. Evaluation of glucose transport and its regulation by insulin in human monocytes using flow cytometry. *Cytom. A* **2005**, *64*, 27–33. [CrossRef]
41. Tumova, S.; Kerimi, A.; Porter, K.E.; Williamson, G. Transendothelial glucose transport is not restricted by extracellular hyperglycaemia. *Vascul. Pharmacol.* **2016**, *87*, 219–229. [CrossRef] [PubMed]
42. Dludla, P.V.; Dias, S.C.; Obonye, N.; Johnson, R.; Louw, J.; Nkambule, B.B. A Systematic Review on the Protective Effect of N-Acetyl Cysteine Against Diabetes-Associated Cardiovascular Complications. *Am. J. Cardiovasc. Drugs* **2018**, *18*, 283–298. [CrossRef] [PubMed]
43. Juni, R.P.; Al-Shama, R.; Kuster, D.W.D.; van der Velden, J.; Hamer, H.M.; Vervloet, M.G.; Eringa, E.C.; Koolwijk, P.; van Hinsbergh, V.W.M. Empagliflozin restores chronic kidney disease-induced impairment of endothelial regulation of cardiomyocyte relaxation and contraction. *Kidney Int.* **2021**, *99*, 1088–1101. [CrossRef] [PubMed]

44. Sukhanov, S.; Higashi, Y.; Yoshida, T.; Mummidi, S.; Aroor, A.R.; Jeffrey Russell, J.; Bender, S.B.; DeMarco, V.G.; Chandrasekar, B. The SGLT2 inhibitor Empagliflozin attenuates interleukin-17A-induced human aortic smooth muscle cell proliferation and migration by targeting TRAF3IP2/ROS/NLRP3/Caspase-1-dependent IL-1beta and IL-18 secretion. *Cell Signal* **2021**, *77*, 109825. [CrossRef] [PubMed]
45. Park, S.H.; Belcastro, E.; Hasan, H.; Matsushita, K.; Marchandot, B.; Abbas, M.; Toti, F.; Auger, C.; Jesel, L.; Ohlmann, P.; et al. Angiotensin II-induced upregulation of SGLT1 and 2 contributes to human microparticle-stimulated endothelial senescence and dysfunction: Protective effect of gliflozins. *Cardiovasc. Diabetol.* **2021**, *20*, 65. [CrossRef]
46. Albertoni Borghese, M.F.; Majowicz, M.P.; Ortiz, M.C.; Passalacqua Mdel, R.; Sterin Speziale, N.B.; Vidal, N.A. Expression and activity of SGLT2 in diabetes induced by streptozotocin: Relationship with the lipid environment. *Nephron. Physiol.* **2009**, *112*, p45–p52. [CrossRef]
47. Umino, H.; Hasegawa, K.; Minakuchi, H.; Muraoka, H.; Kawaguchi, T.; Kanda, T.; Tokuyama, H.; Wakino, S.; Itoh, H. High Basolateral Glucose Increases Sodium-Glucose Cotransporter 2 and Reduces Sirtuin-1 in Renal Tubules through Glucose Transporter-2 Detection. *Sci. Rep.* **2018**, *8*, 6791. [CrossRef]
48. Katsurada, K.; Nandi, S.S.; Sharma, N.M.; Patel, K.P. Enhanced Expression and Function of Renal SGLT2 (Sodium-Glucose Cotransporter 2) in Heart Failure: Role of Renal Nerves. *Circ. Heart Fail.* **2021**, *14*, e008365. [CrossRef]
49. Malide, D.; Davies-Hill, T.M.; Levine, M.; Simpson, I.A. Distinct localization of GLUT-1, -3, and -5 in human monocyte-derived macrophages: Effects of cell activation. *Am. J. Physiol.* **1998**, *274*, E516–E526. [CrossRef]
50. Huang, Y.; Lei, L.; Liu, D.; Jovin, I.; Russell, R.; Johnson, R.S.; Di Lorenzo, A.; Giordano, F.J. Normal glucose uptake in the brain and heart requires an endothelial cell-specific HIF-1alpha-dependent function. *Proc. Natl. Acad. Sci. USA* **2012**, *109*, 17478–17483. [CrossRef]
51. Ganbaatar, B.; Fukuda, D.; Shinohara, M.; Yagi, S.; Kusunose, K.; Yamada, H.; Soeki, T.; Hirata, K.I.; Sata, M. Empagliflozin ameliorates endothelial dysfunction and suppresses atherogenesis in diabetic apolipoprotein E-deficient mice. *Eur. J. Pharmacol.* **2020**, *875*, 173040. [CrossRef]
52. Mucka, S.; Miodonska, M.; Jakubiak, G.K.; Starzak, M.; Cieslar, G.; Stanek, A. Endothelial Function Assessment by Flow-Mediated Dilation Method: A Valuable Tool in the Evaluation of the Cardiovascular System. *Int. J. Environ. Res. Public Health* **2022**, *19*, 11242. [CrossRef]
53. Mone, P.; Lombardi, A.; Kansakar, U.; Varzideh, F.; Jankauskas, S.S.; Pansini, A.; Marzocco, S.; De Gennaro, S.; Famiglietti, M.; Macina, G.; et al. Empagliflozin Improves the MicroRNA Signature of Endothelial Dysfunction in Patients with Heart Failure with Preserved Ejection Fraction and Diabetes. *J. Pharmacol. Exp. Ther.* **2023**, *384*, 116–122. [CrossRef]
54. Cornuault, L.; Rouault, P.; Duplaa, C.; Couffinhal, T.; Renault, M.A. Endothelial Dysfunction in Heart Failure With Preserved Ejection Fraction: What are the Experimental Proofs? *Front. Physiol.* **2022**, *13*, 906272. [CrossRef]
55. Miyosawa, K.; Iwata, H.; Minami-Takano, A.; Hayashi, H.; Tabuchi, H.; Sekita, G.; Kadoguchi, T.; Ishii, K.; Nozaki, Y.; Funamizu, T.; et al. Enhanced monocyte migratory activity in the pathogenesis of structural remodeling in atrial fibrillation. *PLoS ONE* **2020**, *15*, e0240540. [CrossRef]
56. Das, N.A.; Carpenter, A.J.; Belenchia, A.; Aroor, A.R.; Noda, M.; Siebenlist, U.; Chandrasekar, B.; DeMarco, V.G. Empagliflozin reduces high glucose-induced oxidative stress and miR-21-dependent TRAF3IP2 induction and RECK suppression, and inhibits human renal proximal tubular epithelial cell migration and epithelial-to-mesenchymal transition. *Cell Signal* **2020**, *68*, 109506. [CrossRef]
57. Spengler, K.; Kryeziu, N.; Grosse, S.; Mosig, A.S.; Heller, R. VEGF Triggers Transient Induction of Autophagy in Endothelial Cells via AMPKalpha1. *Cells* **2020**, *9*, 687. [CrossRef]
58. Strutz, J.; Cvitic, S.; Hackl, H.; Kashofer, K.; Appel, H.M.; Thuringer, A.; Desoye, G.; Koolwijk, P.; Hiden, U. Gestational diabetes alters microRNA signatures in human feto-placental endothelial cells depending on fetal sex. *Clin. Sci.* **2018**, *132*, 2437–2449. [CrossRef]
59. Tchaikovski, V.; Tchaikovski, S.; Olieslagers, S.; Waltenberger, J. Monocyte dysfunction as a previously unrecognized pathophysiological mechanism in ApoE-/- mice contributing to impaired arteriogenesis. *Int. J. Cardiol.* **2015**, *190*, 214–216. [CrossRef]
60. Godfrey, R.; Arora, D.; Bauer, R.; Stopp, S.; Muller, J.P.; Heinrich, T.; Bohmer, S.A.; Dagnell, M.; Schnetzke, U.; Scholl, S.; et al. Cell transformation by FLT3 ITD in acute myeloid leukemia involves oxidative inactivation of the tumor suppressor protein-tyrosine phosphatase DEP-1/PTPRJ. *Blood* **2012**, *119*, 4499–4511. [CrossRef]

Disclaimer/Publisher's Note: The statements, opinions and data contained in all publications are solely those of the individual author(s) and contributor(s) and not of MDPI and/or the editor(s). MDPI and/or the editor(s) disclaim responsibility for any injury to people or property resulting from any ideas, methods, instructions or products referred to in the content.

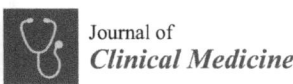 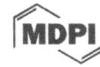

Article

Sex Differences in Cardiovascular Prevention in Type 2: Diabetes in a Real-World Practice Database

Anna Ramírez-Morros [1,2], Josep Franch-Nadal [3,4], Jordi Real [3,4], Mònica Gratacòs [3] and Didac Mauricio [3,4,5,6,*]

[1] DAP-Cat Group, Unitat de Suport a la Recerca de la Catalunya Central, Institut Universitari d'Investigació en Atenció Primària Jordi Gol (IDIAP Jordi Gol), 08272 Sant Fruitós de Bages, Spain; amramirez.cc.ics@gencat.cat
[2] Gerència Territorial de la Catalunya Central, Institut Català de la Salut, 08272 Sant Fruitós de Bages, Spain
[3] DAP-Cat Group, Unitat de Suport a la Recerca de Barcelona, Institut Universitari d'Investigació en Atenció Primària Jordi Gol (IDIAP Jordi Gol), 08007 Barcelona, Spain; josepfranch@gmail.com (J.F.-N.); jreal@idiapjgol.info (J.R.); monica.gratacos@gmail.com (M.G.)
[4] Center for Biomedical Research on Diabetes and Associated Metabolic Diseases (CIBERDEM), Instituto de Salud Carlos III, 08907 Barcelona, Spain
[5] Department of Endocrinology and Nutrition, Hospital de la Santa Creu i Sant Pau and Sant Pau Biomedical Research Institute (IIB Sant Pau), 08041 Barcelona, Spain
[6] Department of Medicine, University of Vic and Central University of Catalonia, 08500 Vic, Spain
* Correspondence: didacmauricio@gmail.com; Tel.: +34-93-556-5661

Abstract: Women with type 2 diabetes mellitus (T2DM) have a 40% excess risk of cardiovascular diseases (CVD) compared to men due to the interaction between sex and gender factors in the development, risk, and outcomes of the disease. Our aim was to assess differences between women and men with T2DM in the management and degree of control of cardiovascular risk factors (CVRF). This was a matched cross-sectional study including 140,906 T2DM subjects without previous CVD and 39,186 T2DM subjects with prior CVD obtained from the System for the Development of Research in Primary Care (SIDIAP) database. The absolute and relative differences between means or proportions were calculated to assess sex differences. T2DM women without previous CVD showed higher levels of total cholesterol (12.13 mg/dL (0.31 mmol/L); 95% CI = 11.9–12.4) and low-density lipoprotein cholesterol (LDL-c; 5.50 mg/dL (0.14 mmol/L); 95% CI = 5.3–5.7) than men. The recommended LDL-c target was less frequently achieved by women as it was the simultaneous control of different CVRF. In secondary prevention, women showed higher levels of total cholesterol (16.89 mg/dL (0.44 mmol/L); 95% CI = 16.5–17.3), higher levels of LDL-c (8.42 mg/dL (0.22 mmol/L); 95% CI = 8.1–8.8), and higher levels of triglycerides (11.34 mg/dL (0.13 mmol/L); 95% CI = 10.3–12.4) despite similar rates of statin prescription. Recommended targets were less often achieved by women, especially LDL-c < 100 mg/dL (2.59 mmol/L). The composite control was 22% less frequent in women than men. In conclusion, there were substantial sex differences in CVRF management of people with diabetes, with women less likely than men to be on LDL-c target, mainly those in secondary prevention. This could be related to the treatment gap between genders.

Keywords: risk factors; cardiovascular diseases; diabetes mellitus; type 2; gender

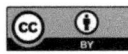

1. Introduction

According to the International Diabetes Federation (IDF), the global age-standardized prevalence of diabetes in subjects 20–79 years in 2019 was similar between men and women (9.6% and 9%, respectively) [1]. However, there were more diabetes-associated deaths among women than in men (2.3 vs. 1.9 million) [1].

Large-scale meta-analyses have consistently shown that type 2 diabetes (T2DM) confers a greater excess risk of macrovascular complications in women compared with men. The relative risk of coronary heart disease (CHD) is estimated to be 44% higher in women; the risk of stroke is 27% higher, the occlusive vascular mortality rate is nearly 50% higher, and the risk of vascular dementia is 19% higher [2–4]. Regarding microvascular complications, it has been reported that the risk of end-stage renal disease is 38% higher in women than in men [2–4]. These disparities have been attributed to the interaction between sex and gender factors in the development, risk, and outcomes of diabetes [3]. Sex differences refer to biology-linked variations, such as sex hormones levels, body composition, and glucose and fat metabolism. Gender differences arise from inequalities in sociocultural processes (e.g., environmental influences, nutritional patterns, lifestyle, or attitudes toward treatment and prevention) [3].

The mechanisms underpinning the biological disparities in the likelihood of developing diabetes-related vascular complications between sexes are not entirely understood. Women develop diabetes at a higher body mass index (BMI) than men, and one of the proposed explanations is that they usually have lower visceral and ectopic fat, which may lead to a slower transition to insulin resistance and diabetes. As a result, women might be exposed longer to hyperglycemia or a suboptimal glucose level state, resulting in greater vascular damage and deterioration of the cardiovascular risk factors (CVRFs) [2–4]. In addition to these sex-specific differences, gender dissimilarities in diabetes management and healthcare provision may partially contribute to the diabetes-related increased CVD risk. For instance, although the recommendations on prevention, management, and treatment of diabetes and diabetes-related complications are similar for both sexes, women are less likely than men to receive guideline-recommended care [4]. Indeed, some studies have reported that women are less likely than men to be monitored for foot and eye complications, and they receive less effective management and screening of CV risk factors such as blood pressure (BP), BMI, or smoking status [2,5]. Additionally, the odds of receiving statins, antihypertensive, and antiplatelet medications differ between genders [6,7].

In Spain, a recent observational, prospective study reported that women with T2DM have threefold higher odds of CV death than men [8]. Additionally, previously published cross-sectional and population-based studies indicated a poorest control of CVRF in primary and secondary prevention among Spanish women [9–12]. In all of these studies, the proportion of women was substantially lower than men, and, most importantly, the baseline characteristics differed significantly between cohorts. For instance, women were on average 2.5–4 years older than men, the duration of T2DM was nearly 1 year longer, they were less likely to smoke, and the prevalence of diabetes-related micro- and macrovascular complications was different between genders. Although these and other differences largely exist in real-life clinical practice, they may limit the interpretation of research findings when traditional cohort matching strategies, stratified analyses, or regression covariate adjustments are used to consider heterogeneity [13]. In contrast, when patients are matched with propensity modeling technologies, the cohorts have a balanced distribution of covariates, thus allowing for equivalent comparisons between groups that can provide inferences about causal effects in observational studies [13].

In Catalonia (Spain), the healthcare system is public and universal. The primary care centers provide first contact and continuing care for persons with any health concerns, and they are usually the principal place where T2DM is diagnosed and managed. The antidiabetic treatment is free of charge for those retired and severely ill people, while active subjects pay just a small part of the cost of the drugs [14]. Briefly, the primary care physicians are responsible for prescribing medications through an electronic prescription that the patient can pick up at the pharmacy. To assess prescribing practices concerning the appropriate use of drugs, the Health Institute of Catalonia uses a quality indicator system created in 2003, the Pharmaceutical Prescription Quality Standard (EQPF) [15]. This study aimed to evaluate whether the pharmacological management of T2DM and the degree of CVRF control in primary care differ between sexes in primary and secondary prevention using a propensity score matching method to balance the inequality of confounding covariates.

2. Materials and Methods

2.1. Study Design

This was a matched, cross-sectional study including data from patients with T2DM available from the SIDIAP population-based database. This database contains anonymized patient information from the computerized medical records stored in the Electronic Clinical station in Primary Care (eCAP). SIDIAP includes data from about 80% of the Catalonia population (5.835 million subjects) distributed within the 279 primary care centers belonging to the Catalan Health Institute (ICS) [16]. The overall T2DM population has been previously described [17], and this dataset was further used to apply the propensity score method.

The investigation conformed with the principles outlined in the Declaration of Helsinki. The study was approved by the Ethics Committee of the Primary Healthcare University Research Institute (IDIAP) Jordi Gol (P14/018) and registered at ClinicalTrials.gov (NCT04653805).

2.2. Study Variables

We used data extracted data from patients aged 31 to 90 years with a diagnosis of T2DM (International Classification of Disease 10 [ICD-10] codes E11 and E14) as at 30 June 2013 who had at least one visit registered with the primary care team in the previous 12 months. For this study, the following variables were used: age, gender, time since diagnosis (years), smoking habit, number of visits with the primary care team in the previous 12 months, estimated glomerular filtration rate (eGFR) with the MDRD (modification of diet in renal disease) formula, presence of diabetic retinopathy (ICD-10 codes E11.3 and H36.0), albumin/creatinine ratio, BMI, glycated hemoglobin (HbA1c), lipid profile (i.e., total cholesterol levels, high-density lipoprotein cholesterol (HDL-c), low-density lipoprotein cholesterol (LDL-c), and triglycerides (TGs)), presence of dyslipidemia (defined as receiving medication for this condition), prescription of glucose-lowering drugs, lipid-lowering drugs (statins or other), blood pressure (BP) (diastolic (dBP) and systolic (sBP)), hypertension (defined as receiving medication for this condition), prescription of hypertension-lowering drugs, and antiplatelet and anticoagulant therapy. Chronic kidney disease was assumed in patients with eGFR < 60 mL/min and/or albumin/creatinine ratio > 300 mg/g. The most recent value registered was used in all cases. For those with a previous CVD, diagnostic codes for macrovascular diseases were collected, including coronary artery disease (CAD; ICD-10 codes I20-I24), cerebrovascular disease (ICD-10 codes I63, I64, G45 or G46), and peripheral artery disease (PAD; ICD-10 code I73.9).

Variables to assess the degree of CVRF control and treatment goals achievement were based on local guidelines [18], i.e., HbA1c $\leq$ 7% (53 mmol/mol), BP $\leq$ 140/90 mmHg, and LDL-c < 130 mg/dL (3.37 mmol/L) for primary prevention and <100 mg/dL (2.59 mmol/L) for secondary prevention. Additionally, the same variables were assessed according to the threshold stated by our institution (ICS): HbA1c $\leq$ 8% (64 mmol/mol), BP $\leq$ 130/80 mmHg, and LDL-c < 100 mg/dL for primary prevention and LDL-c < 70 mg/dL (1.81 mmol/L) for secondary prevention.

2.3. Propensity Score Matching Method

Propensity score matching (PSM) was used to create subpopulations of women and men with T2DM that were balanced in terms of baseline conditions, namely, age, duration of T2DM, number of visits to the primary care team, presence of comorbidities (i.e., hypertension, dyslipidemia, and diabetic retinopathy), eGFR value, albumin/creatinine ratio, and smoking in primary prevention. For the analyses of those in secondary prevention, subjects were also matched for previous macrovascular diseases. Matched groups (male versus female group) were performed (1:1) using the one-to-one nearest neighbor algorithm (with a caliper of 0.1 of the SD of the propensity score on the logit scale) and no replacement. To evaluate PSM quality, we assessed the balance in covariates comparing the absolute difference before and after the matching procedure.

2.4. Statistical Analysis

We summarized data as the mean (standard deviation) for continuous variables and number (percentage) for categorical variables by groups. To assess the association between clinical variables and gender, we computed the absolute difference in the means or proportions (Dif) between groups, and we estimated their 95% confidence interval (95% CI). To assess the magnitude of the gender differences, we calculated the relative percentage difference (rDif) between groups. Dif was calculated by subtracting the mean or proportion for women from the mean or proportion for men, and rDif was calculated as the absolute difference divided by the reference value (mean or proportion value of men) multiplied by 100. We performed graphical analyses with smoothing line plots to evaluate whether the potential differences remained over all age ranges. We performed a complete-case analysis excluding missing information for each quantitative variable. All analyses were performed using the R free software environment for statistical computing (v3.5.1) and the "MatchIt" library for the PSM [19].

3. Results

A total of 343,969 patients with T2DM were identified in the database. After the matching procedure, there were 70,453 subjects in each primary prevention group and 19,593 in each secondary prevention group (Figure 1). Baseline characteristics in these populations were well balanced (Figures S1 and S2).

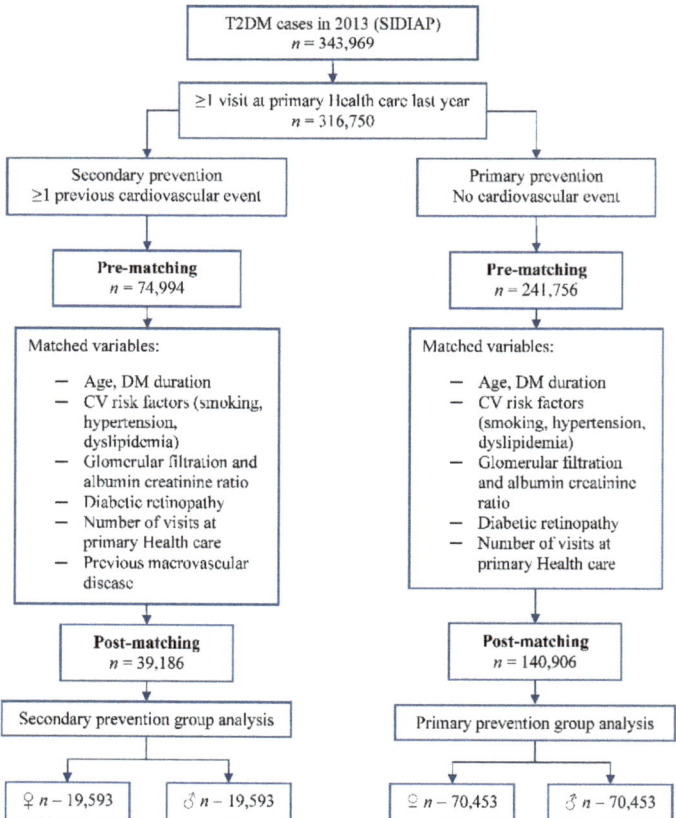

Figure 1. Flow chart of the propensity score matching procedure.

3.1. Primary Prevention

The baseline characteristics of the matched women and men in primary prevention are shown in Table 1. The mean age of the overall population was 66.2 years (SD = 12.2), and the mean duration of diabetes 7.1 years (SD = 5.4) years. Dyslipidemia was present in 52.3% of the patients, hypertension was present in 66.7% of the patients, diabetic retinopathy was present in 6.3% of the patients, and renal impairment was present in 15.9% of the patients.

Table 1. Baseline characteristics of matched women and men with T2DM in primary prevention by gender.

Variable	N Subjects	Women	N Subjects	Men	Dif	95% CI	
Age (years), mean ± SD *	70,453	66.57 ± 12.22	70,453	65.88 ± 12.20	0.69	0.63	0.75
Diabetes duration (years), mean ± SD *		7.10 ± 5.40		7.01 ± 5.34	0.09	0.07	0.12
Number of visits, mean ± SD *,†		6.39 ± 4.66		6.18 ± 5.08	0.21	0.19	0.24
Smoking habit, n (%) *	69,001		69,119				
Nonsmoker		51,753 (75.00)		51,118 (73.96)	1.04	0.67	1.42
Smoker		7684 (11.14)		5934 (8.59)	2.55	2.29	2.81
Former smoker		9564 (13.86)		12,067 (17.46)	−3.60	−3.90	−3.30
BMI (kg/m^2), mean ± SD	48,047	31.09 ± 5.80	47,287	29.34 ± 4.47	1.75	1.72	1.78
HbA1c (%), mean ± SD	54,055	7.24 ± 1.37	53,476	7.22 ± 1.37	0.02	0.01	0.03
Dyslipidemia, n (%) *	70,453	37,367 (53.04)	70,453	36,264 (51.47)	1.57	1.13	2.00
Lipid profile (mg/dL), mean ± SD							
Total cholesterol	54,561	199.02 ± 37.71	53,976	186.89 ± 37.16	12.13	11.91	12.35
HDL-c	49,918	53.76 ± 13.35	48,986	47.53 ± 12.15	6.23	6.15	6.31
LDL-c		116.10 ± 32.62		110.60 ± 31.29	5.50	5.30	5.70
TGs	51,514	152.23 ± 90.36	50,830	153.70 ± 110.82	−1.47	−2.09	−0.85
Hypertension, n (%) *	70,453	47,968 (68.09)	70,453	45,949 (65.22)	2.87	2.46	3.27
Blood Pressure (mmHg), mean ± SD	59,795		59,067				
dBP		75.95 ± 8.35		76.44 ± 8.62	−0.49	−0.54	−0.44
sBP		133.83 ± 13.25		134.86 ± 12.56	−1.03	−1.10	−0.96
Diabetic retinopathy, n (%) *	70,453	4418 (6.27)	70,453	4485 (6.37)	−0.10	−0.29	0.10
Renal disease, n (%) *,$	53,782	8617 (16.02)	53,493	8409 (15.72)	0.30	−0.06	0.66

95% CI, 95% confidence interval; BMI, body mass index; dBP, diastolic blood pressure; HbA1c, glycated hemoglobin; HDL-c, high-density lipoprotein cholesterol; LDL-c, low-density lipoprotein cholesterol; Dif, difference between groups; sBP, systolic blood pressure; SD, standard deviation; TGs, triglycerides. * Variables matched between study groups. † Number of visits with the primary care team in the previous 12 months. $ Renal disease, including eGFR < 60 mL/min and/or albumin/creatinine ratio > 300 mg/g.

In this primary prevention population, women had higher BMI than men (Dif = 1.75 kg/m^2; 95% CI = 1.7 to 1.8) but similar values of HbA1c (Dif = 0.02%; 95% CI = 0.01 to 0.03) and BP (dBP Dif = −0.49 mmHg; 95% CI= −0.5 to −0.4 and sBP Dif = −1.03 mmHg; 95% CI = −1.1 to 0.9). Although the plasmatic TG concentration was comparable between genders, total cholesterol, HDL-c, and LDL-c were higher in women than men (Dif = 12.13 mg/dL, 95% CI = 11.9 to 12.3; Dif = 6.23, 95% CI = 6.1–6.3; Dif = 5.50 mg/dL, 95% CI = 5.3 to 5.7, respectively). Moreover, this sex-difference in total cholesterol and LDL-c was observed across all age ranges (Figure 2A).

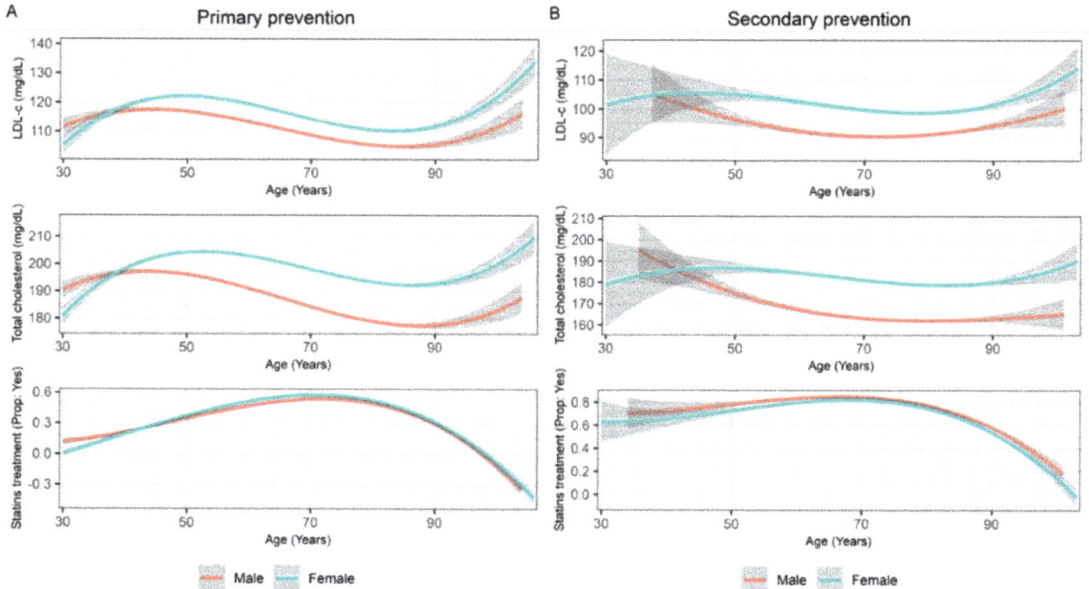

Figure 2. Smoothing line charts with changes in LDL-c, total cholesterol, and statin treatment across age in subjects on primary prevention (**A**) and secondary prevention (**B**) by gender (LDL-c, low-density lipoprotein cholesterol).

Differences by gender in the pharmacological management of T2DM and degree of CVRF control are shown in Table 2 and Figure 3. As for lipid control, statins were more frequently prescribed to women (rDif = 4.7%; Figure 3A). Regarding BP treatment, the prescription of diuretics, beta-blockers, and two antihypertensive drugs was substantially higher in women relative to men (rDif = 16.5%, 10.3%, and 8.1%, respectively). Lastly, women received antiplatelet therapy less often than men (rDif = −15.0%).

Table 2. Pharmacological treatment and cardiovascular risk factor control in matched women and men with T2DM in primary prevention by gender.

Variable	N Subjects	Women	N Subjects	Men	Dif (95% CI)
Lipid-lowering treatment, n (%) *	37,367		36,264		
Statins		34,933 (93.49)		32,374 (89.27)	4.22 (3.91/4.52)
Other		4653 (12.45)		6430 (17.73)	−5.28 (−5.69/−4.87)
Antihypertensive treatment, n (%) †	47,968		45,949		
ACEI/ARBII		38,757 (80.80)		39,492 (85.95)	−5.15 (−5.54/−4.76)
CCBs		13,477 (28.10)		14,352 (31.23)	−3.13 (−3.60/−2.68)
Beta-blockers		9893 (20.62)		8586 (18.69)	1.93 (1.53/2.34)
Diuretics		31,429 (65.52)		25,836 (56.23)	9.29 (8.80/9.79)
Other		2570 (5.36)		4054 (8.82)	−3.46 (−3.69/−3.24)
Number of drugs					
1		16,124 (33.61)		16,404 (35.70)	−2.09 (−2.61/−1.57)
2		18,593 (38.76)		16,479 (35.86)	2.90 (2.40/3.40)
≥3		13,251 (27.62)		13,066 (28.44)	−0.82 (−1.27/−0.35)

Table 2. Cont.

Variable	N Subjects	Women	N Subjects	Men	Dif (95% CI)
Antiplatelet therapy, n (%)	70,453	14,993 (21.28)	70,453	17,645 (25.05)	−3.77 (−4.12/−3.41)
Target CVRF achievement, n (%)					
BP ≤ 130/80 mmHg	59,795	20,442 (34.19)	59,067	18,558 (31.42)	2.77 (2.32/3.22)
BP ≤ 140/90 mmHg		44,555 (74.51)		42,955 (72.72)	1.79 (1.38/2.21)
LDL-c ≤ 130 mg/dL	49,918	34,707 (69.53)	48,986	36,831 (75.19)	−5.66 (−6.14/−5.18)
LDL-c ≤ 100 mg/dL		16,661 (33.38)		19,213 (39.22)	−5.84 (−6.35/−5.34)
HbA1c, %	54,055		53,476		
≤7		30,262 (55.98)		30,152 (56.38)	−0.40 (−0.91/0.11)
≤8		43,269 (80.05)		42,767 (79.97)	0.08 (−0.32/0.47)
>8		10,786 (19.95)		10,709 (20.03)	−0.08 (−0.47/0.32)
HbA1c ≤ 7%, BP ≤ 140/90 mmHg, LDL-c < 130 mg/dL	43,956	13,173 (29.97)	42,788	13,863 (32.40)	−2.43 (−2.96/−1.90)
HbA1c ≤ 7%, BP ≤ 140/90 mmHg, LDL-c < 100 mg/dL		5935 (13.50)		6787 (15.86)	−2.36 (−2.74/−1.98)

95% CI, 95% confidence interval; ACEI/ARBII, angiotensin-converting enzyme inhibitors/angiotensin II receptor blockers; BP, blood pressure; CCB, calcium channel blockers; CVRF, cardiovascular risk factor; HbA1c, glycated hemoglobin; LDL-c, low-density lipoprotein cholesterol; Dif, difference between groups. * Lipid-lowering treatment, proportion data calculated on the basis of those with dyslipidemia. † Antihypertensive treatment, proportion data calculated on the basis of those with hypertension.

The proportion of women who achieved BP target levels was greater in women for both the ≤130/80 mmHg and the ≤140/90 mmHg goals (rDif = 8.8% and 2.5%, respectively). Despite women being more frequently treated with statins than men, fewer women attained the LDL-c ≤ 130 and ≤100 mg/dL thresholds relative to men (rDif = −7.5% and rDif = −14.8%, respectively) (Figure 3B). Regarding glycemic control, the gender differences in the proportion of subjects below the HbA1c ≤ 7 and 8% target was negligible (rDif = −0.7% and 0.1%, respectively). Lastly, the combined achievement of HbA1c, BP, and LDL-c goals was poorest in women relative to men (rDif = −7.4% for LDL-c target < 130 mg/dL and rDif = −14.9% for target ≤ 100 mg/dL).

3.2. Secondary Prevention

Baseline characteristics of the matched women and men with T2DM in secondary prevention are shown in Table 3. Overall, subjects were 74.9 years old (SD = 9.9) with a mean diabetes duration of 9.3 years (SD = 6.4). A significant proportion of patients had dyslipidemia (78.8%), and almost all had hypertension (92.6%). Moreover, 11.7% and 35.6% of subjects presented diabetic retinopathy and renal impairment, respectively. Regarding macrovascular diseases, CAD was the most common prior complication (59.9%), followed by cerebrovascular disease (37.6%) and PAD (13.9%).

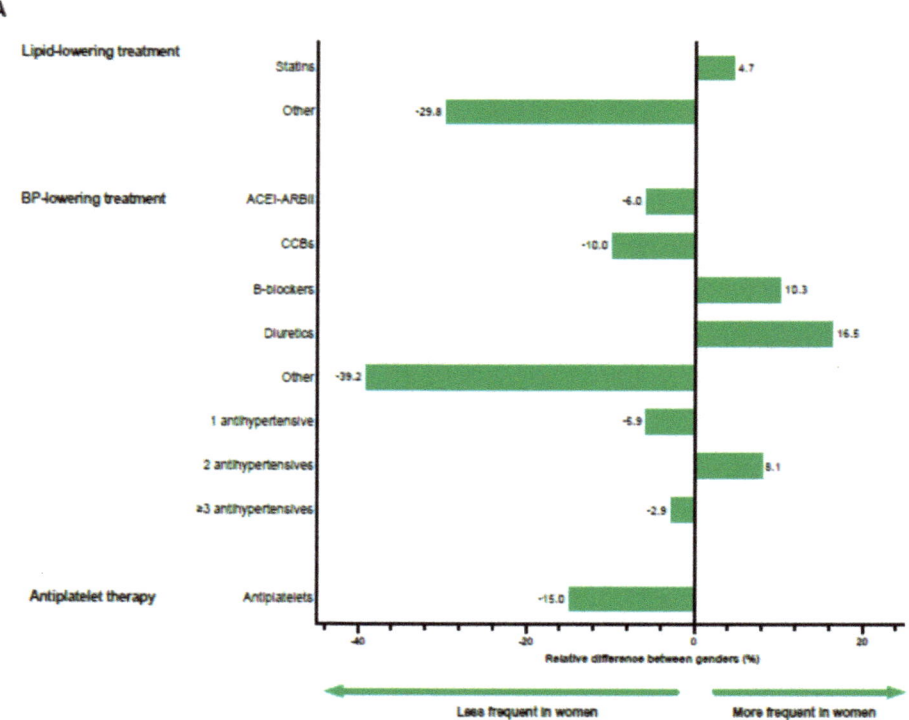
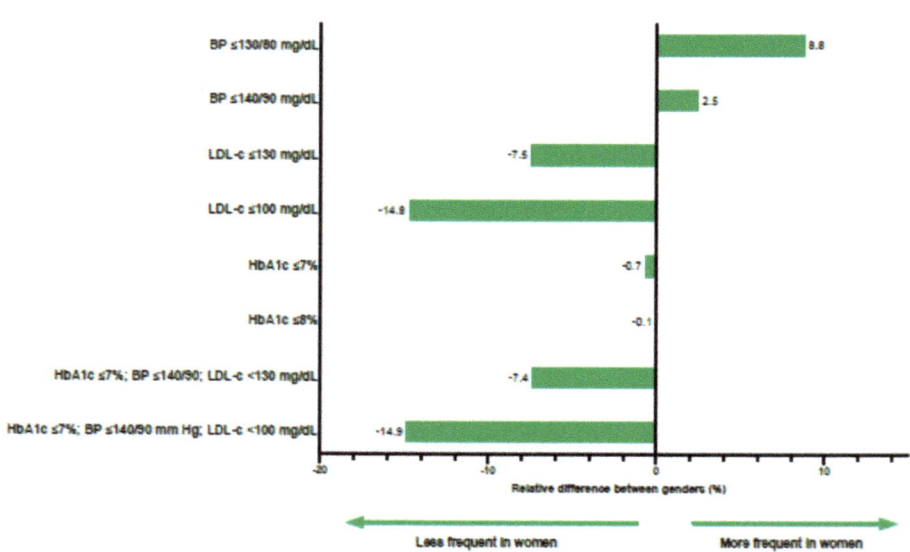

Figure 3. Plot of the relative percent difference between genders for treatments prescribed (**A**) and target achievement (**B**) in the population in primary prevention (ACEI/ARBII, angiotensin-converting enzyme inhibitors/angiotensin II receptor blockers; BP, blood pressure; CCB, calcium channel blockers; HbA1c, glycated hemoglobin; LDL-c, low-density lipoprotein cholesterol; OAD, oral antidiabetic drug).

Table 3. Baseline characteristics of matched women and men with T2DM in secondary prevention by gender.

Variable	N Subjects	Women	N Subjects	Men	Dif	95% CI	
Age (years), mean ± SD *	19,593	75.39 ± 9.99	19,593	74.38 ± 9.73	1.01	0.91	1.11
Diabetes duration (years), mean ± SD *		9.41 ± 6.50		9.19 ± 6.27	0.22	0.16	0.29
Number of visits, mean ± SD *,†		8.58 ± 5.99		8.34 ± 6.45	0.24	0.03	0.30
Smoking habit, n (%) *	19,324		19,342				
Nonsmoker		16,389 (84.81)		16,230 (83.91)	0.90	0.26	1.54
Smoker		958 (4.96)		740 (3.83)	1.13	0.79	1.48
Former smoker		1977 (10.23)		2372 (12.26)	−2.03	−2.57	−1.50
BMI (kg/m^2), mean ± SD	13,022	30.52 ± 5.65	13,181	28.83 ± 4.22	1.69	1.63	1.75
HbA1c (%), mean ± SD	14,738	7.31 ± 1.35	14,494	7.20 ± 1.29	0.11	0.10	0.13
Dyslipidemia, n (%) *	19,593	15,046 (76.79)	19,593	15,814 (80.71)	−3.92	−4.67	−3.17
Lipid profile (mg/dL), mean ± SD							
Total cholesterol	15,142	180.71 ± 39.53	14,914	163.82 ± 35.82	16.89	16.46	17.32
HDL-c	13,854	50.87 ± 12.94	13,772	45.10 ± 11.77	5.77	5.62	5.92
LDL-c		100.16 ± 32.80		91.74 ± 29.62	8.42	8.05	8.79
TGs	14,339	152.88 ± 87.11	14,128	141.54 ± 92.12	11.34	10.30	12.38
Hypertension, n (%) *	19,593	18,113 (92.45)	19,593	18,152 (92.65)	−0.20	−0.64	0.24
Blood pressure (mmHg), mean ± SD	17,381		17,326				
dBP		72.15 ± 8.85		71.62 ± 8.76	0.53	0.44	0.62
sBP		134.84 ± 14.51		133.84 ± 13.69	1.00	0.85	1.15
Diabetic retinopathy, n (%) *	19,593	2330 (11.89)	19,593	2254 (11.50)	0.39	−0.16	0.95
Renal disease, n (%) *,$	15,067	5456 (36.21)	14,969	5223 (34.89)	1.32	0.255	2.384
Macrovascular disease, n (%) *	19,593		19,593				
CAD		11,512 (58.76)		11,942 (60.95)	−2.19	−3.12	−1.27
Cerebrovascular disease		7532 (38.44)		7199 (36.74)	1.70	0.79	2.61
PAD		3512 (17.92)		3881 (19.81)	−1.89	−2.58	−1.19
≥2 macrovascular complications		2771 (14.14)		3157 (16.11)	−1.97	−2.53	−1.35

95% CI, 95% confidence interval; BMI, body mass index; CAD, coronary artery disease; dBP, diastolic blood pressure; Dif, difference of means between groups; HbA1c, glycated hemoglobin; HDL-c, high-density lipoprotein cholesterol; LDL-c, low-density lipoprotein cholesterol; PAD, peripheral artery disease; rDif, relative percentage difference between sexes; sBP, systolic blood pressure; SD, standard deviation; TGs, triglycerides. * Variables matched between study groups. † Number of visits with the primary care team in the previous 12 months. $ Renal disease, including eGFR < 60 mL/min and/or albumin/creatinine ratio > 300 mg/g.

Similar to what was observed in primary prevention patients, women had higher BMI than men (Dif = 1.69 kg/m^2, 95% CI = 1.6 to 1.8) but there were no clinically significant differences in HbA1c levels (Dif = 0.11%, 95% CI = 0.09 to 0.1) and BP values (dBP Dif = 0.53 mmHg, 95% CI = 0.4 to 0.6; sBP Dif = 1.00 mmHg, 95% CI = 0.9 to 1.1). Regarding the lipid profile, TG levels in women were comparable to those observed in primary prevention while they were considerably lower in men, which widened the difference between genders (Dif = 11.34 mg/dL; 95% CI = 10.3 to 12.4). All other parameters, such as total cholesterol, HDL-c, and LDL-c were lower than those observed in primary prevention subjects, particularly in men, and all substantially higher among women (Dif = 16.89 mg/dL; 95% CI = 16.5 to 17.3; Dif = 5.77, 95% CI = 5.6 to 5.9; Dif = 8.42 mg/dL; 95% CI = 8.1 to 8.8, respectively). As shown in Figure 2B, these higher total cholesterol and LDL-c levels in women were observed from 40 years onward and persisted in all age groups. In comparison, values in men progressively decreased until around 80 years of age.

Differences by gender in the pharmacological management of T2DM and degree of CVRF control are shown in Table 4 and Figure 4. The proportion of patients prescribed statins was similar between genders (rDif = −0.5%), but treatment with diuretics and three antihypertensive drugs was more frequent in women relative to men (rDif = 18.5% and rDif = 5.3%, respectively) (Figure 4A). Moreover, women received less often antiplatelet and anticoagulant therapy (rDif = −5.7% and −4.0%, respectively). Although the proportion of patients treated with glucose-lowering drugs was similar between groups (rDif = −1%), women were less often prescribed one or more oral antidiabetic drugs (OAD) than men (rDif = −3.8% for one and −18.6% for more than one OAD). Moreover, women were more frequently treated with either insulin alone (rDif = 19.6%) or combined with one or more OAD (rDif =32.2% with one OAD and 8.2% with more than one OAD).

Table 4. Pharmacological treatment and cardiovascular risk factor control of matched women and men with T2DM in secondary prevention by gender.

Variable	N Subjects	Women	N Subjects	Men	Dif (95% CI)
Lipid-lowering treatment, n (%) *	15,046		15,814		
Statins		14,592 (96.98)		15,407 (97.43)	−0.45 (−0.75/−0.14)
Other		1952 (12.97)		2185 (13.82)	−0.85 (−1.53/−0.16)
Antihypertensive treatment, n (%) †	18,113		18,152		
ACEI/ARBII		14,549 (80.32)		14,581 (80.33)	−0.01 (−0.75/0.75)
CCB		7584 (41.87)		7427 (40.92)	0.95 (−0.03/1.93)
Betablockers		9314 (51.42)		9850 (54.26)	−2.84 (−3.84/−1.85)
Diuretics		12,805 (70.70)		10,831 (59.67)	11.03 (10.10/11.95)
Other		1988 (10.98)		2867 (15.79)	−4.81 (−5.42/−4.22)
Number of drugs					
1		3037 (16.77)		3400 (18.73)	−1.96 (−2.67/−1.26)
2		5652 (31.20)		5779 (31.84)	−0.64 (−1.54/0.28)
≥3		9424 (52.03)		8973 (49.43)	2.60 (1.60/3.59)
Antiplatelet therapy, n (%)	19,593	15,203 (77.59)	19,593	16,127 (82.31)	−4.72 (−5.45/−3.99)
Anticoagulant therapy, n (%)	19,593	2895 (14.78)	19,593	3018 (15.40)	−0.62 (−1.23/0.03)
Diabetes treatment, n (%)	16,896		17,066		
OAD					
1		6220 (36.81)		6528 (38.25)	−1.44 (−2.44/−0.44)
>1		4093 (24.22)		5076 (29.74)	−5.52 (−6.41/−4.63)
Insulin and 1 OAD		2893 (17.12)		2210 (12.95)	4.17 (3.48/4.87)
Insulin and combined OAD		1532 (9.07)		1430 (8.38)	0.69 (0.17/1.21)
Insulin		2158 (12.77)		1822 (10.68)	2.09 (1.48/2.71)
Target CVRF achievement, n (%)					
BP ≤ 130/80 mmHg	17,381	6228 (35.83)	17,326	6666 (38.47)	−2.64 (−3.62/−1.66)
BP ≤ 140/90 mmHg		12,372 (71.18)		12,840 (74.11)	−2.93 (−3.82/−2.04)
LDL-c < 100 mg/dL	13,854	7669 (55.36)	13,772	9161 (66.52)	−11.16 (−12.31/−10.02)
LDL-c < 70 mg/dL		2245 (16.20)		3087 (22.42)	−6.22 (−7.07/−5.35)
LDL-c < 55 mg/dL		762 (5.50)		1068 (7.75)	−2.25 (−2.74/−1.77)
HbA1c, %	14,738		14,494		
≤7		7634 (51.80)		7905 (54.54)	−2.74 (−3.88/−1.60)
≤8		11,391 (77.29)		11,607 (80.08)	−2.79 (−3.68/−1.90)
>8		3347 (22.71)		2887 (19.92)	2.79 (1.90/3.68)
HbA1c ≤ 7%, BP ≤ 140/90 mmHg, LDL-c < 100 mg/dL	12,365	2593 (20.97)	12,239	3275 (26.76)	−5.79 (−6.82/−4.76)
HbA1c ≤ 7%, BP ≤ 140/90 mmHg, LDL-c < 70 mg/dL		767 (6.20)		1083 (8.85)	−2.65 (−3.20/−2.09)
HbA1c ≤ 7%, BP ≤ 140/90 mmHg, LDL-c < 55 mg/dL		262 (2.12)		379 (3.10)	−0.98 (−1.28/−0.67)
Statin treatment and LDL cholesterol target, n (%)	13,854		13,772		
LDL-c < 100 mg/dL and statins		6500 (46.92)		7897 (57.34)	−10.42 (−11.60/−9.24)
LDL-c < 100 mg/dL and no statins		1014 (7.32)		1090 (7.91)	−0.59 (−1.13/−0.06)
LDL-c ≥ 100 mg/dL and statins		4223 (30.48)		3168 (23.00)	7.48 (6.46/8.50)
LDL-c ≥ 100 mg/dL and no statins		2117 (15.28)		1617 (11.74)	3.54 (2.79/4.29)

95% CI, 95% confidence interval; ACEI/ARBII, angiotensin-converting enzyme inhibitors/angiotensin II receptor blockers; BP, blood pressure; CCB, calcium channel blockers; CVRF, cardiovascular risk factor; Dif, difference between groups; HbA1c, glycated hemoglobin; LDL-c, low-density lipoprotein cholesterol; OAD, oral antidiabetic drug; rDif, relative percentage difference between sexes. * Lipid-lowering treatment, proportion data calculated on the basis of those with dyslipidemia. † Antihypertensive treatment, proportion data calculated on the basis of those with hypertension.

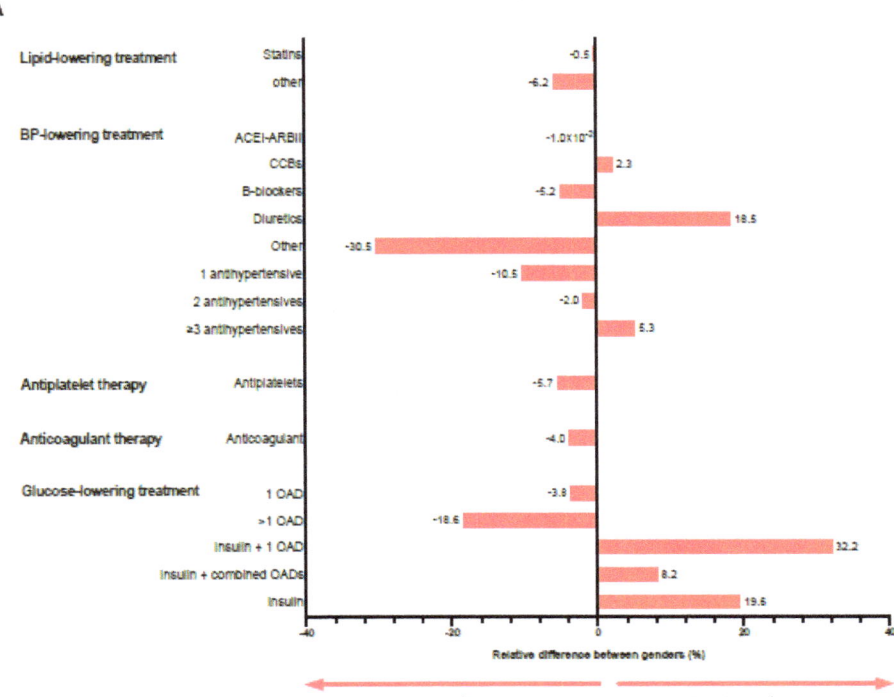

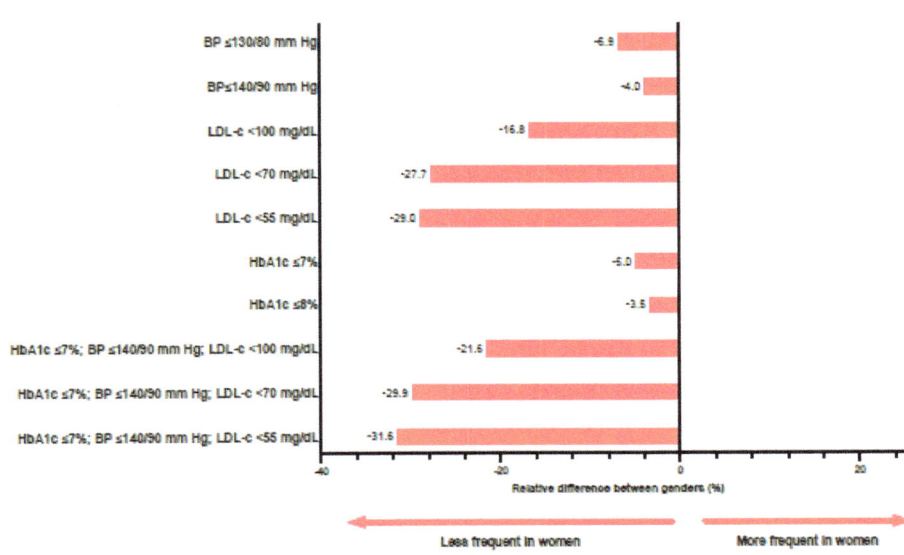

Figure 4. Plot of the relative percentage difference between genders for treatments prescribed (**A**) and target achievement (**B**) in the population in secondary prevention (ACEI/ARBII, angiotensin-converting enzyme inhibitors/angiotensin II receptor blockers; BP, blood pressure; CCB, calcium channel blockers; HbA1c, glycated hemoglobin; LDL-c, low-density lipoprotein cholesterol; OAD, oral antidiabetic drug).

Despite women receiving more intensive antihypertensive treatment, they achieved BP control less frequently than men, either at the ≤130/80 mmHg or at the ≤140/90 mmHg goal (rDif = −6.9% and rDif = −4%, respectively) (Figure 4B). Although the proportion of patients prescribed lipid-lowering treatments was similar between sexes, the targets LDL < 100 mg/dL and <70 mg/dL were less often reached among women (rDif = −16.8% and rDif = −27.7%). Regarding glycemic goals, women showed slightly worse control relative to men (rDif = −5.0% for HbA1c ≤ 7% and −3.5% for HbA1c ≤ 8%). In accordance, the combined target goals of glycemia (HbA1c ≤ 7%), blood pressure (BP ≤ 140/90 mmHg), and LDL-c were less frequently achieved by women than men (rDif = −21.6% for LDL-c < 100 mg/dL and rDif = −29.9% for LDL-c < 70 mg/dL).

4. Discussion

The results of this propensity score-matched analysis in patients with T2DM showed that both genders exhibited comparable BP and HbA1c levels, but women had higher BMI and a significantly poorer lipid profile than men. Moreover, there were sex disparities in treatment prescription. Women were more frequently above recommended treatment goals, particularly LDL-c, and the worst overall CVRF control was more pronounced in secondary prevention patients.

The disparities in baseline characteristics between groups were observed in both the primary and secondary prevention cohorts and agree with previous observational studies conducted in Spain and other international large cohort studies assessing sex differences in T2DM risk and management [2,9–12,20]. Indeed, it has been estimated that women have a BMI nearly 2 kg/m^2 higher than men at T2DM diagnosis despite similar levels of HbA1c [21,22]. This discrepancy has mainly been attributed to the physiological fat distribution in women, which is characterized by more subcutaneous fat mass and less liver and visceral fat, in addition to greater glucose sensitivity compared with men [20]. Thus, women need to gain more weight and accumulate adiposity to establish a diagnosis of diabetes, which extends the prediabetes state with a result of impairment of CVRF [23].

In our study, women had a worse overall lipid profile relative to men, mainly from approximately 40 years onward. These results agree with recent studies reporting that women with T2DM, particularly after menopause, have higher total cholesterol, LDL-c, and HDL-c than men with T2DM [19,24]. This disparity would lead to a more atherogenic lipid and proinflammatory profile in women with T2DM, in turn linked with an increased cardiometabolic risk [25].

Most notably, our findings confirm inequalities between genders in the pharmacological treatment of T2DM and the ability to reach guideline-recommended targets [2]. The unfavorable lipid profile and difficulties in reaching LDL-c levels below treatment goals among T2DM women regardless of statin treatment are well documented [10,12,19,26]. Although the prescription of statins in our study was slightly more frequent in women in primary prevention and used at similar rates in both genders in secondary prevention, a considerably higher proportion of women were not able to reach the corresponding LDL-c targets relative to men in either condition. One explanation for this disparity could be that women are less likely to receive high-intensity statins than men [27,28]. Other factors may interfere, such as an inadequate adherence to statins (estimated to be 10% greater in women than in men [29]), worse tolerance to this drug class, and less likelihood than men to believe that statins are safe or effective [28].

Although there are divergences in the literature, most studies reported no differences between sexes regarding HbA1c control [2]. Our findings show that the degree of glycemic control was similar in both groups in primary prevention, but it was a little worse among women in secondary prevention. However, women were more likely to be prescribed insulin, alone or in combination. A large population-based study conducted in 415,294 Italian patients with T2DM reported that insulin was more frequently used in women than men when off the HbA1c target [26]. Moreover, that study found a wider use of diuretics in women than men and a slightly higher likelihood of reaching the BP target < 130/80 mmHg [26]. We also found that women received more intense antihypertensive treatment, particularly diuretics, but they were more frequently on BP target only in the case of primary prevention. This agrees with a previous study conducted in our population [10], but contrasts two observational studies conducted in the Netherlands, where stratified analyses found no gender differences in the percentage of patients with or without CVD receiving antihypertensive medication and attaining BP control [20,30]. The discrepancy between studies may be more related to sociodemographic factors than sex-specific differences. For instance, one of the Dutch studies found that women with lower educational level had a higher likelihood of receiving antihypertensive medication when systolic BP > 140 mmHg and were at a higher CVD risk than men [20].

As a result of the suboptimal management of individual CVRF among women (particularly LDL-c levels in primary prevention, and LDL-c and BP levels in secondary prevention), the simultaneous attainment of glucose, lipid, and BP recommended goals was considerably less satisfactory among women even when more intensely treated than men. It has been reported that this gap in CV risk burden is due to the existence of additive factors beyond biological dissimilarities, such as lifestyle, cultural and/or socioeconomic factors, and physician biases [2]. For instance, physical activity levels are lower in women with T2DM than their male counterparts [31], and men were more successful in reducing and maintaining weight than women in most studies [32]. Furthermore, there is still a widespread belief among health professionals that CVD is more prevalent in men, leading to underestimation of the problem among women and, consequently, to undertreatment [23]. Moreover, the intensified multifactorial treatment approach, including nonpharmacological (lifestyle recommendations and close monitoring of laboratory and clinical parameters) and pharmacological treatment, have demonstrated a remarkable benefit for reducing the risk of major cardiovascular events (MACEs) and mortality in high-risk diabetic kidney disease [33]

The main strength of this study is the use of real-world data from a large dataset of primary healthcare services in Catalonia that includes urban and rural areas. Moreover, we used a propensity score matching method to homogenize the sample with a satisfactory reduction in absolute differences of potential confounding variables between genders after the matching procedure. Some studies examined the performance of several methods using PSM for the estimation of different measures of association, showing that the PSM approach estimates with less bias than other regression techniques [34–36]. However, the findings of this study must be seen in light of some limitations. Firstly, the cross-sectional design did not allow establishing a causal relationship between the variables. Secondly, we had no data on variables known to contribute to the observed sex dimorphism in diabetes risk and outcome, such as psychosocial risk factors (e.g., socioeconomic status, social support, or educational level) or health behavior (e.g., diet, physical activity, alcohol consumption). Thirdly, we had no data on the doses of the prescribed drugs and whether there were any contraindications (allergies, comorbidities, etc.) that could partially explain gender differences in the disease management. Moreover, we could not assess adherence to the prescribed medications, which may have partly contributed to the observed disparity in CVRF control between sexes. Fourthly, it is not known which comes first, the specific laboratory result (total cholesterol, LDL-c, HDL-c, TGs, and HbA1c) or the particular drug prescription. However, this bias would be present in both groups. Moreover, we did not use the CV risk classification from the 2019 ESC/EASD Guidelines (i.e., moderate, high, or very high CV risk) as the data used predated this recommendation, and the applicable stratification at that time was the requirement of primary vs. secondary prevention. A large population-based study conducted on 373,185 type 2 diabetic subjects in Catalonia reported that at least 50% of them were at very high risk of CV events according to ESC/EASD 2019 classification, and approximately 26% presented with previous CVD [37]. This figure is similar to the proportion of subjects with prior CVD that we included in the secondary prevention group in our study (21.8%). However, categorizing and treating patients according to their CV risk as per the new recommendations will probably provide a more comprehensive and tailored T2DM management than if we only consider the primary/secondary approach [38]. Lastly, we cannot discard that the physician's sex might have somehow influenced the patient's assessment and care.

5. Conclusions

It is essential that, in the process of care, healthcare professionals, from nurses to physicians and researchers, know and consider that CVD is not only a male issue. Inequalities in the management and control of CVRF in women with T2DM may contribute to an increased risk of CVD compared with men. While more research is needed to elucidate the causes of these inequalities, there is a need to implement gender-sensitive strategies to minimize the existing treatment gap. These should include more stringent follow-up implementing an intensified multifactorial treatment approach to achieve optimal risk factor management and educational programs for healthcare professionals and patients to give visibility and cope with gender disparities.

Supplementary Materials: The following supporting information can be downloaded at https://www.mdpi.com/article/10.3390/jcm11082196/s1: Figure S1. Absolute differences between patients with T2DM according gender in primary prevention (DaysDM, days since type 2 diabetes mellitus diagnosis; Smoke: n/d, smoking status not known; ExSmoke, former smoker; HTA, hypertension; DSL, dyslipidemia; Nvis_m, number of visits done in primary healthcare last year; FG_cat62, glomerular filtration rate < 15 mL/min; FG_cat63, glomerular filtration rate 15–30 mL/min; FG_cat64, glomerular filtration rate 31–44 mL/min; FG_cat65, glomerular filtration rate 45–59 mL/min; FG_cat69, glomerular filtration rate > 60 mL/min; QAC_cat2, urinary albumin creatinine ratio < 30 mg/g; QAC_cat3, urinary albumin creatinine ratio 30–300 mg/g; QAC_cat4, urinary albumin creatinine ratio > 300 mg/g; RD, diabetic retinopathy); Figure S2. Absolute differences between patients with T2DM according gender in secondary prevention (DaysDM, days since type 2 diabetes mellitus diagnosis; Smoke: n/d, smoking status not known; ExSmoke, former smoker; HTA, hypertension; DSL, dyslipidemia; Nvis_m, number of visits done in primary healthcare last year; FG_cat62, glomerular filtration rate < 15 mL/min; FG_cat63, glomerular filtration rate 15–30 mL/min; FG_cat64, glomerular filtration rate 31–44 mL/min; FG_cat65, glomerular filtration rate 45–59 mL/min; FG_cat69, glomerular filtration rate > 60 mL/min; QAC_cat2, urinary albumin creatinine ratio < 30 mg/g; QAC_cat3, urinary albumin creatinine ratio 30–300 mg/g; QAC_cat4, urinary albumin creatinine ratio > 300 mg/g; RD, diabetic retinopathy; artper, peripheral artery disease; ci, coronary disease; avc, cerebrovascular disease; ic, heart failure).

Author Contributions: Conceptualization, D.M. and J.F.-N.; methodology, D.M., J.F.-N., J.R. and A.R.-M.; data curation, J.R. and A.R.-M.; investigation, D.M., J.F.-N., J.R. and A.R.-M.; formal analysis, J.R.; writing—original draft preparation, A.R.-M.; writing—review and editing, D.M., J.F.-N., J.R., M.G. and A.R.-M.; validation, D.M., J.F.-N., J.R., M.G. and A.R.-M.; visualization, D.M., J.F.-N., J.R., M.G. and A.R.-M.; supervision, D.M. and J.F.-N. All authors have read and agreed to the published version of the manuscript.

Funding: This research received no external funding.

Institutional Review Board Statement: The investigation conformed with the principles outlined in the Declaration of Helsinki. The study was approved by the Ethics Committee of the Primary Healthcare University Research Institute (IDIAP) Jordi Gol (P14/018) and registered in the ClinicalTrials.gov (NCT04653805).

Informed Consent Statement: Not applicable.

Data Availability Statement: The data presented in this study are available from the corresponding author upon reasonable request.

Acknowledgments: The authors acknowledge Helena Kruyer for language editing and proofreading and the Territorial Management of Central Catalonia of Institut Català de la Salut (ICS) for the grant for research training and doctoral completion in primary healthcare.

Conflicts of Interest: The authors declare no conflict of interest.

References

1. International Diabetes Federation (IDF). IDF Diabetes Atlas: Ninth Edition 2019. Available online: https://www.diabetesatlas.org (accessed on 2 March 2020).
2. de Ritter, R.; de Jong, M.; Vos, R.C.; van der Kallen, C.J.H.; Sep, S.J.S.; Woodward, M.; Stehouwer, C.D.A.; Bots, M.L.; Peters, S.A.E. Sex Differences in the Risk of Vascular Disease Associated with Diabetes. *Biol. Sex Differ.* **2020**, *11*, 1. [CrossRef] [PubMed]
3. Kautzky-Willer, A.; Harreiter, J.; Pacini, G. Sex and Gender Differences in Risk, Pathophysiology and Complications of Type 2 Diabetes Mellitus. *Endocr. Rev.* **2016**, *37*, 278–316. [CrossRef] [PubMed]
4. Peters, S.A.E.; Woodward, M. Sex Differences in the Burden and Complications of Diabetes. *Curr. Diab. Rep.* **2018**, *18*, 33. [CrossRef] [PubMed]
5. Huebschmann, A.G.; Huxley, R.R.; Kohrt, W.M.; Zeitler, P.; Regensteiner, J.G.; Reusch, J.E.B. Sex Differences in the Burden of Type 2 Diabetes and Cardiovascular Risk across the Life Course. *Diabetologia* **2019**, *62*, 1761–1772. [CrossRef] [PubMed]
6. Hyun, K.K.; Redfern, J.; Patel, A.; Peiris, D.; Brieger, D.; Sullivan, D.; Harris, M.; Usherwood, T.; MacMahon, S.; Lyford, M.; et al. Gender Inequalities in Cardiovascular Risk Factor Assessment and Management in Primary Healthcare. *Heart* **2017**, *103*, 492–498. [CrossRef] [PubMed]
7. Eapen, Z.J.; Liang, L.; Shubrook, J.H.; Bauman, M.A.; Bufalino, V.J.; Bhatt, D.L.; Peterson, E.D.; Hernandez, A.F. Current Quality of Cardiovascular Prevention for Million Hearts: An Analysis of 147,038 Outpatients from The Guideline Advantage. *Am. Heart J.* **2014**, *168*, 398–404. [CrossRef]
8. Ares Blanco, J.; Valdés Hernández, S.; Botas, P.; Rodríguez-Rodero, S.; Morales Sánchez, P.; Díaz Naya, L.; Menéndez-Torre, E.; Delgado, E. Diferencias de Género en la Mortalidad de Personas con Diabetes Tipo 2: Estudio Asturias 2018. *Gac. Sanit.* **2019**, *34*, 442–448. [CrossRef]
9. Vinagre, I.; Mata-Cases, M.; Hermosilla, E.; Morros, R.; Fina, F.; Rosell, M.; Castell, C.; Franch-Nadal, J.; Bolíbar, B.; Mauricio, D. Control of Glycemia and Cardiovascular Risk Factors in Patients with Type 2 Diabetes in Primary Care in Catalonia (Spain). *Diabetes Care* **2012**, *35*, 774–779. [CrossRef]
10. Franch-Nadal, J.; Mata-Cases, M.; Vinagre, I.; Patitucci, F.; Hermosilla, E.; Casellas, A.; Bolivar, B.; Mauricio, D. Differences in the Cardiometabolic Control in Type 2 Diabetes According to Gender and the Presence of Cardiovascular Disease: Results from the Econtrol Study. *Int. J. Endocrinol.* **2014**, *2014*, 131709. [CrossRef]
11. Gómez García, M.C.; Franch-Nadal, J.; Millaruelo Trillo, J.M.; Cos-Claramunt, F.X.; Avila Lachica, L.; Buil Cosiales, P. Control Glucémico y de los Factores de Riesgo Cardiovascular en los Pacientes Con Diabetes Tipo 2 con Enfermedad Cardiovascular en España, y su Patrón de Tratamiento, en Función del Género: Estudio CODICE. *Med. Fam. Semer.* **2019**, *46*, 125–135. [CrossRef]
12. Gómez García, M.C.; Millaruelo Trillo, J.M.; Avila Lachica, L.; Cos-Claramunt, F.X.; Franch-Nadal, J.; Cortés Gil, X. Estudio ESCRYTO. Diabetes sin Enfermedad Cardiovascular y Grado de Control. *Med. Fam. Semer.* **2019**, *46*, 261–269. [CrossRef] [PubMed]
13. Rosenbaum, P.R. The Central Role of the Propensity Score in Observational Studies for Causal Effects. *Biometrika* **1983**, *70*, 41–55. [CrossRef]
14. Mata-Cases, M.; Vlacho, B.; Real, J.; Puig-Treserra, R.; Bundó, M.; Franch-Nadal, J.; Mauricio, D. Trends in the Degree of Control and Treat ment of Cardiovascular Risk Factors in People With Type 2 Diabetes in a Primary Care Setting in Catalonia During 2007–2018. *Front. Endocrinol.* **2022**, *12*, 810757. [CrossRef] [PubMed]
15. Institut Català de la Salut. Estàndard de Qualitat de Prescripció Farmacèutica 2021. Available online: http://ics.gencat.cat/web/web/.content/documents/assistencia/31052021_EQPF-2021-GLOBAL-i-MFiC-versio-4.pdf (accessed on 4 April 2022).
16. Bolíbar, B.; Fina Avilés, F.; Morros, R.; del Mar Garcia-Gil, M.; Hermosilla, E.; Ramos, R.; Rosell, M.; Rodríguez, J.; Medina, M.; Calero, S.; et al. Base de Datos SIDIAP: La Historia Clínica Informatizada de Atención Primaria como Fuente de Información para la Investigación Epidemiológica. *Med. Clin.* **2012**, *138*, 617–621. [CrossRef]
17. Mata-Cases, M.; Franch-Nadal, J.; Real, J.; Mauricio, D. Glycaemic Control and Antidiabetic Treatment Trends in Primary Care Centres in Patients with Type 2 Diabetes Mellitus during 2007–2013 in Catalonia: A Population-Based Study. *BMJ Open* **2016**, *6*, e012463. [CrossRef]
18. Mata-Cases, M.; Cos, F.X.; Morros, R.; Diego, L.; Barrot, J.; Berengué, M.; Brugada, M.; Carrera, T.; Cano, J.F.; Estruch, M.; et al. *Abordatge de la Diabetis Mellitus Tipus 2*, 2nd ed.; Guies de pràctica clínica i material docent, núm 15; Institut Català de la Salut: Barcelona, Spain, 2013. Available online: http://hdl.handle.net/11351/4514 (accessed on 2 March 2022).
19. Ho, D.E.; Imai, K.; King, G.; Stuart, E.A. MatchIt: Nonparametric Preprocessing for Parametric Causal Inference. *J. Stat. Softw.* **2011**, *42*, 8. [CrossRef]
20. de Jong, M.; Oskam, M.J.; Sep, S.J.S.; Ozcan, B.; Rutters, F.; Sijbrands, E.J.G.; Elders, P.J.M.; Siegelaar, S.E.; DeVries, J.H.; Tack, C.J.; et al. Sex Differences in Cardiometabolic Risk Factors, Pharmacological Treatment and Risk Factor Control in Type 2 Diabetes: Findings from the Dutch Diabetes Pearl Cohort. *BMJ Open Diabetes Res. Care* **2020**, *8*, e001365. [CrossRef]
21. Logue, J.; Walker, J.J.; Colhoun, H.M.; Leese, G.P.; Lindsay, R.S.; McKnight, J.A.; Morris, A.D.; Pearson, D.W.; Petrie, J.R.; Philip, S.; et al. Scottish Diabetes Research Network Epidemiology Group. Do Men Develop Type 2 Diabetes at Lower Body Mass Indices than Women? *Diabetologia* **2011**, *54*, 3003–3006. [CrossRef]
22. Paul, S.; Thomas, G.; Majeed, A.; Khunti, K.; Klein, K. Women Develop Type 2 Diabetes at a Higher Body Mass Index than Men. *Diabetologia* **2012**, *55*, 1556–1557. [CrossRef]
23. Woodward, M.; Peters, S.A.E.; Huxley, R.R. Diabetes and the Female Disadvantage. *Womens. Health* **2015**, *11*, 833–839. [CrossRef]

24. Ambrož, M.; de Vries, S.T.; Vart, P.; Dullaart, R.P.F.; Roeters van Lennep, J.; Denig, P.; Hoogenberg, K. Sex Differences in Lipid Profile across the Life Span in Patients with Type 2 Diabetes: A Primary Care-Based Study. *J. Clin. Med.* **2021**, *10*, 1775. [CrossRef] [PubMed]
25. Mascarenhas-Melo, F.; Marado, D.; Palavra, F.; Sereno, J.; Coelho, Á.; Pinto, R.; Teixeira-Lemos, E.; Teixeira, F.; Reis, F. Diabetes Abrogates Sex Differences and Aggravates Cardiometabolic Risk in Postmenopausal Women. *Cardiovasc. Diabetol.* **2013**, *12*, 61. [CrossRef] [PubMed]
26. Rossi, M.C.; Cristofaro, M.R.; Gentile, S.; Lucisano, G.; Manicardi, V.; Mulas, M.F.; Napoli, A.; Nicolucci, A.; Pellegrini, F.; Suraci, C.; et al. Sex Disparities in the Quality of Diabetes Care: Biological and Cultural Factors May Play a Different Role for Different Outcomes: A Cross-Sectional Observational Study from the AMD Annals Initiative. *Diabetes Care* **2013**, *36*, 3162–3168. [CrossRef] [PubMed]
27. Virani, S.S.; Woodard, L.D.; Ramsey, D.J.; Urech, T.H.; Akeroyd, J.M.; Shah, T.; Deswal, A.; Bozkurt, B.; Ballantyne, C.M.; Petersen, L.A. Gender Disparities in Evidence-Based Statin Therapy in Patients with Cardiovascular Disease. *Am. J. Cardiol.* **2015**, *115*, 21–26. [CrossRef]
28. Nanna, M.G.; Wang, T.Y.; Xiang, Q.; Goldberg, A.C.; Robinson, J.G.; Roger, V.L.; Virani, S.S.; Wilson, P.W.F.; Louie, M.J.; Koren, A.; et al. Sex Differences in the Use of Statins in Community Practice: Patient and provider assessment of lipid management registry. *Circ. Cardiovasc. Qual. Outcomes* **2019**, *12*, e005562. [CrossRef]
29. Lewey, J.; Shrank, W.H.; Bowry, A.D.K.; Kilabuk, E.; Brennan, T.A.; Choudhry, N.K. Gender and Racial Disparities in Adherence to Statin Therapy: A Meta-Analysis. *Am. Heart J.* **2013**, *165*, 665–678.e1. [CrossRef]
30. de Jong, M.; Vos, R.C.; de Ritter, R.; van der Kallen, C.J.; Sep, S.J.; Woodward, M.; Stehouwer, C.D.A.; Bots, M.L.; Peters, S.A. Sex Differences in Cardiovascular Risk Management for People with Diabetes in Primary Care: A Cross-Sectional Study. *BJGP Open* **2019**, *3*, bjgpopen19X101645. [CrossRef]
31. The Look AHEAD Research Group. Cardiovascular Effects of Intensive Lifestyle Intervention in Type 2 Diabetes. *N. Engl. J. Med.* **2013**, *369*, 145–154. [CrossRef]
32. Harreiter, J.; Kautzky-Willer, A. Sex and Gender Differences in Prevention of Type 2 Diabetes. *Front. Endocrinol.* **2018**, *9*, 220. [CrossRef]
33. Sasso, F.C.; Pafundi, P.C.; Simeon, V.; De Nicola, L.; Chiodini, P.; Galiero, R.; Rinaldi, L.; Nevola, R.; Salvatore, T.; Sardu, C.; et al. Efficacy and Durability of Multifactorial Intervention on Mortality and MACEs: A Randomized Clinical Trial in Type-2 Diabetic Kidney Disease. *Cardiovasc. Diabetol.* **2021**, *20*, 145. [CrossRef]
34. Austin, P.C. The Performance of Different Propensity Score Methods for Estimating Marginal Hazard Ratios. *Stat. Med.* **2013**, *32*, 2837–2849. [CrossRef] [PubMed]
35. Austin, P.C. The Performance of Different Propensity-Score Methods for Estimating Relative Risks. *J. Clin. Epidemiol.* **2008**, *61*, 537–545. [CrossRef] [PubMed]
36. Austin, P.C. The Performance of Different Propensity Score Methods for Estimating Marginal Odds Ratios. *Stat. Med.* **2007**, *26*, 3078–3094. [CrossRef] [PubMed]
37. Cebrián-Cuenca, A.M.; Mata-Cases, M.; Franch-Nadal, J.; Mauricio, D.; Orozco-Beltrán, D.; Consuegra-Sánchez, L. Half of Patients with Type 2 Diabetes Mellitus Are at Very High Cardiovascular Risk According to the ESC/EASD: Data from a Large Mediterranean Population. *Eur. J. Prev. Cardiol.* **2022**, *28*, e32–e34. [CrossRef] [PubMed]
38. Garcia-Moll, X.; Barrios, V.; Franch-Nadal, J. Moving from the Stratification of Primary and Secondary Prevention of Cardiovascular Risk in Diabetes towards a Continuum of Risk: Need for a New Paradigm. *Drugs Context* **2021**, *10*, 2021-6-3. [CrossRef] [PubMed]

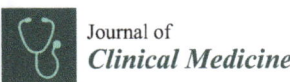

Article

Development of a Complex Intervention for Effective Management of Type 2 Diabetes in a Developing Country

Tigestu Alemu Desse [1,*], Kevin Mc Namara [2,3], Helen Yifter [4] and Elizabeth Manias [1]

1. School of Nursing and Midwifery, Centre for Quality and Patient Safety Research, Institute for Health Transformation, Faculty of Health, Deakin University, Geelong, VIC 3217, Australia; emanias@deakin.edu.au
2. Deakin Rural Health, School of Medicine, Faculty of Health, Deakin University, Geelong, VIC 3217, Australia; kevin.mcnamara@deakin.edu.au
3. Deakin Health Economics, Institute for Healthcare Transformation, Deakin University, Geelong, VIC 3217, Australia
4. Department of Internal Medicine, College of Health Sciences, Addis Ababa University, Addis Ababa 9086, Ethiopia; helenefbr@gmail.com
* Correspondence: talemu@deakin.edu.au; Tel.: +61-481574066

Abstract: There has been little focus on designing tailored diabetes management strategies in developing countries. The aim of this study is to develop a theory-driven, tailored and context-specific complex intervention for the effective management of type 2 diabetes at a tertiary care setting of a developing country. We conducted interviews and focus groups with patients, health professionals, and policymakers and undertook thematic analysis to identify gaps in diabetes management. The results of our previously completed systematic review informed data collection. We used the United Kingdom Medical Research Council framework to guide the development of the intervention. Results comprised 48 interviews, two focus groups with 11 participants and three co-design panels with 24 participants. We identified a lack of structured type 2 diabetes education, counselling, and collaborative care of type 2 diabetes. Through triangulation of the evidence obtained from data collection, we developed an intervention called VICKY (patient-centred collaborative care and structured diabetes education and counselling) for effective management of type 2 diabetes. VICKY comprised five components: (1) patient-centred collaborative care; (2) referral system for patients across transitions of care between different health professionals of the diabetes care team; (3) tools for the provision of collaborative care and documentation of care; (4) diabetes education and counselling by trained diabetes educators; and (5) contextualised diabetes education curriculum, educational materials, and documentation tools for diabetes education and counselling. Implementation of the intervention may help to promote evidence-based, patient-centred, and contextualised diabetes care for improved patient outcomes in a developing country.

Keywords: type 2 diabetes; complex intervention; behaviour change intervention; co-design; continuity of care; developing country; Ethiopia; patient participation; patient transfer

1. Introduction

Type 2 diabetes is a global public health problem and an economic burden to nations, particularly developing countries [1]. It contributes to cardiovascular complications, such as ischemic heart disease, heart failure, and renal disorders [2–4].

Ineffective management of type 2 diabetes has been associated with poor clinical outcomes, which include disease progression, and increased health services utilisation, such as repeated hospitalisations and high all-cause mortality [5–7]. In Sub-Saharan Africa (SSA) [8–10] including Ethiopia [11–13], there exists a high rate of diabetes-related morbidity and mortality, high cost of diabetes care, and poor quality of life for patients with type 2 diabetes. Excessive levels of diabetes-related problems and high cost of type 2 diabetes care in SSA are attributed to widespread lack of treatment success, stemming from inadequate organisational involvement and delivery of care [8,9,14]. Multiple contributing factors exist in the region, such as a lack of contextually tailored diabetes management approaches, inadequate diabetes training of health professionals, and low levels of collaborative care and effective shared treatment plans developed by patients and health professionals [10,14–16]. In Ethiopia, similar factors contributing to ineffective management of type 2 diabetes exist, including inadequate collaborative care among pharmacists, physicians, and nurses; lack of structured diabetes education; and high levels of medication therapy problems and diabetes complications [13,17–23].

Patient-centred collaborative care and the use of culturally tailored interventions, including behavioural interventions, can improve diabetes care in low-income countries [14,24,25]. Evidence indicates that SSA nations require evidence-based type 2 diabetes management strategies tailored to the context and aimed at reducing diabetes-related morbidity and mortality and high healthcare costs [10,16,26]. However, there has been little focus on designing contextually tailored type 2 diabetes management strategies in this region. While evidence suggests that structured diabetes education and counselling and collaborative care by pharmacists, physicians, nurses, and other health professionals can improve health outcomes and cost of type 2 diabetes treatment [27–30], implementation needs for such elements of care are not readily understood for type 2 diabetes in Ethiopia [21,22,31,32]. Furthermore, studies examining type 2 diabetes in Ethiopia are mainly observational and focused on the rate of glycemic control, magnitude of diabetes-related complications, quality of care, and mortality. Moreover, there has been no focus on designing appropriately tailored interventions to improve diabetes care [12,13,18,33–38]. To the authors' knowledge, there has been no pragmatic study undertaken to explore the dynamics of current management for type 2 diabetes at a micro- or meso-level or devise much-needed diabetes management strategies tailored to SSA [10,14,16,39,40].

The aim of this study was to develop a theory-driven, tailored, and context-specific complex intervention for the effective management of type 2 diabetes at a tertiary care setting of a developing country.

2. Materials and Methods

The study was undertaken at the diabetes centre of a tertiary teaching hospital (Tikur Anbessa Specialised Hospital) in Addis Ababa, Ethiopia. Diabetes care is provided at the diabetes centre of the hospital by endocrinologists, endocrinology fellows, internal medicine residents, and nurses [41]. Each month, the diabetes centre serves about 1200 ambulatory patients with type 2 diabetes [42].

The United Kingdom Medical Research Council (UK MRC) [43] framework was used to guide the development of a complex intervention. The MRC framework comprises detailed information about the systematic development of interventions. It utilises the best available evidence and appropriate theory to develop an intervention using a carefully phased approach [43]. The framework has four key elements (Figure 1) [43]: developing a complex intervention, feasibility and piloting, evaluation, and implementation.

2.1. Developing a Complex Intervention

Developing a complex intervention involves three steps (Figure 1): (1) identifying the evidence base, (2) identifying and developing an appropriate theory of the intervention, and (3) modelling the process and outcomes of a complex intervention [43]. This study used all three steps throughout the development of the intervention.

2.2. Identifying the Evidence Base

The first stage in the development of a complex intervention is to identify an existing, relevant evidence base [43]. We undertook a systematic review on the effectiveness of clinical pharmacy interventions on health and economic outcomes of patients with type 2 diabetes [30]. We also completed semi-structured interviews and focus groups with adult patients with type 2 diabetes, health professionals, and policymakers of Tikur Anbessa Specialised Hospital (TASH) and the Ministry of Health of Ethiopia to generate evidence and identify gaps in the management of type 2 diabetes at the hospital. We brought all the relevant evidence obtained through the systematic review [30], interviews, and focus groups together to understand the issues relating to effective and ineffective management of type 2 diabetes and the relevant behaviours that could be targeted for the intervention.

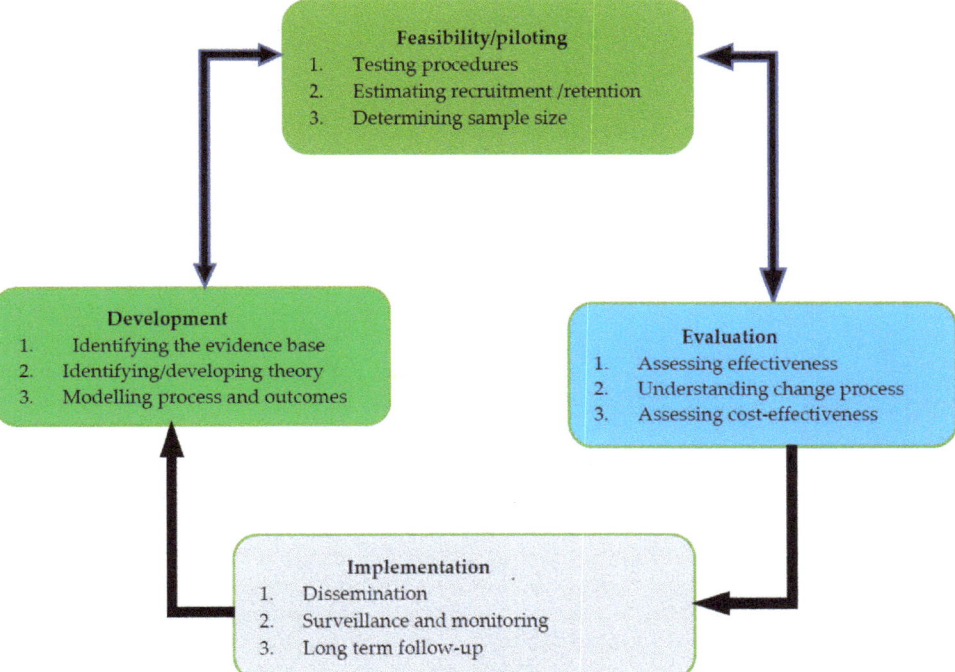

Figure 1. Key elements of the development and evaluation process (Craig et al., 2008). Reproduced with permission of the UK Medical Research Council.

2.3. Identifying and Developing Theory

Identification and development of appropriate theory in intervention design is key to understanding the possible processes of change [43,44]. The use of a theoretical approach in the design of healthcare interventions has been demonstrated to improve the effectiveness of the interventions [44–46]. In this study, the Behaviour Change Wheel (BCW) framework [46,47] was used as a guide to develop an evidence-based behaviour change intervention for the effective management of type 2 diabetes. Use of the BCW supplements the MRC framework to design effective complex interventions to change behaviour in a healthcare system [44,48]. The framework can be used to develop interventions at any level (individuals, groups, and organisations) in healthcare systems [47]. The BCW framework has been effectively implemented in developing behaviour change interventions in healthcare [49–53]. The theory of the complex intervention for this study focused on designing an organisational level intervention, as this approach has been demonstrated to improve the effectiveness of type 2 diabetes management in previous studies [54–56].

We used a co-design panel comprising patients, health professionals, and policymakers at TASH and the Ministry of Health of Ethiopia with a representative of the Ethiopian Diabetes Association and incorporated the findings from the systematic review [30], interviews, and focus groups to inform the initial stages of development of the theory of the complex intervention. We conducted three consecutive co-design workshops with the co-design panel to help with the first two stages of the BCW [47] (Figure 2).

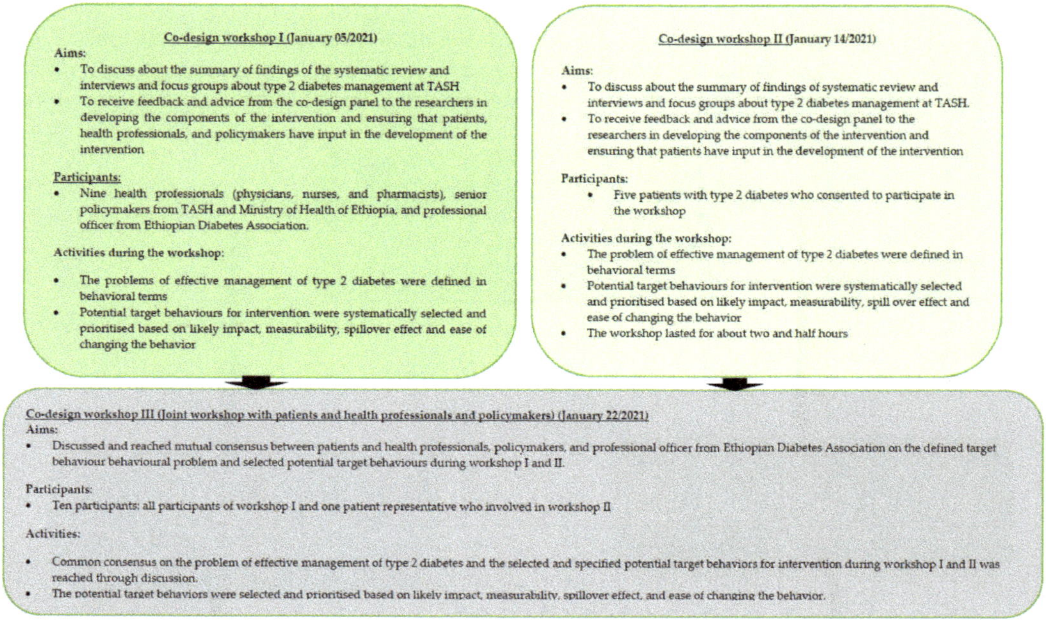

Co-design workshop I (January 05/2021)

Aims:
- To discuss about the summary of findings of the systematic review and interviews and focus groups about type 2 diabetes management at TASH
- To receive feedback and advice from the co-design panel to the researchers in developing the components of the intervention and ensuring that patients, health professionals, and policymakers have input in the development of the intervention

Participants:
- Nine health professionals (physicians, nurses, and pharmacists), senior policymakers from TASH and Ministry of Health of Ethiopia, and professional officer from Ethiopian Diabetes Association.

Activities during the workshop:
- The problems of effective management of type 2 diabetes were defined in behavioral terms
- Potential target behaviours for intervention were systematically selected and prioritised based on likely impact, measurability, spillover effect and ease of changing the behavior

Co-design workshop II (January 14/2021)

Aims:
- To discuss about the summary of findings of systematic review and interviews and focus groups about type 2 diabetes management at TASH.
- To receive feedback and advice from the co-design panel to the researchers in developing the components of the intervention and ensuring that patients have input in the development of the intervention

Participants:
- Five patients with type 2 diabetes who consented to participate in the workshop

Activities during the workshop:
- The problem of effective management of type 2 diabetes were defined in behavioral terms
- Potential target behaviours for intervention were systematically selected and prioritised based on likely impact, measurability, spill over effect and ease of changing the behavior
- The workshop lasted for about two and half hours

Co-design workshop III (Joint workshop with patients and health professionals and policymakers) (January 22/2021)

Aims:
- Discussed and reached mutual consensus between patients and health professionals, policymakers, and professional officer from Ethiopian Diabetes Association on the defined target behaviour behavioural problem and selected potential target behaviours during workshop I and II.

Participants:
- Ten participants: all participants of workshop I and one patient representative who involved in workshop II

Activities:
- Common consensus on the problem of effective management of type 2 diabetes and the selected and specified potential target behaviors for intervention during workshop I and II was reached through discussion.
- The potential target behaviors were selected and prioritised based on likely impact, measurability, spillover effect, and ease of changing the behavior.

Figure 2. Activities undertaken in the co-design workshops.

2.3.1. Workshop I

The first co-design workshop involved health professionals, policymakers from TASH and the Ministry of Health of Ethiopia, and a professional officer from the Ethiopian Diabetes Association (Figure 2). During the workshop, we sought to define the problems affecting the effective management of type 2 diabetes in behavioural terms and selected potential target behaviours deemed to improve the management of type 2 diabetes. The co-design panel also discussed the findings of interviews and focus groups and validated that they truly reflected the existing challenges of diabetes care at the diabetes centre of TASH. The panel then defined the problem of suboptimal management of type 2 diabetes in behavioural terms and identified potential target behaviours for the intervention that would help to improve the management of type 2 at TASH using the findings from the systematic review [30], interviews, and focus groups [42]. The identification of potential target behaviour based on impact, measurability, changeability, and spillover effect was undertaken by rating each list of potential target behaviours identified via interviews and focus groups as unacceptable, unpromising but worth considering, promising, and very promising, by each participant of the co-design panel [47].

2.3.2. Workshop II

We conducted the second co-design workshop with patients with type 2 diabetes (Figure 2). The purpose of undertaking workshop II was to incorporate the views and experiences of patients and engage them in the intervention design. In this workshop, patients discussed the findings of the systematic review [30], interviews and focus groups, and validated these findings; they defined the problem related to facilitating effective management of type 2 diabetes in behavioural terms; and selected potential target behaviours deemed to address the problem. In this workshop, each co-design panel member rated and identified potential target behaviours as described for workshop I. The panel also elected and assigned one patient amongst the group who participated in the third co-design workshop.

2.3.3. Workshop III

A joint workshop was undertaken with a nominated patient, health professionals, policymakers, and a professional officer from the Ethiopian Diabetes Association. The workshop involved examining the defined problem related to the effective management of type 2 diabetes and the selected potential target behaviours during the two separate workshops (workshop I and II). The workshop panel members specified the target behaviours that were agreed upon. In workshop III, the panel members discussed and reached a consensus on the defined problem related to effective management of type 2 diabetes and the selected potential target behaviours at workshops I and II (Figure 2). The criteria for prioritisation and selection of the potential target behaviours for the intervention in workshop III followed the same procedures used in workshops I and III. The co-design panel in the third workshop specified the potential target behaviours for the intervention in terms of the following:

- Who needs to perform the behaviour?
- What do they need to do differently to achieve the desired change?
- When do they need to do it?
- Where do they need to do it?
- How often do they need to do it?
- With whom do they need to do it?

The co-design panel worked through stage one to stage three of the behaviour change intervention design process [47]. The steps in the BCW (Figure 3) were sequentially explored by the co-design panel throughout the three workshops, to both ensure that the appropriate behaviours were targeted, and the intervention functions were achievable and practical in the context of TASH.

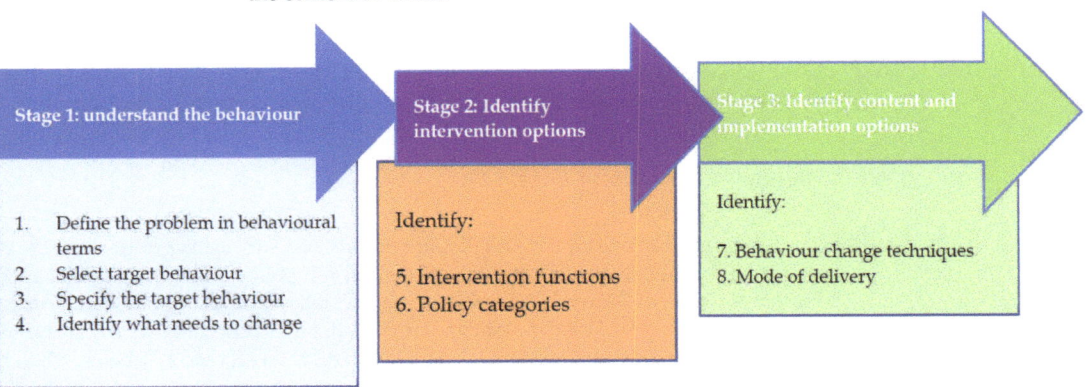

Figure 3. Behaviour change intervention design process (Michie et al., 2014).

Stage One

This stage involved four steps (Figure 3) [47]. Step I involved defining the problem in behavioural terms (i.e., being specific about the target individual, group, or population involved in the behaviour and the behaviour itself). Step II comprised selecting the target behaviour for the intervention among a list of behaviours [47]. Step III involved specifying the target behaviour. Step IV comprised identifying what needs to change for the behaviour to change in terms of capability, opportunity, and/or motivation in the target population, group, or individual [47].

Stage Two

This stage involves the use of the behavioural diagnosis [47] to:

a. Decide what 'intervention functions' to apply: education, persuasion, incentivisation, coercion, training, restriction, environmental restructuring, modelling, and enablement;

b. Select implementation strategy: fiscal policy, legislation, regulation, environmental planning, communications, service provision, and guidelines development.

Stage Three

The focus of the third stage is to:

a. Develop a detailed intervention plan by selecting from among a range of specific behaviour change techniques (BCTs) [57]. Michie identified 93 BCTs within 16 groupings. We used Michie's BCTs [57] to characterise components for the behavioural intervention in this study;
b. Create the detailed intervention specification covering all aspects of content and delivery of the intervention structured around the chosen BCTs and modes of delivery.

Appropriate intervention functions, BCTs, and intervention contents were determined through discussion between the co-design panel and the research team and using the APEASE criteria [47]. The APEASE criteria refer to affordability, practicability, effectiveness, acceptability, safety/side effects, and equity [47].

2.4. Modelling and Creating a Complex Intervention

Modelling of a complex intervention [43] helps to precisely describe and comprehend the interaction of individual intervention components, and perceive possible effects of the intervention [58]. The careful design of a model of a complex intervention is a critical step in designing tailored and contextualised interventions in healthcare systems and choosing appropriate outcomes so that the benefits and risks of the interventions are demonstrated effectively [58].

In this study, we operationalised the intervention functions and BCTs into a complex intervention to improve the effectiveness of type 2 diabetes management. The researchers collaborated with the co-design panels in operationalising the intervention functions and BCTs into the mode of care delivery using the BCW framework [47]. We used the Revised Standards for Quality Improvement Reporting Excellence: (SQUIRE 2.0) publication guidelines [59] to report the findings of this study (Supplementary Materials Table S1).

3. Results

3.1. Study Participants

We undertook interviews with 48 participants and two focus groups (n = 11) with patients with type 2 diabetes, health professionals, and policymakers from TASH and the Ministry of Health of Ethiopia [42] comprising an overall sample of 59 participants; three co-design workshops (n = 24); and a systematic review on the effectiveness of clinical pharmacy interventions on health and economic outcome of patients with type 2 diabetes [30] to help with the intervention design.

3.2. Step One: Define the Health Problem in Behavioural Terms

Evidence from the interviews and focus groups we have undertaken, previous findings [11–13,60], feedback from the co-design workshops, and the context of the hospital enabled identification of the health problem. We identified that improving the effectiveness of type 2 diabetes management for patients with type 2 diabetes was the specific problem existing at the diabetes centre of TASH.

3.3. Step Two: Select the Target Behaviour

We identified through interviews, focus groups, and co-design workshops that had challenges for the effective management of type 2 diabetes related to:

1. Lack of resources, such as medications, laboratory, and diagnostic tests;
2. Lack of continuity of care, such as prolonged follow up clinic visits;
3. Lack of knowledge and awareness of patients about type 2 diabetes and its complications;
4. Lack of self-care activities;

5. Low level of type 2 diabetes education and counselling services;
6. Low competence and experience of health professionals providing diabetes care;
7. Inefficient collaboration among health professionals (nurses, physicians, and pharmacists) in the care of type 2 diabetes;
8. Absence of involvement of clinical pharmacists, dietitians or nutritionists, and psychologists in the care of type 2 diabetes.

Our findings from interviews and focus groups demonstrated that the problem of the effective management of type 2 diabetes can be addressed through multiple behaviours targeted in a complex intervention. These include: ensuring continuity of care; enabling provision of structured type 2 diabetes education and counselling by competent health professionals; providing collaborative care of type 2 diabetes, involving clinical pharmacists, dietitians or nutritionists, and psychologists in type 2 diabetes care; improving health professionals' competency, commitment and professional ethics; and improving the referral system of patients with type 2 diabetes between TASH and other health institutions [42]. The co-design panels in workshop I and II discussed the identified list of potential target behaviours for the intervention that helped with improving the effective management of type 2 diabetes at TASH.

During the co-design workshop, the co-design panel prioritised the potential target behaviours, out of which the four potential target behaviours are listed from highest to lowest priority:

1. Provide structured diabetes education and counselling with competent health professionals;
2. Enable collaborative care of type 2 diabetes;
3. Involve clinical pharmacists, dietitians or nutritionists, and psychologists in the care of type 2 diabetes as members of the collaborative care team;
4. Improve health professionals' competency, commitment, and professional ethics through trainings.

Similarly, the co-design panel in workshop II identified and prioritised the following potential target behaviours for intervention in descending order of priority.

1. Ensure continuous availability of medications;
2. Ensure continuous availability of laboratory and diagnostic tests;
3. Involve clinical pharmacists, dietitians or nutritionists, and psychologists in the care of type 2 diabetes as members of the collaborative care team;
4. Enable collaborative care of type 2 diabetes;
5. Integrate all type 2 diabetes care services at the diabetes centre.

Given the evidence from the interviews, focus groups, and previous findings [22,30,61], based on the context of the hospital, and the "less is more approach" of the BCW [47], it was beneficial to start the intervention with few behaviours and build upon these incrementally [47]. The panels in the co-design workshop III then identified and agreed that the effective management of type 2 diabetes at TASH may most likely be improved through the provision of structured diabetes education, counselling, and collaborative care (involving clinical pharmacists, dietitians or nutritionists, and psychologists) of type 2 diabetes. The panels agreed that these behaviours could easily be changed, measured, and be shared by other health professionals and health facilities with the available resources.

The co-design panels confirmed that there was no involvement of clinical pharmacists, dietitians or nutritionists, and psychologists in the provision of type 2 diabetes care. It was found that there was a profound deficiency of the collaborative care of type 2 diabetes at the diabetes centre of TASH. A collaboratively working care team is more likely to be responsive, efficient, and provide improved care [61]. As multiple behaviours interact and play a role in the provision of structured diabetes education and counselling and collaborative care of type 2 diabetes [62–65], the co-design panel and the research team targeted changing the behaviours of the health professionals (physicians, nurses, and pharmacists, and dietitians or nutritionists) to improve the care of type 2 diabetes at TASH.

3.4. Step Three: Specify the Target Behaviour

After the selection of the potential target behaviours for intervention, the co-design panel in workshop III specified the two target behaviours, namely to enable the provision of structured type 2 diabetes education, counselling, and collaborative care of type 2 diabetes. These details are found in the table of Supplementary Materials (Table S2).

The findings of the interviews, focus groups, and co-design panel workshops indicated the need for the involvement of physicians, nurses, clinical pharmacists, dietitians or nutritionists, psychologists, and peer diabetes educators in the provision of structured diabetes education and counselling with patients or family members (caregivers) to improve the care of type 2 diabetes at TASH. The structured diabetes education involved the education of patients with type 2 diabetes about the condition, its complications, and management and self-care activities (Table S2).

In enabling the collaborative care of type 2 diabetes, physicians, nurses, clinical pharmacists, dietitians or nutritionists, and psychologists would work in coordination with patients and their families (caregivers), administrative bodies of the hospital, and the Ministry of Health of Ethiopia. A collaborative care team would be organised at the diabetes centre of TASH. The duties and activities of each member of the diabetes care team are described in the table of Supplementary Materials (Table S2).

3.5. Step Four: Identify What Needs to Change

We used the COM-B system [47] to identify health professionals' and policymakers' capabilities (C), opportunities (O), and motivations (M) for providing or not providing structured diabetes education, counselling, and collaborative care of type 2 diabetes (Table S3). The research team performed behavioural diagnosis through triangulation of the findings of the interviews, focus groups, the systematic review [30]; and feedback from the co-design panels and the research team discussions. This information was used to determine what needed to change to enable health professionals to provide structured type 2 diabetes education, counselling, and collaborative care of type 2 diabetes at TASH.

3.5.1. Structured Type 2 Diabetes Education and Counselling

The provision of structured diabetes education and counselling at TASH was hampered by a lack of availability and involvement of trained and qualified multidisciplinary health professionals in diabetes education and counselling (C). Insufficient time for the consultation of patients (O) and inadequate space (O) led to a lack of physical opportunity to provide structured diabetes education and counselling about type 2 diabetes. Patient adherence to diabetes educations sessions (O) negatively affected the provision of type 2 diabetes education at TASH. A triangulation of evidence from the interviews, focus groups, systematic review [30], co-design workshops, and the research team discussions and behavioural analysis ensured that there is a need to change the psychological capability, physical and social opportunity, and reflective and automatic motivation of health professionals to achieve the provision of structured type 2 diabetes education and counselling of type 2 diabetes at TASH (Table S3).

3.5.2. Collaborative Care

Time shortages and inappropriate space (O), poor communication among health professionals (O), lack of commitment and motivation of health professionals and policymakers (M), and absence of policies and guidelines for collaboration (O) contributed to a lack of collaborative care of type 2 diabetes at TASH. We triangulated the findings from interviews, focus groups, the co-design panel workshops, and the research team discussions and performed the behavioural analysis using the COM-B [47]. We analysed that the psychological capability, physical and social opportunity, and reflective and automatic motivation of health professionals have to be changed in order to provide collaborative care of type 2 diabetes at TASH (Table S3).

3.6. Step Five: Identify Intervention Functions

Intervention functions appropriate to the context of TASH and that help to improve the management of type 2 diabetes were determined using the APEASE criteria [47] (Table S4).

3.6.1. Intervention Functions for the COM-B Components of the Target Behaviour Provision of Structured Diabetes Education and Counselling

We used the BCW [47] mapping matrix to link the identified COM-B components; namely, psychological capability, physical and social opportunity, automatic and reflective motivation for the target behaviour, and provision of structured diabetes education and counselling with intervention functions. Based on the results of the APEASE criteria [47], we identified five intervention functions (Table S4); namely, education, training, environmental restructuring, modelling, and enablement that help with the intervention to bring about change in the targeted behaviour [47].

3.6.2. Intervention Functions for the COM-B Components of The Target Behaviour in Collaborative Care of Type 2 Diabetes

We linked the COM-B components of the collaborative care of type 2 diabetes (psychological capability, physical and social opportunity, and automatic and reflective motivation) with intervention functions using the BCW [47] mapping matrix to identify intervention functions for the collaborative care of type 2 diabetes. We identified that education, incentivisation, training, environmental restructuring, modelling, and enablement were the most appropriate and pertinent intervention functions to the existing context of TASH in helping to change the target behaviour (collaborative care) (Table S4).

3.7. Step Six: Identifying Policy Categories for the Target Behaviours' Provision of Structured Diabetes Education, Counselling, and Collaborative Care of Type 2 Diabetes

After identification of the intervention functions, we evaluated the appropriate policy categories that support the delivery of the intervention functions using the APEASE criteria [47]. Guidelines, environmental/social planning, and service provision were deemed appropriate to our context to support the intervention functions for the target behaviour provision of structured diabetes education and counselling. To support the delivery of the intervention functions for the target behaviour provision of the collaborative care of type 2 diabetes, guidelines, regulation, environmental/social planning, and service provision were the policy categories identified that were deemed appropriate to our context (Table S4).

3.8. Step Seven: Identifying Behaviour Change Techniques

Behaviour change techniques are active components of an intervention designed to change behaviour [57] that help to characterise the active components of the healthcare intervention [66]. We specified BCTs deemed to be the most effective and feasible in our context of improving the provision of structured diabetes education, counselling, and collaborative care of type 2 diabetes through the triangulation of a literature review; findings of the interviews, focus groups, and the systematic review [30]; and using the APEASE criteria [47]. We linked the intervention functions identified in step five with the most commonly used BCTs described in the Behaviour Change Technique Taxonomy version 1 (BCTTv1) [57] and identified the following 12 BCTs for the target behaviour provision of structured diabetes education and counselling (Table S5):

1. Feedback on behaviour;
2. Self-monitoring of behaviour;
3. Prompt/cues;
4. Salience of consequences;
5. Instruction on how to perform the behaviour;
6. Demonstration of the behaviour;
7. Restructuring the physical environment;
8. Restructuring the social environment;

9. Adding objects to the environment;
10. Goal setting behaviour;
11. Action planning;
12. Social support (unspecified).

3.9. Step Eight: Mode of Delivery and Development of the Complex Intervention

We operationalised the identified BCTs and identified modes of delivery for the provision of structured education and counselling with trained diabetes educators and collaborative care of type 2 diabetes and developed a complex intervention (Table S6). We created a complex intervention called VICKY (Patient-centred collaborative care and evidence-based structured diabetes education and counselling supported with educational materials) to improve the management of type 2 diabetes at TASH. Figure 4 summarises the development of the complex intervention according to the first stage of the UK MRC framework [43].

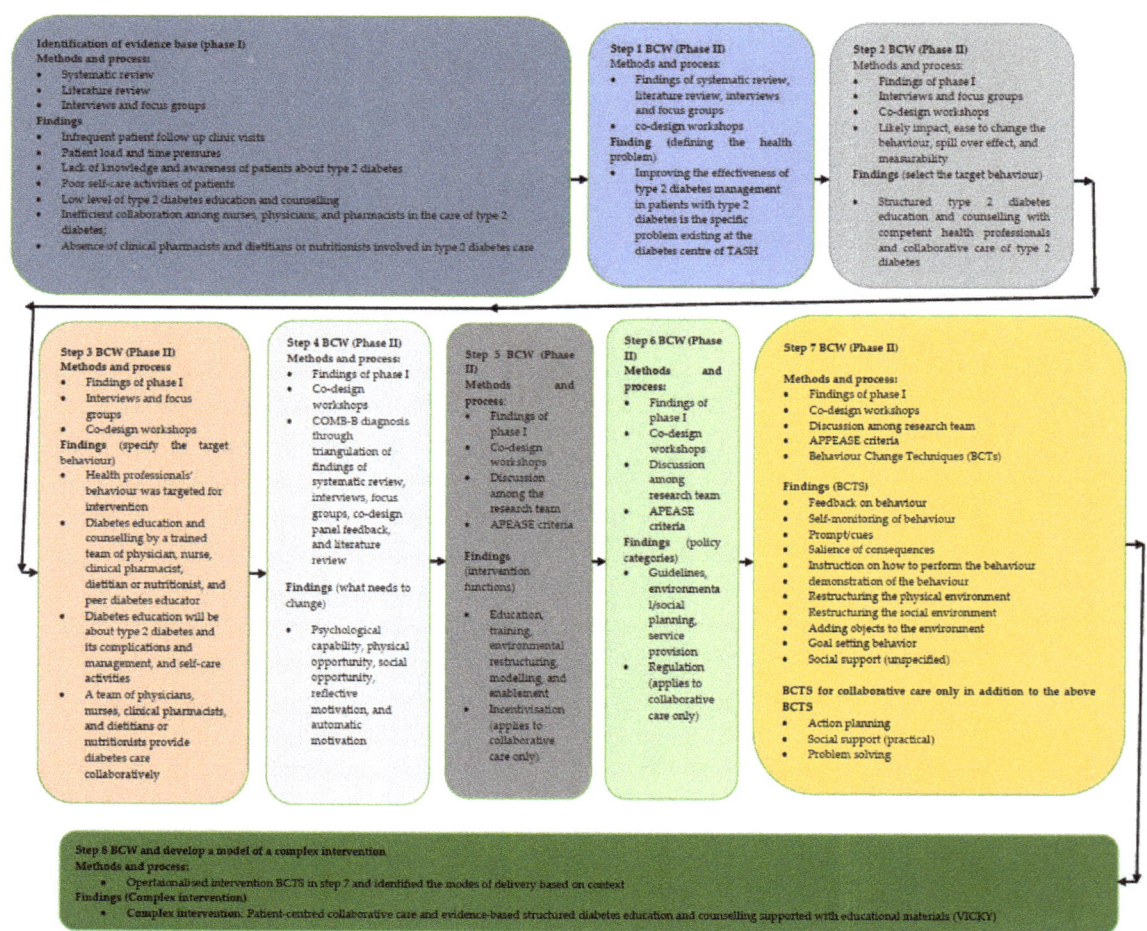

Figure 4. The processes involved in modelling and creating the complex intervention.

The complex intervention (VICKY) consisted of five components (Table 1).

Table 1. Components and intervention plan of the complex (VICKY) intervention.

	Components of the Complex Intervention (VICKY)	Intervention Plan and Activities
1	Patient-centred collaborative care by a team of physicians, clinical pharmacists, nurses, dietitians or nutritionists, psychologists, and policymakers.	• Establish a multidisciplinary collaborative care team of physicians, nurses, clinical pharmacists, dietitians or nutritionists, psychologists, policymakers, and trained diabetes educators • Educational meetings, refresher trainings, discussion forums and refreshments, and feedback mechanisms for the collaborative care team
2	Referral system for patients across transition of care between different health professionals of the diabetes care team (physicians, clinical pharmacists, nurses, dietitians or nutritionists, psychologists, and policymakers).	• Training of the collaborative care team about collaborative care through practical clinic attachments, role plays, and videos. • Organise a separate working room for clinical pharmacists for the provision of clinical pharmacy services. • Mentorship and supervision of junior health professionals by senior professionals. • Establish a referral system for patients during transition of care between health professionals.
3	Tools for provision of collaborative care and documentation for the care provided.	• Protocol that guides the diabetes care team for the provision of collaborative care and referral systems across transition of care between health professionals. • Develop checklists to document the services provided by the collaborative care team to ensure collaborative care was provided • Checklists and documentation tools such as clinical pharmacy services documentation forms that support the provision of collaborative care activities.
4	Evidence-based structured diabetes education and counselling by a team of trained physician, nurse, clinical pharmacist, dietitian or nutritionist, and expert patient.	• A multidisciplinary team of individuals comprising nurses, clinical pharmacists, physicians, dietitians or nutritionists, peer diabetes educators, and policymakers will be established as a team of diabetes educators at the diabetes centre of TASH. • Diabetes educators' training tailored to the context of the hospital and the country will be provided to the multidisciplinary team of nurses, clinical pharmacists, physicians, dietitians or nutritionists, peer diabetes educators, and policymakers to produce trained diabetes educators at the diabetes centre.
5	Educational materials and documentation tools for structured diabetes education and counselling.	• Context-specific diabetes education manual and educational materials such as brochures, leaflets, audio-visuals. • Design computerised patient referral forms for patients that require diabetes education and counselling. • Contextualised diabetes education checklist and patient diary will be developed.

The following 13 BCTs were linked to the intervention functions for the target behaviour in the collaborative care of type 2 diabetes (Table S5).

1. Self-monitoring of behaviour;
2. Prompt/cues;
3. Feedback on behaviour;
4. Instruction on how to perform the behaviour;
5. Restructuring the physical environment;
6. Restructuring the social environment;
7. Adding objects to the environment;
8. Demonstration of the behaviour;
9. Goal setting behaviour;
10. Action planning;
11. Social support (unspecified);
12. Social support (practical);
13. Problem solving.

We used the logic model (Figure 5) to link the context of the healthcare system, such as study setting, the resources, intervention activities, theory, and assumptions underlying the intervention, and the intervention plan, in a logical order [67,68].

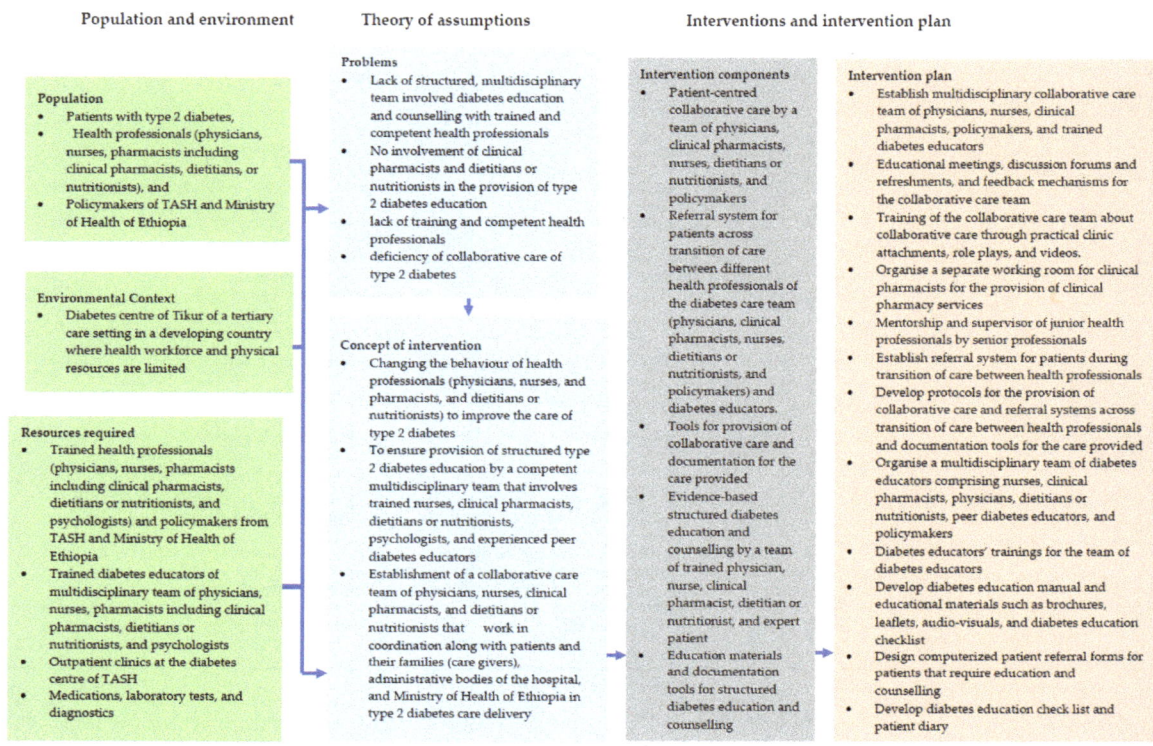

Figure 5. Logic Model linking context of the healthcare system, resources, and intervention activities (Conrad et al., 1999).

4. Discussion

This paper describes a systematic development of a tailored complex intervention to improve the effectiveness of the management of type 2 diabetes in a tertiary care setting of a developing country. To our knowledge, the complex intervention is the first theory-driven and context-specific intervention designed using the first stage of the UK MRC framework and the BCW and co-design approaches for the management of type 2 diabetes in Ethiopia.

Our intervention addresses an organisational level intervention that involves multiple stakeholders and multifaceted approaches, such as the training of health professionals, provision of educational materials, collaborative care, and patient involvement in the care process. Multifaceted approaches have been demonstrated to be successful in improving healthcare in resource-limited settings, including SSA [69–72]. Moreover, multi-level involvement comprising patient and healthcare provider-targeted interventions are likely to be successful in improving healthcare [73–75].

Implementation science offers opportunities to design novel healthcare approaches to ensure the utilisation of resources for evidence-based healthcare delivery in developing countries, including SSA [76,77]. Efforts have also been undertaken to enhance the use of implementation science in SSA [76,78,79] in view of the feasibility and effectiveness of implementation science in the healthcare intervention in this setting [70,76,80]. The resources available for healthcare in SSA are limited, which therefore requires the design, testing, and implementation of novel approaches for healthcare [81,82]. In this study, a novel approach for diabetes care that is based on the context of the available resources of a tertiary care setting in a developing country [22,31,32,41,83–85], has been designed. The intervention developed in this study may be of value in improving the quality and outcomes of diabetes care at the study setting and to tailor similar diabetes care strategies in other healthcare settings in the country [84,86]. The evidence also indicated that healthcare implementation strategies in low-income countries, such as SSA, would be feasible, sustainable, and of interest to policymakers if they are designed based on the contexts of the settings in these countries [71,76,80].

The MRC framework [43] guided the identification of an evidence base, development of theory, and modelling processes and outcomes. The BCW [47] was used to develop a theory-driven intervention, identify intervention strategies, and create elements of the complex intervention tailored to the context of the setting. We used the BCW, as it is a comprehensive framework that considers the context in intervention design [47]. Theory-driven interventions designed for patients with diabetes have been demonstrated to improve care delivery and patient outcomes [44]. Complex interventions are likely to work best if tailored to local contexts [43]. A systematic review of behavioural interventions to improve glycemic control in patients with diabetes indicated that tailored behavioural interventions improved glycemic control of patients with type 2 diabetes [87].

There have been tailored complex interventions [44,48] designed using the UK MRC [43] framework and the BCW [47] for diabetes care in developed countries. Previously developed interventions [44,48] lacked the triangulation of multiple data sources, such as interviews, focus groups, and a co-design approach in their intervention design. The distinguishing feature of our intervention design is the use of multifaceted data sources, such as consumers, health professionals of various disciplines and key policymakers, a literature review, and systematic review [30], and extensive feedback from the co-design panels comprising individuals of diverse backgrounds in contextualising the intervention. Our intervention addresses a tailored and evidence-based strategy in diabetes care delivery in a resource-limited setting.

We designed an organisational level intervention to improve the effectiveness of type 2 diabetes management. There is a broad range of evidence internationally in support of organisational interventions to improve the care of type 2 diabetes and patient outcomes [54–56]. Similarly, health system interventions that involved patient-centred collaborative care with multiple health professionals and diabetes education have shown effectiveness in improving the glycemic control of patients with type 2 diabetes in both developing and developed countries [56,88,89]. As multiple behaviours interact and play a role in the provision of structured diabetes education, counselling, and collaborative care of type 2 diabetes [75–78], the intervention was targeted at changing the health professionals' behaviour involved in diabetes care delivery. Similar interventions that targeted changing health professional behaviour were found to be effective in improving diabetes care and patient outcomes [44,48,90–92]. In a systematic review of behaviour change interventions, such as education, training, collaborative care including physicians, nurses, and pharmacists, audit and feedback targeted at health professionals were effective in improving healthcare delivery and patient outcomes [93]. Successful management and the improved outcome of diabetes requires interaction and implementation of multiple behaviours of different health professionals, such as motivation and commitment, diabetes management knowledge and skills, interprofessional or intraprofessional communications, and compassion [62–65,91,94]. As a result, modifying multiple behaviours of professionals of various disciplines helps to improve the management of diabetes and patient outcomes [62–65,94].

Diabetes care models of developed countries are evidence-based, patient-centred, team-based, and guided by contextually tailored diabetes management guidelines and educational materials, where diabetes education by trained diabetes educators are essential elements of care [95–97]. Studies demonstrated a lack of collaborative care of diabetes, diabetes training of health professionals, diabetes guidelines, and diabetes education in SSA [8–10,98], including in Ethiopia [22]. This situation is partly attributed to the lack of facility-specific evidence about contextual factors, such as the socio-economic factors of diabetes care in SSA and the failure to tailor the diabetes care approach to the context of the SSA setting [10,42]. Therefore, it is essential to understand the specific context of a SSA diabetes care setting and design an evidence-based diabetes care strategy tailored to the context of this setting [9,99].

Our proposed intervention involves the collaborative care of diabetes, diabetes training of health professionals, and diabetes education by a trained team of health professionals. Evidence also indicates that the diabetes care team needs to incorporate a multidisciplinary group involving physicians, nurses, clinical pharmacists, dietitians or nutritionists, and psychologists [62–65]. Expanding diabetes management to several healthcare team disciplines helps patients receive the most optimal and cost-effective diabetes care and achieve better treatment outcomes [65,100,101]. Structured diabetes education is also a key component of the intervention in this study, which has been previously demonstrated to improve diabetes care delivery and treatment outcomes [30,102–105]. The evidence also indicates that multicomponent educational interventions significantly improved the glycemic control of patients with type 2 diabetes [106]. In general, our intervention, which focuses on collaborative care and structured diabetes education, will fill the gaps identified in diabetes management in SSA in general, and Ethiopia in particular [8–10,22,98].

This study has some limitations. We did not include the views of nutritionists or dietitians, psychologists, and laboratory personnel in the intervention design. The intervention was designed at a single healthcare setting, requiring feasibility and piloting prior to evaluation and implementation. Nevertheless, the information obtained can be transferred to other similar settings.

5. Conclusions

This paper indicated the usability and applicability of the UK MRC framework and the BCW to designing tailored and evidence-informed behaviour change interventions in SSA. We developed the UK MRC-guided intervention called patient-centred collaborative care and structured diabetes education and counselling (VICKY) using the BCW. VICKY, which is a tailored intervention to the context of a tertiary care setting of a developing country, is a complex intervention for diabetes management to be tested for feasibility and effectiveness in later phases of this project. This intervention will help to manage diabetes effectively by addressing the current practice gap existing at the hospital, and the country in general. VICKY is a comprehensive diabetes care model co-designed by key stakeholders involving consumers, healthcare providers of various disciplines, and policymakers using multiple evidence sources. This model, if found effective, may serve as a springboard to design similar tailored interventions for other non-communicable diseases in the country.

Supplementary Materials: The following supporting information can be downloaded at: https://www.mdpi.com/article/10.3390/jcm11051149/s1, Table S1: Revised Standards for Quality Improvement Reporting Excellence: (SQUIRE 2.0) publication guidelines, Table S2: Behavioral specification to improve the management of type 2 diabetes at the diabetes centre of a tertiary teaching hospital, Table S3: COM-B diagnosis using the Behaviour Change Wheel for the identified target behaviours, Table S4: Linking intervention functions to COM-B components using the Behaviour Change Wheel linking Matrix, Table S5: COM-B diagnosis, intervention functions, policy categories, and behaviour change techniques for the identified target behaviours for intervention, and Table S6: Mode of delivery structured diabetes education.

Author Contributions: Conceptualisation, T.A.D., K.M.N. and E.M.; methodology, T.A.D.; software, T.A.D.; validation, T.A.D., K.M.N. and E.M.; formal analysis, T.A.D.; investigation, T.A.D., K.M.N. and E.M.; resources, T.A.D.; data curation, T.A.D.; writing—original draft preparation, T.A.D.; writing—review and editing, T.A.D., K.M.N., H.Y. and E.M. visualisation, T.A.D.; supervision, T.A.D., K.M.N., H.Y. and E.M.; project administration, T.A.D., K.M.N., H.Y. and E.M. All authors have read and agreed to the published version of the manuscript.

Funding: This research received no external funding.

Institutional Review Board Statement: The study was conducted according to the guidelines of the Declaration of Helsinki and approved by the ethics committee (the Institutional Review Board) of Deakin University Human Ethics Advisory Group (HEAG-H 102_2019) and the Institutional Review Board of Addis Ababa University (092/19/SoP).

Informed Consent Statement: Written informed consent was obtained from all participants involved in the study.

Data Availability Statement: The data presented in this study are available on request from the corresponding author.

Acknowledgments: We would like to thank the patients, health professionals, and policymakers for participating in the co-design workshops, providing valuable feedback throughout the intervention design, and co-designing the intervention. We also thank the patients, health professionals, and policymakers for volunteering to undertake interviews and focus groups that helped with generating evidence for the intervention design.

Conflicts of Interest: The authors declare no conflict of interest.

References

1. Hu, F.B. Globalisation of diabetes: The role of diet, lifestyle, and genes. *Diabetes Care* **2011**, *34*, 1249–1257. [CrossRef] [PubMed]
2. Bloomgarden, Z.T. Cardiovascular disease in diabetes. *Diabetes Care* **2008**, *31*, 1260–1266. [CrossRef]
3. International Diabetes Federation. *International Diabetes Federation Diabetes Atlas*, 8th ed.; International Diabetes Federation: Brussels, Belgium, 2017.
4. International Diabetes Federation. *IDF Diabetes Atlas*, 9th ed.; International Diabetes Federation: Brussels, Belgium, 2019.
5. Kim, S. Burden of shospitalisations primarily due to uncontrolled diabetes: Implications of inadequate primary health care in the United States. *Diabetes Care* **2007**, *30*, 1281–1282. [CrossRef] [PubMed]
6. Cramer, J.A.; Benedict, Á.; Muszbek, N.; Keskinaslan, A.; Khan, Z.M. The significance of compliance and persistence in the treatment of diabetes, hypertension and dyslipidaemia: A review. *Int. J. Clin. Pr.* **2007**, *62*, 76–87. [CrossRef] [PubMed]
7. Inzucchi, S.E.; Bergenstal, R.M.; Buse, J.; Diamant, M.; Ferrannini, E.; Nauck, M.; Peters, A.; Tsapas, A.; Wender, R.; Matthews, D.R. Management of hyperglycaemia in type 2 diabetes: A patient-centered approach. Position statement of the American Diabetes Association (ADA) and the European Association for the Study of Diabetes (EASD). *Diabetologia* **2012**, *55*, 1577–1596. [CrossRef]
8. Azevedo, M.; Alla, S. Diabetes in Sub-Saharan Africa: Kenya, Mali, Mozambique, Nigeria, South Africa and Zambia. *Int. J. Diabetes Dev. Ctries.* **2008**, *28*, 101–108. [CrossRef]
9. Gill, G.V.; Mbanya, J.-C.; Ramaiya, K.L.; Tesfaye, S. A sub-Saharan African perspective of diabetes. *Diabetologia* **2009**, *52*, 8–16. [CrossRef]
10. Pastakia, S.D.; Pekny, C.R.; Manyara, S.M.; Fischer, L. Diabetes in sub-Saharan Africa—From policy to practice to progress: Targeting the existing gaps for future care for diabetes. *Diabetes Metab. Syndr. Obes.* **2017**, *10*, 247–263. [CrossRef]
11. Shimels, T.; Abebaw, M.; Bilal, A.I.; Tesfaye, T. Treatment Pattern and Factors Associated with Blood Pressure and Fasting Plasma Glucose Control among Patients with Type 2 Diabetes Mellitus in Police Referral Hospital in Ethiopia. *Ethiop. J. Health Sci.* **2018**, *28*, 461–472. [CrossRef]
12. Gudina, E.K.; Amade, S.T.; Tesfamichael, F.A.; Ram, R. Assessment of quality of care given to diabetic patients at Jimma University Specialized Hospital diabetes follow-up clinic, Jimma, Ethiopia. *BMC Endocr. Disord.* **2011**, *11*, 19. [CrossRef]
13. Yigazu, D.M.; Desse, T.A. Glycemic control and associated factors among type 2 diabetic patients at Shanan Gibe Hospital, Southwest Ethiopia. *BMC Res. Notes* **2017**, *10*, 597. [CrossRef] [PubMed]
14. Atun, R.; Davies, J.I.; Gale, E.A.M.; Bärnighausen, T.; Beran, D.; Kengne, A.P.; Levitt, N.; Mangugu, F.W.; Nyirenda, M.J.; Ogle, G.D.; et al. Diabetes in sub-Saharan Africa: From clinical care to health policy. *Lancet Diabetes Endocrinol.* **2017**, *5*, 622–667. [CrossRef]
15. Mobula, L.M.; Sarfo, F.S.; Carson, K.A.; Burnham, G.; Arthur, L.; Ansong, D.; Sarfo-Kantanka, O.; Plange-Rhule, J.; Ofori-Adjei, D. Predictors of glycemic control in type-2 diabetes mellitus: Evidence from a multicenter study in Ghana. *Transl. Metab. Syndr. Res.* **2018**, *1*, 1–8. [CrossRef]
16. Nuche-Berenguer, B.; Kupfer, L.E. Readiness of Sub-Saharan Africa Healthcare Systems for the New Pandemic, Diabetes: A Systematic Review. *J. Diabetes Res.* **2018**, *2018*, 9262395. [CrossRef]
17. Bhagavathula, A.S.; Gebreyohannes, E.A.; Abegaz, T.M.; Abebe, T.B. Perceived Obstacles Faced by Diabetes Patients Attending University of Gondar Hospital, Northwest Ethiopia. *Front. Public Health* **2018**, *6*, 81. [CrossRef] [PubMed]
18. Nigatu, T. Epidemiology, complications and management of diabetes in Ethiopia: A systematic review. *J. Diabetes* **2012**, *4*, 174–180. [CrossRef]
19. Yimama, M.; Jarso, H.; Desse, T.A. Determinants of drug-related problems among ambulatory type 2 diabetes patients with hypertension comorbidity in Southwest Ethiopia: A prospective cross sectional study. *BMC Res. Notes* **2018**, *11*, 679. [CrossRef]
20. Kiflie, Y.; Jira, C.; Nigussie, D. The quality of care provided to patients with chronic non-communicable diseases: A Retrospective multi-set up study in Jimma Zone, southwest Ethiopia. *Ethiop. J. Health Sci.* **2011**, *21*, 119–130. [CrossRef]
21. Bekele, A.; Getachew, T.; Amenu, K.; Defar, A.; Teklie, H.; Gelibo, T.; Taddesse, M.; Assefa, Y.; Kebede, A.; Feleke, Y. Service availability and readiness for diabetes care at health facilities in Ethiopia. *Ethiop. J. Health Dev.* **2017**, *31*, 110–118.
22. Habte, B.M.; Kebede, T.; Fenta, T.G.; Boon, H. Ethiopian patients' perceptions of anti-diabetic medications: Implications for diabetes education. *J. Pharm. Policy Pr.* **2017**, *10*, 14. [CrossRef] [PubMed]

23. Ali, M.; Alemu, T.; Sada, O. Medication adherence and its associated factors among diabetic patients at Zewditu Memorial Hospital, Addis Ababa, Ethiopia. *BMC Res. Notes* **2017**, *10*, 676. [CrossRef]
24. Esterson, Y.B.; Carey, M.; Piette, J.D.; Thomas, N.; Hawkins, M. A Systematic Review of Innovative Diabetes Care Models in Low-and Middle-Income Countries (LMICs). *J. Health Care Poor Underserved* **2014**, *25*, 72–93. [CrossRef] [PubMed]
25. Glazier, R.H.; Bajcar, J.; Kennie, N.R.; Willson, K. A Systematic Review of Interventions to Improve Diabetes Care in Socially Disadvantaged Populations. *Diabetes Care* **2006**, *29*, 1675–1688. [CrossRef] [PubMed]
26. Pinchevsky, Y.; Butkow, N.; Chirwa, T.; Raal, F. Treatment Gaps Found in the Management of Type 2 Diabetes at a Community Health Centre in Johannesburg, South Africa. *J. Diabetes Res.* **2017**, *2017*, 9536025. [CrossRef] [PubMed]
27. Atlantis, E.; Fahey, P.; Foster, J. Collaborative care for comorbid depression and diabetes: A systematic review and meta-analysis. *BMJ Open* **2014**, *4*, e004706. [CrossRef]
28. Powers, M.A.; Bardsley, J.K.; Cypress, M.; Funnell, M.M.; Harms, D.; Hess-Fischl, A.; Hooks, B.; Isaacs, D.; Mandel, E.D.; Maryniuk, M.D.; et al. Diabetes Self-management Education and Support in Adults with Type 2 Diabetes: A Consensus Report of the American Diabetes Association, the Association of Diabetes Care and Education Specialists, the Academy of Nutrition and Dietetics, the American Academy of Family Physicians, the American Academy of PAs, the American Association of Nurse Practitioners, and the American Pharmacists Association. *J. Am. Assoc. Nurse Pr.* **2020**, *43*, 1636–1649.
29. Beck, J.; Greenwood, D.A.; Blanton, L.; Bollinger, S.T.; Butcher, M.K.; Condon, J.E.; Cypress, M.; Faulkner, P.; Fischl, A.H.; Francis, T.; et al. 2017 National Standards for Diabetes Self-Management Education and Support. *Diabetes Care* **2017**, *40*, 1409–1419. [CrossRef] [PubMed]
30. Desse, T.A.; Vakil, K.; Mc Namara, K.; Manias, E. Impact of clinical pharmacy interventions on health and economic outcomes in type 2 diabetes: A systematic review and meta-analysis. *Diabet. Med.* **2021**, *38*, e14526. [CrossRef]
31. Habte, B.M.; Kebede, T.; Fenta, T.G.; Boon, H. Barriers and facilitators to adherence to anti-diabetic medications: Ethiopian patients' perspectives. *Afr. J. Prim. Health Care Fam. Med.* **2017**, *9*, 9. [CrossRef]
32. Ethiopian Public Health Institute. *Services Availability and Readiness Assessment (SARA)*; Ethiopian Public Health Institute: Addis Ababa, Ethiopia, 2018.
33. Cheneke, W.; Suleman, S.; Yemane, T.; Abebe, G. Assessment of glycemic control using glycated hemoglobin among diabetic patients in Jimma University sspecialised hospital, Ethiopia. *BMC Res. Notes* **2016**, *9*, 96. [CrossRef]
34. Abebe, N.; Kebede, T.; Addise, D. Diabetes in Ethiopia 2000–2016—Prevalence and related acute and chronic complications; a systematic review. *Afr. J. Diabetes Med.* **2017**, *25*, 7–12.
35. Fiseha, T.; Alemayehu, E.; Kassahun, W.; Adamu, A.; Gebreweld, A. Factors associated with glycemic control among diabetic adult out-patients in Northeast Ethiopia. *BMC Res. Notes* **2018**, *11*, 316. [CrossRef] [PubMed]
36. Tekalegn, Y.; Addissie, A.; Kebede, T.; Ayele, W. Magnitude of glycemic control and its associated factors among patients with type 2 diabetes at Tikur Anbessa Specialized Hospital, Addis Ababa, Ethiopia. *PLoS ONE* **2018**, *13*, e0193442. [CrossRef] [PubMed]
37. Desse, T.A.; Eshetie, T.C.; Gudina, E.K. Predictors and treatment outcome of hyperglycemic emergencies at Jimma University Specialized Hospital, southwest Ethiopia. *BMC Res. Notes* **2015**, *8*, 553. [CrossRef]
38. Reba, K.; Argaw, Z.; Walle, B.; Gutema, H. Health-related quality of life of patients with diagnosed type 2 diabetes in Felege Hiwot Referral Hospital, North West Ethiopia: A cross-sectional study. *BMC Res. Notes* **2018**, *11*, 544. [CrossRef]
39. Zimmermann, M.; Bunn, C.; Namadingo, H.; Gray, C.M.; Lwanda, J. Experiences of type 2 diabetes in sub-Saharan Africa: A scoping review. *Glob. Health Res. Policy* **2018**, *3*, 25. [CrossRef]
40. Godman, B.; Basu, D.; Pillay, Y.; Mwita, J.C.; Rwegerera, G.M.; Paramadhas, B.D.A.; Tiroyakgosi, C.; Okwen, P.M.; Niba, L.L.; Nonvignon, J.; et al. Review of Ongoing Activities and Challenges to Improve the Care of Patients With Type 2 Diabetes Across Africa and the Implications for the Future. *Front. Pharmacol.* **2020**, *11*, 108. [CrossRef]
41. Yifter, H.; Reja, A.; Ahmed, A.; Narayan, K.M.V.; Amogne, W. Achievement of diabetes care goals at Tikur Anbessa Specialized Hospital, Addis Ababa, Ethiopia. *Ethiop. Med. J.* **2020**, *58*, 125–130.
42. Desse, T.A.; Namara, K.M.; Yifter, H.; Manias, E. Current practices and future preferences of type 2 diabetes care in a developing country: A qualitative study of patient, health professional, and policymaker perspectives. 2021.
43. Craig, P.; Dieppe, P.; Macintyre, S.; Michie, S.; Nazareth, I.; Petticrew, M. Developing and evaluating complex interventions: An introduction to the new Medical Research Council guidance. *Evid.-Based Public Health* **2009**, *337*, a1655. [CrossRef]
44. Murphy, M.E.; Byrne, M.; Zarabzadeh, A.; Corrigan, D.; Fahey, T.; Smith, S.M. Development of a complex intervention to promote appropriate prescribing and medication intensification in poorly controlled type 2 diabetes mellitus in Irish general practice. *Implement. Sci.* **2017**, *12*, 115. [CrossRef]
45. Francis, J.J.; Eccles, M.P.; Johnston, M.; Whitty, P.; Grimshaw, J.M.; Kaner, E.F.; Smith, L.; Walker, A. Explaining the effects of an intervention designed to promote evidence-based diabetes care: A theory-based process evaluation of a pragmatic cluster randomised controlled trial. *Implement. Sci.* **2008**, *3*, 50. [CrossRef] [PubMed]
46. Michie, S.; Van Stralen, M.M.; West, R. The behaviour change wheel: A new method for characterising and designing behaviour change interventions. *Implement. Sci.* **2011**, *6*, 42. [CrossRef]
47. Michie, S.; Atkins, L.; West, R. *The Behaviour Change Wheel. A Guide to Designing Interventions*; Silverback Publishing: Sutton, UK, 2014.
48. Sinnott, C.; Mercer, S.W.; Payne, R.A.; Duerden, M.; Bradley, C.P.; Byrne, M. Improving medication management in multimorbidity: Development of the MultimorbiditY COllaborative Medication Review And DEcision Making (MY COMRADE) intervention using the Behaviour Change Wheel. *Implement. Sci.* **2015**, *10*, 132. [CrossRef] [PubMed]

49. Smits, S.; McCutchan, G.; Wood, F.; Edwards, A.; Lewis, I.; Robling, M.; Paranjothy, S.; Carter, B.; Townson, J.; Brain, K. Development of a Behavior Change Intervention to Encourage Timely Cancer Symptom Presentation Among People Living in Deprived Communities Using the Behavior Change Wheel. *Ann. Behav. Med.* **2018**, *52*, 474–488. [CrossRef] [PubMed]
50. Sargent, L.; McCullough, A.; Del Mar, C.; Lowe, J. Using theory to explore facilitators and barriers to delayed prescribing in Australia: A qualitative study using the Theoretical Domains Framework and the Behaviour Change Wheel. *BMC Fam. Pr.* **2017**, *18*, 20. [CrossRef] [PubMed]
51. Mangurian, C.; Niu, G.C.; Schillinger, D.; Newcomer, J.W.; Dilley, J.; Handley, M.A. Utilisation of the Behavior Change Wheel framework to develop a model to improve cardiometabolic screening for people with severe mental illness. *Implement. Sci.* **2017**, *12*, 134. [CrossRef]
52. Steinmo, S.; Fuller, C.C.; Stone, S.P.; Michie, S. Characterising an implementation intervention in terms of behaviour change techniques and theory: The 'Sepsis Six' clinical care bundle. *Implement. Sci.* **2015**, *10*, 111. [CrossRef]
53. Jackson, C.; Eliasson, L.; Barber, N.; Weinman, J. Applying COM-B to medication adherence: A suggested framework for research and interventions. *Eur. Health Psychol.* **2014**, *16*, 7–17.
54. Leykum, L.K.; Pugh, J.; Lawrence, V.; Parchman, M.; Noël, P.H.; Cornell, J.; McDaniel, R.R. Organisational interventions employing principles of complexity science have improved outcomes for patients with Type II diabetes. *Implement. Sci.* **2007**, *2*, 8. [CrossRef] [PubMed]
55. Murphy, M.E.; Byrne, M.; Galvin, R.; Boland, F.; Fahey, T.; Smith, S. Improving risk factor management for patients with poorly controlled type 2 diabetes: A systematic review of healthcare interventions in primary care and community settings. *BMJ Open* **2017**, *7*, e015135. [CrossRef] [PubMed]
56. Renders, C.M.; Valk, G.D.; Griffin, S.J.; Wagner, E.H.; Eijk van, J.T.; Assendelft, W.J. Interventions to Improve the Management of Diabetes in Primary Care, Outpatient, and Community Settings. *Diabetes Care* **2001**, *24*, 1821–1833. [CrossRef]
57. Michie, S.; Richardson, M.; Johnston, M.; Abraham, C.; Francis, J.; Hardeman, W.; Eccles, M.P.; Cane, J.; Wood, C.E. The Behavior Change Technique Taxonomy (v1) of 93 Hierarchically Clustered Techniques: Building an International Consensus for the Reporting of Behavior Change Interventions. *Ann. Behav. Med.* **2013**, *46*, 81–95. [CrossRef]
58. Rowlands, G.; Sims, J.; Kerry, S. A lesson learnt: The importance of modelling in srandomised controlled trials for complex interventions in primary care. *Fam. Pract.* **2005**, *22*, 132–139. [CrossRef]
59. Ogrinc, G.; Davies, L.; Goodman, D.; Batalden, P.; Davidoff, F.; Stevens, D. SQUIRE 2.0 (Standards for QUality Improvement Reporting Excellence): Revised publication guidelines from a detailed consensus process. *BMJ Qual. Saf.* **2016**, *25*, 986. [CrossRef]
60. Yimam, M.; Desse, T.A.; Hebo, H.J. Glycemic control among ambulatory type 2 diabetes patients with hypertension Co-morbidity in a developing country: A cross sectional study. *Heliyon* **2020**, *6*, e05671. [CrossRef] [PubMed]
61. Schmitt, M.; Blue, A.; Aschenbrener, C.A.; Viggiano, T.R. Core competencies for interprofessional collaborative practice: Reforming health care by transforming health professionals' education. *Acad. Med.* **2011**, *86*, 1351. [CrossRef] [PubMed]
62. Gucciardi, E.; Espin, S.; Morganti, A.; Dorado, L. Exploring interprofessional collaboration during the integration of diabetes teams into primary care. *BMC Fam. Pr.* **2016**, *17*, 12. [CrossRef] [PubMed]
63. Erturkmen, G.B.; Yuksel, M.; Sarigul, B.; Arvanitis, T.N.; Lindman, P.; Chen, R.; Zhao, L.; Sadou, E.; Bouaud, J.; Traore, L.; et al. A Collaborative Platform for Management of Chronic Diseases via Guideline-Driven Individualized Care Plans. *Comput. Struct. Biotechnol. J.* **2019**, *17*, 869–885. [CrossRef]
64. Phelps, K.W.; Howell, C.D.; Hill, S.G.; Seemann, T.S.; Lamson, A.L.; Hodgson, J.L.; Smith, D.A. A collaborative care model for patients with Type-2 diabetes. *Fam. Syst. Health* **2009**, *27*, 131–140. [CrossRef]
65. Johnson, J.; Carragher, R. Interprofessional collaboration and the care and management of type 2 diabetic patients in the Middle East: A systematic review. *J. Interprof. Care* **2018**, *32*, 621–628. [CrossRef]
66. Presseau, J.; Ivers, N.M.; Newham, J.J.; Knittle, K.; Danko, K.J.; Grimshaw, J.M. Using a behaviour change techniques taxonomy to identify active ingredients within trials of implementation interventions for diabetes care. *Implement. Sci.* **2015**, *10*, 55. [CrossRef] [PubMed]
67. Bartholomew, L.K.; Mullen, P.D. Five roles for using theory and evidence in the design and testing of behavior change interventions. *J. Public Health Dent.* **2011**, *71*, S20–S33. [CrossRef]
68. Michie, S.; Johnston, M.; Francis, J.; Hardeman, W.; Eccles, M. From Theory to Intervention: Mapping Theoretically Derived Behavioural Determinants to Behaviour Change Techniques. *Appl. Psychol.* **2008**, *57*, 660–680. [CrossRef]
69. Whitford, D.L.; Roberts, S.H.; Griffin, S. Sustainability and effectiveness of comprehensive diabetes care to a district population. *Diabet. Med.* **2004**, *21*, 1221–1228. [CrossRef] [PubMed]
70. Barrera-Cancedda, A.E.; Riman, K.A.; Shinnick, J.E.; Buttenheim, A.M. Implementation strategies for infection prevention and control promotion for nurses in Sub-Saharan Africa: A systematic review. *Implement. Sci.* **2019**, *14*, 111. [CrossRef]
71. Opiyo, N.; Ciapponi, A.; Dudley, L.; Gagnon, M.-P.; Herrera, C.; Lewin, S.; Martí, S.G.; Oxman, A.D.; Paulsen, E.; Penaloza, B.; et al. Implementation strategies for health systems in low-income countries: An overview of systematic reviews. *Cochrane Database Syst. Rev.* **2014**, *9*, CD011086. [CrossRef]
72. Johnson, L.G.; Armstrong, A.; Joyce, C.M.; Teitelman, A.M.; Buttenheim, A.M. Implementation strategies to improve cervical cancer prevention in sub-Saharan Africa: A systematic review. *Implement. Sci.* **2018**, *13*, 28. [CrossRef]

73. Elwyn, G.; Scholl, I.; Tietbohl, C.; Mann, M.; Edwards, A.G.K.; Clay, C.; Légaré, F.; Van Der Weijden, T.; Lewis, C.L.; Wexler, R.M.; et al. "Many miles to go ... ": A systematic review of the implementation of patient decision support interventions into routine clinical practice. *BMC Med. Inform. Decis. Mak.* **2013**, *13*, S14. [CrossRef] [PubMed]
74. Scholl, I.; LaRussa, A.; Hahlweg, P.; Kobrin, S.; Elwyn, G. Organizational- and system-level characteristics that influence implementation of shared decision-making and strategies to address them—A scoping review. *Implement. Sci.* **2018**, *13*, 40. [CrossRef]
75. Joseph-Williams, N.; Lloyd, A.; Edwards, A.; Stobbart, L.; Tomson, D.; Macphail, S.; Dodd, C.; Brain, K.; Elwyn, G.; Thomson, R. Implementing shared decision making in the NHS: Lessons from the MAGIC programme. *BMJ* **2017**, *357*, j1744. [CrossRef]
76. Yapa, H.M.; Bärnighausen, T. Implementation science in resource-poor countries and communities. *Implement. Sci.* **2018**, *13*, 154. [CrossRef] [PubMed]
77. Eccles, M.P.; Mittman, B.S. Welcome to Implementation Science. *Implement. Sci.* **2006**, *1*, 13. [CrossRef]
78. Kalbarczyk, A.; Davis, W.; Kalibala, S.; Geibel, S.; Yansaneh, A.; Martin, N.A.; Weiss, E.; Kerrigan, D.; Manabe, Y.C. Research Capacity Strengthening in Sub-Saharan Africa: Recognising the Importance of Local Partnerships in Designing and Disseminating HIV Implementation Science to Reach the 90-90-90 Goals. *AIDS Behav.* **2019**, *23* (Suppl. 2), 206–213. [CrossRef]
79. Osanjo, G.O.; Oyugi, J.O.; Kibwage, I.O.; Mwanda, W.O.; Ngugi, E.N.; Otieno, F.C.; Ndege, W.; Child, M.; Farquhar, C.; Penner, J.; et al. Building capacity in implementation science research training at the University of Nairobi. *Implement. Sci.* **2015**, *11*, 30. [CrossRef]
80. Iwelunmor, J.; Blackstone, S.; Veira, D.; Nwaozuru, U.; Airhihenbuwa, C.; Munodawafa, D.; Kalipeni, E.; Jutal, A.; Shelley, D.; Ogedegbe, G. Toward the sustainability of health interventions implemented in sub-Saharan Africa: A systematic review and conceptual framework. *Implement. Sci.* **2015**, *11*, 43. [CrossRef]
81. World Bank Group. *Africa's Pulse, No. 16*; World Bank: Washington, DC, USA, 2017.
82. WHO. *The Abuja Declaration: Ten Years On*; WHO: Geneva, Switzerland, 2011.
83. The Federal Democratic Republic of Ethiopia Ministry of Health. *Health Sector Transformation Plan: 2015/16–2019/20*; The Federal Democratic Republic of Ethiopia Ministry of Health: Addis Ababa, Ethiopia, 2015.
84. Ministry of Health of Ethiopia. *Ethiopian National Health Care Quality Strategy: 2016–2020*; Ministry of Health of Ethiopia: Addis Ababa, Ethiopia, 2016.
85. Ministry of Health of Ethiopia. *Essential Health Services Package of Ethiopia*; Ministry of Health of Ethiopia: Addis Ababa, Ethiopia, 2019.
86. Manyazewal, T.; Matlakala, M. Implementing health care reform: Implications for performance of public hospitals in central Ethiopia. *J. Glob. Health* **2018**, *8*, 010403. [CrossRef]
87. Walker, R.J.; Smalls, B.L.; Bonilha, H.S.; Campbell, J.A.; Egede, L.E. Behavioral interventions to improve glycemic control in African Americans with type 2 diabetes: A systematic review. *Ethn. Dis.* **2013**, *23*, 401–408.
88. Flood, D.; Hane, J.; Dunn, M.; Brown, S.J.; Wagenaar, B.H.; Rogers, E.A.; Heisler, M.; Rohloff, P.; Chopra, V. Health system interventions for adults with type 2 diabetes in low- and middle-income countries: A systematic review and meta-analysis. *PLoS Med.* **2020**, *17*, e1003434. [CrossRef] [PubMed]
89. Tricco, A.C.; Ivers, N.M.; Grimshaw, J.; Moher, D.; Turner, L.; Galipeau, J.; Halperin, I.; Vachon, B.; Ramsay, T.; Manns, B.; et al. Effectiveness of quality improvement strategies on the management of diabetes: A systematic review and meta-analysis. *Lancet* **2012**, *379*, 2252–2261. [CrossRef]
90. Murphy, A.L.; Gardner, D.M.; Kutcher, S.P.; Martin-Misener, R. A theory-informed approach to mental health care capacity building for pharmacists. *Int. J. Ment. Health Syst.* **2014**, *8*, 46. [CrossRef]
91. Hood, K.K.; Hilliard, M.; Piatt, G.A.; Ievers-Landis, C.E. Effective strategies for encouraging behavior change in people with diabetes. *Diabetes Manag.* **2015**, *5*, 499–510. [CrossRef]
92. Cadogan, C.A.; Ryan, C.; Francis, J.J.; Gormley, G.J.; Passmore, P.; Kerse, N.; Hughes, C.M. Improving appropriate polypharmacy for older people in primary care: Selecting components of an evidence-based intervention to target prescribing and dispensing. *Implement. Sci.* **2015**, *10*, 161. [CrossRef] [PubMed]
93. Chauhan, B.F.; Jeyaraman, M.; Mann, A.S.; Lys, J.; Skidmore, B.; Sibley, K.M.; Abou-Setta, A.M.; Zarychanksi, R. Behavior change interventions and policies influencing primary healthcare professionals' practice—An overview of reviews. *Implement. Sci.* **2017**, *12*, 3. [CrossRef] [PubMed]
94. Nielsen, K.; Abildgaard, J.S. Organisational interventions: A research-based framework for the evaluation of both process and effects. *Work Stress* **2013**, *27*, 278–297. [CrossRef]
95. Clement, M.; Filteau, P.; Harvey, B.; Jin, S.; Laubscher, T.; Mukerji, G.; Sherifali, D. Organization of Diabetes Care. *Can. J. Diabetes* **2018**, *42*, S27–S35. [CrossRef] [PubMed]
96. American Association of Diabetes Educators. An Effective Model of Diabetes Care and Education: Revising the AADE7 Self-Care Behaviors®. *Diabetes Educ.* **2020**, *46*, 139–160. [CrossRef] [PubMed]
97. Jones, A.; Bardram, J.E.; Bækgaard, P.; Cramer-Petersen, C.L.; Skinner, T.; Vrangbæk, K.; Starr, L.; Nørgaard, K.; Lind, N.; Christensen, M.B.; et al. Integrated spersonalised diabetes management goes Europe: A multi-disciplinary approach to innovating type 2 diabetes care in Europe. *Prim. Care Diabetes* **2021**, *15*, 360–364. [CrossRef]
98. Mercer, T.; Chang, A.C.; Fischer, L.; Gardner, A.; Kerubo, I.; Tran, D.N.; Laktabai, J.; Pastakia, S. Mitigating The Burden Of Diabetes in Sub-Saharan Africa Through an Integrated Diagonal Health Systems Approach. *Diabetes Metab. Syndr. Obes. Targets Ther.* **2019**, *12*, 2261–2272. [CrossRef]

99. Mohan, V.; Khunti, K.; Chan, S.P.; Filho, F.F.; Tran, N.Q.; Ramaiya, K.; Joshi, S.; Mithal, A.; Mbaye, M.N.; Nicodemus, N.J.; et al. Management of Type 2 Diabetes in Developing Countries: Balancing Optimal Glycaemic Control and Outcomes with Affordability and Accessibility to Treatment. *Diabetes Ther.* **2020**, *11*, 15–35. [CrossRef]
100. Hellquist, K.; Bradley, R.; Grambart, S.; Kapustin, J.; Loch, J. Collaborative Practice Benefits Patients: An Examination of Interprofessional Approaches to Diabetes Care. *Health Interprof. Pract.* **2012**, *1*, eP1017. [CrossRef]
101. Lankhof, B. Perceptions of Collaboration and Mutual Respect Among Members of Interprofessional Teams. Ph.D. Thesis, Walden University, Minneapolis, MN, USA, 2018.
102. Yorke, E.; Atiase, Y. Impact of structured education on glucose control and hypoglycaemia in Type-2 diabetes: A systematic review of srandomised controlled trials. *Ghana Med. J.* **2018**, *52*, 41–60. [CrossRef] [PubMed]
103. Chrvala, C.A.; Sherr, D.; Lipman, R.D. Diabetes self-management education for adults with type 2 diabetes mellitus: A systematic review of the effect on glycemic control. *Patient Educ. Couns.* **2016**, *99*, 926–943. [CrossRef] [PubMed]
104. Zhang, Y.; Chu, L. Effectiveness of Systematic Health Education Model for Type 2 Diabetes Patients. *Int. J. Endocrinol.* **2018**, *2018*, 6530607. [CrossRef] [PubMed]
105. Mohamed, A.; Staite, E.; Ismail, K.; Winkley, K. A systematic review of diabetes self-management education interventions for people with type 2 diabetes mellitus in the Asian Western Pacific (AWP) region. *Nurs. Open* **2019**, *6*, 1424–1437. [CrossRef] [PubMed]
106. Do Rosario Pinto, M.; Parreira, P.; Basto, M.L.; Dos Santos Mendes Monico, L. Impact of a structured multicomponent educational intervention program on metabolic control of patients with type 2 diabetes. *BMC Endocr. Disord.* **2017**, *17*, 77. [CrossRef]

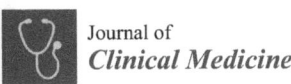

Article

Sex-Related Disparities in the Prevalence of Depression among Patients Hospitalized with Type 2 Diabetes Mellitus in Spain, 2011–2020

Ana Lopez-de-Andres [1], Rodrigo Jimenez-Garcia [1,*], Javier de Miguel-Díez [2], Valentin Hernández-Barrera [3], Jose Luis del Barrio [3], David Carabantes-Alarcon [1], Jose J. Zamorano-Leon [1] and Concepcion Noriega [4]

1. Department of Public Health and Maternal & Child Health, Faculty of Medicine, Universidad Complutense de Madrid, Instituto de Investigación Sanitaria del Hospital Clínico San Carlos (IdISSC), 28040 Madrid, Spain
2. Respiratory Department, Hospital General Universitario Gregorio Marañón, Facultad de Medicina, Universidad Complutense de Madrid, Instituto de Investigación Sanitaria Gregorio Marañón (IiSGM), 28007 Madrid, Spain
3. Preventive Medicine and Public Health Teaching and Research Unit, Health Sciences Faculty, Universidad Rey Juan Carlos, 28922 Alcorcón, Spain
4. Department of Nursery and Physiotherapy, Faculty of Medicine and Health Sciences, University of Alcalá, Alcalá de Henares, 28801 Madrid, Spain
* Correspondence: rodrijim@ucm.es; Tel.: +34-913-941-520

Abstract: (1) Background: Recent reports suggest a decrease in the prevalence of depression among people with diabetes and important sex-differences in the association between these conditions, however data from Spain is sparse. We aim to assess trends in the prevalence of depression and in-hospital outcomes among patients with type 2 diabetes (T2DM) hospitalized (2011–2020) identifying sex-differences. (2) Methods: Using the Spanish national hospital discharge database we analysed the prevalence of depression globally, by sex, and according to the conditions included in the Charlson comorbidity index (CCI). We tested factors associated with the presence of depression and with in-hospital mortality (IHM). Time trends in the prevalence of depression and variables independently associated with IHM were analyzed using multivariable logistic regression. (3) Results: From 2011 to 2020, we identified 5,971,917 hospitalizations of patients with T2DM (5.7% involved depression). The prevalence of depression decreased significantly between 2011 and 2020. The adjusted prevalence of depression was 3.32-fold higher in women than in men (OR 3.32; 95%CI 3.3–3.35). The highest prevalence of depression among men and women with T2DM was found among those who also had a diagnosis of obesity, liver disease, and COPD. Older age, higher CCI, pneumonia, and having been hospitalized in 2020 increased the risk of IHM in patients with T2DM and depression. Obesity was a protective factor for IHM in both sexes, with no differences detected for IHM between men and women. Among patients hospitalized with T2DM, concomitant depression was associated with lower IHM than among patients without depression (depression paradox). (4) Conclusions: The prevalence of depression decreased over time in both sexes. The prevalence of depression was over three-fold higher in women. Female sex and depression were not associated with higher IHM. Based on our results we recommend that clinicians screen regularly for depression in patients with T2DM, particularly women, younger patients, and those with multiple comorbidities.

Keywords: type 2 diabetes; depression; sex; in-hospital mortality; hospitalization

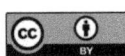

1. Introduction

Diabetes is one of the largest global public health problems, is among the top 10 causes of death globally, and has the second biggest negative total effect on reducing global health adjusted life expectancy worldwide [1]. The Global Burden of Disease (GBD) has demonstrated a large and inexorably increasing burden of diabetes in the world since 1990 [1]. In Spain, according to the GBD, the prevalence and Disability-Adjusted Life

Years (DALYs) have increased from 2000 to 2019 from 8.90% to 11.26% and from 3.80% to 4.15% [2].

In year 2019 depressive disorders ranked 13th among the leading causes of burden worldwide with a significant greater burden in females than males [3]. Worldwide, the prevalence of depression among adults has been estimated to be between 15% and 18%, and an increase in the burden of this disease worldwide is projected in the coming decades [4]. In our country the time trend (2000–2019) has shown an increase in the prevalence from 3.57% to 4.24% among men with equivalent figures of 5.72% to 7.71% among women. For both sexes, the DALYs also rose from 2.64% to 3.70% [2].

Like other chronic diseases, type 2 diabetes (T2DM) predisposes to depression [5–7]. The presence of complications, including depression, increases the risk of hospitalization among people with T2DM [8]. Depression as a comorbidity of T2DM can alter glycaemic control, reduce adherence to treatment, increase the risk of cardiac complications, health care utilization, costs, and increased mortality risk [9]. In their meta-analysis, Nouwen et al. [10] found that the presence of complications in patients with diabetes increased the likelihood of incident depressive disorder (hazard ratio [HR] 1.14; 95% confidence interval [95% CI]: 1.07–1.21). However, other authors, after adjusting for the presence of comorbidities such as coronary heart disease, found no significant association between T2DM and depression [11,12].

The association between depression and T2DM is thought to be bidirectional [13,14]; however, the role of the factors that modulate this association remains controversial [15]. Depression is associated with inadequate lifestyles (sedentary lifestyle, poor diet, obesity), with increased hypothalamic-pituitary-adrenal axis activity, and with increased levels of stress hormones and proinflammatory cytokines [16]. All these factors may affect insulin resistance and subsequently the presence of T2DM [17].

Recognizing and addressing depression among patients with diabetes is an important step in improving outcomes and reducing the growing burden of diabetes care [18]. Studies conducted in the last decades of the past century and first years of the current century showed that the prevalence of depression among people with diabetes was increasing in our country and elsewhere [17–20]. However, more recent investigations suggest that a change in the time trend may be taking place [21–23]. The lack of recent reports in our country makes necessary to confirm if this new tendency is also happening.

In patients with T2DM and depression, sex differences may play a critical role in the incidence and outcomes of hospitalizations, and meta-analyses have concluded that women with T2DM have a higher prevalence of depression than men with T2DM [24,25]. In 2015, the results of a population study in Spain found that the prevalence of depression was over 2.7 times higher in women with T2DM than in men with T2DM [19]. The probability of being diagnosed with depression in patients with T2DM differs by sex [26–28].

There is very little information on the consequences of diabetes-depression comorbidity in the hospital outcomes in Spain [19]. Furthermore, even if no doubt exists regarding the sex-differences in the prevalence of depression among people with diabetes the frequency of other comorbid conditions and how these conditions affect the hospital outcomes among men and women has not been analysed in our country so far.

Therefore, the objective of our study, which was based on national administrative data, was to describe trends in the prevalence of depression in patients with T2DM hospitalized in Spain from 2011 to 2020. Furthermore, we analyzed sex differences in the prevalence of depression among women and men with T2DM according to specific hospital admission diagnoses and the effect of depression on hospital outcomes.

2. Materials and Methods

We conducted a population-based cohort study using data from a registry of hospital discharges in Spain (Register of Specialized Care–Basic Minimum Database, RAE-CMBD) collected from 1 January 2011 to 31 December 2020.

The methodological characteristics of the RAE-CMBD have been described elsewhere [29]. Coding in this database was with the International Classification of Diseases

(ICD), Ninth Revision, for the period between 2011 and 2015 (ICD-9), and the Tenth Revision (ICD-10) from the year 2016 onwards.

The study population included patients aged ≥35 years with a T2DM code in any diagnostic position (see ICD codes in Table S1). Patients with T1DM were excluded.

To respond to the objective of the study, the study population was stratified according to the presence of ICD codes for depression (Table S1) in any diagnostic position in the RAE-CMBD. All analyses were subsequently stratified according to sex.

To determine the prevalence of depression based on the most frequent hospital admission diagnoses, we used the conditions included in the Charlson Comorbidity Index (CCI) in any diagnostic position, excluding diabetes [30,31]. The presence of codes for obesity and pneumonia was also analysed. Table S1 shows the ICD-9 and ICD-10 codes corresponding to the diagnoses included in our investigation.

Regarding hospital outcomes, we analysed length of hospital stay (LOHS) and in-hospital mortality (IHM).

2.1. Statistical Analysis

For all the study years, we calculated the total prevalence of depression in patients with T2DM. The prevalence of depression was stratified by sex, age group, and the above-mentioned clinical diagnoses.

Prevalence was calculated by dividing the number of cases of depression in each year by the number of patients with T2DM in each year and subgroup analysed.

The results of the descriptive statistical analysis are expressed as total frequencies with percentages and means with standard deviations for categorical variables and as medians with interquartile range for continuous variables.

The trend was analysed using the Cochran-Mantel-Haenszel statistic or Cochran-Armitage test in the case of categorical variables and a linear regression t test or Jonckheere-Terpstra test in the case of continuous variables.

Categorical variables were compared using the Fisher exact test. Continuous variables were compared using the t test or the Wilcoxon rank sum test, as required.

We used multivariable logistic regression to analyse factors associated with the presence of depression, taking into account the effect of sex. We also identified the variables associated with IHM in men and women with T2DM and depression.

Finally, we used logistic regression to assess the effect of depression on IHM in both men and women with T2DM. Models were constructed for the concomitant clinical conditions included in the CCI, obesity, and pneumonia.

The results were presented using the odds ratio (OR) and 95% CI.

We used version 14 of Stata to perform the statistical analysis (Stata, College Station, TX, USA). Statistical significance was set at $p < 0.05$ (2-tailed).

2.2. Ethics

To carry out this study, it was not necessary to request the informed consent of the patients or approval by an ethics committee, since the RAE-CMBD is anonymous and can be requested from the Spanish Ministry of Health [32].

3. Results

During the period 2011–2020 in Spain, there were 5,971,917 hospitalizations of patients aged ≥ 35 years who had an ICD diagnostic code corresponding to T2DM. Of these, 333,226 (5.57%) had an ICD code for depression.

The overall prevalence of depression among patients hospitalized with T2DM in Spain decreased significantly between 2011 and 2020 (5.72% vs. 5.04%; $p < 0.05$); however, it should be noted that the prevalence increased between 2011 and 2015, before decreasing from 2016 to 2020 (Table 1).

Regarding the distribution of the study population according to sex, the proportion of women decreased (71.25% in 2011 vs. 67.89% in 2020; $p < 0.05$), whereas that of men increased (28.75% in 2011 vs. 32.11% in 2020; $p < 0.05$). The mean age of patients with depression, as well as the associated comorbidity based on the CCI, increased significantly throughout the study period (Table 1).

Between 2011 and 2020, the prevalence of depression coded as the primary diagnosis decreased (1.23% in 2011 vs. 0.96% in 2020; $p < 0.05$) (Table 1).

In men with T2DM, the prevalence of depression decreased significantly throughout the study period (2.97% in 2011 vs. 2.75% in 2020). Significant increases were also observed during 2011–2020 for mean age (69.96 years vs. 72.67 years), the presence of associated comorbidity (mean CCI 2.82 vs. 3.3), and a diagnosis of obesity (11.11% vs. 15.25%).

The crude IHM increased significantly between 2011 and 2020 (5.93% vs. 8.89%) (Table 2).

The trend for women with T2DM was similar to that of men regarding prevalence (9.15% in 2011 vs. 8.32% in 2020), mean age (73.42 years vs. 76.51 years), comorbidity (mean CCI 2.35 vs. 2.86), and the presence of obesity (21.74% vs. 24.08%). The crude IHM almost doubled (4.88% vs. 8.58%) over the 10 years analysed (Table 2).

Table 3 shows the prevalence of depression among people with T2DM who also had other specific diagnoses. The highest prevalence of depression among men and women with T2DM was found among those who also had a diagnosis of obesity, liver disease, and COPD. A remarkable finding was the very high prevalence of depression among obese women with diabetes, ranging from 10% to 12% over the study period.

The prevalence of depression decreased significantly between 2011 and 2020, in men and women with T2DM who also had kidney disease, liver disease, cancer, and obesity. However, in patients with peripheral vascular disease and COPD, the prevalence of depression increased significantly.

Throughout the study period and for all specific hospital admission diagnoses, the prevalence of depression was higher in women with T2DM than in men with T2DM ($p < 0.05$).

For all the specific hospital admission diagnoses analysed, IHM was significantly lower in women with T2DM and depression than in women without depression. This association was also found in men with T2DM and depression, except for those with acute myocardial infarction and cancer (Table 4).

Table 5 presents the results of the multivariable analysis to identify the factors associated with the presence of depression and with IHM in men and women with T2DM and depression. Older age and the most recent years of hospital admission (years 2018, 2019, and 2020) were associated with a lower risk of depression. However, the prevalence of depression increased significantly during the years 2013, 2014, and 2015 in both men and women with T2DM. The presence of more comorbid conditions based on the CCI and obesity was associated with a higher probability of a code for depression in both men and women. In the T2DM population, and after adjusting for age and all the comorbid conditions, women were 3.32-fold more likely to have a code for depression in their discharge report than men (OR 3.32; 95%CI 3.3–3.35).

Table 1. Characteristics of the patients hospitalized with type 2 diabetes suffering concomitant depression according to year (2011–2020).

	2011	2012	2013	2014	2015	2016	2017	2018	2019	2020
Depression, n	31,101	32,236	34,471	36,401	37,684	30,669	34,680	32,218	33,475	30,291
Depression, prevalence (%) *	5.72	5.79	6.05	6.19	6.21	5.41	5.57	4.94	5.03	5.04
Men, n (%) *	8941 (28.75)	9260 (28.73)	10,132 (29.39)	10,323 (28.36)	11,042 (29.3)	9500 (30.98)	10,477 (30.21)	10,026 (31.12)	10,572 (31.58)	9727 (32.11)
Women, n (%) *	22,160 (71.25)	22,976 (71.27)	24,339 (70.61)	26,078 (71.64)	26,642 (70.7)	21,169 (69.02)	24,203 (69.79)	22,192 (68.88)	22,903 (68.42)	20,564 (67.89)
Age, mean (SD) *	72.42 (11.41)	72.81 (11.36)	72.9 (11.43)	73.08 (11.44)	73.55 (11.45)	74.14 (11.39)	74.51 (11.34)	74.89 (11.26)	75.12 (11.22)	75.28 (11.28)
CCI, mean (SD) *	2.49 (1.65)	2.51 (1.65)	2.55 (1.69)	2.55 (1.69)	2.55 (1.65)	2.8 (1.8)	2.84 (1.81)	2.9 (1.87)	2.98 (1.91)	3 (1.94)
Depression as first diagnosis, n (%) *	382 (1.23)	398 (1.23)	382 (1.11)	372 (1.02)	404 (1.07)	344 (1.12)	344 (0.99)	382 (1.19)	323 (0.96)	291 (0.96)

CCI: Charlson Comorbidity Index. * $p < 0.05$ (time trend analysis).

Table 2. Prevalence of depression, distribution by age and clinical characteristics and in-hospital outcomes among men and women hospitalized with type 2 diabetes in Spain 2011–2020.

		2011	2012	2013	2014	2015	2016	2017	2018	2019	2020
Men	Depression, n (Prevalence) *	8941 (2.97)	9260 (2.99)	10,132 (3.16)	10,323 (3.12)	11,042 (3.21)	9500 (2.94)	10,477 (2.93)	10,026 (2.65)	10,572 (2.73)	9727 (2.75)
	Age, mean (SD) *	69.96 (11.73)	70.16 (11.70)	70.17 (11.74)	70.51 (11.87)	70.92 (11.78)	71.28 (11.83)	71.77 (11.60)	72.17 (11.54)	72.63 (11.34)	72.67 (11.48)
	35–59 year, n (%) *	1824 (3.72)	1810 (3.72)	2068 (4.14)	2061 (4.09)	1974 (3.90)	1708 (3.68)	1685 (3.44)	1513 (3.01)	1491 (2.97)	1413 (3.02)
	60–69 year, n (%) *	2177 (2.94)	2322 (3.03)	2552 (3.19)	2522 (3.08)	2766 (3.35)	2218 (2.88)	2612 (3.07)	2413 (2.70)	2449 (2.70)	2182 (2.64)
	70–79 year, n (%) *	2833 (2.74)	2922 (2.81)	3013 (2.86)	3025 (2.80)	3299 (2.96)	2851 (2.74)	3088 (2.71)	3040 (2.46)	3352 (2.57)	3110 (2.63)
	≥80 year, n (%) *	2107 (2.82)	2206 (2.73)	2499 (2.94)	2715 (2.98)	3003 (3.03)	2723 (2.84)	3092 (2.83)	3060 (2.65)	3280 (2.82)	3022 (2.85)
	CCI, mean (SD) *	2.82 (1.82)	2.83 (1.80)	2.86 (1.83)	2.86 (1.82)	2.83 (1.78)	3.14 (1.96)	3.18 (1.97)	3.23 (2)	3.29 (2.06)	3.3 (2.09)
	Obesity, n (%) *	993 (11.11)	1001 (10.81)	1167 (11.52)	1275 (12.35)	1440 (13.04)	1316 (13.85)	1507 (14.38)	1469 (14.65)	1550 (14.66)	1483 (15.25)
	LHS, median (IQR)	6 (8)	6 (8)	6 (8)	6 (7)	6 (7)	6 (8)	6 (8)	6 (8)	6 (8)	6 (8)
	IHM, n (%) *	530 (5.93)	526 (5.68)	583 (5.75)	542 (5.25)	626 (5.67)	561 (5.91)	691 (6.60)	687 (6.85)	736 (6.96)	865 (8.89)
Women	Depression, n (Prevalence) *	22,160 (9.15)	22,976 (9.33)	24,339 (9.75)	26,078 (10.16)	26,642 (10.14)	21,169 (8.71)	24,203 (9.13)	22,192 (8.11)	22,903 (8.23)	20,564 (8.32)
	Age, mean (SD) *	73.42 (11.12)	73.88 (11.04)	74.03 (11.11)	74.1 (11.10)	74.64 (11.14)	75.42 (10.95)	75.7 (11.02)	76.13 (10.91)	76.27 (10.97)	76.51 (10.97)
	35–59 year, n (%) *	2802 (12.14)	2732 (12.03)	2831 (12.14)	2981 (12.33)	2858 (12.14)	2084 (9.62)	2271 (9.87)	1927 (8.26)	1936 (7.93)	1695 (7.81)
	60–69 year, n (%) *	4315 (11.21)	4530 (11.60)	4727 (11.81)	5129 (12.66)	4990 (12.50)	3638 (10.19)	4237 (10.78)	3709 (9.26)	3828 (9.51)	3300 (9.24)
	70–79 year, n (%) *	7718 (9.65)	7675 (9.78)	8032 (10.36)	8351 (10.80)	8458 (11.05)	6616 (9.46)	7278 (9.97)	6683 (8.79)	6921 (8.81)	6286 (9.14)
	≥80 year, n (%) *	7325 (7.28)	8039 (7.58)	8749 (8.04)	9617 (8.39)	10,336 (8.42)	8831 (7.64)	10,417 (8.02)	9873 (7.36)	10,218 (7.57)	9283 (7.67)
	CCI, mean (SD) *	2.35 (1.56)	2.38 (1.57)	2.43 (1.61)	2.42 (1.62)	2.43 (1.59)	2.65 (1.70)	2.69 (1.72)	2.75 (1.79)	2.83 (1.81)	2.86 (1.86)

Table 2. Cont.

	2011	2012	2013	2014	2015	2016	2017	2018	2019	2020
Obesity, n (%) *	4817 (21.74)	4858 (21.14)	5427 (22.30)	5772 (22.13)	5957 (22.36)	5093 (24.06)	5730 (23.67)	5010 (22.58)	5567 (24.31)	4951 (24.08)
LHS, median (IQR)	6 (8)	6 (7)	6 (7)	6 (7)	6 (7)	6 (7)	6 (7)	6 (7)	6 (7)	6 (7)
IHM, n (%) *	1081 (4.88)	1185 (5.16)	1209 (4.97)	1266 (4.85)	1423 (5.34)	1221 (5.77)	1473 (6.09)	1398 (6.3)	1467 (6.41)	1764 (8.58)

Prevalence: Prevalence of depression among patients hospitalized with type 2 diabetes. CCI: Charlson Comorbidity Index. LHS: length of hospital stay. IQR interquartile range. IHM: in-hospital mortality. * $p < 0.05$ (time trend analysis).

Table 3. Prevalence of depression among men and women hospitalized with type 2 diabetes, according to the presence of selected concomitant conditions in Spain from year 2011 to year 2020.

		2011	2012	2013	2014	2015	2016	2017	2018	2019	2020
Acute myocardial infarction, n (%)	Men *	697 (2.5)	620 (2.25)	724 (2.65)	664 (2.48)	703 (2.6)	870 (2.48)	969 (2.36)	1032 (2.25)	1117 (2.28)	998 (2.22)
	Women *	862 (6.8)	834 (6.69)	846 (6.79)	948 (8.02)	866 (7.61)	957 (6.74)	1219 (7.58)	1175 (6.76)	1237 (6.71)	1176 (7)
Congestive heart failure, n (%)	Men *	1212 (2.41)	1296 (2.46)	1427 (2.57)	1466 (2.57)	1568 (2.57)	1656 (2.73)	1829 (2.69)	1853 (2.48)	1971 (2.51)	1770 (2.52)
	Women *	4154 (7.84)	4278 (7.74)	4545 (8.16)	4734 (8.24)	4918 (8.21)	4725 (8.17)	5432 (8.51)	5051 (7.53)	5433 (7.76)	4612 (7.65)
Peripheral vascular disease, n (%)	Men *	789 (2.25)	854 (2.37)	947 (2.43)	961 (2.44)	977 (2.41)	1022 (2.63)	1145 (2.64)	1153 (2.51)	1219 (2.5)	1093 (2.39)
	Women *	808 (6.69)	821 (6.77)	916 (7.21)	929 (7.48)	924 (7.25)	835 (7.46)	951 (7.73)	822 (6.76)	951 (7.05)	861 (6.9)
Cerebrovascular disease, n (%)	Men	1142 (3.48)	1251 (3.65)	1296 (3.69)	1287 (3.54)	1383 (3.73)	1282 (3.73)	1453 (3.77)	1382 (3.43)	1512 (3.59)	1345 (3.49)
	Women *	2415 (9.05)	2571 (9.6)	2716 (9.86)	2828 (10.26)	2816 (10.18)	2325 (9.18)	2751 (9.97)	2280 (8.19)	2622 (8.9)	2298 (8.69)
COPD, n (%)	Men *	2286 (3.04)	2443 (3.17)	2581 (3.29)	2734 (3.37)	2887 (3.4)	2535 (3.34)	2868 (3.42)	2607 (3)	2808 (3.19)	2389 (3.2)
	Women *	3528 (9.95)	3821 (10.26)	4253 (10.97)	4489 (10.89)	4755 (11.08)	3829 (11.75)	4339 (11.88)	3600 (10.09)	3834 (10.29)	3258 (10.37)
Renal disease, n (%)	Men *	1162 (2.33)	1257 (2.3)	1528 (2.56)	1574 (2.46)	1716 (2.45)	1951 (2.77)	2279 (2.81)	2222 (2.5)	2358 (2.5)	2254 (2.6)
	Women *	2435 (6.57)	2725 (6.77)	3089 (7.1)	3404 (7.23)	3785 (7.42)	3979 (7.77)	4794 (8.05)	4612 (7.27)	4934 (7.37)	4541 (7.5)
Liver disease, n (%)	Men *	805 (3.02)	902 (3.29)	1016 (3.47)	1043 (3.4)	1114 (3.52)	966 (3.33)	1131 (3.4)	1143 (3.12)	1173 (2.97)	1072 (2.91)
	Women *	1376 (10.28)	1497 (10.54)	1592 (10.8)	1857 (11.79)	1854 (11.61)	1480 (10.58)	1895 (11.63)	1758 (10.03)	1897 (9.95)	1817 (10.23)
Cancer, n (%)	Men *	1440 (2.72)	1421 (2.58)	1577 (2.74)	1574 (2.64)	1630 (2.68)	1536 (2.62)	1691 (2.56)	1563 (2.23)	1685 (2.3)	1528 (2.31)
	Women *	2090 (8.45)	2125 (8.25)	2368 (8.95)	2489 (9.07)	2577 (9.45)	2027 (7.77)	2287 (7.88)	2227 (7.34)	2325 (7.33)	2100 (7.26)
Obesity, n (%)	Men *	993 (3.41)	1001 (3.21)	1167 (3.42)	1275 (3.51)	1440 (3.74)	1316 (3.56)	1507 (3.51)	1469 (3.12)	1550 (3.1)	1483 (3.03)
	Women *	4817 (12.15)	4858 (11.73)	5427 (12.55)	5772 (12.72)	5957 (12.79)	5093 (11.54)	5730 (11.5)	5010 (9.94)	5567 (10.4)	4951 (10.26)
Pneumonia, n (%)	Men	735 (3.13)	808 (3.28)	818 (3.43)	841 (3.21)	974 (3.37)	719 (3.43)	779 (3.24)	763 (2.96)	789 (3.13)	644 (3.08)
	Women *	1318 (8.34)	1460 (8.77)	1409 (8.96)	1604 (9.19)	1921 (9.7)	1201 (9.34)	1381 (9.48)	1359 (8.7)	1295 (8.61)	1014 (8.67)

COPD: chronic obstructive pulmonary disease. Liver disease: moderate or severe. * $p < 0.05$ (time trend analysis).

Table 4. In-hospital mortality among men and women hospitalized with type 2 diabetes, according to selected concomitant condition and to the presence of depression in Spain for the period 2011–2020.

	IHM Men			IHM Women		
	Without Depression	With Depression	p-Value	Without Depression	With Depression	p-Value
Acute myocardial infarction, n (%)	25,562 (7.43)	587 (6.99)	0.132	14,672 (10.99)	904 (8.93)	<0.001
Congestive heart failure, n (%)	62,701 (10.23)	1525 (9.5)	0.003	64,516 (11.68)	4220 (8.81)	<0.001
Peripheral vascular disease, n (%)	28,165 (7)	656 (6.46)	0.034	11,607 (10.1)	700 (7.94)	<0.001
Cerebrovascular disease, n (%)	37,223 (10.45)	1104 (8.28)	<0.001	32,625 (13.19)	2352 (9.18)	<0.001
COPD, n (%)	58,614 (7.52)	1737 (6.65)	<0.001	23,433 (7.11)	1877 (4.73)	<0.001
Renal disease, n (%)	66,215 (9.44)	1535 (8.39)	<0.001	53,524 (11.1)	3254 (8.5)	<0.001
Liver disease, n (%)	25,559 (8.23)	636 (6.14)	<0.001	12,184 (8.6)	990 (5.82)	<0.001
Cancer, n (%)	76,108 (12.59)	1973 (12.61)	0.946	34,828 (13.65)	2866 (12.67)	<0.001
Obesity, n (%)	16,404 (4.29)	474 (3.59)	<0.001	23,860 (5.83)	2218 (4.17)	<0.001
Pneumonia, n (%)	36,745 (15.56)	1134 (14.41)	0.006	24,602 (17.41)	1760 (12.61)	<0.001

IHM: in-hospital mortality. COPD: chronic obstructive pulmonary disease.

Table 5. Multivariate analysis of the factors associated with the presence of depression among men and women hospitalized with type 2 diabetes and factors associated with in-hospital mortality among patients with type 2 diabetes and concomitant depression., Spain 2011–2020.

	Presence of Depression			IHM of Patients with T2DM and Depression		
	Men	Women	Both Sexes	Men	Women	Both Sexes
	OR (95%CI)	OR (95%CI)	OR (95%CI)	OR (95%CI)	OR (95%CI)	OR (95%CI)
Year 2011	1	1	1	1	1	1
Year 2012	1.01 (0.98–1.04)	1.03 (1.01–1.05)	1.02 (1–1.04)	0.95 (0.83–1.07)	1.03 (0.94–1.12)	1 (0.93–1.07)
Year 2013	1.07 (1.04–1.1)	1.08 (1.06–1.1)	1.07 (1.06–1.09)	0.95 (0.84–1.08)	0.97 (0.89–1.05)	0.96 (0.9–1.03)
Year 2014	1.05 (1.02–1.08)	1.13 (1.11–1.15)	1.11 (1.09–1.12)	0.86 (0.75–0.97)	0.93 (0.86–1.01)	0.91 (0.85–0.97)
Year 2015	1.09 (1.06–1.12)	1.13 (1.11–1.16)	1.12 (1.1–1.14)	0.92 (0.81–1.03)	1 (0.92–1.09)	0.97 (0.91–1.04)
Year 2016	1 (0.97–1.03)	0.96 (0.94–0.98)	0.97 (0.96–0.99)	0.87 (0.77–0.98)	1 (0.91–1.09)	0.95 (0.89–1.02)
Year 2017	1 (0.97–1.02)	1.02 (1–1.04)	1.01 (0.99–1.03)	0.97 (0.86–1.1)	1.03 (0.95–1.12)	1.01 (0.95–1.08)
Year 2018	0.9 (0.87–0.92)	0.9 (0.88–0.91)	0.9 (0.88–0.91)	0.98 (0.87–1.1)	1.01 (0.93–1.1)	1 (0.94–1.07)
Year 2019	0.93 (0.9–0.96)	0.91 (0.89–0.93)	0.92 (0.9–0.93)	0.96 (0.86–1.09)	1.01 (0.93–1.1)	1 (0.93–1.07)
Year 2020	0.94 (0.91–0.97)	0.92 (0.91–0.94)	0.93 (0.91–0.94)	1.3 (1.15–1.45)	1.4 (1.3–1.52)	1.37 (1.28–1.46)
Age, 35–59 years	1	1	1	1	1	1
Age, 60–69 years	0.84 (0.82–0.85)	1.08 (1.06–1.1)	0.98 (0.96–0.99)	1.67 (1.48–1.88)	1.41 (1.26–1.58)	1.52 (1.4–1.65)
Age, 70–79 years	0.78 (0.76–0.79)	0.98 (0.96–0.99)	0.9 (0.89–0.91)	2.31 (2.07–2.58)	2.19 (1.98–2.42)	2.23 (2.07–2.41)
Age, ≥80 year	0.82 (0.8–0.83)	0.79 (0.78–0.8)	0.78 (0.77–0.79)	4.02 (3.61–4.48)	4.39 (3.98–4.83)	4.29 (3.99–4.61)
CCI	1.13 (1.11–1.16)	1.03 (1.01–1.05)	1.07 (1.06–1.09)	1.3 (1.28–1.31)	1.34 (1.33–1.35)	1.33 (1.32–1.34)
Obesity	1.14 (1.12–1.16)	1.33 (1.32–1.35)	1.29 (1.27–1.3)	0.66 (0.6–0.73)	0.78 (0.74–0.82)	0.75 (0.72–0.79)
Pneumonia	0.97 (0.94–1.02)	0.95 (0.91–1.01)	0.96 (0.93–1.01)	2.48 (2.31–2.66)	2.37 (2.24–2.51)	2.41 (2.31–2.52)
Women			3.32 (3.3–3.35)			0.97 (0.94–1.01)

IHM: In-Hospital Mortality. T2DM: Type 2 diabetes. CCI: Charlson Comorbidity Index. OR: Odds Ratio.CI: Confidence interval.

Older age, the presence of comorbidity (CCI), the presence of pneumonia, and having been hospitalized in 2020 increased the risk of IHM in men and women with T2DM and depression (Table 5). However, obesity was a protective factor for IHM in both men and women. Sex was not associated with IHM in patients with depression and T2DM (OR for women 0.97; 95% CI 0.94–1.01).

Finally, after multivariable adjustment by year, age and CCI, among men with T2DM and cerebrovascular disease, kidney disease, and liver disease, the presence of depression was associated with a lower risk of dying in hospital (Table S2). For all the specific hospital admissions analysed (except for cancer) in women with T2DM, the presence of depression had a protective effect on IHM (Table S3).

4. Discussion

The results of this nationwide population-based observational study of almost six million patients with T2DM hospitalized in Spain during 2011–2020 reveals several key findings. First, a decrease in the prevalence of depression was observed in men and women with T2DM between 2011 and 2020. Second, the prevalence of depression was 3.32 times higher in women with T2DM than in men. Third, IHM among people with T2DM and depression increased throughout the study period, although IHM was lower in patients with depression than in those without depression. Finally, we found no sex differences in IHM among people hospitalized with T2DM and depression.

Epidemiological studies over the last two decades have reported a global increase in the prevalence of depression in persons with diabetes [20]. As in a previous report, we found an increase in the prevalence of depression in patients hospitalized with T2DM from 2011 to 2015 [19]; however, since 2016, the prevalence of depression has been decreasing. Our results could indicate that care and treatment of people with depression, particularly those with diabetes, is improving. Screening for depression in clinical practice, particularly among people with diabetes, may be a useful first step in identifying patients at high risk of this disease. The change in the time trend of prevalence has been reported in various studies [21–23]. In a population-based study in Norway, Bojanic et al. [21] found a general decrease in depressive symptoms in men with diabetes and relatively stable symptoms in women with this condition between 1995-97 and 2017-19, concluding that this change could be explained in part by awareness of these psychological conditions and improvements in treatment. Similarly, a decrease in prevalence was observed in a population-based study of Mexican adults with diabetes (age $\geq$ 50 years) between 2001 and 2015 [33].

As has been described in the literature, the prevalence of depression is higher in women with diabetes than in men [19,24,25]. In a recent study of 123,232 patients with diabetes mellitus between 1997 and 2014, Deischinger et al. [28] concluded that a diagnosis of depression is more likely in women than in men between age 30 and 69 years (OR 1.37; 95% CI: 1.32–1.43). Various factors seem to contribute to the difference between men and women regarding depression. The prevalence of depression is higher in women owing to biological factors and the fact that the psychological burden of having the disease is greater [27]. Men, on the other hand, are thought to visit their doctor less frequently, potentially leading to underdiagnosis of T2DM and depression. This effect might be even more prominent in a multimorbid condition such as diabetes, which requires more extensive medical care [34].

Furthermore, differences between women and men in psychological reactions following cardiovascular events have been addressed in the literature. In a meta-analysis investigating depression after diagnosis of cardiovascular disease/events, Buckland et al. [35] suggested that women experience a higher level of depression after a coronary event than men.

In our study, obesity was associated with the presence of depression. A recent meta-analysis concluded that persons with T2DM and obesity have a 1.63-fold greater risk of depression than those with T2DM without obesity [36]. A strong relationship between obesity and depression has been described in the literature, especially in women [37]. Vittengl et al. [38] indicate that this relationship can be explained by somatic, behavioural, and psychosocial mechanisms, including physical deterioration, social dysfunction (discrimination based on weight, low participation in social life or little social support), and emotional eating, which are more frequent in women.

Diabetes and depression are chronic diseases in which ageing, and the presence of concomitant medical conditions are crucial factors [13]. However, our results are in line with the literature, showing that depression affects younger people more than older people [6,19,25,39], because younger people find the onset of T2DM more difficult and need a longer period of adaptation to their disease [40].

The presence of depression in persons with diabetes was recently associated with a 2.16-fold increased risk of dying [41]. In our study, IHM increased over time, with particularly high values in 2020 because of COVID-19.

The main risk factors associated with IHM in patients with T2DM diagnosed with depression are older age, comorbidity, the presence of pneumonia, and having been hospitalized in 2020, as reported in the literature [19,41]. However, obesity was a protective factor for IHM, thus confirming the obesity paradox, as described elsewhere [42].

In our study, female sex was not associated with higher IHM in patients with depression, even though depression is more prevalent in women. In a population-based study of 64,177 Norwegian adults, Naicker et al. [26] found that the presence of depression increased the risk of mortality only in men with diabetes (HR 2.47; 95% CI 1.47–4.17) and not in women with diabetes, suggesting that men were more likely to be diagnosed later with depression and treated in more advanced stages of the disease. Consequently, they would present greater functional impairment than women. Sex differences in the prevalence of depressive disorders are well documented, although few studies to date have examined sex differences in outcomes in patients hospitalized with depression.

Finally, we found that among men and women with T2DM who also experienced depression, the risk of dying in hospital was similar to or even lower than among men and women without depression. This unexpected result has also been reported elsewhere [43–45]. In their population-based study comparing 38,537 diabetic patients with depression and 154,148 diabetic patients without depression, Wu et al. [43] concluded that there were no statistically significant differences in mortality from cardiovascular diseases. Patients with depression adhered slightly better to antidiabetic medication and slightly more underwent screening tests, thus potentially explaining the authors' results. Pino et al. [44] studied patients in the general population hospitalized for ST-elevation myocardial infarction and found that, paradoxically, the probability of dying in hospital was lower among patients with a clinically co-occurring depression and/or anxiety than those without. As an explanation for this "depression paradox", the authors suggested potentially underdiagnosed mental health issues surrounding major cardiovascular events, and indeed, chronic disease as a whole. Depression has also been associated with lower in-hospital mortality in patients undergoing colorectal surgery [45]. Another possible reason is that T2DM patients with depression are hospitalized with less severe acute or chronic conditions, thus increasing their probability of surviving. More studies are needed to understand the factors underlying this paradox and whether information or selection bias is responsible for the association.

The strengths of our study are the use of a national population database (RAE-CMBD), the 10-year study period, and the fact that our methodology has been used elsewhere [19]. However, our study is also subject to a series of limitations. The RAE-CMBD collects practically all hospitalizations in Spain; however, it is an administrative database and does not collect all the variables included in the clinical history. Therefore, we have no data on disease severity, glycaemic control, disease duration, or medication for diabetes or depression.

The decreased frequency of depression as of 2016 could be explained by the change in coding in the RAE-CMBD. Consequently, the results should be interpreted with caution. In addition, given that the RAE-CMBD provides anonymous patient data, we cannot know whether a patient has been admitted more than once during the same year or whether he/she has been transferred to another hospital, in which case he/she could appear twice. However, the use of hospital discharge records and administrative databases for the diagnosis of psychiatric illnesses, including depression, has been shown to be sufficiently sensitive and specific for epidemiological investigations [46,47]. Finally, in year 2020 the COVID19 pandemic had a very important impact in the Spanish health services and hospitals were collapsed by patients with this infection. This may have resulted in underdiagnose of depression that year. However, the decreasing trend in the prevalence of depression among patients with T2DM was also observed in the years immediately before 2020.

5. Conclusions

The prevalence of depression in men and women with T2DM decreased between 2011 and 2020. Our data highlight major sex differences, indicating that the prevalence of depression is more than three times higher in women than in men. However, female sex and depression are not associated with higher IHM than male sex. Older age, associated comorbidity, the presence of pneumonia, and having been hospitalized in 2020 are predictors of IHM in men and women with T2DM and depression, with obesity being a protective factor. IHM is lower in patients with T2DM and depression than in patients without depression. Future studies should analyse the possible existence of a depression paradox for in-hospital mortality among people with diabetes.

Based on our results we recommend that clinicians screen regularly for depression in patients with T2DM, particularly women, younger patients, and those with multiple comorbidities.

Supplementary Materials: The following supporting information can be downloaded at: https://www.mdpi.com/article/10.3390/jcm11216260/s1, Table S1: Diagnosis analyzed with their corresponding ICD-9-CM and ICD10 codes; Table S2: Multivariate analysis of the factors associated with in-hospital mortality in men with type 2 diabetes and selected concomitant conditions in Spain, 2011–2020; Table S3: Multivariate analysis of the factors associated with in-hospital mortality in women with type 2 diabetes and selected concomitant conditions in Spain, 2011–2020.

Author Contributions: Conceptualization, A.L.-d.-A., R.J.-G. and C.N.; methodology J.J.Z.-L. and J.L.d.B.; validation, D.C.-A.; data curation, V.H.-B.; Formal analysis, V.H.-B. and J.d.M.-D.; Funding: A.L.-d.-A. and R.J.-G.; Writing—original draft, A.L.-d.-A., R.J.-G. and C.N.; Writing—review & editing, J.J.Z.-L., D.C.-A., J.L.d.B. and J.d.M.-D. All authors have read and agreed to the published version of the manuscript.

Funding: This study is a part of the research funded by: Convenio V-PRICIT de la Comunidad de Madrid y la Universidad Complutense de Madrid ("Programa de Excelencia para el Profesorado Universitario" INV.AY.20.2021.1E126). And by: Universidad Complutense de Madrid. Grupo de Investigación en Epidemiología de las Enfermedades Crónicas de Alta Prevalencia en España (970970). And by: FIS (Fondo de Investigaciones Sanitarias—Health Research Fund, Instituto de Salud Carlos III) and co-financed by the European Union through the Fondo Europeo de Desarrollo Regional (FEDER, "Una manera de hacer Europa"): grant no. PI20/00118.

Institutional Review Board Statement: Not applicable.

Informed Consent Statement: Not applicable.

Data Availability Statement: According to the contract signed with the Spanish Ministry of Health and Social Services, which provided access to the databases from the Spanish National Hospital Database (RAE-CMBD, Registro de Actividad de Atención Especializada. Conjunto Mínimo Básico de Datos, Registry of Specialized Health Care Activities. Minimum Basic Data Set), we cannot share the databases with any other investigator, and we have to destroy the databases once the investigation has concluded. Consequently, we cannot upload the databases to any public repository. However, any investigator can apply for access to the databases by filling out the questionnaire available at https://www.sanidad.gob.es/estadEstudios/estadisticas/estadisticas/estMinisterio/SolicitudCMBD.htm. (accessed on 20 October 2022). All other relevant data are included in the paper.

Conflicts of Interest: The authors declare no conflict of interest.

References

1. Lin, X.; Xu, Y.; Pan, X.; Xu, J.; Ding, Y.; Sun, X.; Song, X.; Ren, Y.; Shan, P.F. Global, regional, and national burden and trend of diabetes in 195 countries and territories: An analysis from 1990 to 2025. *Sci. Rep.* **2020**, *10*, 14790. [CrossRef] [PubMed]
2. Institute for Health Metrics and Evaluation. GBD Results. Available online: https://www.healthdata.org/data-visualization/gbd-results (accessed on 17 October 2022).
3. GBD 2019 Mental Disorders Collaborators. Global, regional, and national burden of 12 mental disorders in 204 countries and territories, 1990-2019: A systematic analysis for the Global Burden of Disease Study 2019. *Lancet Psychiatry* **2022**, *9*, 137–150. [CrossRef]
4. Malhi, G.S.; Mann, J.J. Depression. *Lancet* **2018**, *392*, 2299–2312. [CrossRef]
5. Farr, S.L.; Hayes, D.K.; Bitsko, R.H.; Bansil, P.; Dietz, P.M. Depression, diabetes, and chronic disease risk factors among US women of reproductive age. *Prev. Chronic. Dis.* **2011**, *8*, A119. [PubMed]
6. Dogan, B.; Oner, C.; Akalin, A.A.; Ilhan, B.; Caklili, O.T.; Oguz, A. Psychiatric symptom rate of patients with Diabetes Mellitus: A case control study. *Diabetes Metab. Syndr.* **2019**, *13*, 1059–1063. [CrossRef] [PubMed]

7. Zheng, Y.; Ley, S.H.; Hu, F.B. Global aetiology and epidemiology of type 2 diabetes mellitus and its complications. *Nat. Rev. Endocrinol.* **2018**, *14*, 88–98. [CrossRef] [PubMed]
8. Greenberg, P.E.; Fournier, A.A.; Sisitsky, T.; Pike, C.T.; Kessler, R.C. The economic burden of adults with major depressive disorder in the United States (2005 and 2010). *J. Clin. Psychiatry* **2015**, *76*, 155–162. [CrossRef]
9. Farooqi, A.; Khunti, K.; Abner, S.; Gillies, C.; Morriss, R.; Seidu, S. Comorbid depression and risk of cardiac events and cardiac mortality in people with diabetes: A systematic review and meta-analysis. *Diabetes Res. Clin. Pract.* **2019**, *156*, 107816. [CrossRef]
10. Nouwen, A.; Adriaanse, M.C.; van Dam, K.; Iversen, M.M.; Viechtbauer, W.; Peyrot, M.; Caramlau, I.; Kokoszka, A.; Kanc, K.; de Groot, M.; et al. Longitudinal associations between depression and diabetes complications: A systematic review and meta-analysis. *Diabet. Med* **2019**, *36*, 1562–1572. [CrossRef]
11. Brown, L.C.; Majumdar, S.R.; Newman, S.C.; Johnson, J.A. Type 2 diabetes does not increase risk of depression. *CMAJ* **2006**, *175*, 42–46. [CrossRef]
12. Icks, A.; Kruse, J.; Dragano, N.; Broecker-Preuss, M.; Slomiany, U.; Mann, K.; Jöckel, K.H.; Erbel, R.; Giani, G.; Heinz Nixdorf Recall Study Investigator Group; et al. Are symptoms of depression more common in diabetes? Results from the Heinz Nixdorf Recall study. *Diabet. Med.* **2008**, *25*, 1330–1336. [CrossRef] [PubMed]
13. Tabák, A.G.; Akbaraly, T.N.; Batty, G.D.; Kivimäki, M. Depression and type 2 diabetes: A causal association? *Lancet Diabetes Endocrinol.* **2014**, *2*, 236–245. [CrossRef]
14. Moulton, C.D.; Pickup, J.C.; Ismail, K. The link between depression and diabetes: The search for shared mechanisms. *Lancet Diabetes Endocrinol.* **2015**, *3*, 461–471. [CrossRef]
15. Alzoubi, A.; Abunaser, R.; Khassawneh, A.; Alfaqih, M.; Khasawneh, A.; Abdo, N. The Bidirectional Relationship between Diabetes and Depression: A Literature Review. *Korean J. Fam. Med.* **2018**, *39*, 137–146. [CrossRef] [PubMed]
16. Champaneri, S.; Wand, G.S.; Malhotra, S.S.; Casagrande, S.S.; Golden, S.H. Biological basis of depression in adults with diabetes. *Curr. Diab. Rep.* **2010**, *10*, 396–405. [CrossRef] [PubMed]
17. van Dooren, F.E.; Nefs, G.; Schram, M.T.; Verhey, F.R.; Denollet, J.; Pouwer, F. Depression and risk of mortality in people with diabetes mellitus: A systematic review and meta-analysis. *PLoS ONE* **2013**, *8*, e57058. [CrossRef] [PubMed]
18. Chima, C.C.; Salemi, J.L.; Wang, M.; Mejia de Grubb, M.C.; Gonzalez, S.J.; Zoorob, R.J. Multimorbidity is associated with increased rates of depression in patients hospitalized with diabetes mellitus in the United States. *J. Diabetes Complicat.* **2017**, *31*, 1571–1579. [CrossRef] [PubMed]
19. Lopez-de-Andrés, A.; Jiménez-Trujillo, M.I.; Hernández-Barrera, V.; de Miguel-Yanes, J.M.; Méndez-Bailón, M.; Perez-Farinos, N.; de Burgos Lunar, C.; Cárdenas-Valladolid, J.; Salinero-Fort, M.Á.; Jiménez-García, R.; et al. Trends in the prevalence of depression in hospitalized patients with type 2 diabetes in Spain: Analysis of hospital discharge data from 2001 to 2011. *PLoS ONE* **2015**, *10*, e0117346. [CrossRef]
20. Chaturvedi, S.K.; Manche Gowda, S.; Ahmed, H.U.; Alosaimi, F.D.; Andreone, N.; Bobrov, A.; Bulgari, V.; Carrà, G.; Castelnuovo, G.; de Girolamo, G.; et al. More anxious than depressed: Prevalence and correlates in a 15-nation study of anxiety disorders in people with type 2 diabetes mellitus. *Gen. Psychiatr.* **2019**, *32*, e100076. [CrossRef]
21. Bojanić, I.; Sund, E.R.; Sletvold, H.; Bjerkeset, O. Prevalence trends of depression and anxiety symptoms in adults with cardiovascular diseases and diabetes 1995-2019: The HUNT studies, Norway. *BMC Psychol.* **2021**, *9*, 130. [CrossRef] [PubMed]
22. Jonson, M.; Sigström, R.; Hedna, K.; Rydberg Sterner, T.; Falk Erhag, H.; Wetterberg, H.; Fässberg, M.M.; Waern, M.; Skoog, I. Time trends in depression prevalence among Swedish 85-year-olds: Repeated cross-sectional population-based studies in 1986, 2008, and 2015. *Psychol. Med.* **2021**, 1–10. [CrossRef] [PubMed]
23. Kendrick, T.; Stuart, B.; Newell, C.; Geraghty, A.W.; Moore, M. Changes in rates of recorded depression in English primary care 2003-2013: Time trend analyses of effects of the economic recession, and the GP contract quality outcomes framework (QOF). *J. Affect Disord.* **2015**, *180*, 68–78. [CrossRef]
24. Ali, S.; Stone, M.A.; Peters, J.L.; Davies, M.J.; Khunti, K. The prevalence of co-morbid depression in adults with Type 2 diabetes: A systematic review and meta-analysis. *Diabet. Med.* **2006**, *23*, 1165–1173. [CrossRef] [PubMed]
25. Khaledi, M.; Haghighatdoost, F.; Feizi, A.; Aminorroaya, A. The prevalence of comorbid depression in patients with type 2 diabetes: An updated systematic review and meta-analysis on huge number of observational studies. *Acta Diabetol.* **2019**, *56*, 631–650. [CrossRef] [PubMed]
26. Naicker, K.; Johnson, J.A.; Skogen, J.C.; Manuel, D.; Øverland, S.; Sivertsen, B.; Colman, I. Type 2 Diabetes and Comorbid Symptoms of Depression and Anxiety: Longitudinal Associations with Mortality Risk. *Diabetes Care* **2017**, *40*, 352–358. [CrossRef] [PubMed]
27. Kuehner, C. Why is depression more common among women than among men? *Lancet Psychiatry* **2017**, *4*, 146–158. [CrossRef]
28. Deischinger, C.; Dervic, E.; Leutner, M.; Kosi-Trebotic, L.; Klimek, P.; Kautzky, A.; Kautzky-Willer, A. Diabetes mellitus is associated with a higher risk for major depressive disorder in women than in men. *BMJ Open Diabetes Res. Care* **2020**, *8*, e001430. [CrossRef]
29. Ministerio de Sanidad, Servicios Sociales e Igualdad. Real Decreto 69/2015, de 6 de febrero, por el que se regula el Registro de Actividad de Atención Sanitaria Especializada. (Spanish National Hospital Discharge Database). *BOE* **2015**, *35*, 10789–10809. Available online: https://www.mscbs.gob.es/estadEstudios/estadisticas/docs/BOE_RD_69_2015_RAE_CMBD.pdf (accessed on 31 May 2022).

30. Sundararajan, V.; Henderson, T.; Perry, C.; Muggivan, A.; Quan, H.; Ghali, W.A. New ICD-10 version of the Charlson comorbidity index predicted in-hospital mortality. *J. Clin. Epidemiol.* **2004**, *57*, 1288–1294. [CrossRef]
31. Quan, H.; Sundararajan, V.; Halfon, P.; Fong, A.; Burnand, B.; Luthi, J.C.; Saunders, L.D.; Beck, C.A.; Feasby, T.E.; Ghali, W.A. Coding algorithms for defining comorbidities in ICD-9-CM and ICD-10 administrative data. *Med. Care* **2005**, *43*, 1130–1139. [CrossRef]
32. Ministerio de Sanidad, Consumo y Bienestar Social. Solicitud de Extracción de Datos–Extraction Request (Spanish National Hospital Discharge Database). Available online: https://www.mscbs.gob.es/estadEstudios/estadisticas/estadisticas/estMinisterio/SolicitudCMBDdocs/2018_Formulario_Peticion_Datos_RAE_CMBD.pdf (accessed on 31 May 2022).
33. Alvarez-Cisneros, T.; Roa-Rojas, P.; Garcia-Peña, C. Relación longitudinal de diabetes y síntomas depresivos en adultos mayores de México: Un análisis de datos secundarios. *BMJ Open Diabetes Res. Care* **2020**, *8*, e001789. [CrossRef] [PubMed]
34. Cavanagh, A.; Wilson, C.J.; Kavanagh, D.J.; Caputi, P. Differences in the Expression of Symptoms in Men Versus Women with Depression: A Systematic Review and Meta-analysis. *Harv. Rev. Psychiatry* **2017**, *25*, 29–38. [CrossRef]
35. Buckland, S.A.; Pozehl, B.; Yates, B. Depressive Symptoms in Women with Coronary Heart Disease: A Systematic Review of the Longitudinal Literature. *J. Cardiovasc. Nurs.* **2019**, *34*, 52–59. [CrossRef] [PubMed]
36. González-Castro, T.B.; Escobar-Chan, Y.M.; Fresan, A.; López-Narváez, M.L.; Tovilla-Zárate, C.A.; Juárez-Rojop, I.E.; Ble-Castillo, J.L.; Genis-Mendoza, A.D.; Arias-Vázquez, P.I. Higher risk of depression in individuals with type 2 diabetes and obesity: Results of a meta-analysis. *J. Health Psychol.* **2021**, *26*, 1404–1419. [CrossRef] [PubMed]
37. Pereira-Miranda, E.; Costa, P.R.F.; Queiroz, V.A.O.; Pereira-Santos, M.; Santana, M.L.P. Overweight and Obesity Associated with Higher Depression Prevalence in Adults: A Systematic Review and Meta-Analysis. *J. Am. Coll. Nutr.* **2017**, *36*, 223–233. [CrossRef] [PubMed]
38. Vittengl, J.R. Mediation of the bidirectional relations between obesity and depression among women. *Psychiatry Res.* **2018**, *264*, 254–259. [CrossRef] [PubMed]
39. Lopez-Herranz, M.; Jiménez-García, R.; Ji, Z.; de Miguel-Diez, J.; Carabantes-Alarcon, D.; Maestre-Miquel, C.; Zamorano-León, J.J.; López-de-Andrés, A. Mental Health among Spanish Adults with Diabetes: Findings from a Population-Based Case-Controlled Study. *Int. J. Environ. Res. Public Health* **2021**, *18*, 6088. [CrossRef] [PubMed]
40. Schieman, S.; Van Gundy, K.; Taylor, J. The relationship between age and depressive symptoms: A test of competing explanatory and suppression influences. *J. Aging Health* **2002**, *14*, 260–285. [CrossRef] [PubMed]
41. Prigge, R.; Wild, S.H.; Jackson, C.A. Depression, diabetes, comorbid depression and diabetes and risk of all-cause and cause-specific mortality: A prospective cohort study. *Diabetologia* **2022**, *65*, 1450–1460. [CrossRef] [PubMed]
42. Engelmann, J.; Manuwald, U.; Rubach, C.; Kugler, J.; Birkenfeld, A.L.; Hanefeld, M.; Rothe, U. Determinants of mortality in patients with type 2 diabetes: A review. *Rev. Endocr. Metab. Disord.* **2016**, *17*, 129–137. [CrossRef] [PubMed]
43. Wu, C.S.; Hsu, L.Y.; Wang, S.H. Association of depression and diabetes complications and mortality: A population-based cohort study. *Epidemiol. Psychiatr. Sci.* **2020**, *29*, e96. [CrossRef] [PubMed]
44. Pino, E.C.; Zuo, Y.; Borba, C.P.; Henderson, D.C.; Kalesan, B. Clinical depression and anxiety among ST-elevation myocardial infarction hospitalizations: Results from Nationwide Inpatient Sample 2004-2013. *Psychiatry Res.* **2018**, *266*, 291–300. [CrossRef] [PubMed]
45. Oduyale, O.K.; Eltahir, A.A.; Stem, M.; Prince, E.; Zhang, G.Q.; Safar, B.; Efron, J.E.; Atallah, C. What Does a Diagnosis of Depression Mean for Patients Undergoing Colorectal Surgery? *J. Surg. Res.* **2021**, *260*, 454–461. [CrossRef] [PubMed]
46. Castillo, E.G.; Olfson, M.; Pincus, H.A.; Vawdrey, D.; Stroup, T.S. Electronic health records in mental health research: A framework for developing valid research methods. *Psychiatr. Serv.* **2015**, *66*, 193–196. [CrossRef] [PubMed]
47. Spiranovic, C.; Matthews, A.; Scanlan, J.; Kirkby, K.C. Increasing knowledge of mental illness through secondary research of electronic health records: Opportunities and challenges. *Adv. Ment. Health* **2016**, *14*, 14–25. [CrossRef]

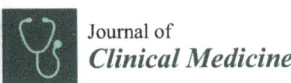 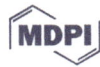

Article

Hospital Readmission Risk and Risk Factors of People with a Primary or Secondary Discharge Diagnosis of Diabetes

Daniel J. Rubin [1,*], Naveen Maliakkal [2], Huaqing Zhao [3] and Eli E. Miller [1]

[1] Section of Endocrinology, Diabetes, and Metabolism, Lewis Katz School of Medicine, Temple University, 3322 N. Broad Street, Suite 205, Philadelphia, PA 19140, USA
[2] Department of Medicine, Temple University Hospital, Philadelphia, PA 19140, USA
[3] Department of Biomedical Education and Data Science, Lewis Katz School of Medicine, Temple University, 3322 N. Broad Street, Suite 205, Philadelphia, PA 19140, USA
* Correspondence: daniel.rubin@tuhs.temple.edu; Tel.: +1-215-707-4746; Fax: +1-215-707-5599

Abstract: Hospital readmission among people with diabetes is common and costly. A better understanding of the differences between people requiring hospitalization primarily for diabetes (primary discharge diagnosis, 1°DCDx) or another condition (secondary discharge diagnosis, 2°DCDx) may translate into more effective ways to prevent readmissions. This retrospective cohort study compared readmission risk and risk factors between 8054 hospitalized adults with a 1°DCDx or 2°DCDx. The primary outcome was all-cause hospital readmission within 30 days of discharge. The readmission rate was higher in patients with a 1°DCDx than in patients with a 2°DCDx (22.2% vs. 16.2%, $p < 0.01$). Several independent risk factors for readmission were common to both groups including outpatient follow up, length of stay, employment status, anemia, and lack of insurance. C-statistics for the multivariable models of readmission were not significantly different (0.837 vs. 0.822, $p = 0.15$). Readmission risk of people with a 1°DCDx was higher than that of people with a 2°DCDx of diabetes. Some risk factors were shared between the two groups, while others were unique. Inpatient diabetes consultation may be more effective at lowering readmission risk among people with a 1°DCDx. These models may perform well to predict readmission risk.

Keywords: diabetes; readmission; risk factors

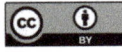

1. Introduction

Readmission to the hospital is an undesirable outcome. Thus, there is widespread interest in reducing readmission risk to improve both the patient health and control costs [1–3]. It has been established that diabetes is an independent risk factor for readmission [4,5]. Furthermore, the sheer number of readmissions and their associated costs among people with diabetes are staggering. In the U.S., there were more than eight million hospital discharges of patients with diabetes, accounting for nearly 30% of all discharges in 2018 [6,7]. At that time, 10.5% of the U.S. population had diabetes, a difference that reflects the overall hospitalization risk associated with diabetes [8]. Given the 16.0 to 20.4% rate of readmission within 30 days of discharge (30-day readmission) [9,10], the annual cost of such readmissions is $20–25 billion in the U.S. alone. Of note, most hospitalized patients with diabetes have type 2 diabetes, reflecting the underlying prevalence of type 2 diabetes in the general population [7].

Over the past several years, there have been multiple efforts to determine the risk factors for readmission among patients with diabetes [9,10]. Many risk factors across several domains have been identified including sociodemographics, diabetic complications, comorbidity burden, abnormal laboratory values, multiple hospitalizations, and hospital length of stay. Patients with diabetes, however, are a heterogeneous population that can be categorized as requiring hospitalization primarily for diabetes (primary discharge diagnosis) or another condition (secondary discharge diagnosis of diabetes). One study found that hospitalized patients with a primary diagnosis of diabetes had a higher risk of readmission than patients with a secondary diagnosis of diabetes [11], suggesting that the readmission risk factors of these two populations may be different. Whether or not the risk factors for readmission vary by the primary or secondary discharge diagnosis of diabetes is unknown. A better understanding of the differences between these populations may translate into more effective ways to prevent readmissions.

To compare the readmission risk and risk factors between patients with a primary or secondary discharge diagnosis of diabetes, we performed a secondary analysis of a previously described cohort [12].

2. Methods

2.1. Study Sample

This retrospective cohort study was based on electronic medical records of 17,284 patients with 44,203 hospital discharges between 1 January 2004 and 1 December 2012 at Boston Medical Center, an urban academic medical center in Boston, MA, as previously described [12]. The inclusion criteria were a diagnosis of diabetes defined by a hospital discharge associated with an International Classification of Diseases, Ninth Revision, Clinical Modification (ICD-9-CM) code of 250.xx or preadmission documentation of a diabetes medication. Patients were excluded for the following: age less than 18 years on the day of an admission, discharge by transfer to another hospital, discharge from an obstetric service, inpatient death, outpatient death within 30 days of discharge, missing data, or lack of follow-up 30 days after discharge. A readmission within 8 h after an index discharge was considered as a false positive and merged with the index discharge to avoid counting an in-hospital transfer as a readmission. Among the discharges with a primary diagnosis of diabetes, simple random sampling was used to select one discharge per patient, without replacement, yielding 4027 discharges. Among the patients with only secondary discharge diagnoses of diabetes, 4027 discharges were randomly selected, one discharge per patient. A post-hoc analysis was performed in the subgroup of 3674 patients who had an HbA1c value available. The Temple University Institutional Review Board approved the protocol.

2.2. Definition of Variables and Outcomes

A total of 49 sociodemographic, clinical, and administrative variables linked with hospital discharges were evaluated for their association with all-cause hospital readmission within 30 days of discharge, as previously described [12]. The first value of each variable up to 24 h before the admission was analyzed so that the related outpatient and emergency department visits were included. The most extreme blood glucose level was based on capillary point-of-care or venous values during the entire hospitalization. The most extreme value was placed into one of three categories: 70–180 mg/dL (3.9–10 mmol/L), 40–69 or 181–300 mg/dL (2.2–3.8 or 10.1–16.7 mmol/L), or <40 or >300 mg/dL (<2.2 or >16.7 mmol/L). The most common ICD-9-CM codes within each cohort were grouped by condition or organ system and sorted by frequency. Inpatient consultation by the diabetes management team was assessed as present or absent. These consultations were requested by primary hospital providers. The team consisted of a nurse practitioner/certified diabetes educator, an endocrinology fellow, and an endocrinology attending with expertise in diabetes. Consultations may have consisted of a single visit or intermittent or daily follow-up visits with co-management throughout the hospital stay including recommendations for diabetes management upon discharge.

2.3. Statistical Analyses

Summaries of the categorical variables included the counts and percentages. For continuous variables, the means and standard deviations or medians and interquartile ranges were used accordingly after the assessment of normality. The characteristics of patients with a primary diagnosis of diabetes were compared to the characteristics of those with a secondary diagnosis of diabetes. In addition, readmitted and non-readmitted patients were compared among those with a primary diagnosis of diabetes and among those with a secondary diagnosis of diabetes. For the categorical variables, these comparisons were conducted by χ^2 tests. For continuous variables, 2-sample t tests or Wilcoxon rank sum tests were used. For multivariable modeling, non-normally distributed continuous variables (admission serum creatinine and length of stay) were log transformed. Univariate analyses identified variables associated with 30-day readmission. Variables with $p < 0.1$ in the univariate analyses were selected to undergo multivariable modeling. To determine the adjusted associations of the variables with all-cause 30-day readmission, multivariable logistic regression with generalized estimating equations and the best subset selection was performed [13,14]. The threshold for retention in the multivariable models was an association with 30-day all-cause readmission at $p < 0.05$. A p-value < 0.05 was considered statistically significant. To explore the performance of the models for readmission prediction, c-statistics, a measure of discrimination representing the area under the receiver operating characteristic curve [15], were calculated with 95% confidence intervals and calibration plots were drawn [16]. All analyses were performed using SAS version 9.4 (SAS Institute, Cary, NC, USA).

3. Results

A total of 8054 patients were analyzed: 4027 with a primary discharge diagnosis of diabetes and 4027 with a secondary discharge diagnosis of diabetes (Table 1). The cohort was ethnically diverse (40.4% Black, 24.3% White, 12.5% Hispanic), well-distributed across four age brackets, and balanced for sex (47.1% female). Most of the patients were unmarried, educated at a high-school level or greater, not employed, insured by Medicare or Medicaid, and lived within 5 miles of the hospital. Nearly 40% of patients had at least one microvascular diabetic complication and almost 50% had at least one macrovascular complication. The most common comorbidities other than diabetic complications were hypertension, anemia, and depression. The median hospital length of stay was 3.3 days.

Table 1. Characteristics of the hospitalized patients by the primary or secondary discharge diagnosis of diabetes.

Variable	All Patients N = 8054	Primary Diabetes Dx N = 4027	Secondary Diabetes Dx N = 4027	p Value
Age, N (%)				<0.0001
<50 years	2246 (27.9)	1557 (38.7)	689 (17.1)	
50–59 years	1890 (23.5)	972 (24.1)	918 (22.8)	
60–69 years	1808 (22.4)	771 (19.1)	1037 (25.8)	
70+ years	2110 (26.2)	727 (18.1)	1383 (34.3)	
Female, N (%)	3796 (47.1)	1757 (43.6)	2039 (50.6)	0.0004
Marital status, [a] N (%)				<0.0001
Married	2337 (29.0)	948 (23.5)	1389 (34.5)	
Single	5558 (69.0)	3018 (74.9)	2540 (63.1)	
Race/ethnicity, [a] N (%)				<0.0001
Black	3254 (40.4)	1990 (49.4)	1264 (31.4)	
Hispanic	1008 (12.5)	509 (12.6)	499 (12.4)	
White	1956 (24.3)	785 (19.5)	1171 (29.1)	
Not recorded	1522 (18.9)	616 (15.3)	906 (22.5)	
English speaking, N (%)	6569 (81.6)	3409 (84.7)	3160 (78.5)	<0.0001
Insurance status, N (%)				<0.0001
Medicaid	1592 (19.8)	948 (23.5)	644 (16.0)	
Medicare	2935 (36.4)	1366 (33.9)	1569 (39.0)	
None	469 (5.8)	334 (8.3)	135 (3.4)	
Private	1614 (20.0)	780 (19.4)	834 (20.7)	
Not recorded	1444 (17.9)	599 (14.9)	845 (21.0)	

Table 1. *Cont.*

Variable	All Patients N = 8054	Primary Diabetes Dx N = 4027	Secondary Diabetes Dx N = 4027	p Value
Home zip code < 5 mi. from hospital, N (%)	5688 (70.6)	3121 (77.5)	2567 (63.7)	<0.0001
Educational level, N (%)				<0.0001
Less than high school	1039 (12.9)	503 (12.5)	536 (13.3)	
Any high school	4465 (55.4)	2366 (58.8)	2099 (52.1)	
Some college	535 (6.6)	294 (7.3)	241 (6.0)	
College graduate	1261 (15.7)	571 (14.2)	690 (17.1)	
Not recorded	754 (9.4)	293 (7.3)	461 (11.4)	
Employment,[a] N (%)				<0.0001
Disabled	1742 (21.6)	1033 (25.7)	709 (17.6)	
Employed	885 (11.0)	410 (10.2)	475 (11.8)	
Retired	2536 (31.5)	941 (23.4)	1595 (39.6)	
Unemployed	2635 (32.7)	1551 (38.5)	1084 (26.9)	
Pre-admission sulfonylurea use, N (%)	1066 (13.2)	408 (10.1)	658 (16.3)	<0.0001
Pre-admission metformin use, N (%)	2029 (25.2)	753 (18.7)	1276 (31.7)	<0.0001
Pre-admission insulin use, N (%)	3404 (42.3)	2216 (55.0)	1188 (29.5)	<0.0001
Steroids at admission	595 (7.4)	222 (5.5)	373 (9.3)	<0.0001
Most extreme blood glucose level,[b] N (%)				<0.0001
40–69 or 181–300 mg/dL	3008 (37.3)	1238 (30.7)	1770 (44.0)	
70–180 mg/dL	2182 (27.1)	502 (12.5)	1680 (41.7)	
<40 or >300 mg/dL	2864 (35.6)	2287 (56.8)	577 (14.3)	
Diabetes inpatient consultation, N (%)	1854 (23.0)	1438 (35.7)	416 (10.3)	<0.0001
Current or prior DKA or HHS, N (%)	1471 (18.3)	1416 (35.2)	55 (1.4)	<0.0001
Microvascular complications,[c] N (%)				<0.0001
0	5099 (63.3)	1938 (48.1)	3161 (78.5)	
1	1781 (22.1)	1164 (28.9)	617 (15.3)	
2	781 (9.7)	588 (14.6)	193 (4.8)	
3	393 (4.9)	337 (8.4)	56 (1.4)	
Macrovascular complications,[d] N (%)				<0.0001
0	4207 (52.2)	2346 (58.3)	1861 (46.2)	
1	2126 (26.4)	967 (24.0)	1159 (28.8)	
2	1228 (15.2)	447 (11.1)	781 (19.4)	
3	393 (4.9)	217 (5.4)	176 (4.4)	
4	100 (1.2)	50 (1.2)	50 (1.2)	
Pre-admission blood pressure meds, N (%)				<0.0001
None	2743 (34.1)	1521 (37.8)	1222 (30.3)	
ACE-i or ARB	3699 (45.9)	1789 (44.4)	1910 (47.4)	
Non-ACE or ARB	1612 (20.0)	717 (17.8)	895 (22.2)	
Pre-admission statin use, N (%)	3389 (42.1)	1462 (36.3)	1927 (47.9)	<0.0001
Admission white blood cell count, N (%)				<0.0001
Low < 4 K/µL	387 (4.8)	218 (5.4)	169 (4.2)	
Normal 4–11 K/µL	6278 (77.9)	3228 (80.2)	3050 (75.7)	
High > 11 K/µL	1389 (17.2)	581 (14.4)	808 (20.1)	
Admission serum albumin, N (%)				<0.0001
4+ g/dL	3116 (38.7)	1722 (42.8)	1394 (34.6)	
<4 g/dL	4088 (50.8)	1984 (49.3)	2104 (52.2)	
Unknown	850 (10.6)	321 (8.0)	529 (13.1)	
Admission serum sodium, N (%)				<0.0001
Low < 135 mmol/L	914 (11.3)	533 (13.2)	381 (9.5)	
Normal 135–145 mmol/L	7078 (87.9)	3470 (86.2)	3608 (89.6)	
High > 145 mmol/L	62 (0.8)	24 (0.6)	38 (0.9)	
Admission serum potassium, N (%)				<0.0001
Low < 3.1 mmol/L	95 (1.2)	46 (1.1)	49 (1.2)	
Normal 3.1–5.3 mmol/L	7196 (89.3)	3473 (86.2)	3723 (92.5)	
High > 5.3 mmol/L	763 (9.5)	508 (12.6)	255 (6.3)	
Admission creatinine (mg/dL), median (IQR)	0.9 (0.7–1.3)	1.0 (0.8–1.4)	0.9 (0.7–1.3)	0.0012
Discharged 90 d before index admission, N (%)	2390 (29.7)	1335 (33.2)	1055 (26.2)	<0.0001

Table 1. *Cont.*

Variable	All Patients N = 8054	Primary Diabetes Dx N = 4027	Secondary Diabetes Dx N = 4027	p Value
Year of discharge, N (%)				<0.0001
2004	805 (10.0)	411 (10.2)	394 (9.8)	
2005	844 (10.5)	464 (11.5)	380 (9.4)	
2006	878 (10.9)	496 (12.3)	382 (9.5)	
2007	1048 (13.0)	574 (14.3)	474 (11.8)	
2008	951 (11.8)	507 (12.6)	444 (11.0)	
2009	1037 (12.9)	494 (12.3)	543 (13.5)	
2010	1047 (13.0)	482 (12.0)	565 (14.0)	
2011	788 (9.8)	321 (8.0)	467 (11.6)	
2012	656 (8.1)	278 (6.9)	378 (9.4)	
Length-of-stay (days), median (IQR)	3.3 (2.1–5.8)	3.1 (2.0–5.1)	3.6 (2.1–6.2)	<0.0001
Urgent or emergent admission, N (%)				<0.0001
No	955 (11.9)	318 (7.9)	637 (15.8)	
Yes	7099 (88.1)	3709 (92.1)	3390 (84.2)	
Yes	1395 (17.3)	717 (17.8)	678 (16.8)	
No	6659 (82.7)	3310 (82.2)	3349 (83.2)	
Blood transfusion given, N (%)				<0.0001
Yes	885 (11.0)	319 (7.9)	566 (14.1)	
No	7169 (89.0)	3708 (92.1)	3461 (85.9)	
Parenteral or enteral nutrition, N (%)				<0.0001
Yes	180 (2.2)	43 (1.1)	137 (3.4)	
No	7874 (97.8)	3984 (98.9)	3890 (96.6)	
Discharge status of index admission, [a] N (%)				0.0024
Home	4909 (61.0)	2475 (61.5)	2434 (60.4)	
Home with nursing care	1550 (19.2)	786 (19.5)	764 (19.0)	
Sub-acute facility	1363 (16.9)	628 (15.6)	735 (18.3)	
Against medical advice	190 (2.4)	121 (3.0)	69 (1.7)	
Discharge 1 year prior to index admission, N (%)				<0.0001
Home	2852 (35.4)	1562 (38.8)	1290 (32.0)	
Home with nursing care	923 (11.5)	473 (11.7)	450 (11.2)	
Sub-acute facility	774 (9.6)	383 (9.5)	391 (9.7)	
Against medical advice	133 (1.7)	90 (2.2)	43 (1.1)	
No discharge recorded	3372 (41.9)	1519 (37.7)	1853 (46.0)	
Body mass index, N (%)				<0.0001
<18.5 kg/m^2	182 (2.3)	113 (2.8)	69 (1.7)	
18.5–24.9 kg/m^2	1587 (19.7)	971 (24.1)	616 (15.3)	
25.0–29.9 kg/m^2	2223 (27.6)	1082 (26.9)	1141 (28.3)	
≥30.0 kg/m^2	4062 (50.4)	1861 (46.2)	2201 (54.7)	
Depression or psychosis ever, N (%)	2438 (30.3)	1358 (33.7)	1080 (26.8)	0.0002
Gastroparesis ever, N (%)	683 (8.5)	596 (14.8)	87 (2.2)	<0.0001
Pancreatitis ever, N (%)	410 (5.1)	246 (6.1)	164 (4.1)	0.037
Hypertension ever, N (%)	5630 (69.9)	2631 (65.3)	2999 (74.5)	<0.0001
COPD or asthma ever, N (%)	1551 (19.3)	625 (15.5)	926 (23.0)	<0.0001
Cardiac dysrhythmias ever, N (%)	1431 (17.8)	492 (12.2)	939 (23.3)	<0.0001
Malignant neoplasm ever, N (%)	596 (7.4)	140 (3.5)	456 (11.3)	<0.0001
Drug abuse, N (%)				<0.0001
Never	6262 (77.8)	2990 (74.2)	3272 (81.3)	
History	1403 (17.4)	786 (19.5)	617 (15.3)	
Current	389 (4.8)	251 (6.2)	138 (3.4)	
Current complication of device, graft, or implant, N (%)				<0.0001
Yes	208 (2.6)	53 (1.3)	155 (3.8)	
Current fluid or electrolyte disorder, N (%)	1695 (21.0)	969 (24.1)	726 (18.0)	<0.0001
Charlson comorbidity index, N (%)				<0.0001
0	1271 (15.8)	1269 (31.5)	2 (0.0)	
1–2	2211 (27.5)	914 (22.7)	1297 (32.2)	

Table 1. Cont.

Variable	All Patients N = 8054	Primary Diabetes Dx N = 4027	Secondary Diabetes Dx N = 4027	p Value
3–4	1503 (18.7)	508 (12.6)	995 (24.7)	
5–6	791 (9.8)	370 (9.2)	421 (10.5)	
>6	2278 (28.3)	966 (24.0)	1312 (32.6)	
Outpatient visit, N (%)				<0.0001
Yes	3683 (45.7)	1820 (45.2)	1863 (46.3)	
No	2303 (28.6)	1239 (30.8)	1064 (26.4)	
Unknown	2068 (25.7)	968 (24.0)	1100 (27.3)	

[a] "Other" category not shown; [b] See text for SI units; [c] Retinopathy, neuropathy, nephropathy; [d] Coronary artery disease, heart failure, stroke, peripheral vascular disease; ACE-i = Angiotensin-converting enzyme inhibitor; ARB = Angiotensinogen receptor blocker; COPD = Chronic Obstructive Pulmonary Disease; DKA = Diabetic ketoacidosis; Ever = current or prior; IQR = Interquartile range; HHS = Hyperglycemic Hyperosmolar Syndrome; No = not recorded.

Out of the 49 characteristics analyzed, 44 were statistically significantly different between patients with a primary and secondary discharge diagnosis of diabetes (Table 1). There were no statistically significant differences in preadmission thiazolidinedione use, admission hematocrit, intensive care unit admission, a diagnosis of anemia ever, or current infection during the admission.

The readmission rate was higher in patients with a primary discharge diagnosis of diabetes than in patients with a secondary discharge diagnosis of DM (22.2% vs. 16.2%, $p < 0.01$). Several independent risk factors for readmission were common to both a primary and a secondary discharge diagnosis of diabetes, specifically, a lack of an outpatient visit within 30 days of discharge, length of stay, being unemployed, being discharged within 90 days before admission, and a diagnosis of anemia (Figures 1 and 2). Being uninsured was associated with lower readmission risk. There were also multiple independent readmission risk factors unique to patients with a primary discharge diagnosis of diabetes (Figure 3): the Charlson comorbidity index, education level, gastroparesis, higher serum creatinine, and lower hematocrit. Inpatient diabetes consultation and preadmission TZD use were associated with lower odds of readmission in this group. Similarly, there were several independent readmission risk factors unique to those with a secondary discharge diagnosis of diabetes (Figure 4): discharge against medical advice, discharge home with nursing care, pancreatitis, abnormal serum sodium, urgent or emergent admission, and low serum albumin.

C-statistics for the multivariable models of readmission indicated very good discrimination and were not significantly different between the study groups (0.837 [0.823–0.851] 95% CI vs. 0.822 [0.807–0.837] 95% CI, $p = 0.15$). Calibration of the primary discharge diagnosis model was excellent, while calibration of the secondary discharge diagnosis model was fair (Figures 5 and 6).

Many of the most frequent reasons for hospital admission based on primary ICD-9-CM code among patients with a secondary discharge diagnosis of diabetes were also frequent secondary ICD-9-CM codes among those with a primary discharge diagnosis of diabetes (i.e., cardiovascular disease, infection, lung disease, procedure or postoperative complications, and disorders of fluid electrolyte or acid–base balance, Tables S1 and S2). Other common reasons for admission in the patients with a secondary discharge diagnosis of diabetes were ischemic stroke, alteration of consciousness, hallucinations, syncope, convulsions, dizziness, fever, or malaise, overweight, obesity and other hyperalimentation, and pancreatitis (Table S2).

In the subgroup analysis performed among patients with an HbA1c value, the mean HbA1c in the primary discharge diagnosis group was 10.7 ± 3.0% and in the secondary discharge diagnosis group, it was 7.8 ± 2.0% ($p < 0.001$). When HbA1c was added to the models for readmission, there was no association of HbA1c with readmission in either group of patients (Tables S3 and S4). Although two and three of the variables in each model were no longer statistically significant, the direction of the odds ratios above or below 1 remained the same.

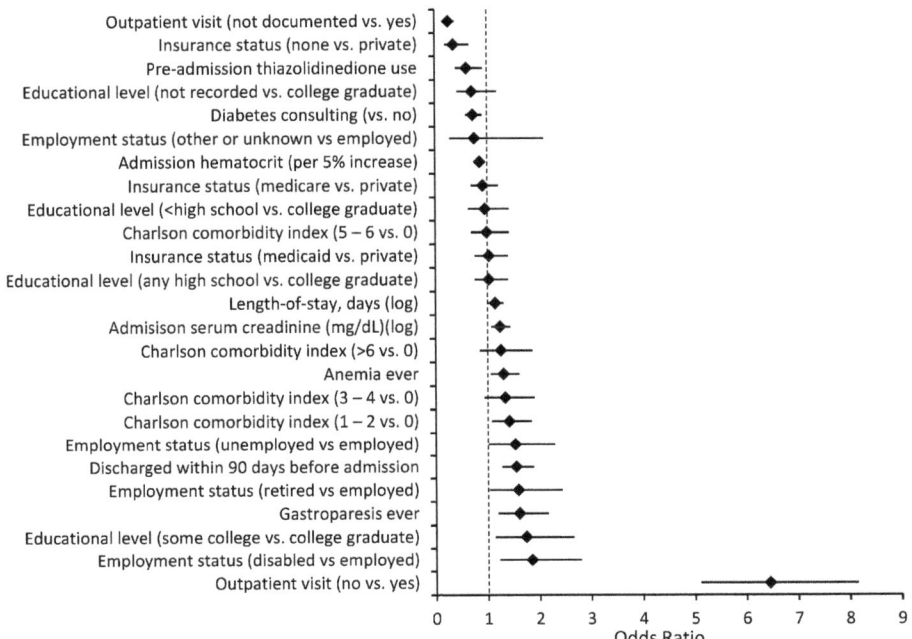

Figure 1. Risk factors for all-cause 30-day readmission among 4027 patients with primary discharge diagnosis of diabetes in multivariable logistic regression model, OR (95% CI), adjusted for year of discharge. ♦ = Odds ratio.

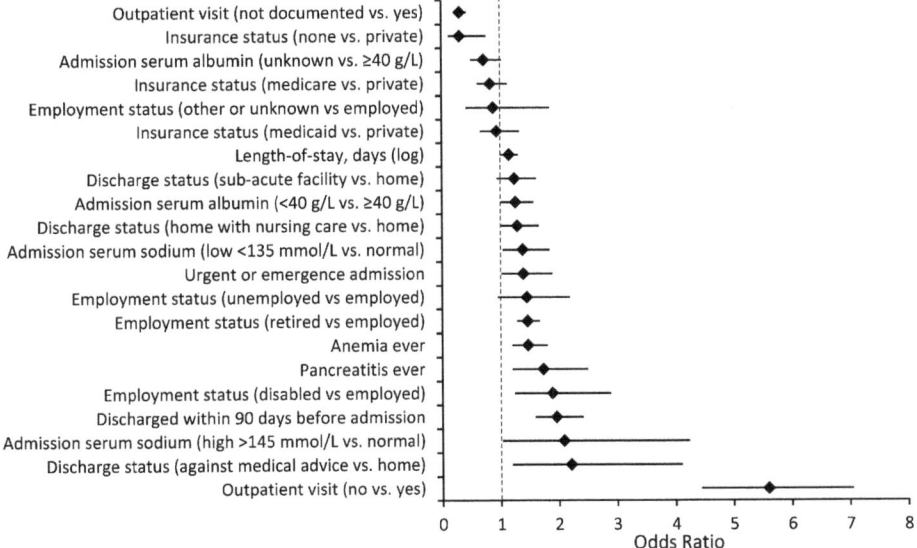

Figure 2. Risk factors for all-cause 30-day readmission among 4027 patients with secondary discharge diagnosis of diabetes in the multivariable logistic regression model, OR (95% CI). Adjusted for year of discharge. ♦ = Odds ratio.

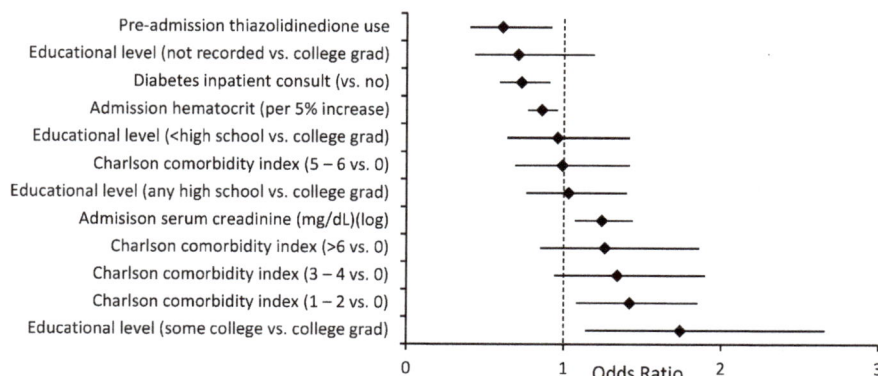

Figure 3. Risk factors for readmission unique to primary discharge diagnosis of diabetes, OR (95% CI). ♦ = Odds ratio.

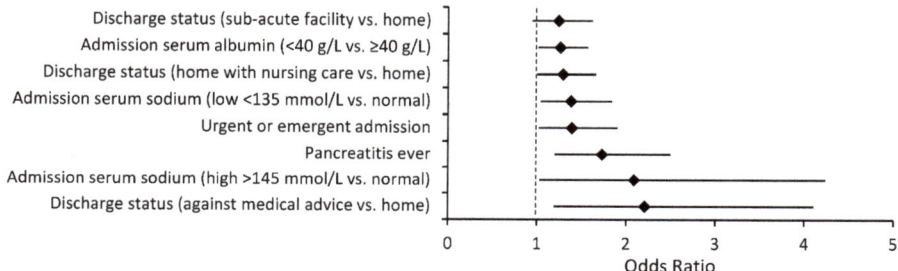

Figure 4. Risk factors for readmission unique to the secondary discharge diagnosis of diabetes, OR (95% CI). ♦ = Odds ratio.

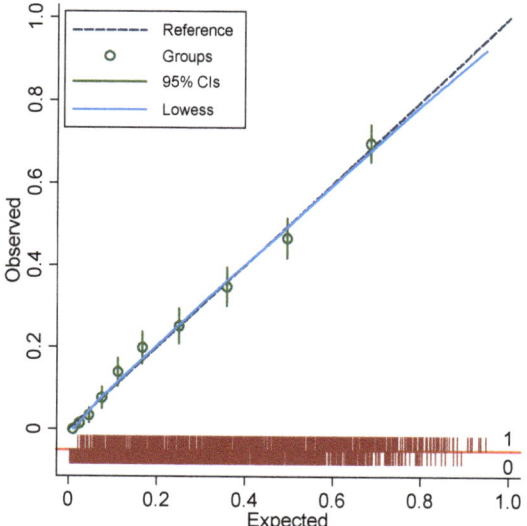

Figure 5. Calibration plot for the multivariable logistic regression model in people with primary discharge diagnosis of diabetes. Each decile is denoted by a circle with a short intersecting line to indicate the corresponding 95% confidence interval. The diagonal smooth line (Lowess) indicates excellent agreement between the observed and expected values.

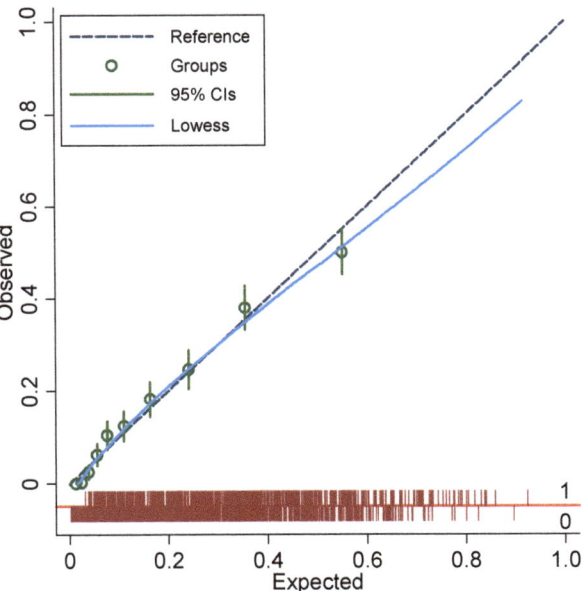

Figure 6. Calibration plot for the multivariable logistic regression model in people with secondary discharge diagnosis of diabetes. Each decile is denoted by a circle with a short intersecting line to indicate the corresponding 95% confidence interval. The diagonal smooth line (Lowess) indicates fair agreement between the observed and expected values.

4. Discussion

In this retrospective cohort study of 8054 hospitalized patients with either a primary or secondary diagnosis of diabetes, 49 socioeconomic, demographic, clinical, and administrative variables were evaluated for associations with all-cause 30-day readmission. Multivariable analysis revealed several independent risk factors for readmission, some of which were shared between the two study groups and some of which were not. Both models performed well in terms of discrimination (c-statistics 0.834 and 0.822), suggesting very good performance for prediction, with no statistically significant difference between them. Post-hoc analysis in the subgroup of patients with an HbA1c value found no association of HbA1c with readmission and did not substantively change the model in either group. The loss of statistical significance in a few of the variables in the models was attributable to the markedly smaller sample sizes. Finally, patients with a primary discharge diagnosis of diabetes had a significantly higher readmission rate than those with a secondary discharge diagnosis of diabetes.

The higher readmission rate of patients with a primary discharge diabetes diagnosis was consistent with the existing literature as well as our clinical experience. In a study of 16,266 people with diabetes, Sonmez and others reported 30-day readmission rates of 16.5% and 13.6% among those with a primary or secondary discharge diagnosis of diabetes, respectively [11]. Another study of adults with type 1 diabetes hospitalized for diabetic ketoacidosis (DKA) reported a readmission rate of 19.4% [17]. It has been speculated, and we agree, that the higher readmission rate of those with a primary discharge diagnosis of diabetes may be related to the more extreme metabolic abnormalities (e.g., diabetic ketoacidosis, hyperglycemic hyperosmolar state, severe hyper and hypoglycemia) that patients tend to have relative to those for whom diabetes is a secondary diagnosis [11]. Sonmez and colleagues called for studies to reveal the causes for the observed difference in readmission rates between the two populations. We are not aware of studies besides ours that compared the multiple risk factors between patients with a primary or secondary discharge diagnosis of diabetes.

The difference in readmission rates between patients with a primary or secondary diabetes diagnosis may be at least partly attributable to the risk factors that were unique to each subgroup. Most notably, inpatient consultation by a diabetes management service was associated with lower odds of readmission in people with a primary discharge diagnosis of diabetes. This association has been reported in other studies of hospitalized patients with diabetes including one randomized controlled trial [18–21]. These studies, however, did not distinguish between those with a primary or secondary discharge diagnosis of diabetes. The literature, our findings, and clinical intuition considered together suggest that inpatient diabetes team consultation is more effective at reducing readmission risk among patients primarily admitted for diabetes than in patients with diabetes admitted for another condition.

Risk factors unique to patients with a secondary discharge diagnosis of diabetes include being discharged against medical advice, being discharged home with nursing care, and urgent or emergent admission. In contrast to inpatient diabetes consultation, these factors are not diabetes specific. Given that diabetes is not the central issue among those with a secondary diagnosis, it is logical that non-specific risk factors are more important than among those with a primary diagnosis of diabetes. For secondary diabetes diagnosis patients, it appears that the circumstances around the hospital admission and discharge are more important for determining the readmission risk than for primary diabetes diagnosis patients.

It is worth noting that the risk factors common to both primary and secondary diabetes diagnosis patients (i.e., lack of an outpatient visit within 30 days of discharge, length of stay, being unemployed, lacking health insurance, being discharged within 90 days before admission, and a diagnosis of anemia) are also not specific to diabetes per se. In addition, the only modifiable factors on this list are outpatient follow-up and insurance status. There is some support from randomized controlled trials for the hypothesis that in-person outpatient follow-up reduces readmission risk in people with diabetes [22,23], although another trial has provided conflicting evidence [24], and the nature of follow-up and the study population characteristics vary across the few trials that have examined this. Whether follow-up by telephone and specific components of outpatient follow-up such as education and medication adjustment contribute to readmission risk reduction has been reviewed elsewhere recently and was beyond the scope of the current study [9]. Lack of health insurance was strongly and inversely associated with readmission risk in both groups of patients. Previously, we reported this association in a larger study of the parent cohort from which the current sample was drawn [12]. We speculate that patients who lack insurance delay seeking care to avoid paying medical bills. The association of hospital length of stay with readmission has been widely reported [9,10], and likely represents a marker of illness severity rather than a causal factor. It is unclear why a diagnosis of anemia is the only condition among all the diagnoses evaluated to be shared as a risk factor for readmission in both primary and secondary diabetes diagnosis patients. Additional research to both confirm and explore reasons for this association is warranted.

There is some commonality and some differences between the risk factors reported here and a study of adults with type 1 diabetes hospitalized with DKA [17]. Common risk factors were Charlson comorbidity index and kidney disease. Risk factors identified in the other study not identified in ours among patients with a primary discharge diagnosis of diabetes include age, sex, income, large hospital bed size, smoking, discharge against medical advice, obesity, and hypertension. These differences likely reflect differences in the data available as well as the study populations. The other study used a national sample of much younger patients and did not include much patient-level data such as laboratory results and medication use.

The c-statistics of the two models presented here suggest very good prediction of readmissions and compare favorably to other models that predict readmission risk in people with diabetes, for which the c-statistics ranged from 0.63 to 0.97 [9]. We previously published a model using the parent cohort of people with diabetes without stratifying the sample by discharge diagnosis, which had a comparable c-statistic of 0.82 [12]. These two studies indicate that developing separate models for patients with either a primary or secondary discharge diagnosis of diabetes did not yield better performance than a single model developed in a unified cohort. They also reinforced the conclusion that using more variables, especially variables based on data available on or after discharge, enabled stronger prediction than models based only on variables available at the time of admission such as the Diabetes Early Readmission Risk Indicator (DERRI®), which had a c-statistic of 0.69 [25]. It remains unknown whether models might perform better when stratified by other characteristics such as the type of diabetes.

It is difficult to speculate how the readmission risk factors among people with diabetes may have changed since the appearance of COVID-19. Given that the pandemic exacerbated health disparities [26], it is possible that the associations related to access to care such as outpatient visits, employment status, and insurance were strengthened. While several studies have identified diabetes as a risk factor for readmission among people hospitalized for COVID-19 [27], we are unaware of any studies that have examined COVID-19 as a risk factor for readmission among people with diabetes.

The strengths of this study are a moderately large sample size, a diverse population, and analysis of multiple socioeconomic, demographic, administrative, and clinical factors. These strengths are tempered by some limitations. Because the sample came from one urban academic medical center, the results may not be generalizable to other settings and populations. Additionally, readmissions that may have occurred at other hospitals could not be assessed. However, given that the readmission rate of 20.4% in the parent cohort is at the higher end of the range reported for people with diabetes [9,10], it seems unlikely that a substantial number of people were readmitted at other hospitals. Post-discharge mortality data were not available, and different mortality rates between the two groups may have influenced the observed readmission rates. Data on other potentially important risk factors or confounders such as A1c (due to lack of collection in about half the cohort), diabetes type (for which the accuracy of ICD-9-CM codes is suboptimal) [28], inpatient management, and classification of primary teams as medical or surgical were not available to analyze. Furthermore, the study period ended before FDA approval of SGLT2-inhibitors and the widespread use of GLP1-receptor agonists, which are drug classes that may influence the risk of hospitalization and readmission. Finally, the observational nature of this study precludes causal inference.

In conclusion, this retrospective observational study of patients with a primary or secondary discharge diagnosis of diabetes identified shared unique risk factors for all-cause 30-day readmission while confirming the higher readmission risk of patients with a primary diabetes diagnosis. The results suggest that inpatient diabetes consultation may be more effective at lowering the readmission risk among patients with a primary diabetes diagnosis than those with a secondary diabetes diagnosis. Given the burden incurred and imposed by hospital readmissions among people with diabetes, identifying those at greater risk of readmission offers the potential to allocate resources more efficiently and effectively to reduce readmission risk. These models may perform well to predict readmission risk, although additional study is needed to validate their performance. Randomized controlled trials are needed to test the strategy of linking readmission risk prediction with interventions for reducing such risk.

Supplementary Materials: The following supporting information can be downloaded at: https://www.mdpi.com/article/10.3390/jcm12041274/s1, Table S1. Most common secondary ICD-9-CM codes among 4027 patients with a primary discharge diagnosis of diabetes; Table S2. Most common reasons for hospital admission based on primary ICD-9-CM code among 4027 patients with a secondary discharge diagnosis of diabetes; Table S3. Risk factors for readmission in subgroup of patients with a primary discharge diagnosis of diabetes and an HbA1c value (n = 2182), OR (95% CI);

Table S4. Risk factors for readmission in subgroup of patients with a secondary discharge diagnosis of diabetes and an HbA1c value (n = 1492), OR (95% CI).

Author Contributions: Conceptualization, D.J.R.; Methodology, D.J.R. and H.Z.; Formal analysis, H.Z.; Investigation, D.J.R. and E.E.M.; Writing—original draft preparation, N.M. and E.E.M.; Writing—review and editing, D.J.R. and H.Z.; Visualization, N.M. and E.E.M.; Funding acquisition, D.J.R. All authors have read and agreed to the published version of the manuscript.

Funding: This research was funded by the National Institute of Diabetes and Digestive and Kidney Diseases of the National Institutes of Health, grant numbers K23DK102963 and R01DK122073. The content is solely the responsibility of the authors and does not necessarily represent the official views of the National Institutes of Health. The APC was funded by Temple University.

Institutional Review Board Statement: The study was conducted in accordance with the Declaration of Helsinki and approved by the Institutional Review Board of Temple University (protocol code 20658, approved on 5 November 2018) for studies involving humans.

Informed Consent Statement: Patient consent was waived due to the lack of direct patient interaction required to collect the retrospective EHR data, de-identification of the data, and the impracticality of obtaining consent from thousands of patients.

Data Availability Statement: Data are available on request due to institutional privacy restrictions on data use.

Conflicts of Interest: The authors declare no conflict of interest. The funders had no role in the design of the study; in the collection, analyses, or interpretation of data; in the writing of the manuscript; or in the decision to publish the results.

References

1. Benbassat, J.; Taragin, M. Hospital readmissions as a measure of quality of health care: Advantages and limitations. *Arch. Intern. Med.* **2000**, *160*, 1074–1081. [CrossRef] [PubMed]
2. Kocher, R.P.; Adashi, E.Y. Hospital readmissions and the affordable care act: Paying for coordinated quality care. *JAMA* **2011**, *306*, 1794–1795. [CrossRef] [PubMed]
3. McIlvennan, C.K.; Eapen, Z.J.; Allen, L.A. Hospital readmissions reduction program. *Circulation* **2015**, *131*, 1796–1803. [CrossRef]
4. Enomoto, L.M.; Shrestha, D.P.; Rosenthal, M.B.; Hollenbeak, C.S.; Gabbay, R.A. Risk factors associated with 30-day readmission and length of stay in patients with type 2 diabetes. *J Diabetes Complicat.* **2017**, *31*, 122–127. [CrossRef]
5. Ostling, S.; Wyckoff, J.; Ciarkowski, S.L.; Pai, C.W.; Choe, H.M.; Bahl, V.; Gianchandani, R. The relationship between diabetes mellitus and 30-day readmission rates. journal article. *Clin. Diabetes Endocrinol.* **2017**, *3*, 3. [CrossRef]
6. AHRQ. Healthcare Cost and Utilization Project (HCUP) National Inpatient Sample (NIS) 2018. Available online: https://hcupnet.ahrq.gov/#setup (accessed on 27 January 2022).
7. Fingar, K.R.; Reid, L.D. *Diabetes-Related Inpatient Stays, 2018*; Agency for Healthcare Research and Quality (US): Rockville, MD, USA, 2021.
8. Centers for Disease Control and Prevention. *National Diabetes Statistics Report*; U.S. Dept of Health and Human Services: Atlanta, GA, USA, 2020.
9. Rubin, D.J.; Shah, A.A. Predicting and Preventing Acute Care Re-Utilization by Patients with Diabetes. *Curr. Diabetes Rep.* **2021**, *21*, 34. [CrossRef] [PubMed]
10. Rubin, D.J. Hospital Readmission of Patients with Diabetes. *Curr. Diabetes Rep.* **2015**, *15*, 17. [CrossRef]
11. Sonmez, H.; Kambo, V.; Avtanski, D.; Lutsky, L.; Poretsky, L. The readmission rates in patients with versus those without diabetes mellitus at an urban teaching hospital. *J. Diabetes Complicat.* **2017**, *31*, 1681–1685. [CrossRef]
12. Karunakaran, A.; Zhao, H.; Rubin, D.J. Predischarge and Postdischarge Risk Factors for Hospital Readmission Among Patients With Diabetes. *Med. Care* **2018**, *56*, 634–642. [CrossRef]
13. Furnival, G.M.; Wilson, R.W., Jr. Regressions by Leaps and Bounds. *Technometrics* **1974**, *16*, 499–511. [CrossRef]
14. Hanley, J.A.; Negassa, A.; Edwardes, M.D.; Forrester, J.E. Statistical Analysis of Correlated Data Using Generalized Estimating Equations: An Orientation. *Am. J. Epidemiol.* **2003**, *157*, 364–375. [CrossRef] [PubMed]
15. Hanley, J.A.; McNeil, B.J. The meaning and use of the area under a receiver operating characteristic (ROC) curve. *Radiology* **1982**, *143*, 29–36. [CrossRef] [PubMed]
16. Steyerberg, E.W.; Vickers, A.J.; Cook, N.R.; Gerds, T.; Gonen, M.; Obuchowski, N.; Pencina, M.J.; Kattan, M. Assessing the performance of prediction models: A framework for traditional and novel measures. Research Support, Non-U.S. Gov't. *Epidemiology* **2010**, *21*, 128–138. [CrossRef]

17. Shaka, H.; Aguilera, M.; Aucar, M.; El-Amir, Z.; Wani, F.; Muojieje, C.C.; Kichloo, A. Rate and Predictors of 30-day Readmission Following Diabetic Ketoacidosis in Type 1 Diabetes Mellitus: A US Analysis. *J. Clin. Endocrinol. Metab.* **2021**, *106*, 2592–2599. [CrossRef]
18. Koproski, J.; Pretto, Z.; Poretsky, L. Effects of an intervention by a diabetes team in hospitalized patients with diabetes. *Diabetes Care*. **1997**, *20*, 1553–1555. [CrossRef]
19. Wang, Y.J.; Seggelke, S.; Hawkins, R.M.; Gibbs, J.; Lindsay, M.; Hazlett, I.; Wang, C.C.L.; Rasouli, N.; Young, K.A.; Draznin, B. Impact of glucose management team on outcomes of hospitalizaron in patients with type 2 diabetes admitted to the medical service. *Endocr. Pract.* **2016**, *22*, 1401–1405. [CrossRef]
20. Mandel, S.R.; Langan, S.; Mathioudakis, N.N.; Sidhaye, A.R.; Bashura, H.; Bie, J.Y.; Mackay, P.; Tucker, C.; Demidowich, A.P.; Simonds, W.F.; et al. Retrospective study of inpatient diabetes management service, length of stay and 30-day readmission rate of patients with diabetes at a community hospital. *J. Community Hosp. Intern. Med. Perspect.* **2019**, *9*, 64–73. [CrossRef]
21. Bansal, V.; Mottalib, A.; Pawar, T.K.; Abbasakoor, N.; Chuang, E.; Chaudhry, A.; Sakr, M.; Gabbay, R.A.; Hamdy, O. Inpatient diabetes management by specialized diabetes team versus primary service team in non-critical care units: Impact on 30-day readmission rate and hospital cost. *BMJ Open Diabetes Res. Care* **2018**, *6*, e000460. [CrossRef]
22. Bhalodkar, A.; Sonmez, H.; Lesser, M.; Leung, T.; Ziskovich, K.; Inlall, D.; Murray-Bachmann, R.; Krymskaya, M.; Poretsky, L. The Effects of a Comprehensive Multidisciplinary Outpatient Diabetes Program on Hospital Readmission Rates in Patients with Diabetes: A Randomized Controlled Prospective Study. *Endocr. Pract.* **2020**, *26*, 1331–1336. [CrossRef]
23. Seggelke, S.A.; Hawkins, R.M.; Gibbs, J.; Rasouli, N.; Wang, C.; Draznin, B. Transitional care clinic for uninsured and medicaid-covered patients with diabetes mellitus discharged from the hospital: A pilot quality improvement study. *Hosp. Pract.* **2014**, *42*, 46–51. [CrossRef]
24. Magny-Normilus, C.; Nolido, N.V.; Borges, J.C.; Brady, M.; Labonville, S.; Williams, D.; Soukup, J.; Lipsitz, S.; Hudson, M.; Schnipper, J.L. Effects of an Intensive Discharge Intervention on Medication Adherence, Glycemic Control, and Readmission Rates in Patients With Type 2 Diabetes. *J. Patient Saf.* **2021**, *17*, 73–80. [CrossRef]
25. Rubin, D.J.; Handorf, E.A.; Golden, S.H.; Nelson, D.B.; McDonnell, M.E.; Zhao, H. Development and Validation of a Novel Tool to Predict Hospital Readmission Risk Among Patients With Diabetes. *Endocr. Pract.* **2016**, *22*, 1204–1215. [CrossRef] [PubMed]
26. Nana-Sinkam, P.; Kraschnewski, J.; Sacco, R.; Chavez, J.; Fouad, M.; Gal, T.; AuYoung, M.; Namoos, A.; Winn, R.; Sheppard, V.; et al. Health disparities and equity in the era of COVID-19. *J. Clin. Transl. Sci.* **2021**, *5*, e99. [CrossRef] [PubMed]
27. Subramaniam, A.; Lim, Z.J.; Ponnapa Reddy, M.; Shekar, K. Systematic review and meta-analysis of the characteristics and outcomes of readmitted <scp>COVID</scp> -19 survivors. *Intern. Med. J.* **2021**, *51*, 1773–1780. [CrossRef] [PubMed]
28. Klompas, M.; Eggleston, E.; McVetta, J.; Lazarus, R.; Li, L.; Platt, R. Automated Detection and Classification of Type 1 Versus Type 2 Diabetes Using Electronic Health Record Data. *Diabetes Care* **2013**, *36*, 914–921. [CrossRef]

Disclaimer/Publisher's Note: The statements, opinions and data contained in all publications are solely those of the individual author(s) and contributor(s) and not of MDPI and/or the editor(s). MDPI and/or the editor(s) disclaim responsibility for any injury to people or property resulting from any ideas, methods, instructions or products referred to in the content.

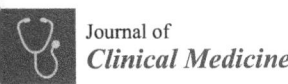

Review

COVID-19 and Diabetes

Virginia Bellido [1] and Antonio Pérez [2,3,*]

[1] Endocrinology and Nutrition Department, Hospital Universitario Virgen del Rocío, 41013 Sevilla, Spain; virginiabellido@gmail.com
[2] Endocrinology and Nutrition Department, Hospital de la Santa Creu i Sant Pau, Institut d'Investigació Bio-Mèdica Sant Pau, 08041 Barcelona, Spain
[3] Centro de Investigación Biomédica en Red de Diabetes y Enfermedades Metabólicas Asociadas (CIBERDEM), Universitat Autònoma de Barcelona, 08193 Barcelona, Spain
* Correspondence: aperez@santpau.cat

Abstract: Diabetes mellitus (DM) is one of the most common comorbid conditions in persons with COVID-19 and a risk factor for poor prognosis. The reasons why COVID-19 is more severe in persons with DM are currently unknown although the scarce data available on patients with DM hospitalized because of COVID-19 show that glycemic control is inadequate. The fact that patients with COVID-19 are usually cared for by health professionals with limited experience in the management of diabetes and the need to prevent exposure to the virus may also be obstacles to glycemic control in patients with COVID-19. Effective clinical care should consider various aspects, including screening for the disease in at-risk persons, education, and monitoring of control and complications. We examine the effect of COVID-19 on DM in terms of glycemic control and the restrictions arising from the pandemic and assess management of diabetes and drug therapy in various scenarios, taking into account factors such as physical exercise, diet, blood glucose monitoring, and pharmacological treatment. Specific attention is given to patients who have been admitted to hospital and critically ill patients. Finally, we consider the role of telemedicine in the management of DM patients with COVID-19 during the pandemic and in the future.

Keywords: diabetes mellitus; COVID-19; hyperglycemia; glycemic control; blood glucose monitoring; telemedicine

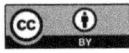

1. Diabetes and COVID-19

Diabetes mellitus (DM) is a medical condition that can have a considerable impact on affected persons and on society owing to the high costs associated with its care, especially those arising from complications. The situation becomes more serious during a pandemic, such as that of COVID-19, as having DM entails a greater risk of extended hospital stay and death. In addition to the direct effects on health, the absence of regular care owing to closure of outpatient clinics and social isolation—combined with changes in diet, physical activity, and personal care—favors deterioration of disease control and hampers detection of complications. All of the above factors could prove responsible for poorer clinical outcomes in patients with DM

This study examines the impact of the COVID-19 pandemic on persons with DM and covers implications for health in the short and long terms. It also examines how to address the threat to persons with DM arising from more limited health services and changes in lifestyle resulting from the pandemic.

2. COVID-19 in Persons with Diabetes

2.1. Impact of Diabetes on COVID-19

DM is one of the most common comorbid conditions in persons with COVID-19, and while the presence of DM does not seem to increase the risk of infection [1], it is a risk factor for poor prognosis [2,3]. The prevalence of DM in persons with COVID-19 varies widely according to published series, from 7% to 30% [4]. A meta-analysis by Fadini et al. [1] in Italy examined 12 studies performed in China and, including outpatients and hospitalized patients, found the prevalence of DM to be 10.3%, which overlapped with or was even slightly inferior to the prevalence of DM in the Chinese population adjusted for age. In the whole-population study by Barron et al. [5] in England, which included 61,414,470 live individuals registered in primary care, 0.4% had been diagnosed with type 1 diabetes (T1D), 4.7% had a diagnosis of type 2 diabetes (T2D), and 0.1% had other types of DM. The odds ratios (ORs) for in-hospital COVID-19-related death were 3.51 (95% CI, 3.16–3.90) in people with type 1 diabetes and 2.03 (1.97–2.09) in people with type 2 diabetes after adjustment for age, sex, deprivation, ethnicity, and geographical region. These effects were attenuated, reaching ORs of 2.86 (2.58–3.18) for type 1 diabetes and 1.80 (1.75–1.86) for type 2 diabetes when also adjusted for previous hospital admissions with coronary heart disease, cerebrovascular disease, and heart failure. Various studies have shown that DM is present in approximately 20% of persons infected by type 2 coronavirus causing severe acute respiratory syndrome (SARS-CoV-2) and that it is one of the most common comorbid conditions together with arterial hypertension, obesity, and cardiovascular disease [6–8].

Once COVID-19 is acquired, DM might increase the severity and mortality of the disease to the extent that patients with uncontrolled hyperglycemia or DM have a greater risk of respiratory failure and cardiac complications and more than double the probability of being admitted to the intensive care unit (ICU). Moreover, mortality is 3-fold greater than in patients without DM or uncontrolled hyperglycemia [2,3,5,9,10]. In the study by Barron et al. [5], 30% of deaths from COVID-19 were in persons with DM, and the risk of death was almost 3-fold greater for persons with T1D and almost double for those with T2D than in those who did not have DM. In addition to the impact on health, the COVID-19 pandemic considerably affects the use of health care resources and costs. In the USA, the average direct medical cost during the course of the infection was estimated to double or triple in patients with comorbid conditions, such as DM [11].

The reasons why COVID-19 is more severe in persons with DM are currently unknown [12]. Potential pathophysiological mechanisms that contribute to the increase in morbidity and mortality include presence of an underlying chronic inflammatory state in DM, impaired immune response, and coagulation abnormalities. The high prevalence of DM in severe cases of COVID-19 could reflect the greater prevalence of T2D in elderly people. Furthermore, DM in the elderly is associated with cardiovascular diseases and obesity, which in themselves go some way to explaining the association with the fatal outcome of COVID-19. However, the association between DM and a poorer prognosis is maintained in non-hypertensive younger patients [9]. Current studies have shown that hyperglycemia at admission to hospital is a predictor of death and other severe outcomes of COVID-19 [13,14]. The Spanish registry of the Spanish Society of Internal Medicine for COVID-19 [14], which included 11,312 patients (18.9% with previous DM) hospitalized with COVID-19 in 109 hospitals, showed that patients who were not critically ill but presented with hyperglycemia at admission, irrespective of whether they had previously had DM or not, were more likely to develop complications and die and that this risk increased with the grade of hyperglycemia (blood glucose >180 mg/dL (>10 mmol/L); HR for mortality, 1.50; 95% CI, 1.31–1.73; and blood glucose 140–180 mg/dL (7.8–10 mmol/L); HR, 1.48; 95% CI, 1.29–1.70). A retrospective study of 1544 patients with COVID-19 from 91 hospitals in the USA [13] showed that both hyperglycemia and hypoglycemia were associated with poor outcomes in patients with COVID-19. In addition, although clearly insufficient, available data support the fact that optimal control of glycemia during hospital stay could prove to be beneficial in terms of clinical outcomes in patients with DM and COVID-19. A study of 59 patients with COVID-19 admitted to two Italian hospitals [15] showed that treatment with insulin infusion until blood glucose levels of <140 mg/dL (<7.8 mmol/L) were reached in 15 subjects with hyperglycemia and improved their prognosis with respect to patients who had not received an insulin infusion. Furthermore, levels of interleukin 6 and D-dimer decreased once hyperglycemia was treated.

Specific mechanisms with a potential role in COVID-19 infection include angiotensin II–converting enzyme (ACE2) and dipeptidyl peptidase 4 (DPP4) [12,16]. ACE2 has been identified as a coronavirus surface protein receptor. COVID-19 reduces expression of ACE2, thus inducing cell damage, hyperinflammation, and respiratory failure. Acute hyperglycemia upregulates expression of ACE2 in cells, thus potentially facilitating the entry of viral cells [3,17]. However, we know that chronic hyperglycemia negatively regulates expression of ACE2, leaving cells vulnerable to the effects of the virus [18]. Cell studies have identified DPP4 as a functional receptor for human coronavirus–Erasmus Medical Center (HCoV-EMC) and antibodies targeting DPP4 inhibited infection of primary cells by HCoV-EMC [16]. At present, it is unknown whether these mechanisms can also be applied to COVID-19 and whether treatment of DM with DPP4 inhibitors in clinical practice affects the course of the infection.

2.2. Impact of COVID-19 on Diabetes

DM is not only a risk factor for greater severity of COVID-19; in fact, the disease affects persons with DM directly, as in other viral infections (by worsening previous DM and even inducing new-onset DM), or indirectly, as a consequence of the restrictions arising from lockdown during the COVID-19 pandemic.

2.2.1. Effects of COVID-19 on Glycemic Control

The scarce data available on patients with DM hospitalized because of COVID-19 show that glycemic control is inadequate [19,20]. A study that analyzed glycemic outcomes during admission found that 39.1% of values were over 180 mg/dL (10 mmol/L) and that the mean blood glucose level was over 180 mg/dL (10 mmol/L) for 37.8% of hospital stay [19]. In a study carried out in the USA [13], more than half of patients admitted to the ICU (56%) and outside the ICU (53%) did not reach their target blood glucose levels during the first two or three days; a study performed in China found that 56.6% of capillary blood glucose test results were higher than the recommended target (140–180 mg/dL) (7.8–10 mmol/L) [20]. In patients who required insulin, SARS-CoV-2 infection was associated with very high insulin requirements, reaching doses of 201 IU/d (2.2 IU/kg/d) [21]; these high values are associated with levels of inflammatory cytokines. Decompensation in the form of diabetic ketoacidosis has been reported in patients with T2D and COVID-19, as is the case in other severe infections. One systematic review reported that 77% of patients with COVID-19 who developed ketoacidosis had underlying T2D, and DM was diagnosed in 10 patients at admission; of these, seven had glycated hemoglobin >9.5% [22]. The pathophysiology of these manifestations of DM is complex and probably goes beyond the well-established stress response associated with severe disease and the toxicity induced by persistently elevated glucose concentrations. The proinflammatory medium induced by COVID-19 can lead to a high degree of insulin resistance, thus increasing insulin requirements. Pancreatic β cells express ACE2, which can lead the virus to enter the pancreatic islets and damage the β cells, thus causing insulin deficiency. This effect worsens the course of DM and causes acute hyperglycemia, even in persons without DM [23]. Insulin deficiency in the setting of marked insulin resistance might also explain the common finding of cases of severe diabetic ketoacidosis and ketosis at admission [24]. Furthermore, drugs that are commonly used in clinical practice for patients with COVID-19, such as systemic corticosteroids and antiviral agents, worsen glycemic control and lead to marked glycemic excursions over a 24-h period [25,26]. In addition, there have been reports of a high number of hypoglycemic episodes at admission, probably favored by the anorexia induced by COVID-19 and without the concomitant adjustment of glucose-lowering drugs [20,27]. Finally, the fact that patients with COVID-19 are cared for by health professionals with limited experience in the management of hyperglycemia and the need to prevent exposure to the virus may also be obstacles to glycemic control in patients with COVID-19. Therefore, impaired glycemic control in patients with DM and hyperglycemia in patients without previous DM is considered a complication of COVID-19.

2.2.2. Effects on Diabetes of the Restrictions Arising from the COVID-19 Pandemic

The COVID-19 pandemic was and continues to be a considerable challenge for people with DM since their normal routines have been interrupted in order to comply with social distancing measures. The immediate consequence is that a patient's ability to gain access to and receive medical care, obtain medication and material for control of DM, and maintain a healthy lifestyle and social connections have been considerably affected. While information on the indirect consequences of the COVID-19 pandemic on DM is limited, we are now seeing data that make it possible to evaluate the impact of the first wave.

Studies in patients with T1D who use continuous glucose monitoring (CGM) or flash glucose monitoring (FGM) have shown that during lockdown, there was no deterioration in glycemic control or even beneficial effects [28,29]. A recent meta-analysis including 3441 individuals with T1D with CGM or FGM showed that, during the lockdown period, time in range 70–180 mg/dL increased by 3.05% (95% CI, 1.67–4.43%; $p < 0.0001$), while time above range (>180 mg/dL and > 250 mg/dL) declined by 3.39% (−5.14 to −1.63%) and 1.96% (−2.51 to −1.42%), respectively ($p < 0.0001$ for both) [30]. It has been speculated that this improvement could be associated with the ability to spend more time monitoring DM, having more regular timetables, and experiencing less stress associated with going to and from work. However, these findings may not be applicable to people with T1D who are less motivated to control their disease, who do not use CGM, or whose social-occupational situation competes for the time spent on managing DM. Of the 763 persons with T1D who participated in the Taking Control of Your Diabetes study in the USA, 46% reported that the pandemic hampered their management of DM. Furthermore, in approximately 25%, there was an increase in the frequency of high blood glucose levels and variations in blood glucose [31]. Finally, of the 603 patients with T1D who participated in a web survey in Spain, two-thirds reported impaired glycemic control, and 4 out of 10 reported weight gain [32].

The T2D population is much more heterogeneous than the T1D population in relevant aspects such as treatment, monitoring, and ability to self-adjust treatment and use remote consultation tools. The results of the survey among the subjects of Taking Control of Your Diabetes (763 persons with T1D and 619 with T2D) show that the impact of lockdown on management of DM was similar in both populations [31]. Patients were mainly non-Hispanic White, were educated to a high level, and had good control of their glycemia. Furthermore, in the case of patients with T2D, 46% received treatment with insulin, and 25% used CGM. A study of 114 patients with T2D followed at a tertiary center in Italy found that lockdown led to poorer metabolic control in the short term in 26% of patients who had previously been well controlled [33]. Given the characteristics of the populations studied and the care setting, these data are not applicable to the general population with T2D, especially in those patients who require care from the health system for monitoring of control and intensification of treatment. In addition, given that published data are very short term and that T2D is progressive, we might expect that the absence of or reduction in monitoring and in intensification of treatment leads to more frequently impaired control in the longer term. Data from the electronic medical records of a cohort of 13,352,550 patients from 1709 primary care centers in the United Kingdom followed between March and April 2020 raise particular concern over the considerable reduction (77–84%) in testing of glycated hemoglobin and in the prescription of metformin and insulin, especially in older persons with T2D [34]. Similar changes in glucose-lowering therapy were reported in patients with T2D in Germany between January and July 2019 ($N = 79,268$) and between January and July 2020 ($N = 85,046$). Compared with 2019, the number of persons with ≥ 1 change in medication fell in 2020, as follows: DPP4 inhibitors, −15%; sodium-glucose co-transporter 2 (SGLT2) inhibitors, −3%; glucagon-like peptide-1 (GLP1) receptor agonists, 0%; other oral hypoglycemic drugs, −6%; and insulin, −21% [35]. Another indirect consequence of the COVID-19 pandemic in T2D patients is the effect on diagnosis of DM, which requires specific diagnostic tests that must be performed in a clinical setting. The first four months of lockdown in the United Kingdom saw a reduction of 70% in new diagnoses of T2D; that is, more than 45,000 diagnoses were either not made or delayed during this period [34]. Taken together, these data are worrying since absence of or delaying diagnosis and monitoring of DM hampers decisions on therapy aimed at improving metabolic control and preventing the development or progression of potentially severe complications in the long term.

3. Treatment of Diabetes during the COVID-19 Pandemic: Disease Management and Drug Therapy in Various Scenarios

3.1. Diabetes Patients without COVID-19: Lockdown and Lack of Physical Exercise

People with DM must be aware of the importance of maintaining good glycemic control during the COVID-19 pandemic since stability of blood glucose levels can help to ensure a milder clinical course if the individual becomes infected [36]. Good glycemic control depends on tailoring therapy to the individual patient's situation. A balanced diet, regular physical exercise, psychological stability, and adequately adjusted treatment are key elements when attempting to achieve objectives for disease control. It is also important to control comorbid conditions associated with DM, such as routine vaccination against pneumococcus and influenza (Table 1) [37]. It is as well a priority for people with diabetes to receive the COVID-19 vaccine. Clinical data have shown a robust neutralizing antibody response in patients with diabetes [38]. However, recent data have shown that hyperglycemia at the time of COVID-19 vaccination worsens the immune response, whereas achieving adequate glycemic control during the post-vaccination period improves the immune response [39]. Therefore, we need to focus on achieving good glycemic control, which can play a role in clinical COVID-19 outcomes and vaccine efficiency

Table 1. General recommendations for the prevention of COVID-19 in persons with diabetes [37].

Hygiene and social Distancing Measures
Lifestyle
• Healthy diet: limit refined sugar and fat; avoid snacks [40,41] • Physical exercise: avoid a sedentary lifestyle; take regular aerobic exercise (walking, cycling, etc.) combined with strength exercise (weights, resistance bands, pushing exercises, etc.) [42,43]. • Avoid smoking; avoid alcohol • Stress management
Glycemic control
• Regular monitoring of blood glucose levels • Continue with regular treatment, except in the case of contraindications • Consider dose adjustment (insulin, sulfonylureas, etc.) depending on diet and physical activity • Ketone level monitoring in T1D, especially if hyperglycemia is persistent (>250 mg/dL), or there are symptoms suggestive of ketoacidosis (nausea, vomiting, abdominal pain, etc.)
Control of comorbid conditions (obesity, blood pressure, dyslipidemia, etc.)
Vaccination (routine vaccination against pneumococcal and seasonal influenza)
Minimize exposure to SARS-CoV-2 (prioritize telemedicine)

SARS-CoV-2, severe acute respiratory syndrome coronavirus 2.

Table 1 summarizes the main recommendations for the prevention of COVID-19 in people with diabetes.

General public health measures issued by health authorities (e.g., social distancing, hand washing, masks, and lockdown) should receive specific emphasis in people with DM. Similarly, telemedicine should be preferred to limit exposure of people with DM while at the same time guaranteeing continuity of care [44].

Greater vigilance is warranted for early detection of signs and symptoms—even atypical ones—of SARS-CoV-2 infection in patients with DM. A lower clinical threshold for suspicion of COVID-19 should be established in order to avoid delays in health care and adverse outcomes in this population [45].

3.2. Patients with Diabetes and COVID-19 Who Have Not Been Admitted to Hospital

Most persons with COVID-19 and DM develop mild disease that can be managed at home according to local guidelines. In these cases, regular contact with and follow-up by health services are crucial for identifying impaired control or clinical status. Similarly, optimization of glycemic control is key if we are to reduce the risk of severe disease. Therefore, blood glucose levels should be monitored frequently, and patients should follow a healthy diet, ensure appropriate fluid intake, and adjust treatment in cases of impaired glycemic control [37]. Integrated management of comorbid conditions and associated cardiovascular risk factors are equally important during this period [37].

Figure 1 shows general recommendations for prevention and management of COVID-19 in people with diabetes.

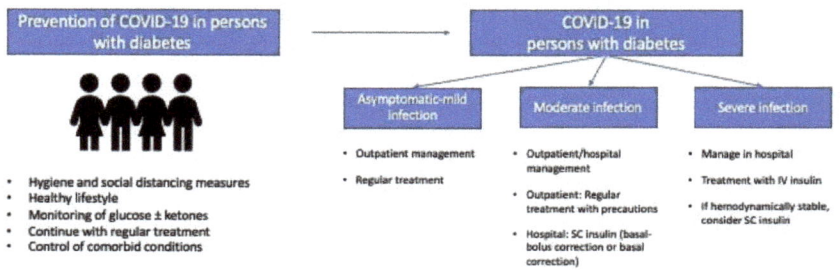

Figure 1. General recommendations for prevention and management of COVID-19 in persons with diabetes.

3.2.1. Objectives of Glycemic Control

The objectives of glycemic control should be tailored according to age, comorbid conditions, complications, and the clinical severity of infection. It is generally recommended to maintain preprandial glucose levels between 70 and 130 mg/dL and postprandial levels <180 mg/dL. In the case of elderly or frail patients, more easily achievable objectives can be set, with priority given to avoiding hypoglycemia [46].

In the case of patients who use CGM, the objective should be to reach time in range (70 to 180 mg/dL) of more than 70%, with time in hypoglycemia (<70 mg/dL) lower than 4%. The values for elderly or frail patients are reaching time in range >50% and time in hypoglycemia <1% [47,48].

3.2.2. Glucose Monitoring

Control of glucose levels is essential if we are to maintain good glycemic control during infection and detect possible hyperglycemic complications or hypoglycemia. The number of checks depends on the type of DM, treatment, and degree of control. However, in the case of COVID-19 infection, the number of daily checks should be increased and the results analyzed. The use of CGM or FGM systems as well as glucose monitors with the option to download data and a cloud connection enables remote monitoring by health professionals.

In the case of CGM, it is important to remember the possible interference of paracetamol with some systems (Dexcom G5, Guardian Connect, Enlite-Guardian Link, Enlite-Guardian 2 Link, Guardian Sensor 3-Guardian Link 3, Eversense, etc.) [49]. In these cases, capillary blood glucose monitoring should be performed before taking paracetamol.

3.2.3. Pharmacologic Treatment

Various glucose-lowering agents (e.g., metformin, DPP4 inhibitors, and GLP1 receptor agonists) have anti-inflammatory action, thus supporting the hypothesis that one or more of these drugs could be particularly useful in persons with T2D and COVID-19 [50].

However, in the absence of prospective randomized controlled trials, there continues to be insufficient evidence for stating whether the use of a specific class of glucose-lowering agents is beneficial or harmful for people with COVID-19 [51]. An analysis of COVID-19 results from 1317 persons with DM (88.5% with T2D) in French hospitals revealed no clear association between glucose-lowering agents and symptom severity [52]. Similarly, no significant association was found between treatment and clinical findings for COVID-19 infection in 1762 persons with T2D in the SEMI-COVID-19 registry in Spain [53].

Patients with mild COVID-19 can generally continue with their usual treatment, providing they maintain adequate oral tolerance with good fluid intake, and there are no contraindications for treatment. Nevertheless, factors such as kidney function, nutritional status, risk of hypoglycemia, severity of infection, and glycemic control itself may require treatment to be adjusted. The main recommendations for antihyperglycemic agents in patients with COVID-19 are summarized in Table 2 [25,37,48,50].

Table 2. Recommendations on the use of antihyperglycemic drugs in patients with diabetes and COVID-19 [37,48,54–57].

Treatment	Clinical Recommendation	Special Considerations in COVID-19
Metformin	Suspend in severe cases, with hemodynamic instability or hypoxia	Risk of lactic acidosis in hypoxia and acute disease Monitor kidney function. Suspend if glomerular filtration <30 mL/min/1.73 m^2
Sulfonylureas	Suspend in cases where food intake is not guaranteed owing to the risk of hypoglycemia	The risk of hypoglycemia may be greater with concomitant use of treatments such as hydroxychloroquine
DPP4i	Continue in outpatients Potential option in hospitalized patients with mild hyperglycemia, combined with basal insulin	Favorable safety profile and possible use in kidney failure
GLP1ra	Suspend in severe cases	Risk of dehydration in the case of severe gastrointestinal adverse effects (nausea, vomiting, etc.) Maintain a regular diet and ensure good hydration
SGLT2i	Suspend in severe cases, or if food/fluid intake cannot be guaranteed	Risk of euglycemic diabetic ketoacidosis induced by dehydration and insulin deficiency Preserving cardiovascular and kidney function is critical for ensuring favorable progress of COVID-19 in persons with diabetes
Glitazones	Suspend in severe cases with hemodynamic instability or heart of liver dysfunction	Risk of fluid retention and heart failure
Insulin	Continue treatment of choice in hospitalized patients. Adjust dose depending on glycemic control, risk of hypoglycemia, severity of infection, and concomitant treatment Requires frequent monitoring of blood glucose (capillary glycemia or CGM/FGM)	Insulin requirements may be very high in hospitalized patients with severe infection

GLP1ra, glucagon-like peptide 1 receptor agonist; DPP4i, dipeptidyl peptidase 4 inhibitor; SGLT2i, sodium-glucose co-transporter-2 inhibitors; CGM, continuous glucose monitoring; FGM, flash glucose monitoring.

3.2.4. Control of Other Cardiovascular Risk Factors

Angiotensin-converting enzyme inhibitors (ACEI) and angiotensin II receptor blockers (ARA2) are essential for management of hypertension, heart failure, and diabetic nephropathy. No clear evidence in favor of or against these agents in persons with T2D at risk of or infected by SARS-CoV-2 has been published to date, despite speculation over possible adverse effects [7]. There are clear risks associated with discontinuation since control of hypertension and protection against kidney disease may be compromised. At present, most international organizations recommend continuation of ACEI/ARA2 unless there are explicit contraindications, such as hypotension or acute kidney injury [58,59].

As for dyslipidemia, there is currently insufficient evidence in favor of or against continuation of statins in patients with DM and COVID-19. Increased liver and muscle enzymes have been associated with the infection [60], and some authors recommend monitoring creatine kinase in affected patients [61]. Decisions should be tailored taking into account the indication for statins as well as possible interactions with antiviral agents.

Risk of thrombosis should also be taken into account. Persons with DM are more likely to experience thrombosis, which is a relatively frequent complication in COVID-19 [60]. Treatment should be continued in patients taking antithrombotic agents. Similarly, in the absence of contraindications, all patients hospitalized with COVID-19 should receive prophylaxis for venous thromboembolism [62].

3.2.5. Special Considerations in T1D

Persons with T1D should never discontinue insulin owing to the high risk of hyperosmolar hyperglycemic syndrome and diabetic ketoacidosis after infection [63]. It is essential to guarantee appropriate fluid intake and frequent monitoring of glucose levels and ketone bodies. Patients should be trained to know when to monitor ketones and be aware of the need for additional doses of insulin. In the case of blood ketone levels higher than 3 mmol/L, patients should consult their health professionals.

3.3. Hospitalized Patients with Diabetes and COVID-19

The COVID-19 pandemic has generated new challenges in hospital management of DM. Good control of glycemia helps to improve clinical outcomes although it also requires frequent contact between health care personnel and patients to ensure appropriate monitoring of blood glucose, administration of insulin, and resolution of hypoglycemia in a situation where it is recommended to minimize interactions with patients in order to avoid exposure to COVID-19 [64]. Table 3 summarizes the main recommendations for management of hyperglycemia in critically ill and non-critically ill patients depending on their clinical status.

Table 3. Management of hyperglycemia in critically ill and non-critically ill patients with COVID-19 [65].

	Blood Glucose Target	Clinical Situation		Insulin Regimen	Glucose Monitoring
Critically ill patients	140–180 mg/dL *	Hemodynamically unstable Parenteral nutrition Varying insulin requirements Treatment with corticosteroids		Continuous intravenous insulin infusion	Every hour
		Hemodynamically stable Stable insulin requirements		Subcutaneous insulin Basal + correction or basal-bolus + correction	Every 4–6 h
Non-critically ill patients	110–180 mg/dL **	T1D T2D with OAD ± insulin	No oral intake	Basal insulin + correction	Every 4–6 h ****
			Oral intake	Basal-bolus insulin + correction	Before meals and at bedtime ****
		T2D with diet DM not known	Glycemia on admission <180 mg/dL	Correction insulin dose before meals or every 6 h ***	Before meals and at bedtime or every 6 h ****
			Glycemia on admission >180 mg/dL	Basal-bolus insulin + correction	Before meals and at bedtime ****

* 110–140 mg/dL may be reasonable for selected patients, providing it can be reached without hypoglycemia. ** 110–140 mg/dL may be reasonable in patients with mild disease and good previous glycemic control. Blood glucose >180 mg/dL may be reasonable for patients with high risk of hypoglycemia or limited life expectancy. *** In order to calculate insulin requirements during the first 24 h. Afterwards, intensify to basal correction or basal-bolus correction regimen. **** Consider using continuous glucose monitoring, if possible, in order to limit the number of capillary blood glucose controls. OAD, oral antidiabetic agents; DM, diabetes mellitus; T1D, diabetes mellitus type 1; T2D, diabetes mellitus type 2.

3.3.1. Management of Hyperglycemia in Critically Ill Patients with COVID-19

Glucose levels should be maintained between 140 and 180 mg/dL in most critically ill patients [66]; more rigorous targets (110–140 mg/dL) could be reasonable for selected patients, providing they can be reached without significant hypoglycemia [67–70].

Insulin should be the treatment of choice for critically ill patients with COVID-19 [71]. The most effective way of reaching glucose targets is continuous intravenous infusion based on validated written or computerized protocols [72,73]. Most protocols require glucose to be monitored at least once hourly, thus necessitating contact with staff. Exposure of health care staff managing hyperglycemia in critically ill patients with COVID-19 should be minimized. In the case of hemodynamically stable patients not receiving parenteral nutrition or high doses of corticosteroids, we recommend using subcutaneous insulin regimens (basal-bolus correction or basal correction) instead of intravenous regimens and monitoring blood glucose four times daily, together with other nursing care, in order to reduce the need to enter the patient's room [65].

Transferring administration of insulin from intravenous to subcutaneous is recommended when the patient is clinically stable. The initial dose of subcutaneous insulin when switching can be calculated as 60–80% of the intravenous dose administered during the previous 24 h. Short-acting insulin can be administered for 1–2 h and long-acting insulin for 2–3 h before interrupting administration of intravenous insulin [74,75].

3.3.2. Management of Hyperglycemia in Non-Critically Ill Patients with COVID-19

Glucose values before meals and after fasting <140 mg/dL with random maximum glucose <180 mg/dL could be appropriate in stable patients with mild disease and strict previous glycemic control, whereas glucose levels >180 mg/dL may be acceptable in patients with a high risk of hypoglycemia or limited life expectancy as a way of minimizing the risk of hypoglycemia [65].

Insulin is still considered the most appropriate drug for effective control of glycemia in hospital. A regimen with basal, prandial, and correctional components is the preferred approach in non-critically ill hospitalized patients with COVID-19 and good nutritional intake; basal insulin or basal insulin with correction doses is the best choice for patients whose oral intake cannot be guaranteed. Prolonged use of sliding-scale rapid-acting insulin as the only treatment for hyperglycemia is not recommended.

DPP4 inhibitors combined with basal insulin can be an alternative in patients with COVID-19 and mild-to-moderate hyperglycemia. The DARE-19 study recently showed that in patients with cardiometabolic risk factors hospitalized with COVID-19, treatment with dapagliflozin did not result in a statistically significant reduction in the risk of organ dysfunction or death. Similarly, it did not result in a significant improvement in clinical recovery although it was well tolerated. Therefore, these findings could support continuation of SGLT2i for patients already receiving them before a COVID-19 diagnosis as long as they are monitored [76].

Treatment of corticosteroid-induced hyperglycemia with insulin corticosteroids can aggravate or induce hyperglycemia in hospitalized patients with COVID-19 with and without DM [65,77]. As for management, some authors have reported their experience adding neutral protamine Hagedorn insulin at doses of 20–30 IU in the morning as well as the usual insulin regimen [71]. In our experience, the best option is to add the calculated increase in the dose of insulin, taking into account body weight, corticosteroid dose, and the patient's usual total dose, which should be distributed according to the insulin regimen and the usual corticosteroid schedule [26].

3.3.3. Glucose Monitoring of Patients with COVID-19 in Hospital

Control of DM in hospital usually requires multiple daily glucose readings. This is challenging for patients who are in isolation. Therefore, the United States Food and Drug Administration (FDA) has authorized self-monitoring of glucose in hospital by patients using their own glucose monitors during the COVID-19 pandemic [78] and is in favor of using CGM in non-critically ill patients [79–81] although this does not imply approval for use in hospital. Dexcom G6 and FreeStyle Libre have proven to reduce the incidence of hypoglycemia in non-critically ill patients [82–84]. Neither requires calibration of capillary glycemia, thus minimizing staff exposure and workload. Similarly, the fact that these devices are not affected by interference with paracetamol is yet another advantage in patients with COVID-19. A pilot study found that Dexcom G6 is feasible in non-critically ill COVID-19 patients, with a MARD of 9.77% [85]. Similar results have been described in critically ill hospitalized patients with COVID-19 [86].

Therefore, CGM and FGM could be considered for non-critically ill hospitalized patients with COVID-19 in order to limit the number of capillary glycemia tests, minimize staff exposure, and optimize glycemic control [64]. Potential candidates include patients with moderate-severe hyperglycemia requiring treatment with multiple doses of insulin, patients with high glycemic variability or risk of hypoglycemia, and patients with hyperglycemia that is difficult to manage, such as corticosteroid-induced hyperglycemia or hyperglycemia induced by artificial nutrition [87]. Similarly, persons using CGM or FGM as outpatients could continue to use their devices in hospital, providing protocols are in place, and there are staff trained in their management [88].

4. Care of Patients with Diabetes during the COVID-19 Pandemic and Afterwards

The pandemic led to unprecedented changes in clinical practice, including the closure of some primary care centers and restructuring of hospitals, with considerable resources aimed at management of patients with COVID-19 and a rapid transition to online care for other conditions. As the government was promoting measures to curb and contain the spread of the disease, health professionals faced the difficult task of managing risks both for patients and for themselves while learning to implement new remote care systems. In this setting, the first challenge was to maintain remote care, mainly by telephone, in order to address urgent situations and patients whose care could not be delayed as well as to adapt management protocols for hospitalized patients with DM to the special circumstances affecting hospitalization of patients with COVID-19. The second challenge was to plan health care after the initial phase in order not to postpone scheduled care and resume previously postponed activity via a face-to-face or remote visit.

New management protocols have been suggested for hospitalized patients with DM or hyperglycemia although information on the safety and efficacy of these protocols and their application is lacking [65]. While waiting for these strategies to be evaluated, and faced with the urgent need to implement effective approaches to glycemic control in hospitalized patients with COVID-19, we recently proposed a series of recommendations on management of hyperglycemia in the critical setting and noncritical care setting, taking into account factors such as the need to prevent staff exposure and the fact that many health professionals caring for patients with COVID-19 may be relatively unfamiliar with management of hyperglycemia [65].

With the sudden outbreak of the COVID-19 pandemic, those working in outpatient care have seen how the struggle against SARS-CoV-2 became a priority for the health system and how care of persons with chronic diseases, such as DM, was interrupted partially or completely. Health professionals responded with rapid and urgent adoption of alternative means of caring for patients, as follows: online visits via video calls and, more commonly, by telephone; easier access to prescription medication via online prescriptions; promotion of structured educational resources online; and the increase in the use of telemedicine tools that make it possible to transfer the results of glucose monitoring to health professionals (limited until relatively recently to patients with T1D). However, many patients had their visits and appointments for analyses and additional testing cancelled. In a survey on the impact of COVID-19 on persons with DM carried out by the Spanish Diabetes Federation (Federación Española de Diabetes (FEDE)) and the Spanish Diabetes Society (Sociedad Española de Diabetes (SED)), 46% of the 335 patients surveyed (59% with T1D) had their visit cancelled, and 40% had an online visit; furthermore, 78% felt that they would experience difficulties making changes to their treatment. An audit of more than 125.8 million primary care visits from the US National Disease and Therapeutic Index showed that visit frequency decreased by 21.4% during the second quarter of 2020 compared with the mean quarterly visit volume for the second quarters of 2018 and 2019, which were not compensated for by remote visits. In addition, evaluation of risk factors was less common during the remote visits than during face-to-face visits [89]. Similarly, changes in care were implemented without clear guidelines or planning and mainly involved glycemia but not other comorbid conditions, such as obesity, hypertension, dyslipidemia, and cardiovascular disease. Moreover, evidence on the efficacy of these strategies in the case of the COVID-19 pandemic is scarce. A meta-analysis of randomized controlled clinical trials that compared telemedicine-based interventions with standard care found that systems enabling adjustments to medication with or without text messages or a web page improved glycosylated hemoglobin but not other clinically relevant outcomes in patients with DM [90]. The most recent meta-analysis, which included eight studies based on remote visits and 34 based on remote monitoring in patients with T1D and T2D, revealed that telemedicine-based interventions were more effective than standard care for control of DM [91].

One positive aspect is that the disruptive effect of the pandemic has led to the rapid disappearance of barriers to the use of remote care tools, thus making telemedicine another option in the care of chronically ill patients in the future. The pandemic has considerably promoted the use of already available but rarely used applications and platforms, which enable patients to upload data from their glucose monitors, CGM devices, or insulin pumps so that their doctors can make decisions on treatment. In addition, health professionals and probably health care organizations have recognized the value of some of these profound changes in a sector such as that of health care, where habits are hard to change. However, there are major limitations to telemedicine becoming a powerful tool in the care of patients with DM. First, efficient use of this approach is currently restricted to patients who are fully able to manage the necessary technology and are seen at centers whose professionals are skilled in the use of this technology. In most cases, remote care is limited to telephone calls. The FEDE/SED survey showed that 41% of patients considered remote visits to be poorly efficient or inefficient, and 57% preferred their future health care to be based on a mix of face-to-face and remote visits. Similarly, many of the tools were used on an improvised basis, without previous cost-effectiveness studies and without changes in the care model to make efficient application easier. Research on telemedicine during the pandemic, while generating some knowledge, has generally been based on small or nonrepresentative samples and limited to analysis of frequency of use although with few data on content and safety and efficacy.

The question many of us ask today is whether this greater use of remote care will be maintained once the health care crisis brought about by COVID-19 has passed. The answer is not easy to predict although it seems foolish not to take advantage of what we have learned from the rapid deployment of telemedicine, especially if we consider that this is a broad area with room for development. Furthermore, while not replacing face-to-face visits, telemedicine can facilitate processes, streamline the system, and provide valuable information for health professionals and their patients. Nevertheless, it is also clear that for telemedicine to become a reality, more widespread adoption as a result of the pandemic is not sufficient, and a series of initiatives will be needed to improve it, as follows:

- Development and broad implementation of remote diagnostic and treatment technologies that make it possible to obtain variables of interest for management of DM from the patient in his/her usual environment;
- General electronic clinical histories in health services that include all the information generated during the patient's lifetime. System standardization and interoperability are essential if we are to ensure real integration and coordination between various care levels;
- Establishment of universal mechanisms and protocols for transferring data on variables of interest independently of where they are generated to the clinical history in

standard format and in such a way that they are easily interpretable. The complexity and poor user-friendliness of the approach use up health professionals' time and are among the main reasons this modality is discontinued. All of these actions are essential so that health professionals spend more time making decisions and less time recording data, thus leading to greater clinical efficacy and reduced resistance to change by professionals;
- In parallel, all those involved should be trained to avoid the digital gap between patients and professionals, and collaboration between professionals and care levels should be encouraged by providing reimbursement for the use of digital technology and models for evaluation and assignment of resources that discourage silo working;
- As for any other medical intervention, it is necessary to generate evidence on use—in terms of cost-effectiveness and implementation challenges—of new telemedicine systems and strategies by comparing them with previously used approaches.

If these aspects are not taken into account, we will probably miss the opportunity brought about by the COVID-19 pandemic to achieve the real goal, that is, to transform our health care model so that it can respond to the challenges the system faces in providing health care to persons with chronic diseases, such as DM.

While the long-term implications of COVID-19 in persons with DM are unknown, available data indicate that even short-term interruption of care could prove catastrophic. The impact is especially important in older persons from disadvantaged areas with reduced ability to self-monitor and self-adjust treatment [30]. Prolongation of the pandemic and restrictions in effective clinical care will worsen the situation. In order to minimize the consequences of this situation, it is necessary to guarantee that patients receive efficient clinical care that takes into account various services, including screening for the disease in at-risk persons, education, and monitoring of control and complications at face-to-face or remote visits as well as adaptation of treatment of DM in the setting of COVID-19.

5. Conclusions

Diabetes is one of the most common comorbidities linked to COVID-19, and there is consistent evidence that diabetes increases the risk of severe COVID-19 disease, including admission to the intensive care unit and death. Socioeconomic disadvantage and higher blood glucose levels are associated with worse COVID-19 outcomes. Tight control of glucose levels could prove crucial in patients with diabetes mellitus to prevent progression to severe COVID-19. However, data on the effect of insulin and non-insulin anti-diabetic drugs are lacking. To minimize the consequences of this situation, it is crucial to guarantee that patients remain engaged with diabetes services and receive efficient clinical care, including screening for the disease, education, and monitoring of control and complications at face-to-face or remote visits. Treatment of diabetes must be adapted appropriately to the COVID-19 setting.

This article summarizes recommendations for management of diabetes in various situations during the COVID-19 pandemic and could serve as a guide for healthcare providers to ensure continuity of care for people with diabetes. More research is needed on the acute and long-term effects of COVID-19 in this population. It is also necessary to assess the impact of these recommendations and the implementation of technological advances in the deployment of telemedicine and management of diabetes in inpatient and outpatient care.

Author Contributions: All named authors meet the International Committee of Medical Journal Editors (ICMJE) criteria for authorship for this article and take responsibility for the integrity of the work. V.B. and A.P. wrote the first draft of the manuscript and critically reviewed the final version. All authors have read and agreed to the published version of the manuscript.

Funding: Support from Sanofi was received for the development of the manuscript, but the opinions represent those of authors and not Sanofi.

Institutional Review Board Statement: Not applicable.

Informed Consent Statement: Not applicable.

Acknowledgments: We thank Content Ed Net for medical writing assistance.

Conflicts of Interest: V.B. has received speaker/advisory honoraria from Abbott, AstraZeneca, Boehringer Ingelheim, Eli Lilly, Esteve, Janssen, Merck, Mundipharma, Novartis, Novo Nordisk, Roche, and Sanofi. A.P. has served as a consultant for or received research support, lecture fees, or travel reimbursement from Sanofi, Almirall, Novo Nordisk, Lilly, MSD, Boehringer Ingel-heim, Esteve, Gilead, Novartis, Abbott, Amgen, Menarini, and Astra Zeneca.

References

1. Fadini, G.P.; Morieri, M.L.; Longato, E.; Avogaro, A. Prevalence and impact of diabetes among people infected with SARS-CoV-2. *J. Endocrinol. Investig.* **2020**, *43*, 867–869. [CrossRef] [PubMed]
2. Roncon, L.; Zuin, M.; Rigatelli, G.; Zuliani, G. Diabetic patients with COVID-19 infection are at higher risk of ICU admission and poor short-term outcome. *J. Clin. Virol.* **2020**, *127*, 104354. [CrossRef] [PubMed]
3. Singh, A.K.; Gupta, R.; Ghosh, A.; Misra, A. Diabetes in COVID-19: Prevalence, pathophysiology, prognosis and practical considerations. *Diabetes Metab. Syndr.* **2020**, *14*, 303–310. [CrossRef] [PubMed]
4. Li, B.; Yang, J.; Zhao, F.; Zhi, L.; Wang, X.; Liu, L.; Bi, Z.; Zhao, Y. Prevalence and impact of cardiovascular metabolic diseases on COVID-19 in China. *Clin. Res. Cardiol.* **2020**, *109*, 531–538. [CrossRef] [PubMed]
5. Barron, E.; Bakhai, C.; Kar, P.; Weaver, A.; Bradley, D.; Ismail, H.; Knighton, P.; Holman, N.; Khunti, K.; Sattar, N.; et al. Associations of type 1 and type 2 diabetes with COVID-19-related mortality in England: A whole-population study. *Lancet Diabetes Endocrinol.* **2020**, *8*, 813–822. [CrossRef]
6. Zhou, F.; Yu, T.; Du, R.; Fan, G.; Liu, Y.; Liu, Z.; Xiang, J.; Wang, Y.; Song, B.; Gu, X.; et al. Clinical course and risk factors for mortality of adult inpatients with COVID-19 in Wuhan, China: A retrospective cohort study. *Lancet* **2020**, *395*, 1054–1062. [CrossRef]
7. Fang, L.; Karakiulakis, G.; Roth, M. Are patients with hypertension and diabetes mellitus at increased risk for COVID-19 infection? *Lancet Respir. Med.* **2020**, *8*, e21. [CrossRef]
8. Moazzami, B.; Chaichian, S.; Kasaeian, A.; Djalalinia, S.; Akhlaghdoust, M.; Eslami, M.; Broumand, B. Metabolic risk factors and risk of COVID-19: A systematic review and meta-analysis. *PLoS ONE* **2020**, *15*, e0243600. [CrossRef]
9. Huang, I.; Lim, M.A.; Pranata, R. Diabetes mellitus is associated with increased mortality and severity of disease in COVID-19 pneumonia. A systematic review, meta-analysis, and meta-regression. *Diabetes Metab. Syndr.* **2020**, *14*, 395–403. [CrossRef]
10. Bloomgarden, Z.T. Diabetes and COVID-19. *J. Diabetes* **2020**, *12*, 347–348. [CrossRef]
11. Bartsch, S.M.; Ferguson, M.C.; McKinnell, J.A.; O'Shea, K.J.; Wedlock, P.T.; Siegmund, S.S.; Lee, B.Y. The potential health care costs and resource use associated with COVID-19 in The United States. *Health Aff.* **2020**, *39*, 927–935. [CrossRef]
12. Muniyappa, R.; Gubbi, S. Covid-19 pandemic, coronaviruses, and diabetes mellitus. *Am. J. Physiol. Endocrinol. Metab.* **2020**, *318*, E736–E741. [CrossRef] [PubMed]
13. Klonoff, D.C.; Messler, J.C.; Umpiérrez, G.E.; Peng, L.; Booth, R.; Crowe, J.; Garrett, V.; McFarland, R.; Pasquel, F.J. Association between achieving inpatient glycemic control and clinical outcomes in hospitalized patients with COVID-19: A multicenter, retrospective hospital-based analysis. *Diabetes Care* **2021**, *44*, 578–585. [CrossRef] [PubMed]
14. Carrasco-Sánchez, F.J.; López-Carmona, M.D.; Martínez-Marcos, F.J.; Pérez-Belmonte, L.M.; Hidalgo-Jiménez, A.; Buonaiuto, V.; Fernández Suárez, C.; Freire Castro, S.J.; Luordo, D.; Pesqueira Fontan, P.M. Admission hyperglycaemia as a predictor of mortality in patients hospitalized with COVID-19 regardless of diabetes status: Data from the Spanish SEMI-COVID-19 Registry. *Ann. Med.* **2021**, *53*, 103–116. [CrossRef] [PubMed]
15. Sardu, C.; D'Onofrio, N.; Balestrieri, M.L.; Barbieri, M.; Rizzo, M.R.; Messina, V.; Maggi, P.; Coppola, N.; Paolisso, G.; Marfella, R. Outcomes in patients with hyperglycemia affected by COVID-19: Can we do more on glycemic control? *Diabetes Care* **2020**, *43*, 1408–1415. [CrossRef]
16. Iacobellis, G. COVID-19 and diabetes: Can DPP4 inhibition play a role? *Diabetes Res. Clin. Pract.* **2020**, *162*, 108125. [CrossRef]
17. Rao, S.; Lau, A.; Hon-Cheong, S. Exploring diseases/traits and blood proteins causally related to expression of ACE2, the putative receptor of SARS-CoV-2: A Mendelian randomization analysis highlights tentative relevance of diabetes-related traits. *Diabetes Care* **2020**, *43*, 1416–14126. [CrossRef]
18. Bindom, S.M.; Lazartigues, E. The sweeter side of ACE2: Physiological evidence for a role in diabetics. *Mol. Cell Endocrinol.* **2009**, *301*, 193–202. [CrossRef]
19. Bode, B.; Garrett, V.; Messler, J.; McFarland, R.; Crowe, J.; Booth, R.; Klonoff, D.C. Glycemic characteristics and clinical outcomes of COVID-19 patients hospitalized in the United States. *J. Diabetes Sci. Technol.* **2020**, *14*, 813–821. [CrossRef] [PubMed]
20. Zhou, J.; Tan, J. Diabetes patients with COVID-19 need better blood glucose management in Wuhan, China. *Metabolism* **2020**, *107*, 154216. [CrossRef]
21. Wu, L.; Girgis, C.M.; Cheung, N.W. COVID-19 and diabetes: Insulin requirements parallel illness severity in critically unwell patients. *Clin. Endocrinol.* **2020**, *93*, 390–393. [CrossRef]
22. Pal, R.; Banerjee, M.; Yadav, U.; Bhattacharjee, S. Clinical profile and outcomes in COVID-19 patients with diabetic ketoacidosis: A systematic review of literature. *Diabetes Metab. Syndr.* **2020**, *14*, 1563–1569. [CrossRef]

23. Yang, J.K.; Lin, S.S.; Ji, X.J.; Guo, L.M. Binding of SARS coronavirus to its receptor damages islets and causes acute diabetes. *Acta Diabetol.* **2010**, *47*, 193–199. [CrossRef]
24. Li, J.; Wang, X.; Chen, J.; Zuo, X.; Zhang, H.; Deng, A. COVID-19 infection may cause ketosis and ketoacidosis. *Diabetes Obes. Metab.* **2020**, *22*, 1935–1941. [CrossRef] [PubMed]
25. Lim, S.; Bae, J.H.; Kwon, H.S.; Nauck, M.A. COVID-19 and diabetes mellitus: From pathophysiology to clinical management. *Nat. Rev. Endocrinol.* **2021**, *17*, 11–30. [CrossRef] [PubMed]
26. Perez, A.; Jansen-Chaparro, S.; Saigi, I.; Bernal-López, M.R.; Miñambres, I.; Gómez-Huelgas, R. Glucocorticoid-induced hyperglycemia. *J. Diabetes* **2014**, *6*, 9–20. [CrossRef] [PubMed]
27. Scheen, A.J.; Marre, M.; Thivolet, C. Prognostic factors in patients with diabetes hospitalized for COVID-19: Findings from the CORONADO study and other recent reports. *Diabetes Metab.* **2020**, *46*, 265–271. [CrossRef]
28. Fernández, E.; Cortázar, A.; Bellido, V. Impact of COVID-19 lockdown on glycemic control in patients with type 1 diabetes. *Diabetes Res. Clin. Pract.* **2020**, *166*, 108348. [CrossRef]
29. Capaldo, B.; Annuzzi, G.; Creanza, A.; Giglio, C.; De Angelis, R.; Lupoli, R.; Masulli, M.; Riccardi, G.; Albarosa Rivellese, A.; Bozzetto, L. Blood glucose control during lockdown for COVID-19: CGM metrics in Italian adults with type 1 diabetes. *Diabetes Care* **2020**, *43*, e88–e89. [CrossRef]
30. Garofolo, M.; Aragona, M.; Rodia, C.; Falcetta, P.; Bertolotto, A.; Campi, F.; Del Prato, S.; Penno, G. Glycaemic control during the lockdown for COVID-19 in adults with type 1 diabetes: A meta-analysis of observational studies. *Diabetes Res. Clin. Pract.* **2021**, *180*, 109066. [CrossRef]
31. Fisher, L.; Polonsky, W.; Asuni, A.; Jolly, Y.; Hessler, D. The early impact of the COVID-19 pandemic on adults with type 1 or type 2 diabetes: A national cohort study. *J. Diabetes Complicat.* **2020**, *34*, 107748. [CrossRef] [PubMed]
32. Tejera-Pérez, C.; Moreno-Pérez, Ó.; Ríos, J.; Reyes-García, R. People living with type 1 diabetes point of view in COVID-19 times (covidT1 study): Disease impact, health system pitfalls and lessons for the future. *Diabetes Res. Clin. Pract.* **2021**, *171*, 108547. [CrossRef] [PubMed]
33. Biancalana, E.; Parolini, F.; Mengozzi, A.; Solini, A. Short-term impact of COVID-19 lockdown on metabolic control of patients with well-controlled type 2 diabetes: A single-centre observational study. *Acta Diabetol.* **2021**, *58*, 431–436. [CrossRef] [PubMed]
34. Carr, M.J.; Wright, A.K.; Leelarathna, L.; Thabit, H.; Milne, N.; Kanumilli, N.; Ashcroft, D.M.; Rutter, M.K. Impact of COVID-19 on diagnoses, monitoring and mortality in people with type 2 diabetes: A UK-wide cohort study involving 14 million people in primary care. *Lancet Diabetes Endocrinol.* **2021**, *9*, 413–415. [CrossRef]
35. Jacob, L.; Rickwood, S.; Rathmann, W.; Kostev, K. Change in glucose-lowering medication regimens in individuals with type 2 diabetes mellitus during the COVID-19 pandemic in Germany. *Diabetes Obes. Metab.* **2020**, *23*, 910–915. [CrossRef]
36. Wang, A.; Zhao, W.; Xu, Z.; Gu, J. Timely blood glucose management for the outbreak of 2019 novel coronavirus disease (COVID-19) is urgently needed. *Diabetes Res. Clin. Pract.* **2020**, *162*, 108118. [CrossRef]
37. Katulanda, P.; Dissanayake, H.A.; Ranathunga, I.; Ratnasamy, V.; Wijewickrama, P.S.A.; Yogendranathan, N.; Gamage, K.K.K.; de Silva, N.L.; Sumanatilleke, M.; Somasundaram, N.; et al. Prevention and management of COVID-19 among patients with diabetes: An appraisal of the literature. *Diabetologia* **2020**, *63*, 1440–1452. [CrossRef]
38. Pal, R.; Bhadada, S.K.; Misra, A. COVID-19 vaccination in patients with diabetes mellitus: Current concepts, uncertainties and challenges. *Diabetes Metab. Syndr.* **2021**, *15*, 505–508. [CrossRef] [PubMed]
39. Marfella, R.; D'Onofrio, N.; Sardu, C.; Scisciola, L.; Maggi, P.; Coppola, N.; Romano, C.; Messina, V.; Turriziani, F.; Siniscalchi, M. Does poor glycaemic control affect the immunogenicity of the COVID-19 vaccination in patients with type 2 diabetes: The CAVEAT study. *Diabetes Obes. Metab.* **2021**. [CrossRef]
40. Pascual Fuster, V.; Pérez Pérez, A.; Carretero Gómez, J.; Caixàs Pedragós, A.; Gómez-Huelgas, R.; Pérez-Martínez, P. Executive summary: Updates to the dietary treatment of prediabetes and type 2 diabetes mellitus. *Clin. Investig. Arterioscler.* **2021**, *33*, 73–84.
41. Reyes-García, R.; Moreno-Pérez, Ó.; Tejera-Pérez, C.; Fernández-García, D.; Bellido-Castañeda, V.; De la Torre Casares, M.L.; Rozas-Moreno, P.; Fernández-García, J.C.; Martínez Marco, A.; Escalada-San Martín, J. Documento de abordaje integral de la diabetes tipo 2. *Endocrinol. Diabetes Nutr.* **2019**, *66*, 443–458. [CrossRef]
42. Marçal, I.R.; Fernandes, B.; Viana, A.A.; Ciolac, E.G. The urgent need for recommending physical activity for the management of diabetes during and beyond COVID-19 outbreak. *Front. Endocrinol.* **2020**, *11*, 584642. [CrossRef]
43. Philippou, A.; Chryssanthopoulos, C.; Maridaki, M.; Dimitriadis, G.; Koutsilieris, M. Exercise metabolism in health and disease. In *Cardiorespiratory Fitness in Cardiometabolic Diseases*; Kokkinos, P., Narayan, P., Eds.; Springer: Berlin/Heidelberg, Germany, 2010. [CrossRef]
44. Koliaki, C.; Tentolouris, A.; Eleftheriadou, I.; Melidonis, A.; Dimitriadis, G.; Tentolouris, N. Clinical management of diabetes mellitus in the era of COVID-19: Practical issues, peculiarities and concerns. *J. Clin. Med.* **2020**, *9*, 2288. [CrossRef]
45. Hussain, A.; Bhowmik, B.; Do Vale Moreira, N.C. COVID-19 and diabetes: Knowledge in progress. *Diabetes Res. Clin. Pract.* **2020**, *162*, 108142. [CrossRef]
46. American Diabetes Association. 6. Glycemic targets-Standards of medical care in diabetes—2021. *Diabetes Care* **2021**, *44* (Suppl. S1), S73–S84. [CrossRef] [PubMed]
47. Battelino, T.; Danne, T.; Bergenstal, R.M.; Amiel, S.A.; Beck, R.; Biester, T.; Bosi, E.; Buckingham, B.A.; Cefalu, W.T.; Close, K.L.; et al. Clinical targets for continuous glucose monitoring data interpretation: Recommendations from the international consensus on time in range. *Diabetes Care* **2019**, *42*, 1593–1603. [CrossRef] [PubMed]

48. Bornstein, S.R.; Rubino, F.; Khunti, K.; Mingrone, G.; Hopkins, D.; Birkenfeld, A.L.; Boehm, B.; Amiel, S.; Holt, R.I.; Skyler, J.S.; et al. Practical recommendations for the management of diabetes in patients with COVID-19. *Lancet Diabetes Endocrinol.* **2020**, *8*, 546–550. [CrossRef]
49. Maahs, D.M.; DeSalvo, D.; Pyle, L.; Ly, T.; Messer, L.; Clinton, P.; Westfall, E.; Wadwa, R.P.; Buckingham, B. Effect of acetaminophen on CGM glucose in an outpatient setting. *Diabetes Care* **2015**, *38*, e158–e159. [CrossRef] [PubMed]
50. Sun, B.; Huang, S.; Zhou, J. Perspectives of antidiabetic drugs in diabetes with coronavirus infections. *Front. Pharmacol.* **2021**, *11*, 592439. [CrossRef]
51. Finan, B.; Yang, B.; Ottaway, N.; Smiley, D.L.; Ma, T.; Clemmensen, C.; Chabenne, J.; Zhang, L.; Habegger, K.M.; Fischer, K.; et al. A rationally designed monomeric peptide triagonist corrects obesity and diabetes in rodents. *Nat. Med.* **2015**, *21*, 27–36. [CrossRef]
52. Cariou, B.; Hadjadj, S.; Wargny, M.; Pichelin, M.; Al-Salameh, A.; Allix, I.; Amadou, C.; Arnault, G.; Baudoux, F.; Bauduceau, B.; et al. Phenotypic characteristics and prognosis of inpatients with COVID-19 and diabetes: The CORONADO study. *Diabetologia* **2020**, *63*, 1500–1515. [CrossRef]
53. Pérez-Belmonte, L.M.; Torres-Peña, J.D.; López-Carmona, M.D.; Ayala-Gutiérrez, M.M.; Fuentes-Jiménez, F.; Huerta, L.J.; Muñoz, J.A.; Rubio-Rivas, M.; Madrazo, M.; Guzmán García, M.; et al. Mortality and other adverse outcomes in patients with type 2 diabetes mellitus admitted for COVID-19 in association with glucose-lowering drugs: A nationwide cohort study. *BMC Med.* **2020**, *18*, 359. [CrossRef]
54. DeFronzo, R.; Fleming, G.A.; Chen, K.; Bicsak, T.A. Metformin-associated lactic acidosis: Current perspectives on causes and risk. *Metabolism* **2016**, *65*, 20–29. [CrossRef]
55. Vitale, R.J.; Valtis, Y.K.; McDonnell, M.E.; Palermo, N.E.; Fisher, N.D.L. Euglycemic diabetic ketoacidosis with COVID-19 infection in patients with type 2 diabetes taking SGLT2 inhibitors. *AACE Clin. Case Rep.* **2021**, *7*, 10–13. [CrossRef]
56. Schwartz, S.; DeFronzo, R.A. Is incretin-based therapy ready for the care of hospitalized patients with type 2 diabetes? The time has come for GLP-1 receptor agonists! *Diabetes Care* **2013**, *36*, 2107–2111. [CrossRef]
57. Longo, M.; Caruso, P.; Maiorino, M.I.; Bellastella, G.; Giugliano, D.; Esposito, K. Treating type 2 diabetes in COVID-19 patients: The potential benefits of injective therapies. *Cardiovasc. Diabetol.* **2020**, *19*, 115. [CrossRef]
58. Vaduganathan, M.; Vardeny, O.; Michel, T.; McMurray, J.J.V.; Pfeffer, M.A.; Solomon, S.D. Renin–angiotensin–aldosterone system inhibitors in patients with Covid-19. *N. Engl. J. Med.* **2020**, *382*, 1653–1659. [CrossRef]
59. Patel, A.B.; Verma, A. COVID-19 and angiotensin-converting enzyme inhibitors and angiotensin receptor blockers: What is the evidence? *JAMA* **2020**, *323*, 1769–1770. [CrossRef]
60. Bangash, M.N.; Patel, J.; Parekh, D. COVID-19 and the liver: Little cause for concern. *Lancet Gastroenterol. Hepatol.* **2020**, *5*, 529–530. [CrossRef]
61. Ceriello, A.; Standl, E.; Catrinoiu, D.; Itzhak, B.; Lalic, N.M.; Rahelic, D.; Schnell, O.; Škrha, J.; Valensi, P. Diabetes and Cardiovascular Disease (D&CVD) EASD Study Group. Issues of cardiovascular risk management in people with diabetes in the COVID-19 era. *Diabetes Care* **2020**, *43*, 1427–1432.
62. Rahimi, L.; Malek, M.; Ismail-Beigi, F.; Khamseh, M.E. Challenging issues in the management of cardiovascular risk factors in diabetes during the COVID-19 pandemic: A review of current literature. *Adv. Ther.* **2020**, *37*, 3450–3462. [CrossRef] [PubMed]
63. Ebekozien, O.A.; Noor, N.; Gallagher, M.P.; Alonso, G.T. Type 1 diabetes and COVID-19: Preliminary findings from a multicenter surveillance study in the U.S. *Diabetes Care* **2020**, *43*, e83–e85. [CrossRef]
64. Korytkowski, M.; Antinori-Lent, K.; Drincic, A.; Hirsch, I.B.; McDonnell, M.E.; Rushakoff, R.; Muniyappa, R. A pragmatic approach to inpatient diabetes management during the COVID-19 pandemic. *J. Clin. Endocrinol. Metab.* **2020**, *105*, 342. [CrossRef]
65. Bellido, V.; Pérez, A. Inpatient hyperglycemia management and COVID-19. *Diabetes Ther.* **2021**, *12*, 121–132. [CrossRef]
66. American Diabetes Association. 15 Diabetes care in the hospital-Standards of medical care in diabetes—2020. *Diabetes Care* **2020**, *43* (Suppl. S1), S193–S202. [CrossRef]
67. Umpiérrez, G.; Cardona, S.; Pasquel, F.; Jacobs, S.; Peng, L.; Unigwe, M.; Newton, C.A.; Smiley-Byrd, D.; Vellanki, P.; Halkos, M.; et al. Randomized controlled trial of intensive versus conservative glucose control in patients undergoing coronary artery bypass graft surgery: GLUCO-CABG Trial. *Diabetes Care* **2015**, *38*, 1665–1672. [CrossRef]
68. Krinsley, J.S.; Preiser, J.C.; Hirsch, I.B. Safety and efficacy of personalized glycemic control in critically ill patients: A 2-year before and after intervention trial. *Endocr. Pract.* **2017**, *23*, 318–330. [CrossRef]
69. Pérez, A.; Ramos, A.; Carreras, G. Insulin therapy in hospitalized patients. *Am. J. Ther.* **2020**, *27*, e71–e78. [CrossRef]
70. Pasquel, F.J.; Umpiérrez, G.E. Individualizing inpatient diabetes management during the coronavirus disease 2019 pandemic. *J. Diabetes Sci. Technol.* **2020**, *14*, 705–707. [CrossRef]
71. Hamdy, O.; Gabbay, R.A. Early observation and mitigation of challenges in diabetes management of COVID-19 patients in critical care units. *Diabetes Care* **2020**, *43*, e81–e82. [CrossRef]
72. Moghissi, E.S.; Korytkowski, M.T.; DiNardo, M.; Einhorn, D.; Hellman, R.; Hirsch, I.B.; Inzucchi, S.E.; Ismail-Beigi, F.; Kirkman, M.S.; Umpierrez, G.E. American Association of Clinical Endocrinologists and American Diabetes Association consensus statement on inpatient glycemic control. *Diabetes Care* **2009**, *32*, 1119–1131. [CrossRef]
73. Pérez Pérez, A.; Conthe Gutiérrez, P.; Aguilar Diosdado, M.; Bertomeu Martínez, V.; Galdos Anuncibay, P.; García de Casasola, G.; Gomis de Bárbara, R.; Palma Gamiz, J.L.; Puig Domingo, M.; Sánchez Rodríguez, A. Hospital management of hyperglycemia. *Med. Clin.* **2009**, *132*, 465–475. [CrossRef]

74. Avanzini, F.; Marelli, G.; Donzelli, W.; Busi, G.; Carbone, S.; Bellato, L.; Colombo, E.L.; Foschi, R.; Riva, E.; Roncaglioni, M.C.; et al. Transition from intravenous to subcutaneous insulin: Effectiveness and safety of a standardized protocol and predictors of outcome in patients with acute coronary syndrome. *Diabetes Care.* **2011**, *34*, 1445–1450. [CrossRef]
75. Ramos, A.; Zapata, L.; Vera, P.; Betbese, A.J.; Pérez, A. Transition from intravenous insulin to subcutaneous long-acting insulin in critical care patients on enteral or parenteral nutrition. *Endocrinol. Diabetes Nutr.* **2017**, *64*, 552–556. [CrossRef]
76. Kosiborod, M.N.; Esterline, R.; Furtado, R.H.M.; Oscarsson, J.; Gasparyan, S.B.; Koch, G.G.; Martinez, F.; Mukhtar, O.; Verma, S.; Chopra, V.; et al. Dapagliflozin in patients with cardiometabolic risk factors hospitalized with COVID-19 (DARE-19): A randomized, double-blind, placebo-controlled, phase 3 trial. *Lancet Diabetes Endocrinol.* **2021**, *9*, 586–594. [CrossRef]
77. Mehta, P.; McAuley, D.F.; Brown, M.; Sánchez, E.; Tattersall, R.S.; Manson, J.J.; HLH Across Specialty Collaboration, UK. COVID-19: Consider cytokine storm syndromes and immunosuppression. *Lancet* **2020**, *395*, 1033–1034. [CrossRef]
78. FDA. FAQs on Home-Use Blood Glucose Meters Utilized within Hospitals during the COVID-19 Pandemic. 2020. Available online: https://www.fda.gov/medical-devices/coronavirus-covid-19-and-medical-devices/using-home-use-blood-glucose-meters-hospitals-during-covid-19-pandemic (accessed on 2 March 2021).
79. Welsh, J.B.; Hu, G.; Walker, T.C.; Sharma, N.; Cherñavvsky, D. Glucose monitoring and diabetes management in the time of coronavirus disease 2019. *J. Diabetes Sci. Technol.* **2020**, *14*, 809–810. [CrossRef]
80. Dexcom. Fact Sheet for Healthcare Providers: Use of Dexcom Continuous Glucose Monitoring Systems during the COVID-19 Pandemic. 2020. Available online: https://www.dexcom.com/hospitalfacts (accessed on 2 March 2021).
81. Abbott. Press release. FreeStyle Libre: Diabetes Care during COVID-19. 2020. Available online: https://www.abbott.com/corpnewsroom/product-and-innovation/freestyle-libre-diabetes-care-during-covid-19.html (accessed on 25 March 2020).
82. Galindo, R.J.; Migdal, A.L.; Davis, G.M.; Urrutia, M.A.; Albury, B.; Zambrano, C.; Vellanki, P.; Pasquel, F.J.; Fayfman, M.; Peng, L.; et al. Comparison of the FreeStyle Libre pro flash continuous glucose monitoring (CGM) system and point-of-care capillary glucose testing in hospitalized patients with type 2 diabetes treated with basal-bolus insulin regimen. *Diabetes Care* **2020**, *43*, 2730–2735. [CrossRef]
83. Fortmann, A.L.; Spierling Bagsic, S.R.; Talavera, L.; García, I.M.; Sandoval, H.; Hottinger, A.; Philis-Tsimikas, A. Glucose as the fifth vital sign: A randomized controlled trial of continuous glucose monitoring in a non-ICU hospital setting. *Diabetes Care* **2020**, *43*, 2873–2877. [CrossRef]
84. Singh, L.G.; Satyarengga, M.; Marcano, I.; Scott, W.H.; Pinault, L.F.; Feng, Z.; Sorkin, J.D.; Umpierrez, G.E.; Spanakis, E.K. Reducing inpatient hypoglycemia in the general wards using real-time continuous glucose monitoring: The glucose telemetry system, a randomized clinical trial. *Diabetes Care* **2020**, *43*, 2736–2743. [CrossRef]
85. Reutrakul, S.; Genco, M.; Salinas, H.; Sargis, R.M.; Paul, C.; Eisenberg, Y.; Fang, J.; Caskey, R.N.; Henkle, S.; Fatoorehchi, S.; et al. Feasibility of inpatient continuous glucose monitoring during the COVID-19 pandemic: Early experience. *Diabetes Care* **2020**, *43*, e137–e138. [CrossRef]
86. Agarwal, S.; Mathew, J.; Davis, G.M.; Shephardson, A.; Levine, A.; Louard, R.; Urrutia, A.; Perez-Guzman, C.; Umpierrez, G.E.; Peng, L.; et al. Continuous glucose monitoring in the intensive care unit during the COVID-19 pandemic. *Diabetes Care* **2021**, *44*, 847–849. [CrossRef] [PubMed]
87. Galindo, R.J.; Aleppo, G.; Klonoff, D.C.; Spanakis, E.K.; Agarwal, S.; Vellanki, P.; Olson, D.E.; Umpierrez, G.E.; Davis, G.M.; Pasquel, F.J. Implementation of continuous glucose monitoring in the hospital: Emergent considerations for remote glucose monitoring during the COVID-19 pandemic. *J. Diabetes Sci. Technol.* **2020**, *14*, 822–832. [CrossRef]
88. Galindo, R.J.; Umpiérrez, G.E.; Rushakoff, R.J.; Basu, A.; Lohnes, S.; Nichols, J.H.; Spanakis, E.K.; Espinoza, J.; Palermo, N.E.; Awadjie, D.G. Continuous glucose monitors and automated insulin dosing systems in the Hospital Consensus Guideline. *J. Diabetes Sci. Technol.* **2020**, *14*, 1035–1064. [CrossRef] [PubMed]
89. Alexander, G.C.; Tajanlangit, M.; Heyward, J.; Mansour, O.; Qato, D.M.; Stafford, R.S. Use and content of primary care office-based vs telemedicine care visits during the COVID-19 pandemic in the US. *JAMA Netw. Open* **2020**, *3*, e2021476. [CrossRef]
90. Faruque, L.I.; Wiebe, N.; Ehteshami-Afshar, A.; Liu, Y.; Dianati-Maleki, N.; Hemmelgarn, B.R.; Manns, B.J.; Tonelli, M.; Alberta Kidney Disease Network. Effect of telemedicine on glycated hemoglobin in diabetes: A systematic review and meta-analysis of randomized trials. *CMAJ* **2017**, *189*, E341–E364. [CrossRef]
91. Tchero, H.; Kangambega, P.; Briatte, C.; Brunet-Houdard, S.; Retali, G.-R.; Rusch, E. Clinical effectiveness of telemedicine in diabetes mellitus: A meta-analysis of 42 randomized controlled trials. *Telemed. J. E Health* **2019**, *25*, 569–583. [CrossRef]

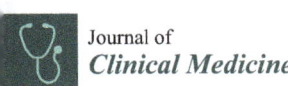

Article

Perceptions about the Management of Patients with DM2 and COVID-19 in the Hospital Care Setting

Ricardo Gómez-Huelgas [1,*] and Fernando Gómez-Peralta [2]

[1] Servicio de Medicina Interna, Hospital Regional Universitario, Instituto de Investigación Biomédica de Málaga (IBIMA), Universidad de Málaga (UMA), 29010 Málaga, Spain
[2] Unidad de Endocrinología y Nutrición, Hospital General, Calle Luis Erik Clavería Neurólogo S/N, 40002 Segovia, Spain; fgomezp@saludcastillayleon.es
* Correspondence: ricardogomezhuelgas@hotmail.com

Abstract: Background: COVID-19 entails a higher rate of complications in subjects with type 2 diabetes mellitus (T2DM). Likewise, COVID-19 infection can cause alterations in glucose metabolism that may lead to worse control. The aim of the study was to analyse the perceptions of a large group of Spanish physicians about the relationship between COVID-19 and T2DM, as well as the management, monitoring, and treatment of both diseases. Methods: A cross-sectional multicenter national project was conducted based on a survey which included opinion, attitude, and behavior (OAB) questions. Physicians specialised in internal medicine or endocrinology, whose usual clinical practices included the management of T2DM, responded to the survey between March and April 2021. Results: A total of 112 participants responded to the survey, from which 64.3% believed that COVID-19 entailed a higher risk of glycaemic decompensation irrespective of the presence of previously known T2DM. Obesity was considered a risk factor for poor control of T2DM by 57.7% and for a worse course of COVID-19 by 61.0%. Treatment intensification in not-on-target patients was considered by 57.1% in the presence of COVID-19 and by 73.2% in the absence of COVID-19. No participants considered the suspension of dipeptidyl peptidase 4 inhibitors (DPP-4i) in ambulatory patients, 85.7% declared that this therapeutic approach in hospitalized patients should be kept, and 88.4% supported the option of maintaining DPP-4i when corticosteroids were prescribed. Conclusion: The physicians involved in the management of T2DM and COVID-19 are aware of the bidirectional relationship between both conditions. However, the monitoring and therapeutic management of patients with T2DM who are infected by SARS-CoV-2 needs improvement through the following of the current recommendations and available evidence.

Keywords: diabetes mellitus; type 2; diabetes complications; coronavirus infections; hypoglycemic agents; hospitalization; ambulatory care; comorbidity

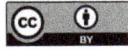

1. Introduction

Diabetes mellitus (DM) is a prevalent condition, affecting 9.3% of the worldwide population. Its prevalence has been constantly growing over the past 20 years, and it is expected to reach 10.9% of the population in 2045 [1,2]. In Spain, the prevalence of DM has been described as being even higher, reaching 13.8% of the inhabitants [3].

Patients with DM are at a higher risk of several infections, such as those of the lower respiratory tract, the urinary tract, and the skin and mucous, than patients without DM [4]. In the particular case of COVID-19, which has caused more than 11 million confirmed cases and 100,000 deaths in Spain [5], no greater risk of being infected by SARS-CoV-2 has yet been described in the population with DM. However, the SEMI-COVID-19 Registry found a higher prevalence of DM in patients hospitalized due to COVID-19 (19.4%) than in the general population [6]. Moreover, patients with DM have a higher rate of complications than subjects without DM when infected with SARS-CoV-2, such as severity, progression, hospital and intensive care unit (ICU) admissions, severe pneumonia, and mortality [7–11]. A plausible explanation for these outcomes is that chronic hyperglycaemia is associated with a chronic inflammatory state that can compromise the immune response [12]. Likewise, patients with SARS-CoV-2 and DM have increased levels of IL-6 and C-reactive protein (CRP), which can favour the systemic inflammatory response accompanying the typical acute respiratory distress syndrome in COVID-19 [10].

The relationship between DM and COVID-19 seems to be bidirectional as SARS-CoV-2 can cause alterations in glucose metabolism that may lead to the appearance of DM [13]. The underlying pathophysiological mechanism for this event might be the binding of SARS-CoV-2 to the ACE2 receptors in the pancreas (mainly in the islet cells), producing the dysfunction of β cells and acute hyperglycaemia [14]. In line with this, a greater risk of pancreatic injury has been observed among those patients with severe COVID-19 than those with a mild condition [14]. Moreover, the infection with COVID-19 can cause a wide range of sequelae, including DM, beyond the acute phase [15].

A proper blood glucose control seems to be important as hyperglycaemia, hypoglycaemia, and glycaemic variability can lead to worse outcomes in patients infected by SARS-CoV-2 [16–21]. In fact, glycaemia at admission due to COVID-19 is a powerful prognostic marker, not only in patients with DM but also in patients without diagnosed DM [21].

The global pandemic caused by the SARS-CoV-2 coronavirus infection has entailed a great impact on the routine care of patients with any chronic condition [22], as is the case with type 2 DM (T2DM). The requirements in terms of the clinical management of diabetes have probably changed after the COVID-19 pandemic: telemedicine, educational programs, strategies to ensure adherence, and glucose testing availability and affordability have become more necessary than ever [23].

In view of these new scenarios, it is crucial to optimise the management of patients with T2DM and COVID-19 in order to improve the prognosis and reduce the burden for health systems. The current study aimed to analyse the perception and experience of a large group of physicians involved in the management of these patients (internal medicine and endocrinology) on the relationship between COVID-19 and T2DM, their management, their monitoring, and their treatment of patients, whether hospitalized or not. Likewise, another objective was to identify potential differences between the current clinical practice and the recommendations of the scientific societies and expert panels and the best available evidence.

2. Materials and Methods

The present study is a cross-sectional multicentre national project based on a survey designed by a dedicated scientific committee, including several opinion, attitude, and behavior (OAB) questions (Appendix SA). This publication shows the results from a selection of 15 OAB questions related to (a) the relationship between T2DM and COVID-19; (b) the management of ambulatory patients with T2DM infected with COVID-19; (c) the management of patients with T2DM hospitalized due to COVID-19; and (d) the management of hyperglycaemia induced by corticosteroids (CS) in patients with COVID-19.

The participants were physicians specialised in internal medicine or endocrinology, whose usual practice included the management of T2DM. They were selected by means of a non-probabilistic directed sampling by conglomerates, according to proportional geographic and demographic distribution criteria. Data collection was out carried between the 15th of March and the 30th of April 2021 using an anonymous online questionnaire, completed by physicians in accordance with their usual practice.

Regarding statistical methods and analysis, the sample was calculated according to a 95% confidence interval for a finite population proportion. The final sample size provided a precision level between ±7% and ±6.5% for a 95% confidence interval. With a reference population of 46,332,614 inhabitants and 217 hospitals with 100 beds or more, a sample of 108 physicians from different regions of Spain was estimated and was intended to be representative of the specialists in internal medicine and endocrinology in Spain.

A descriptive statistical analysis was performed. The variables reported are qualitative and expressed as the values and percentages of multiple choice answers. Due to the exploratory nature of the study, no inferential statistics or regression analyses were performed. There were no missing data as the complete questionnaires were required. Statistical analysis was performed using the statistical program Stata v15.1 (StataCorp LLC, College Station, TX, USA).

3. Results

3.1. Participants

At the end of the field work, 112 invited participants had responded to all the survey items. We evaluated whether the final collected sample followed the estimated random sample, and we found that it was quite similar, although not exact, and supported the appropriateness of our sample. A proportion of 51.8% of them were 45 years old or younger; 67.9% were men. A total of 81.2% were specialists in internal medicine and 18.8% in endocrinology. The percentage of participants who used to work in hospitals with more than 300 beds was 59.8% (Table 1).

Table 1. Characteristics of participants (n = 112).

		n (%)
Age	30–45	58 (51.8)
	46–55	27 (24.1)
	56–65	26 (23.2)
	>65	1 (0.9)
Gender	Women	36 (32.1)
	Men	76 (67.9)
Medical specialty	Internal medicine	91 (81.2)
	Endocrinology	21 (18.8)
Work centre	<100 beds	13 (11.6)
	100–200 beds	18 (16.1)
	201–300 beds	14 (12.5)
	>300 beds	67 (59.8)
Participation in COVID-19/DM data analysis initiatives	None	95 (84.8)
	Collaborative Open-Access Virtual Database for COVID-19 in Diabetes	2 (1.8)
	Others	15 (13.4)
Training/update in the management of COVID-19/DM	Hospital protocols	71 (63.4)
	Clinical sessions	65 (58.0)
	Bibliography	82 (73.2)
	Webinars	70 (62.5)
	Pharmaceutical company initiatives	45 (40.2)
	Courses	48 (42.9)
	Task forces in scientific societies	75 (67.0)

3.2. COVID-19 and Type 2 Diabetes Mellitus Relationship

From the total pool of participants, 64.3% of the participants believed that COVID-19 always entailed a higher risk of glycaemic decompensation, while 14.3% considered it as such only in patients with known previous T2DM (Figure 1). Treatment with corticosteroids (CS), poor control of T2DM, and the presence of comorbidities were pointed to as factors for a higher risk of decompensation by 12.5%, 4.5%, and 4.5% of the participants, respectively.

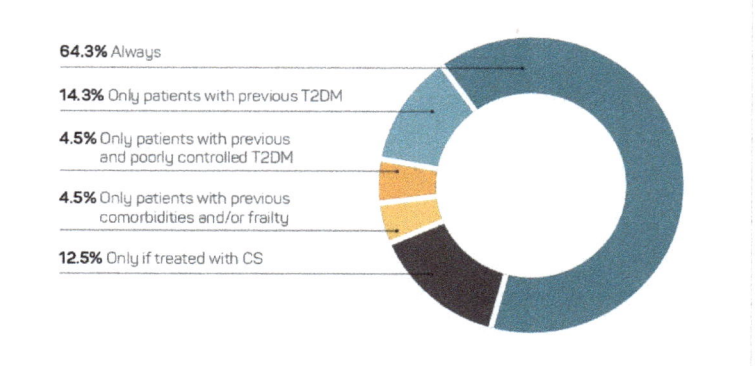

Figure 1. Opinion on whether patients with COVID-19 have a higher risk of glycaemic decompensation (n = 112). CS, Corticosteroids.

Likewise, 71.4% of the sample believed that T2DM was an independent risk factor for a bad prognosis of COVID-19, and 25.9% considered it as such only when T2DM was uncontrolled. The percentage of participants declaring that they had become stricter in terms of the objectives of T2DM control was 62.5%, while 37.5% answered that their clinical practice had not changed due to the appearance of COVID-19 (Figure S1).

The impact of several comorbidities on the control of T2DM and on the course of COVID-19 was inquired about among the participants; obesity was considered as a risk factor for poorer control of T2DM by 57.7% and for a worse course of COVID-19 by 61.0% of the participants. Frailty was considered as such by 13.5% and 10.5% and COPD by 10.6% and 11.4% of the sample, respectively (Table 2).

Table 2. Opinion on the impact of comorbidities on T2DM control or on the course of COVID-19 in patients with both diseases.

Comorbidity	% of Responses	
	Poorer Control of T2DM (n = 104)	Worse Course of COVID-19 (n = 105)
Obesity	57.7	61.0
Frailty	13.5	10.5
COPD	10.6	11.4
Renal insufficiency	7.7	4.8
Heart disease	6.7	8.6
Hypertension	2.9	2.9
Oncohematological disease	1.0	1.0

3.3. Ambulatory Patients with COVID-19 and Type 2 Diabetes Mellitus

With regard to the recommendations about glycaemia monitoring in patients with T2DM and COVID-19 who did not require hospitalization, 73.2% of the participants declared an increase in the frequency of the controls, 25.0% stated that they had maintained it, and 0.9% that they had reduced it (Figure S2). The participants were also asked about the incorporation of new measures for the optimization of glycaemia control. The percentage of participants who responded that they had carried out treatment intensification in not-on-target patients with COVID-19 was 57.1%, and without COVID-19 was 73.2%. Likewise, 42.9% and 64.3% declared that they had insisted on diet and exercise recommendations in those patients with COVID-19 and without COVID-19, respectively (Table 3).

Table 3. Opinion on measures incorporated in clinical practice for the optimization of glycaemic control in ambulatory patients with T2DM (n = 112).

Measures	% of Agreement	
	Patients with COVID-19	Patients without COVID-19
Carry out treatment intensification if the patient is not on target	57.1	73.2
Insist on recommendations about diet and exercise	42.9	64.3
Frequent self-monitoring of glucose	42.0	27.7
Stricter control targets if well tolerated	28.6	33.9
Monitor glycemic variability in controls	25.9	25.9
More frequent HbA1c controls to confirm degree of control	17.7	25.0
Continuous glucose monitoring systems	4.5	5.4

The participants gave their opinion on the therapeutic management of ambulatory patients with T2DM and COVID-19, and 62.5% of the participants indicated that they had maintained the usual treatment. From the 38.4% of participants who declared that they had suspended medication sometimes, 69.8% pointed at sulphonylureas, 51.2% at pioglitazone, and 46.5% at metformin. No participants considered the suspension of dipeptidyl peptidase 4 inhibitors (DPP-4i). From the 19.6% of participants who declared that they had reduced medication dosing sometimes, 59.1% pointed at sulphonylureas and 54.6% at metformin. iDPP4 and sodium-glucose transport protein 2 inhibitors (SGLT2i) were selected by 4.6% and glucagon-like peptide 1 receptor agonists (GLP-1 RA) by none of the participants (Figure 2A). The participants were asked to indicate which warning signs should be considered as an indication for hospital admission. The common warning signs of COVID-19, such as fever, cough, tiredness, and loss of taste or smell were selected by 65.2% of the participants. Impaired glycaemic control and altered ketone bodies values were indicated by 37.5% and 32.1% of the sample, respectively (Figure 2B).

3.4. Patients Hospitalized Due to COVID-19 with Type 2 Diabetes Mellitus

The participants gave answers regarding the patients for whom they thought hyperglycaemia at admission meant a worse prognosis: 68% of them agreed that it was worse in patients with both known and unknown T2DM; 23% stated that it was worse only in patients with known T2DM; and 5% said that it was worse only in patients with unknown T2DM (Figure S3).

In patients with unknown T2DM admitted to hospital due to COVID-19, who presented with hyperglycemia and did not require CS, 57.1% of the participants answered that they had requested a determination of HbA1C if the basal blood glucose was >140 mg/dL and/or the evening blood glucose was> 180 mg/dL. Moreover, 50.0% of them coincided in adding DPP4i and basal insulin if the basal glycaemia exceeded 180 mg/dL (Figure 3).

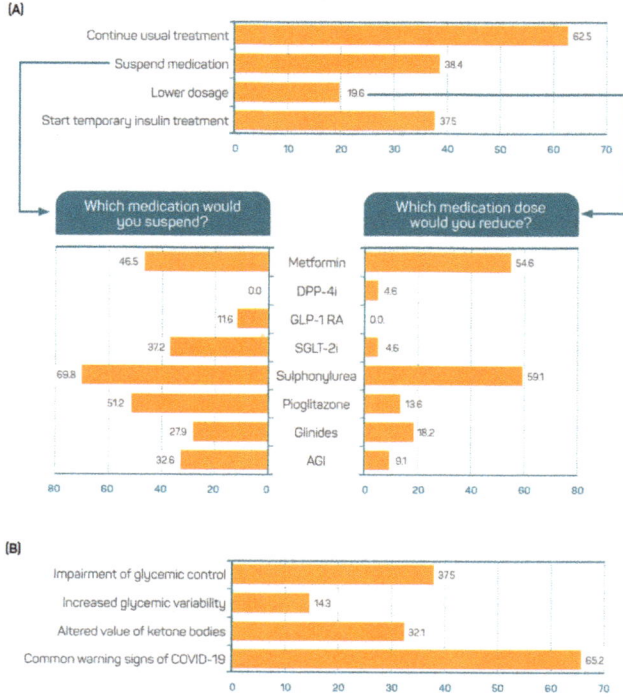

Figure 2. Opinion on management of ambulatory patients with T2DM and COVID-19: (**A**) therapeutic decisions made in these patients; (**B**) specific warning signs of T2DM to indicate hospital admission in these patients (*n* = 112). AGI: Alpha-glucosidase inhibitors; DPP-4i, Dipeptidyl peptidase 4 inhibitors; GLP-1 RA, Glucagon-like peptide 1 receptor agonists; SGLT2i, Sodium-glucose transport protein 2 inhibitors.

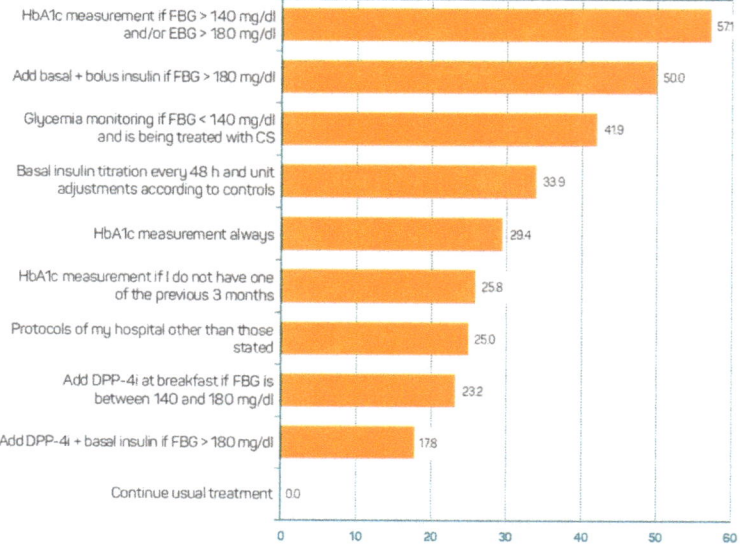

Figure 3. Opinion on therapeutic management of patients with unknown T2DM admitted to hospital due to COVID-19, who presented with hyperglycemia and did not require corticosteroids (*n* = 112. CS, Corticosteroids; DPP-4i, Dipeptidyl peptidase 4 inhibitors; EBG, evening blood glucose; FBG, fasting blood glucose; HbA1c, Glycated haemoglobin.

In the patients with known T2DM admitted to hospital due to COVID-19, the risk of hypoglycemia, the value of glycemia at admission, the presence of comorbidities and conditions, and the risk of ketoacidosis were the four most important factors to consider when a glucose-lowering treatment was prescribed (Figure 4A).

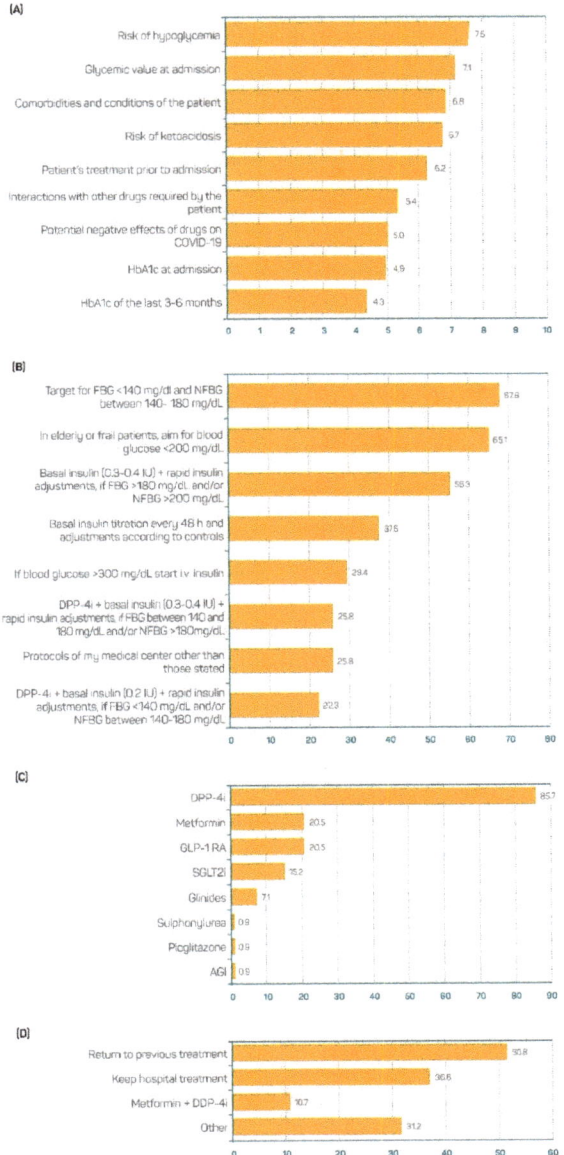

Figure 4. Opinion on clinical practice in patients with known T2DM admitted to hospital due to COVID-19: (**A**) factors to consider when choosing a glucose-lowering treatment; (**B**) criteria to consider when treating hyperglycemia; (**C**) pharmacological class maintained during hospitalization; (**D**) glucose-lowering approach taken at discharge (*n* = 112). AGI: Alpha-glucosidase inhibitors; DPP-4i, Dipeptidyl peptidase 4 inhibitors; FBG, fasting blood glucose; GLP-1 RA, Glucagon-like peptide 1 receptor agonists; HbA1c, Glycated haemoglobin; IU, International units; NFBG, non-fasting blood glucose: SGLT2i, Sodium-glucose transport protein 2 inhibitors.

Considering the patients with T2DM hospitalized due to COVID-19, 67.8% of the participants were in favour of setting a fasting glucose target < 140 mg/dL and 140–180 mg/dL during the rest of the day. The percentage of participants in favour of considering milder goals (<200 mg/dL) in elderly or frail patients was 65.1%. The percentage of participants declaring that they had prescribed basal insulin and rapid insulin corrections when required to patients with basal glycaemia > 180 mg/dL and/or non-basal glycaemia > 200 mg/dL was 55.3% (Figure 4B).

From the total sample, 85.7% chose to keep the current glucose-lowering treatment when this was DPP4i, while other therapeutic options, such as metformin or GLP-1 Ras, were only considered by 20.5%. The maintenance of other options, such as sulfonylurea, pioglitazone, or an alpha-glucosidase inhibitor (AGI), was supported by 0.9% of the participants (Figure 4C). When the participants were asked about what glucose-lowering approach they considered at discharge, 50.8% declared that they had returned to the previous treatment, 36.6% coincided with keeping the treatment prescribed at the hospital, and 10.7% stated that they had prescribed metformin plus DPP-4i (Figure 4D).

3.5. Corticosteroids-Induced Hyperglycaemia in Patients with COVID-19

In those patients with previously known T2DM who were admitted to hospital due to COVID-19 and required treatment with CS, 88.4% of the participants supported the option of maintaining the treatment with DPP-4i; the maintenance of metformin was supported by 18.8% and of GLP-1 RA by 19.6%. None of the participants supported the maintenance of sulphonylureas (Figure 5).

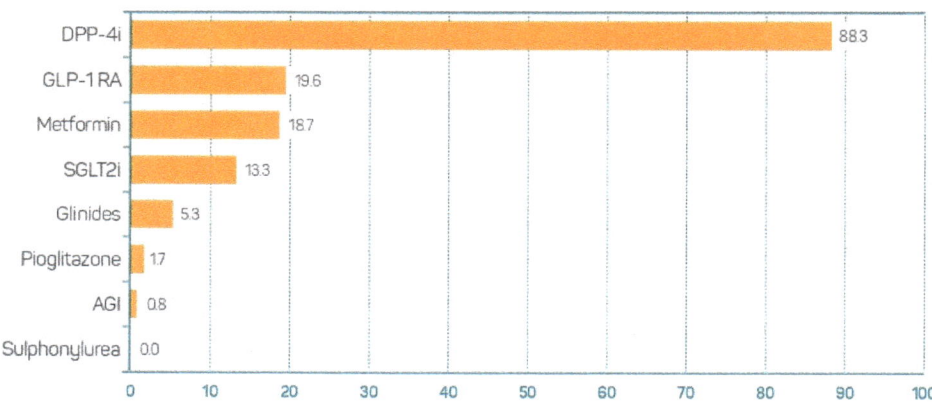

Figure 5. Opinion on pharmacological classes to be maintained in patients with known T2DM admitted to hospital due to COVID-19 and requiring corticosteroids. AGI: Alpha-glucosidase inhibitors; DPP-4i, Dipeptidyl peptidase 4 inhibitors; GLP-1 RA, Glucagon-like peptide 1 receptor agonists; SGLT2i, Sodium-glucose transport protein 2 inhibitors.

The criteria for the treatment of CS-induced hyperglycaemia in patients with COVID-19 were also inquired about. In the patients with unknown T2DM at the time of hyperglycaemia onset, 76.8% considered it critical to control glycaemia within the days after starting the treatment with CS, and 61.6% supported objectives of <140 mg/dL for basal glycaemia and of <200 mg/dL for postprandial glycaemia. These percentages were 86.6% and 57.1% when considering patients with a previous diagnosis of T2DM (Figure S4).

4. Discussion

The current publication provides an overview of the perception and the current clinical practice in patients with T2DM who are infected with SARS-CoV-2 in the Spanish setting. In general terms, the majority of the participants believed that COVID-19 itself entailed a higher risk of T2DM decompensation and T2DM new onset, as has been supported by recent evidence [15]. As previously described, both the SARS-CoV-2 infection and the therapy administered at admission, frequently including CS, increase the risk of glycaemic decompensation [21,24]. A plausible explanation for this is the presence and replication of the virus in the pancreatic islets [25,26] and the inflammation process generated by COVID-19 [27], which could lead to insulin resistance. Some authors have hypothesized that new-onset diabetes in patients with COVID-19 has a multifactorial nature and could stem from factors that induce autoimmunity, β-cell stress, insulin resistance, and local hypoxia and from inflammation that damages β-cells [28]. At the same time, hyperglycemia is associated with the need for mechanical ventilation and ICU admission and with mortality [21] in patients with COVID-19; so, it is important to reduce its risk. Despite these data, and although hyperglycaemia is a factor of bad prognosis in all patients with COVID-19, particularly in those with no diagnosis of T2DM [21,29], nearly 15% of the sample believed that it only affected those patients with previously diagnosed T2DM. A similar percentage of participants believed that the risk of hyperglycaemia was only increased for those patients treated with CS.

DM is one of the most prevalent comorbidities in patients hospitalized due to COVID-19 in Spain, being present in 19.4% of patients with the infection [6]. DM has been described as a risk factor for a bad prognosis of COVID-19 [20,30]. In this study, 71.4% of the sample considered T2DM as an independent risk factor, and the rest took into consideration other conditioning factors, such as poor control, comorbidities, or frailty. The percentage of participants who declared that they had not modified their usual clinical practice in light of this fact was 37.5%, probably meaning a problem of therapeutic inertia when it comes to managing patients with T2DM infected by SARS-CoV-2.

Obesity is a highly prevalent condition in patients with severe manifestations of COVID-19 [31]. In patients with T2DM, obesity also increases the risk of poor glycemic control, and it is probably the comorbidity with the greatest impact on COVID-19 prognosis [32]. However, around 40% of the participants did not identify it as a risk factor for poorer control of T2DM and a worse course of COVID-19 in patients with both diseases. Also remarkable was the low number of participants rating comorbidities such as hypertension or heart disease as reasons for a worse course of COVID-19 in patients with T2DM, even though they have been described as such in populations with T2DM, regardless of COVID-19 disease [33].

The COVID-19 pandemic and the resulting lockdowns and behavioral changes could have exerted an impact on the glycaemic control of patients with T2DM [34], although the data from a large database in the USA showed no differences between HbA1c levels between the pandemic period and the previous year [35]. In the current work, 73.2% of the participants recommended increasing the frequency of glycaemia controls in SARS-CoV-2-infected non-hospitalized patients. With regard to the glucose-lowering treatment of patients who are affected by COVID-19, a large retrospective study conducted in Germany showed a negative impact of the pandemic on T2DM patients' care: the intensification of the treatment with any therapeutic option was reduced. The number of uncontrolled patients who underwent at least one therapeutic regimen change was reduced too [36]. From the measures for the optimization of glycemic control, 73.2% of the participants chose the intensification of patients without COVID-19 who were not on target, and 57.1% chose the patients with COVID-19. Thus, a relevant part of the sample did not agree with this measure, although it is recommended in the main international guidelines [37] and, in the case of patients with COVID-19, it helps to avoid severe manifestations. Moreover, higher levels of HbA1c are associated with systemic inflammation, hypercoagulability, and bad prognosis of COVID-19 [17], and hyperglycemia has also been shown to have a clear negative impact on mortality in hospitalized patients with COVID-19 [21].

The participants also gave their opinion on the use of different glucose-lowering therapeutic options in patients with T2DM and COVID-19. In this regard, GLP1 RA and SGLT2i could be an inappropriate option as they can induce overexpression of angiotensin-converting enzyme 2 (ACE2) [38], the receptor by which SARS-CoV-2 attacks pneumocytes [39]. Moreover, the discontinuation of SGLT2i is recommended at hospital admission, as it can increase the risk of diabetic ketoacidosis, urinary and genital infections, and volume depletion [40]. GLP1 RA should be used with caution, as long as dehydration does not occur, and by always encouraging adequate fluid intake and regular meals [41]. Its discontinuation should be considered in patients with long-term disease and intestinal symptoms [42]. Sulfonylureas increase the risk of hypoglycemia and are discouraged in hospitalized patients with severe disease. The use of metformin possesses a certain risk of lactic acidosis in patients with hypoxia and acute disease [43], and it is consequently contraindicated in patients with respiratory problems and hypoxia. Some authors advise a careful monitoring of kidney disease and also the withdrawal of metformin in dehydrated patients as there is a risk of lactic acidosis [41], and some others state its contraindication in patients hospitalized due to COVID-19 [40]. Different meta-analyses have reported a negative association with DPP-4 inhibitor use and a risk of mortality. DPP-4i may represent a good option for preventing and reducing the complications of SARS-CoV-2 infection [12,44,45]. However, given the observational nature of the available studies, the possible benefits of using any antidiabetic agent should be addressed [12,44]. In line with these previous findings, the proportion of physicians who declared that they had suspended or reduced the treatment with DPP-4i in ambulatory patients was imperceptible, and this therapeutic option was the most valued when the participants were asked about which glucose-lowering drug would be maintained in the case of hospitalization, even in patients requiring CS therapy.

The use of CS in patients with pre-existing T2DM results in a worsening of glycemic control [46], and it is the main cause of hyperglycemic decompensation in hospitalized patients. For this reason, glycaemia needs to be narrowly monitored and treated accordingly in all patients under CS treatment [46,47]. CS is a frequently prescribed medication in patients with COVID-19 because of its effect on hyperinflammation and the potential reduction in mortality [48]. Even so, the percentage of participants who did not agree with controlling glycaemia during the days after introducing CS was 23.2% when it came to patients with known T2DM, and 13.4% with unknown T2DM. Consequently, an important proportion of physicians managing patients with T2DM and COVID-19 might not be following the current recommendations and increasing the risk of hyperglycemia in these patients.

This study entails certain limitations related to its qualitative nature and its design. First, there was not a randomized selection, and this sample might not be representative of the whole population of Spanish physicians specialised in internal medicine or endocrinology. Consequently, the generalizations are limited; another sample may reach different conclusions. However, we used the published data by the Spanish Ministry of Health of 2008 to know the approximate distribution of internists and endocrinologists and the female percentage for both specialties in Spanish hospitals, and by indirect comparison, our sample was not very far from the published data.

Second, the number of specialists in internal medicine was greater than the number of specialists in endocrinology. Once again, the purpose was not to compare results among specialties, but to obtain the global opinion of physicians. Third, the survey was designed with pre-defined answers, which could have made it difficult to contribute with personal ideas or clarifications. In this regard, the inclusion of more answers or an open field would have supposed a higher risk of an excessive dispersion of answers. To counteract this limitation, the survey was designed by a scientific committee including specialists in both internal medicine and endocrinology, thus ensuring the inclusion of those answers considered to be more relevant. Last, but not least, the interpretation of the statements or options of response could have been variable among the participants, but in any case, the questionnaire was reviewed by experts belonging to both endocrinology and internal medicine specialties.

5. Conclusions

The appearance of COVID-19 has impacted on the clinical outcomes of patients with T2DM. Thus, clinical management needs to be adapted to the new reality. Physicians involved in this study seem to be aware of the bidirectional relationship between both T2DM and the COVID-19/coronavirus infection. However, there is still room for improvement in terms of the monitoring and therapeutic management of patients with T2DM who are infected by SARS-CoV-2. It is important to put emphasis on spreading the available evidence, following current recommendations, and favouring practices that ensure an adequate metabolic control and that minimize the risk of complications and the hospitalization of these patients. Although a randomized sample was desirable, the data obtained from this large panel group of Spanish physicians concerning T2DM and COVID-19 management, and the way in which the results are consistent with those suggested by the guidelines or known evidence, can contribute to the identification of key issues and trends to explore in further studies in order to identify strategies aimed at optimizing the clinical practice.

Supplementary Materials: The following supporting information can be downloaded at: https://www.mdpi.com/article/10.3390/jcm11154507/s1, Figure S1: opinion on (a) the consideration of T2DM as an independent risk factor of COVID-19 bad prognosis and (b) its impact in clinical practice (n = 112), Figure S2: opinion on recommendations of blood glucose monitoring of ambulatory patients with DM2 and COVID-19 (n = 112), Figure S3: opinion on which hospitalized patients have a worse prognosis when hyperglycaemia at admission is present (n = 112), Figure S4: opinion on criteria for the treatment of corticosteroid-induced hyperglycaemia in patients with COVID-19 (a) with unknown T2DM and (b) with known T2DM (n = 112).

Author Contributions: Both named authors (R.G.-H. and F.G.-P.) meet the International Committee of Medical Journal Editors (ICMJE) criteria for authorship for this article. All named authors (R.G.-H. and F.G.-P.) take responsibility for the integrity of the work as a whole and have given their approval for this version to be published. Both authors (R.G.-H. and F.G.-P.) have equally collaborated on the design of the study, the interpretation of the data, and the drafting and review of the manuscript. All authors have read and agreed to the published version of the manuscript.

Funding: Financial and logistic support was provided by ESTEVE Pharmaceuticals S.A Barcelona, Spain, including the journal's publication fee. ESTEVE Pharmaceuticals S.A did not influence and was not involved in data interpretation and analysis.

Institutional Review Board Statement: Not applicable. Data were collected by means of anonymous questionnaires in online format, completed by physicians in accordance with their usual practice. Participation was voluntary. The respondents expressed their consent to participate in the survey through logging into the secure online survey platform and actively clicking a consent box.

Informed Consent Statement: Not applicable. The study was based on an on-line survey that did not require data on individual patients to be recorded or involve the participation of patients.

Data Availability Statement: The majority of the data are contained within the article or supplementary material. The datasets generated during and/or analysed during the current study are available from the corresponding author upon reasonable request.

Acknowledgments: The authors would like to especially thank the panel of physicians for their participation; Esteve Pharmaceuticals, S.A. for the support provided to carry out the study; IDEMM-FARMA S.L for the technical and methodological support; Montse Fontboté and Jemina Moretó for their support in the medical writing; and Francisco López for performing the statistical analysis.

Conflicts of Interest: Ricardo Gómez-Huelgas has provided consultancy services and has served as a speaker and has participated as a researcher in studies financed by Boehringer Ingelheim, Eli Lilly, Novo Nordisk, Sanofi, Astra Zeneca, MSD, Janssen, or Esteve. Fernando Gómez-Peralta has provided consulting services for Abbott, Astra Zeneca, Esteve, Novartis, Novo Nordisk, and Sanofi and has participated as an investigator in studies funded by Boehringer Ingelheim, Eli Lilly, Novo Nordisk, and Sanofi; he has served as a speaker for Abbott, Astra Zeneca, Boehringer Ingelheim, Bristol Myers Squibb, Eli Lilly, Esteve, Novartis, Novo Nordisk, and Sanofi. The funders had no role in the design of the study; in the collection, analyses, or interpretation of data; in the writing of the manuscript; or in the decision to publish the results.

References

1. International Diabetes Federation (IDF). *Diabetes Atlas*, 9th ed. 2019. Available online: https://www.diabetesatlas.org/en/ (accessed on 10 May 2021).
2. Saeedi, P.; Petersohn, I.; Salpea, P.; Malanda, B.; Karuranga, S.; Unwin, N.; Colagiuri, S.; Guariguata, L.; Motala, A.A.; Ogurtsova, K.; et al. Global and regional diabetes prevalence estimates for 2019 and projections for 2030 and 2045: Results from the International Diabetes Federation Diabetes Atlas, 9th edition. *Diabetes Res. Clin. Pract.* **2019**, *157*, 107843. [CrossRef]
3. Soriguer, F.; Goday, A.; Bosch-Comas, A.; Bordiú, E.; Calle-Pascual, A.; Carmena, R.; Casamitjana, R.; Castaño, L.; Castell, C.; Catalá, M.; et al. Prevalence of diabetes mellitus and impaired glucose regulation in Spain: The Diabetes Study. *Diabetologia* **2012**, *55*, 88–93. [CrossRef]
4. Muller, L.M.A.J.; Gorter, K.J.; Hak, E.; Goudzwaard, W.L.; Schellevis, F.G.; Hoepelman, A.I.M.; Rutten, G.E.H.M. Increased Risk of Common Infections in Patients with Type 1 and Type 2 Diabetes Mellitus. *Clin. Infect. Dis.* **2005**, *41*, 281–288. [CrossRef] [PubMed]
5. Spain: WHO Coronavirus Disease (COVID-19) Dashboard with Vaccination Data | WHO Coronavirus (COVID-19) Dashboard with Vaccination Data. Available online: https://covid19.who.int/region/euro/country/es (accessed on 22 October 2021).
6. Casas-Rojo, J.M.; Antón-Santos, J.M.; Millán-Núñez-Cortés, J.; Lumbreras-Bermejo, C.; Ramos-Rincón, J.M.; Roy-Vallejo, E.; Artero-Mora, A.; Arnalich-Fernández, F.; García-Bruñén, J.M.; Vargas-Núñez, J.A.; et al. Clinical characteristics of patients hospitalized with COVID-19 in Spain: Results from the SEMI-COVID-19 Registry. *Rev. Clin. Esp.* **2020**, *220*, 480–494. [CrossRef] [PubMed]
7. Yang, X.; Yu, Y.; Xu, J.; Shu, H.; Xia, J.; Liu, H.; Wu, Y.; Zhang, L.; Yu, Z.; Fang, M.; et al. Clinical course and outcomes of critically ill patients with SARS-CoV-2 pneumonia in Wuhan, China: A single-centered, retrospective, observational study. *Lancet Respir. Med.* **2020**, *8*, 475–481. [CrossRef]
8. Guan, W.; Ni, Z.; Hu, Y.; Liang, W.; Ou, C.; He, J.; Liu, L.; Shan, H.; Lei, C.; Hui, D.S.C.; et al. Clinical Characteristics of Coronavirus Disease 2019 in China. *N. Engl. J. Med.* **2020**, *382*, 1708–1720. [CrossRef] [PubMed]
9. de Almeida-Pititto, B.; Dualib, P.M.; Zajdenverg, L.; Dantas, J.R.; de Souza, F.D.; Rodacki, M.; Bertoluci, M.C. Brazilian Diabetes Society Study Group (SBD) Severity and mortality of COVID-19 in patients with diabetes, hypertension and cardiovascular disease: A meta-analysis. *Diabetol. Metab. Syndr.* **2020**, *12*, 75. [CrossRef] [PubMed]
10. Guo, W.; Li, M.; Dong, Y.; Zhou, H.; Zhang, Z.; Tian, C.; Qin, R.; Wang, H.; Shen, Y.; Du, K.; et al. Diabetes is a risk factor for the progression and prognosis of COVID-19. *Diabetes Metab. Res. Rev.* **2020**, *36*, e3319. [CrossRef] [PubMed]
11. Zhou, F.; Yu, T.; Du, R.; Fan, G.; Liu, Y.; Liu, Z.; Xiang, J.; Wang, Y.; Song, B.; Gu, X.; et al. Clinical course and risk factors for mortality of adult inpatients with COVID-19 in Wuhan, China: A retrospective cohort study. *Lancet* **2020**, *395*, 1054–1062. [CrossRef]
12. Iacobellis, G. COVID-19 and diabetes: Can DPP4 inhibition play a role? *Diabetes Res. Clin. Pract.* **2020**, *162*, 108125. [CrossRef]
13. Rubino, F.; Amiel, S.A.; Zimmet, P.; Alberti, G.; Bornstein, S.; Eckel, R.H.; Mingrone, G.; Boehm, B.; Cooper, M.E.; Chai, Z.; et al. New-Onset Diabetes in COVID-19. *N. Engl. J. Med.* **2020**, *383*, 789–790. [CrossRef]
14. Liu, F.; Long, X.; Zhang, B.; Zhang, W.; Chen, X.; Zhang, Z. ACE2 Expression in Pancreas May Cause Pancreatic Damage After SARS-CoV-2 Infection. *Clin. Gastroenterol. Hepatol.* **2020**, *18*, 2128–2130.e2. [CrossRef]
15. Xie, Y.; Al-Aly, Z. Risks and burdens of incident diabetes in long COVID: A cohort study. *Lancet Diabetes Endocrinol.* **2022**, *10*, 311–321. [CrossRef]
16. Sardu, C.; D'Onofrio, N.; Balestrieri, M.L.; Barbieri, M.; Rizzo, M.R.; Messina, V.; Maggi, P.; Coppola, N.; Paolisso, G.; Marfella, R. Outcomes in Patients with Hyperglycemia Affected by COVID-19: Can We Do More on Glycemic Control? *Diabetes Care* **2020**, *43*, 1408–1415. [CrossRef]
17. Wang, Z.; Du, Z.; Zhu, F. Glycosylated hemoglobin is associated with systemic inflammation, hypercoagulability, and prognosis of COVID-19 patients. *Diabetes Res. Clin. Pract.* **2020**, *164*, 108214. [CrossRef]
18. Piarulli, F.; Lapolla, A. COVID-19 and low-glucose levels: Is there a link? *Diabetes Res. Clin. Pract.* **2020**, *166*, 108283. [CrossRef]
19. Zhu, L.; She, Z.-G.; Cheng, X.; Qin, J.-J.; Zhang, X.-J.; Cai, J.; Lei, F.; Wang, H.; Xie, J.; Wang, W.; et al. Association of Blood Glucose Control and Outcomes in Patients with COVID-19 and Pre-existing Type 2 Diabetes. *Cell Metab.* **2020**, *31*, 1068–1077.e3. [CrossRef]
20. Holman, N.; Knighton, P.; Kar, P.; O'Keefe, J.; Curley, M.; Weaver, A.; Barron, E.; Bakhai, C.; Khunti, K.; Wareham, N.J.; et al. Risk factors for COVID-19-related mortality in people with type 1 and type 2 diabetes in England: A population-based cohort study. *Lancet Diabetes Endocrinol.* **2020**, *8*, 823–833. [CrossRef]
21. Carrasco-Sánchez, F.J.; López-Carmona, M.D.; Martínez-Marcos, F.J.; Pérez-Belmonte, L.M.; Hidalgo-Jiménez, A.; Buonaiuto, V.; Fernández, C.S.; Castro, S.J.F.; Luordo, D.; Fontan, P.M.P.; et al. Admission hyperglycaemia as a predictor of mortality in patients hospitalized with COVID-19 regardless of diabetes status: Data from the Spanish SEMI-COVID-19 Registry. *Ann. Med.* **2021**, *53*, 103–116. [CrossRef]
22. Chudasama, Y.V.; Gillies, C.L.; Zaccardi, F.; Coles, B.; Davies, M.J.; Seidu, S.; Khunti, K. Impact of COVID-19 on routine care for chronic diseases: A global survey of views from healthcare professionals. *Diabetes Metab. Syndr.* **2020**, *14*, 965–967. [CrossRef] [PubMed]

23. Caballero, A.E.; Ceriello, A.; Misra, A.; Aschner, P.; McDonnell, M.; Hassanein, M.E.; Ji, L.; Mbanya, J.C.; Fonseca, V.A. COVID-19 in people living with diabetes: An international consensus. *J. Diabetes Complicat.* **2020**, *34*, 107671. [CrossRef] [PubMed]
24. Wake, D.J.; Gibb, F.W.; Kar, P.; Kennon, B.; Klonoff, D.C.; Rayman, G.; Rutter, M.K.; Sainsbury, C.; Semple, R.K. Endocrinology in the time of COVID-19: Remodelling diabetes services and emerging innovation. *Eur. J. Endocrinol.* **2020**, *183*, G67–G77. [CrossRef]
25. Drucker, D.J. Diabetes, obesity, metabolism, and SARS-CoV-2 infection: The end of the beginning. *Cell Metab.* **2021**, *33*, 479–498. [CrossRef]
26. Müller, J.A.; Groß, R.; Conzelmann, C.; Krüger, J.; Merle, U.; Steinhart, J.; Weil, T.; Koepke, L.; Bozzo, C.P.; Read, C.; et al. SARS-CoV-2 infects and replicates in cells of the human endocrine and exocrine pancreas. *Nat. Metab.* **2021**, *32*, 149–165. [CrossRef] [PubMed]
27. Li, G.; Fan, Y.; Lai, Y.; Han, T.; Li, Z.; Zhou, P.; Pan, P.; Wang, W.; Hu, D.; Liu, X.; et al. Coronavirus infections and immune responses. *J. Med. Virol.* **2020**, *92*, 424–432. [CrossRef] [PubMed]
28. Atkinson, M.A.; Powers, A.C. Distinguishing the real from the hyperglycaemia: Does COVID-19 induce diabetes? *Lancet Diabetes Endocrinol.* **2021**, *9*, 328–329. [CrossRef]
29. Bode, B.; Garrett, V.; Messler, J.; McFarland, R.; Crowe, J.; Booth, R.; Klonoff, D.C. Glycemic Characteristics and Clinical Outcomes of COVID-19 Patients Hospitalized in the United States. *J. Diabetes Sci. Technol.* **2020**, *14*, 813–821. [CrossRef] [PubMed]
30. Apicella, M.; Campopiano, M.C.; Mantuano, M.; Mazoni, L.; Coppelli, A.; Del Prato, S. COVID-19 in people with diabetes: Understanding the reasons for worse outcomes. *Lancet Diabetes Endocrinol.* **2020**, *8*, 782–792. [CrossRef]
31. Simonnet, A.; Chetboun, M.; Poissy, J.; Raverdy, V.; Noulette, J.; Duhamel, A.; Labreuche, J.; Mathieu, D.; Pattou, F.; Jourdain, M.; et al. High Prevalence of Obesity in Severe Acute Respiratory Syndrome Coronavirus-2 (SARS-CoV-2) Requiring Invasive Mechanical Ventilation. *Obesity* **2020**, *28*, 1195–1199. [CrossRef] [PubMed]
32. Cariou, B.; Hadjadj, S.; Wargny, M.; Pichelin, M.; Al-Salameh, A.; Allix, I.; Amadou, C.; Arnault, G.; Baudoux, F.; Bauduceau, B.; et al. Phenotypic characteristics and prognosis of inpatients with COVID-19 and diabetes: The CORONADO study. *Diabetologia* **2020**, *63*, 1500–1515. [CrossRef] [PubMed]
33. Información Científica-Técnica, COVID-19 en Distintos Entornos y Grupos de Personas. Available online: https://www.sanidad.gob.es/profesionales/saludPublica/ccayes/alertasActual/nCov/documentos/Documento_GRUPOS_PERSONAS.pdf (accessed on 3 March 2022).
34. Tanji, Y.; Sawada, S.; Watanabe, T.; Mita, T.; Kobayashi, Y.; Murakami, T.; Metoki, H.; Akai, H. Impact of COVID-19 pandemic on glycemic control among outpatients with type 2 diabetes in Japan: A hospital-based survey from a country without lockdown. *Diabetes Res. Clin. Pract.* **2021**, *176*, 108840. [CrossRef] [PubMed]
35. Patel, S.Y.; McCoy, R.G.; Barnett, M.L.; Shah, N.D.; Mehrotra, A. Diabetes Care and Glycemic Control During the COVID-19 Pandemic in the United States. *JAMA Intern. Med.* **2021**, *181*, 1412–1414. [CrossRef] [PubMed]
36. Jacob, L.; Rickwood, S.; Rathmann, W.; Kostev, K. Change in glucose-lowering medication regimens in individuals with type 2 diabetes mellitus during the COVID-19 pandemic in Germany. *Diabetes Obes. Metab.* **2021**, *23*, 910–915. [CrossRef] [PubMed]
37. Buse, J.B.; Wexler, D.J.; Tsapas, A.; Rossing, P.; Mingrone, G.; Mathieu, C.; D'Alessio, D.A.; Davies, M.J. Correction to: 2019 update to: Management of hyperglycaemia in type 2 diabetes, 2018. A consensus report by the American Diabetes Association (ADA) and the European Association for the Study of diabetes (EASD). *Diabetologia* **2020**, *63*, 1667. [CrossRef] [PubMed]
38. Pal, R.; Bhadada, S.K. Should anti-diabetic medications be reconsidered amid COVID-19 pandemic? *Diabetes Res. Clin. Pract.* **2020**, *163*, 108146. [CrossRef]
39. Fang, L.; Karakiulakis, G.; Roth, M. Are patients with hypertension and diabetes mellitus at increased risk for COVID-19 infection? *Lancet Respir. Med.* **2020**, *8*, e21. [CrossRef]
40. Korytkowski, M.; Antinori-Lent, K.; Drincic, A.; Hirsch, I.B.; McDonnell, M.E.; Rushakoff, R.; Muniyappa, R. A Pragmatic Approach to Inpatient Diabetes Management during the COVID-19 Pandemic. *J. Clin. Endocrinol. Metab.* **2020**, *105*, 3076–3087. [CrossRef] [PubMed]
41. Bornstein, S.R.; Rubino, F.; Khunti, K.; Mingrone, G.; Hopkins, D.; Birkenfeld, A.L.; Boehm, B.; Amiel, S.; Holt, R.I.; Skyler, J.S.; et al. Practical recommendations for the management of diabetes in patients with COVID-19. *Lancet Diabetes Endocrinol.* **2020**, *8*, 546–550. [CrossRef]
42. Mirabelli, M.; Chiefari, E.; Puccio, L.; Foti, D.P.; Brunetti, A. Potential Benefits and Harms of Novel Antidiabetic Drugs during COVID-19 Crisis. *Int. J. Environ. Res. Public Health* **2020**, *17*, 3664. [CrossRef] [PubMed]
43. Bellido, V.; Pérez, A. COVID-19 and Diabetes. *J. Clin. Med.* **2021**, *10*, 5341. [CrossRef]
44. Yang, Y.; Cai, Z.; Zhang, J. DPP-4 inhibitors may improve the mortality of coronavirus disease 2019: A meta-analysis. *PLoS ONE* **2021**, *16*, e0251916. [CrossRef] [PubMed]
45. Rakhmat, I.I.; Kusmala, Y.Y.; Handayani, D.R.; Juliastuti, H.; Nawangsih, E.N.; Wibowo, A.; Lim, M.A.; Pranata, R. Dipeptidyl peptidase-4 (DPP-4) inhibitor and mortality in coronavirus disease 2019 (COVID-19)—A systematic review, meta-analysis, and meta-regression. *Diabetes Metab Syndr.* **2021**, *15*, 777–782. [CrossRef] [PubMed]
46. Roberts, A.; James, J.; Dhatariya, K.; Agarwal, N.; Brake, J.; Brooks, C.; Castro, E.; Gregory, R.; Higham, C.; Hobley, L.; et al. Management of hyperglycaemia and steroid (glucocorticoid) therapy: A guideline from the Joint British Diabetes Societies (JBDS) for Inpatient Care group. *Diabet. Med.* **2018**, *35*, 1011–1017. [CrossRef] [PubMed]

47. Perez, A.; Jansen-Chaparro, S.; Saigi, I.; Bernal-Lopez, M.R.; Miñambres, I.; Gomez-Huelgas, R. Glucocorticoid-induced hyperglycemia. *J. Diabetes* **2014**, *6*, 9–20. [CrossRef]
48. Wagner, C.; Griesel, M.; Mikolajewska, A.; Mueller, A.; Nothacker, M.; Kley, K.; Metzendorf, M.-I.; Fischer, A.-L.; Kopp, M.; Stegemann, M.; et al. Systemic corticosteroids for the treatment of COVID-19. *Cochrane Database Syst. Rev.* **2021**, *2021*, CD014963. [CrossRef]

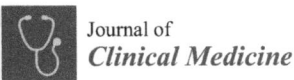 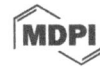

Article

Diabetes Does Not Increase the Risk of Hospitalization Due to COVID-19 in Patients Aged 50 Years or Older in Primary Care—APHOSDIAB—COVID-19 Multicenter Study

Domingo Orozco-Beltrán [1,2,3,†], Juan Francisco Merino-Torres [4,†], Antonio Pérez [2,5,6,7,*], Ana M. Cebrián-Cuenca [8,9,10], Ignacio Párraga-Martínez [11,12], Luis Ávila-Lachica [13,14], Gemma Rojo-Martínez [2,6,15], Francisco J. Pomares-Gómez [16], Fernando Álvarez-Guisasola [11,17], Manuel Sánchez-Molla [18], Felix Gutiérrez [3,19,20], Francisco J. Ortega [21], Manel Mata-Cases [22,23], Enrique Carretero-Anibarro [24], Josep Maria Vilaseca [25] and Jose A. Quesada [3]

1 Health Center Cabo Huertas, Consejeria de Sanidad Univesal y Salud Pública, 03540 Alicante, Spain; dorozco@umh.es
2 Spanish Diabetes Society, 28002 Madrid, Spain; gemma.rojo.m@gmail.com
3 Clinical Medice Department, University Miguel Hernández, 03550 Alicante, Spain; gutierrez_fel@umh.es (F.G.); jquesada@umh.es (J.A.Q.)
4 Endocrinology and Nutrition Service, University of Valencia, Hospital Universitari i Politècnic La Fe, 46026 Valencia, Spain; juan.merino@uv.es
5 Medicine Department, Autonoums University of Barcelona, 08193 Barcelona, Spain
6 Biomedical Research Network in Diabetes and Associated Metabolic Disorders (CIBERDEM), 20029 Madrid, Spain
7 Hospital Santa Creu i Sant Pau, Servicio Catalán de Salud, 08041 Barcelona, Spain
8 Primary Care and Prediabetes Group of the Spanish Diabetes Society, 30201 Cartagena, Spain; anicebrian@gmail.com
9 Health Center Cartagena Casco, Servicio Murciano de Salud, 30201 Cartagena, Spain
10 Primary Care Research Group, Biomedical Research Institute of Murcia (IMIB), 30120 Murcia, Spain
11 Spanish Society of Family and Community Medicine (semFyC), 28004 Madrid, Spain; iparraga@gmail.com (I.P.-M.); faguisasola@gmail.com (F.Á.-G.)
12 Health Center Zone VIII, Servicio de Salud Castilla la Mancha, 02006 Albacete, Spain
13 Secretario GAPP-SED, Grupo DM-semFyC, 28004 Madrid, Spain; carlu91@gmail.com
14 Consultorio de Almáchar, UGC Vélez Norte, 29718 Malaga, Spain
15 Biomedical Research Institute (IBIMA), Endocrinology and Nutrition Clinical Management Unit, Malaga Regional University Hospital, 29010 Malaga, Spain
16 Diabetes Mellitus Plan of the Valencian Community, University Hospital San Juan de Alicante, 03550 Alicante, Spain; pomares_fra@gva.es
17 Health Center Ribera de Órbigo, Consejería de Salud Castilla León, 24280 León, Spain
18 Family Physician, Elche General University Hospital, 03203 Elche, Spain; manuel.sanchezm@umh.es
19 Internal Medicine, Elche General University Hospital, 03203 Elche, Spain
20 CIBER Infectious Diseases, 28029 Madrid, Spain
21 Health Center Campos-Lampreana, Consejería de Salud Castilla y León, 49137 Zamora, Spain; fjortegarios@telefonica.net
22 Primary Care Center La Mina, Sant Adrià de Besòs, Servicio Catalán de Salud, 08930 Barcelona, Spain; manelmatacases@gmail.com
23 Group DAP-Cat, Research Support Unit, Jordi Gol University Institute for Primary Healthcare Research, CIBERDEM, 08036 Barcelona, Spain
24 Health Center José Gallego Arroba, Servicio Andauz de Salud, 14500 Córdoba, Spain; almudenayenrique@yahoo.es
25 Medicine Department, University of Barcelona, 08007 Barcelona, Spain; vilasesca@clinic.cat
* Correspondence: aperez@santpau.cat; Tel.: +34-93-556-56-61
† These authors contributed equally to this work.

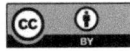

Abstract: The purpose of this study was to identify clinical, analytical, and sociodemographic variables associated with the need for hospital admission in people over 50 years infected with SARS-CoV-2 and to assess whether diabetes mellitus conditions the risk of hospitalization. A multicenter case-control study analyzing electronic medical records in patients with COVID-19 from 1 March 2020 to 30 April 2021 was conducted. We included 790 patients: 295 cases admitted to the hospital and

495 controls. Under half (n = 386, 48.8%) were women, and 8.5% were active smokers. The main comorbidities were hypertension (50.5%), dyslipidemia, obesity, and diabetes (37.5%). Multivariable logistic regression showed that hospital admission was associated with age above 65 years (OR from 2.45 to 3.89, ascending with age group); male sex (OR 2.15, 95% CI 1.47–3.15), fever (OR 4.31, 95% CI 2.87–6.47), cough (OR 1.89, 95% CI 1.28–2.80), asthenia/malaise (OR 2.04, 95% CI 1.38–3.03), dyspnea (4.69, 95% CI 3.00–7.33), confusion (OR 8.87, 95% CI 1.68–46.78), and a history of hypertension (OR 1.61, 95% CI 1.08–2.41) or immunosuppression (OR 4.97, 95% CI 1.45–17.09). Diabetes was not associated with increased risk of hospital admission (OR 1.18, 95% CI 0.80–1.72; p = 0.38). Diabetes did not increase the risk of hospital admission in people over 50 years old, but advanced age, male sex, fever, cough, asthenia, dyspnea/confusion, and hypertension or immunosuppression did.

Keywords: COVID-19; obesity and diabetes mellitus type 2; research; hospitalization; primary care

1. Introduction

Coronavirus type 2 is the cause of severe acute respiratory syndrome (SARS-CoV-2), better known as coronavirus disease 2019 (COVID-19), representing a major global health problem [1]. The infection presents an incubation period of around five days [2,3], after which the most frequent presenting symptoms are fever, dry cough, and fatigue, although other symptoms may also include productive cough, headache, hemoptysis, diarrhea, dyspnea, or lymphopenia [4–6].

Regarding the prognosis of the disease, 80% of cases are mild, 15% severe, and around 5% are critical; the case fatality rate is about 2% [7]. These figures are consistent with a technical document on the clinical management of COVID-19, wherein the Spanish Ministry of Health also estimates that approximately 80% of reported cases are mild [8]. In other countries, a hospitalization rate of 20 per 100,000 population between 1 January and 1 September has been described [9]. Applying this rate to the Spanish population would mean that around 6% of patients with COVID-19 and treated in ambulatory care would require hospitalization, leaving the vast majority of mild COVID-19 cases to be managed in primary care or on an outpatient basis. However, practitioners in these settings need to be able to identify the factors that increase the risk of severity and hospital admission in order to carry out an adequate assessment of the patient's clinical prognosis and management and to assist in healthcare planning.

In that sense, some studies have suggested that diabetes mellitus is associated with a worse clinical prognosis [9], while others with large samples find no such relationship [10]. However, to our knowledge, there is no published information on prognostic variables predicting the need for hospitalization in patients with type 2 diabetes and COVID-19 who are treated in ambulatory care.

The aim of this study is to identify clinical, analytical, and sociodemographic variables associated with the need for hospital admission in people over 50 years of age who are infected with SARS-CoV-2 and followed in ambulatory care, and to specifically assess whether diabetes mellitus conditions the risk of hospitalization.

2. Materials and Methods

This retrospective case-control study was based on the analysis of variables included in the patients' EMRs.

2.1. Selection Criteria

The study included all patients aged 50 and over diagnosed with COVID-19 based on laboratory tests and followed up in 41 participating primary care or outpatient endocrinology units, with home isolation. Patients who did not have laboratory confirmation of COVID-19 were excluded. Cases were defined as patients attended in ambulatory care and later admitted to the hospital due to COVID-19; controls were those who did not require admission.

2.2. Follow-Up Period

Patients were followed up retrospectively from 1 March 2020 until the cure date in cases of full ambulatory follow-up or the date of hospitalization in the admitted patients. The inclusion of patients ended on 30 April 2021.

2.3. Sample Size

The sample size was calculated to identify variables that increased the risk of hospitalization by 50% or more (odds ratio (OR) > 1.5), as described for different pathologies, including diabetes. Each study group required 173 patients, with an increase to account for missing data in an estimated 15% of EMRs. To ensure greater validity and representativeness in the control group, especially in variables with low prevalence, two controls were included for each case. Therefore, the estimated minimum sample size was 597 patients (199 cases and 398 controls).

2.4. Data Collection and Analysis

All data were collected retrospectively from the EMRs.

A descriptive analysis was performed by calculating frequencies for qualitative variables and the minimum, maximum, mean, and standard deviation (SD) for quantitative variables. The factors associated with hospital admission were analyzed using contingency tables, applying the chi-square test for qualitative variables, the Student's t test for comparing means for quantitative variables, or nonparametric tests, as appropriate. To estimate the magnitude of the associations with hospital admission, logistic regression models were fit, using a simple adjustment for age and sex along with a multivariable adjustment. A stepwise variable selection procedure was performed based on the Akaike Information Criterion (AIC). Indicators of goodness-of-fit and predictive indicators such as the area under the receiver operating curve (AUC) are shown. Results are expressed as ORs with their 95% confidence intervals (CIs). Analyses were performed using SPSS (v.26) and R (v.3.6.1) software.

2.5. Ethical Aspects

The study complies with the principles of the Declaration of Helsinki for medical research involving humans and all relevant data protection laws. Data from EMRs were treated anonymously by assigning an individual patient identifier that did not allow linkage to the record number. The treatment, storage, and use of data complied with Organic Law 37/2018, of 5 December, on the Protection of Personal Data, as well as Regulation 2016/679 of the European Parliament and of the Council, of 27 April 2016, regarding the processing of personal data, as well as all applicable regulations and/or legislation. The Ethics Committee of San Juan University Hospital (Alicante) approved the study (code 20/025, dated 20 May 2020).

3. Results

A total of 790 patients throughout Spain were included by 61 researchers who had performed clinical care and follow-up in primary care centers or in outpatient endocrinology clinics (35%) (Supplementary Materials). Of these, 495 who were not hospitalized during follow-up were assigned to the control group, and 295 who were admitted due to SARS-COV-2 were assigned to the case group.

Figure 1 describes the most frequent comorbidities present in the sample of patients studied. Hypertension was the most prevalent (50.5%), followed by dyslipidemia, obesity, and diabetes (37.5%). Just under half the patients ($n = 386$, 48.8%) were women, and 8.5% were active smokers. The distribution by age groups was as follows: <50–55 years, 18.1% ($n = 143$); 55–64 years, 31.9% ($n = 252$); 65–74 years, 24.6% ($n = 194$); 74–84 years, 18.2% ($n = 144$), and >84 years, 7.2% ($n = 57$). Table 1 describes the variables analyzed and their distribution between cases and controls, using a bivariable analysis.

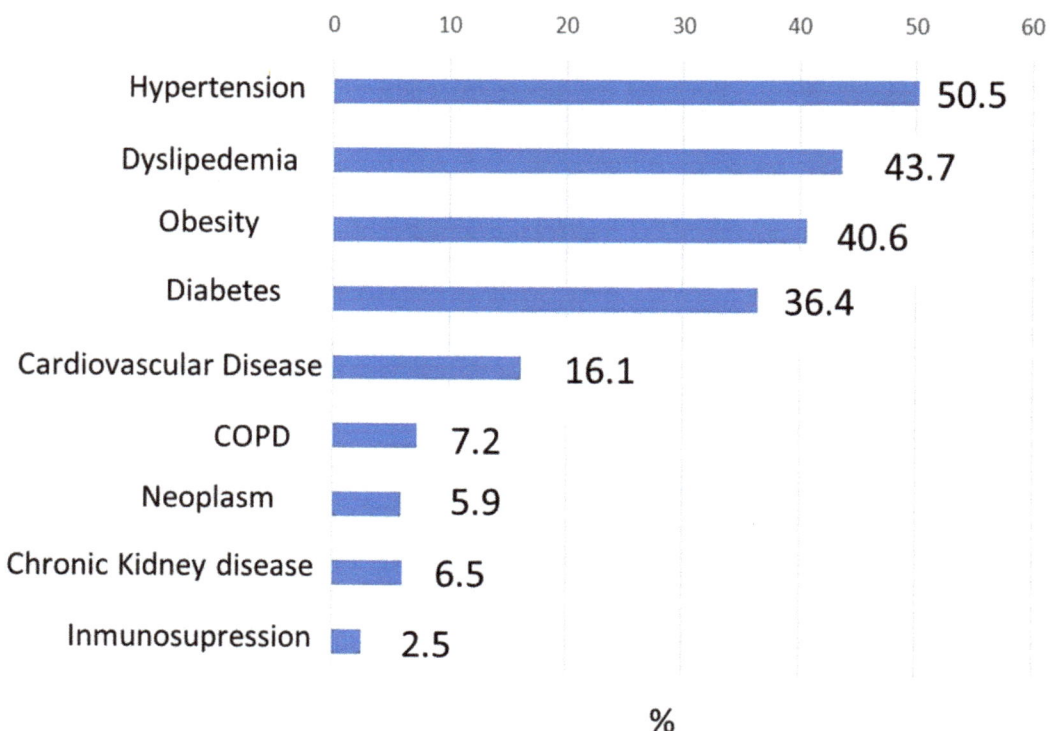

COPD: CHRONIC OBSTRUCTIVE PULMONARY DISEASE

Figure 1. Most frequent comorbidities.

Table 1. Variables associated with hospital admission for COVID-19, bivariable analysis.

	Not Admitted (n = 495)		Admitted (n = 295)		p Value
	n	%	n	%	
Sex					
Female	277	56.0%	109	36.9%	<0.001
Male	218	44.0%	186	63.1%	
Age					
50–54 years	111	22.4%	32	10.8%	<0.001
55–64 years	174	35.2%	78	26.4%	
65–74 years	107	21.6%	87	29.5%	
75–84 years	74	14.9%	70	23.7%	
>84 years	29	5.9%	28	9.5%	
Body mass index					
<25 kg/m^2	65	13.1%	44	14.9%	0.002
25–30 kg/m^2	97	19.6%	71	24.1%	
>30 kg/m^2	94	19.0%	78	26.4%	
Missing	239	48.3%	102	34.6%	

Table 1. *Cont.*

	Not Admitted (n = 495)		Admitted (n = 295)		p Value
	n	%	n	%	
O₂ saturation					
Normal 90–100	204	41.2%	202	68.5%	<0.001
Low <90	1	0.2%	23	7.8%	
Missing	290	58.6%	70	23.7%	
Heart rate					
<60 bpm	6	1.2%	15	5.1%	<0.001
60–100 bpm	220	44.4%	184	62.4%	
>100 bpm	17	3.4%	23	7.8%	
Missing	252	50.9%	73	24.7%	
Systolic blood pressure					
<140 mmHg	217	43.8%	175	59.3%	<0.001
≥140 mmHg	75	15.2%	70	23.7%	
Missing	203	41.0%	50	16.9%	
Diastolic blood pressure					
<90 mmHg	260	52.5%	209	70.8%	<0.001
≥90 mmHg	32	6.5%	36	12.2%	
Missing	203	41.0%	50	16.9%	
Symptoms					
Fever	163	32.9%	222	75.3%	<0.001
Cough	174	35.2%	190	64.4%	<0.001
Asthenia/malaise	177	35.8%	193	65.4%	<0.001
Anorexia	26	5.3%	57	19.3%	<0.001
Myalgia	122	24.6%	103	34.9%	0.002
Dyspnea	47	9.5%	135	45.8%	<0.001
Productive cough	39	7.9%	42	14.2%	0.004
Sore throat	87	17.6%	29	9.8%	0.003
Diarrhea	59	11.9%	62	21.0%	0.001
Nausea/vomiting	31	6.3%	29	9.8%	0.067
Dizziness	17	3.4%	29	9.8%	<0.001
Headache	94	19.0%	66	22.4%	0.25
Shivering	37	7.5%	53	18.0%	<0.001
Loss of taste/smell	66	13.3%	33	11.2%	0.38
Chest tightness	18	3.6%	31	10.5%	<0.001
Confusion	2	0.4%	18	6.1%	<0.001
Comorbidities					
Hypertension	218	44.0%	191	64.7%	<0.001
Diabetes mellitus	158	31.9%	138	46.8%	<0.001
Dyslipidemia	210	42.4%	140	47.5%	0.17
Cardiovascular disease	68	13.7%	63	21.4%	0.005
Cancer	24	4.8%	23	7.8%	0.090

Table 1. Cont.

	Not Admitted (n = 495)		Admitted (n = 295)		p Value
	n	%	n	%	
O_2 saturation					
Chronic kidney disease	27	5.5%	25	8.5%	0.098
Immunosuppression	6	1.2%	14	4.7%	0.002
Gastrointestinal disease	28	5.7%	19	6.4%	0.65
COPD	25	5.1%	35	11.9%	<0.001
Asthma	28	5.7%	15	5.1%	0.73

bpm: beats per minute; COPD: chronic obstructive pulmonary disease.

Table 2a shows the results of the logistic regression adjusted for age and sex, and Table 2b shows a multivariate adjustment performed with a backward variable selection strategy, based on the AIC criterion, to arrive at an optimal model with all significant variables. The multivariable model used had a high explanatory power to assess the risk of hospital admission (AUC 0.860). The warning signs of a patient at risk of hospital admission were confusion, dyspnea, cough, and fever, while sore throat was associated with a lower probability of admission. Patient characteristics conferring a higher risk of hospitalization were age over 65 years and male sex, while the most relevant comorbidities were hypertension and immunosuppression. After adjusting for all other variables analyzed, neither diabetes nor obesity were associated with a higher risk of hospital admission in patients with COVID-19 followed in ambulatory care.

Table 2. (a) Variables associated with hospital admission for COVID-19, multivariable analysis. Adjustment for age and sex. (b) Variables associated with hospital admission for COVID-19, multivariable analysis. Multivariable adjustment.

(a)				
		\multicolumn{3}{c}{Adjustment for Age and Sex}
		OR	95% CI	p
Body mass index	<25 kg/m^2	1		
	25–30 kg/m^2	0.80	(0.48–1.35)	0.41
	>30 kg/m^2	1.03	(0.62–1.72)	0.91
	Missing	0.52	(0.33–0.84)	0.008
Active smoker	No	1		
	Yes	1.07	(0.61–1.88)	0.80
	Missing	1.02	(0.71–1.46)	0.91
O_2 saturation	Normal 90–100%	1		
	Low < 90%	25.05	(3.29–190.63)	0.002
	Missing	0.24	(0.17–0.34)	<0.001
Heart rate	<60 bpm	1		
	60–100 bpm	0.43	(0.15–1.18)	0.10
	>100 bpm	0.76	(0.23–2.52)	0.66
	Missing	0.15	(0.05–0.41)	<0.001
Systolic blood pressure	<140 mmHg	1		
	≥140 mmHg	0.94	(0.63–1.41)	0.77
	Missing	0.30	(0.21–0.45)	<0.001

Table 2. Cont.

		(a)		
			Adjustment for Age and Sex	
		OR	**95% CI**	**p**
Symptoms	Fever	6.68	(4.74–9.41)	<0.001
	Cough	3.48	(2.53–4.78)	<0.001
	Asthenia/malaise	3.58	(2.60–4.92)	<0.001
	Anorexia	4.35	(2.61–7.26)	<0.001
	Myalgia	1.85	(1.32–2.58)	<0.001
	Dyspnea	7.89	(5.31–11.7)	<0.001
	Productive cough	1.72	(1.06–2.80)	0.027
	Sore throat	0.51	(0.32–0.81)	0.004
	Diarrhea	2.01	(1.34–3.02)	0.001
	Nausea/vomiting	2.04	(1.17–3.58)	0.012
	Dizziness	3.18	(1.66–6.06)	<0.001
	Headache	1.43	(0.99–2.08)	0.060
	Shivering	2.80	(1.74–4.49)	<0.001
	Loss of taste/smell	1.00	(0.63–1.60)	>0.99
	Chest tightness	3.47	(1.86–6.48)	<0.001
	Confusion	10.35	(2.33–46.06)	0.002
Comorbidities	Hypertension	1.70	(1.23–2.35)	0.001
	Diabetes mellitus	1.43	(1.05–1.96)	0.024
	Dyslipidemia	0.99	(0.72–1.34)	0.93
	Cardiovascular disease	1.15	(0.77–1.72)	0.50
	Cancer	1.20	(0.64–2.22)	0.57
	Chronic kidney disease	1.10	(0.60–2.01)	0.76
	Immunosuppression	4.02	(1.46–11.07)	0.007
	Gastrointestinal disease	1.02	(0.55–1.91)	0.94
	COPD	1.61	(0.91–2.83)	0.10
	Asthma	0.73	(0.37–1.43)	0.36

		(b)		
	Variables		**Multivariable Adjustment**	
		OR	**95% CI**	**p**
Age	50–54 years	1		
	55–64 years	1.24	(0.69–2.22)	0.47
	65–74 years	2.45	(1.32–4.54)	0.005
	75–84 years	2.95	(1.52–5.73)	0.001
	>84 years	3.89	(1.7–8.9)	0.001
Sex	Female	1		
	Male	2.15	(1.47–3.15)	<0.001
Symptoms	Fever	4.31	(2.87–6.47)	0.000
	Cough	1.89	(1.28–2.80)	0.001
	Asthenia/malaise	2.04	(1.38–3.03)	<0.001
	Dyspnea	4.69	(3.00–7.33)	<0.001
	Sore throat	0.33	(0.18–0.58)	<0.001
Comorbidities	Confusion	8.87	(1.68–46.78)	0.010
	Hypertension	1.61	(1.08–2.41)	0.020
	Dyslipidemia	0.65	(0.44–0.96)	0.031
	Immunosuppression	4.97	(1.45–17.09)	0.011

bpm: beats per minute; COPD: chronic obstructive pulmonary disease. n = 790; N hospital admissions = 295. Likelihood ratio test, multivariable model (chi^2 338.3; p < 0.001); area under the receiver operating curve multivariable model = 0.860 (95% CI 0.835–0.886).

4. Discussion

This study included patients diagnosed with COVID-19 and followed-up in ambulatory care. Its main finding was that the risk of hospital admission was associated with the presence of certain symptoms (cough, fever, dyspnea, and/or confusion) along with male sex, age over 65 years, and comorbidities including hypertension or immunosuppression. However, the presence of diabetes was not independently associated with a higher risk of hospital admission.

Our sample had a rather high prevalence of several comorbidities (hypertension, dyslipidemia, diabetes, and obesity) (Table 1). This was due to its case-control design, where cases were defined by hospital admission. It is thus logical that the group of cases would be older with a higher prevalence of comorbidities than that in the general population. This was not a cross-sectional study, and its objective was not to describe the prevalence of diabetes but rather its possible association with the risk of admission.

One of the first indications regarding the relationship between diabetes and COVID-19 was the finding of a higher prevalence of diabetes among patients infected by COVID-19 [11,12]. Other studies have reported that the prevalence of diabetes is twice as high in people who died of COVID-19 (31%) compared with that in survivors (14%) [13]. In their meta-analysis, Puri et al. [14] identified 66 studies (39 in Asia and 27 in other regions) showing that the proportion of hypertension, diabetes, cardiovascular disease, and chronic kidney disease was significantly higher in patients with severe COVID-19 compared to that in patients with milder cases. However, these were prevalence studies, and the risk of hospitalization was not analyzed.

Other studies have focused on in-hospital mortality, observing that once adjusted for age, sex, degree of deprivation, ethnicity, and geographic region, the risk of in-hospital mortality doubled in people with type 2 diabetes (OR 2.03, 95% CI 1.97–2.09) and tripled in those with type 1 diabetes (OR 3.1, 95% CI 3.16–3.90) [12].

Regarding the risk factors for hospital admission observed internationally, Zhou et al. identified advanced age, the SOFA index (Sequential Organ Failure Assessment), and increased D-dimers as the most important [13]. In a study of 5416 adults in the USA [15], hospitalization rates were higher in patients with at least three comorbidities (aRR5.0, 95% CI 3.9–6.3), morbid obesity (aRR4.4, 95% CI 3.4–5.7), chronic kidney disease (aRR4.0, 95% CI 3.0–5.2), diabetes (aRR3.2, 95% CI 2.5–4.1), obesity (aRR2.9, 95% CI 2.3–3.5), hypertension (aRR2.8, 95% CI 2.3–3.4), and asthma (aRR1.4, 95% CI 1.1–1.7) after adjusting for age, sex, and race/ethnicity. Higher hospitalization rates were also seen in adults aged 65 years or older and in those aged from 45 to 64 years (vs. 18–44 years), in men (vs. women), and in non-Hispanic Black people and other races/ethnicities (versus non-Hispanic whites). Another study found higher rates of hospitalization in Black and Hispanic patients as well as at different poverty levels [16], and two meta-analyses have described increased risk of severe COVID-19 in patients with diabetes [17,18] and obesity [19]. In another study [20], patients with advanced age or comorbidities, including diabetes mellitus (in 28.3% of all patients), also had higher rates of hospitalization. Another meta-analysis presented similar results [21]. In Spain [22], studies in the first months of the pandemic reported that diabetes is associated with an increased risk of hospitalization and death, but the diagnosis of COVID-19 was a clinical suspicion, with no laboratory confirmation. Another study was done in patients with type 1 diabetes, confirmed COVID-19, and ambulatory follow-up showed age over 40 years as the main independent risk factor for hospital admission due to COVID-19, after adjusting for other variables such as HbA1c, sex, race, type of health insurance, and comorbidities [23]. Another study, this time in England [24], analyzed ambulatory EMRs to identify factors associated with COVID-19 mortality, finding that advanced age is the main factor, with risk increasing after age 60; a weaker association is also observed for diabetes. However, the interpretation of these results has been called into question [25].

With specific regard to patients with diabetes, poor glycemic control has been associated with an increased risk of complications in COVID-19 [26,27]. Hyperglycemia on admission also seems to be a risk factor for more complications and higher mortality [28]. As for antidiabetic treatment, a better prognosis has been observed in patients treated with metformin or sulfonyl ureas, while those treated with insulin are more likely to fare poorly [29]. In our subgroup of diabetic patients ($n = 296$), we observed that patients with poor glycemic control were at higher risk of hospitalization, but testing that association was not the objective of the study. Obtaining robust results about the impact of glycemic control on the evolution of the patient would require a larger sample and a specifically articulated research objective. For the same reason, antidiabetic treatments were not included in the analysis, since a larger sample of patients would be required to achieve valid results.

Many studies concluding that diabetes is associated with a worse prognosis in COVID-19 have a major limitation in that they either focus on the hospital setting (emergencies, admissions) or they do not differentiate between patients attended in ambulatory care versus those who are hospitalized or who present to the emergency department. Based on those data, it is impossible to identify the factors associated with the risk of admission in ambulatory patients, who represent approximately 85% of the population with COVID-19.

Another prevalent limitation in the literature is the lack of consideration for variables related to COVID-19 symptoms, though a meta-analysis of 12 studies and 3046 patients from the general population showed that fever, cough, fatigue, and dyspnea are associated with greater severity [30–33].

In our study, the bivariable analysis showed a significant association between the presence of diabetes and the risk of hospital admission, and the prevalence of diabetes was higher in patients who required hospital admission (46.8% vs. 31.9%; $p = 0.001$; Table 1). The same occurred with the presence of obesity (Table 1). However, after adjusting for the other included variables, including the clinical symptoms presented by the patient, the multivariable model could not confirm that diabetes and obesity were associated with an increased risk of hospital admission (Table 2). Rather, these factors were confounded by other variables (certain symptoms, advanced age, male sex, arterial hypertension), which more precisely determined the risk of admission. In fact, our multivariable model had a high explanatory capacity with an AUC of 0.86 (Table 2).

To our knowledge, this is the first study to identify prognostic variables related to the need for hospital admission in patients with COVID-19 followed in ambulatory services, considering both patient characteristics (age, sex, comorbidities) and the symptomatic presentation of COVID-19, which are the two criteria that are usually used in the follow-up of COVID-19 patients in clinical practice. We observed that the symptoms of the disease, as well as age and sex, were the predominant factors determining the risk of admission, outweighing some comorbidities such as diabetes or obesity. This result suggests that patients were not more likely to be admitted because of diabetes but because of advanced age, male sex, and presenting with fever, dyspnea, or confusion, among other symptoms. These data are not incompatible with the results of studies that relate diabetes to severity, since people with diabetes or obesity may present severe symptoms more frequently, but the symptoms and demographic characteristics confer a higher risk than the comorbidities themselves. All of this supports the applicability of these results to ambulatory practice in patients with COVID-19.

Strengths and Limitations

The main strength of this study is the widely representative sample of patients, recruited by 61 researchers (family doctors and endocrinologists) throughout Spain, and the consideration of prognostic variables related to patient characteristics and COVID-19 symptoms (Supplementary Materials). The inclusion of patients with and without diabetes, the confirmation of the diagnosis by laboratory tests, and the quality of the data collected by the attending physicians are also strengths of the study.

Limitations include the lack of data on some analytical parameters for assessing severity, which are routinely collected in the emergency department or during hospital admissions, but not in the ambulatory setting. For this reason, analytical prognostic variables such as neutrophils, lymphopenia, C-reactive protein, interleukin 6, serum ferritin, procalcitonin, or D-dimer were not included, as these tend to be requested only at the hospital level in patients presenting signs of severity in the emergency department or in those who are already admitted.

Finally, this study focused exclusively on assessing the risk of hospital admission. Mortality was not analyzed, since this would require a much larger sample size for the study design we applied. There were three out-of-hospital deaths that were not included in the analysis.

5. Conclusions

In patients over 50 years of age diagnosed with laboratory-confirmed COVID-19 and followed in ambulatory services, the risk of hospitalization was associated with symptoms such as cough, fever, confusion and dyspnea, underlying hypertension and immunosuppression, male sex, and advanced age. All these variables allowed the construction of a patient profile that would indicate a higher risk of admission: male, over 65 years of age, with high blood pressure or immunosuppression, who presented with cough, fever, dyspnea and/or confusion but not a sore throat. Finally, despite the relatively high prevalence of diabetes in included patients with COVID-19, diabetes was not independently associated with a higher risk of admission after adjusting for confounders. Although our findings suggest the potential role of these variables in developing hospitalization risk scores in ambulatory patients with COVID-19, regardless of the presence of diabetes, future studies designed to adequately evaluate their applicability in clinical practice are needed.

Supplementary Materials: The following supporting information can be downloaded at: https://www.mdpi.com/article/10.3390/jcm11082092/s1.

Author Contributions: Conceptualization, D.O.-B., A.P., A.M.C.-C. and J.A.Q.; methodology, software, D.O.-B., A.P., A.M.C.-C. and J.A.Q.; validation, D.O.-B., A.P., A.M.C.-C., I.P.-M., L.Á.-L., G.R.-M. and F.J.P.-G.; formal analysis, J.A.Q.; investigation, D.O.-B., A.P., A.M.C.-C., I.P.-M., L.Á.-L., G.R.-M., F.J.P.-G., F.Á.-G., M.S.-M., F.G., F.J.O., M.M.-C., E.C.-A., J.M.V., J.A.Q. and J.F.M.-T.; resources, D.O.-B., A.P., A.M.C.-C., I.P.-M., L.Á.-L., G.R.-M., F.J.P.-G., F.Á.-G., M.S.-M., F.G., F.J.O., M.M.-C., E.C.-A., J.M.V., J.A.Q. and J.F.M.-T.; data curation, D.O.-B., A.P., A.M.C.-C., I.P.-M., L.Á.-L., G.R.-M., F.J.P.-G., F.Á.-G., M.S.-M., F.G., F.J.O., M.M.-C., E.C.-A., J.M.V., J.A.Q. and J.F.M.-T.; writing—original draft preparation, D.O.-B. and J.A.Q.; writing—review and editing, D.O.-B., A.P., A.M.C.-C., I.P.-M., L.Á.-L., G.R.-M., F.J.P.-G., F.Á.-G., M.S.-M., F.G., F.J.O., M.M.-C., E.C.-A., J.M.V., J.A.Q. and J.F.M.-T.; visualization, F.Á.-G., M.S.-M., F.G., F.J.O., M.M.-C., E.C.-A., J.M.V., J.A.Q. and J.F.M.-T.; supervision, D.O.-B., A.P., A.M.C.-C., I.P.-M., L.Á.-L., G.R.-M. and F.J.P.-G.; project administration, D.O.-B., A.P., A.M.C.-C., I.P.-M., L.Á.-L., G.R.-M. and F.J.P.-G.; funding acquisition D.O.-B., A.P. and J.F.M.-T. All authors have read and agreed to the published version of the manuscript.

Funding: The study was funded through an unrestricted grant from Boehringer Ingelheim to the Spanish Diabetes Society.

Institutional Review Board Statement: The study was conducted in accordance with the Declaration of Helsinki and approved by the Ethics Committee of San Juan University Hospital (Alicante) approved the study (code 20/025, dated 20 May 2020).

Informed Consent Statement: Informed consent was obtained from all subjects involved in the study.

Data Availability Statement: All the data used for this analysis can be confirmed at any time.

Acknowledgments: We provide a list of the researchers participating in Supplementary Materials to whom we thank for their collaboration, as well as the entities that collaborated in it: Spanish Society of Diabetes, Miguel Hernandez University of Elche, Spanish Society of Family and CommunityMedicine.

Conflicts of Interest: The funders had no role in the design of the study; in the collection, analyses, or interpretation of data; in the writing of the manuscript, or in the decision to publish the results.

References

1. Rothan, H.A.; Byrareddy, S.N. The epidemiology and pathogenesis of coronavirus disease (COVID-19) outbreak. *J. Autoimmun.* **2020**, *109*, 102433. [CrossRef] [PubMed]
2. World Health Organization. Report of the WHO-China Joint Mission on Coronavirus Disease 2019 (COVID-19). 2020. Available online: https://www.who.int/docs/default-source/coronaviruse/who-china-joint-mission-on-COVID-19-final-report.pdf (accessed on 18 April 2020).
3. Quesada, J.A.; López-Pineda, A.; Gil-Guillén, V.F.; Arriero-Marín, J.M.; Gutiérrez, F.; Carratala-Munuera, C. Período de incubación de la COVID-19: Revisión sistemática y metaanálisis [Incubation Period of COVID-19: A Systematic Review and Meta-analysis]. *Rev. Clin. Esp.* **2021**, *221*, 109–117. (In Spanish) [CrossRef] [PubMed]
4. Li, Q.; Guan, X.; Wu, P.; Wang, X.; Zhou, L.; Tong, Y.; Ren, R.; Leung, K.S.M.; Lau, E.H.Y.; Wong, J.Y.; et al. Early Transmission Dynamics in Wuhan, China, of Novel Coronavirus—Infected Pneumonia. *N. Engl. J. Med.* **2020**, *382*, 1199–1207. [CrossRef] [PubMed]
5. Huang, C.; Wang, Y.; Li, X.; Ren, L.; Zhao, J.; Hu, Y.; Zhang, L.; Fan, G.; Xu, J.; Gu, X.; et al. Clinical features of patients infected with 2019 novel coronavirus in Wuhan, China. *Lancet* **2020**, *395*, 497–506. [CrossRef]
6. Wang, W.; Tang, J.; Wei, F. Updated understanding of the outbreak of 2019 novel coronavirus (2019-nCoV) in Wuhan, China. *J. Med. Virol.* **2020**, *92*, 441–447. [CrossRef]
7. The Novel Coronavirus Pneumonia Emergency Response Epidemiology Team. Vital Surveillances: The Epidemiological Characteristics of an Outbreak of 2019 Novel Coronavirus Diseases (COVID-19). China CDC Wkly. 2020. Available online: http://weekly.chinacdc.cn/en/article/id/e53946e2-c6c4-41e9-9a9b-fea8db1a8f51 (accessed on 18 April 2020).
8. Ministerio de Sanidad. Documento Técnico. Manejo en Atención Primaria del COVID-19. Available online: https://www.mscbs.gob.es/profesionales/saludPublica/ccayes/alertasActual/nCov-China/documentos/Manejo_primaria.pdf (accessed on 18 April 2020).
9. Nyland, J.E.; Raja-Khan, N.T.; Bettermann, K.; Haouzi, P.A.; Leslie, D.L.; Kraschnewski, J.L.; Parent, L.J.; Grigson, P.S. Diabetes, Drug Treatment, and Mortality in COVID-19: A Multinational Retrospective Cohort Study. *Diabetes* **2021**, *70*, 2903–2916. [CrossRef]
10. Wong, K.C.; Xiang, Y.; Yin, L.; So, H.C. Uncovering Clinical Risk Factors and Predicting Severe COVID-19 Cases Using UK Biobank Data: Machine Learning Approach. *JMIR Public Health Surveill.* **2021**, *7*, e29544. [CrossRef]
11. Moazzami, B.; Chaichian, S.; Kasaeian, A.; Djalalinia, S.; Akhlaghdoust, M.; Eslami, M.; Broumand, B. Metabolic risk factors and risk of COVID-19: A systematic review and meta-analysis. *PLoS ONE* **2020**, *15*, e0243600. [CrossRef]
12. Barron, E.; Bakhai, C.; Kar, P.; Weaver, A.; Bradley, D.; Ismail, H.; Knighton, P.; Holman, N.; Khunti, K.; Sattar, N.; et al. Associations of type 1 and type 2 diabetes with COVID-19-related mortality in England: A whole-population study. *Lancet Diabetes Endocrinol.* **2020**, *8*, 813–822. [CrossRef]
13. Zhou, F.; Yu, T.; Du, R.; Fan, G.; Liu, Y.; Liu, Z.; Xiang, J.; Wang, Y.; Song, B.; Gu, X.; et al. Clinical course and risk factors for mortality of adult inpatients with COVID-19 in Wuhan, China: A retrospective cohort study. *Lancet* **2020**, *395*, 1054–1062, Erratum in *Lancet* **2020**, *395*, 1038. [CrossRef]
14. Puri, A.; He, L.; Giri, M.; Wu, C.; Zhao, Q. Comparison of comorbidities among severe and non-severe COVID-19 patients in Asian versus non-Asian populations: A systematic review and meta-analysis. *Nurs. Open* **2021**, *9*, 733–751. [CrossRef] [PubMed]
15. Ko, J.Y.; Danielson, M.L.; Town, M.; Derado, G.; Greenlund, K.J.; Kirley, P.D.; Alden, N.B.; Yousey-Hindes, K.; Anderson, E.J.; Ryan, P.A.; et al. Risk Factors for Coronavirus Disease 2019 (COVID-19)-Associated Hospitalization: COVID-19-Associated Hospitalization Surveillance Network and Behavioral Risk Factor Surveillance System. *Clin. Infect. Dis.* **2021**, *72*, e695–e703. [CrossRef] [PubMed]
16. Wortham, J.M.; Meador, S.A.; Hadler, J.L.; Yousey-Hindes, K.; See, I.; Whitaker, M.; O'Halloran, A.; Milucky, J.; Chai, S.J.; Reingold, A.; et al. Census tract socioeconomic indicators and COVID-19-associated hospitalization rates-COVID-19-NET surveillance areas in 14 states, March 1–April 30, 2020. *PLoS ONE* **2021**, *16*, e0257622. [CrossRef] [PubMed]
17. Li, X.; Zhong, X.; Wang, Y.; Zeng, X.; Luo, T.; Liu, Q. Clinical determinants of the severity of COVID-19: A systematic review and meta-analysis. *PLoS ONE* **2021**, *16*, e0250602. [CrossRef] [PubMed]
18. Singh, A.K.; Gillies, C.L.; Singh, R.; Singh, A.; Chudasama, Y.; Coles, B.; Seidu, S.; Zaccardi, F.; Davies, M.J.; Khunti, K. Prevalence of co-morbidities and their association with mortality in patients with COVID-19: A systematic review and meta-analysis. *Diabetes Obes. Metab.* **2020**, *22*, 1915–1924. [CrossRef]
19. Cai, Z.; Yang, Y.; Zhang, J. Obesity is associated with severe disease and mortality in patients with coronavirus disease 2019 (COVID-19): A meta-analysis. *BMC Public Health* **2021**, *21*, 1505. [CrossRef]
20. Garg, S.; Kim, L.; Whitaker, M.; O'Halloran, A.; Cummings, C.; Holstein, R.; Prill, M.; Chai, S.J.; Kirley, P.D.; Alden, N.B.; et al. Hospitalization Rates and Characteristics of Patients Hospitalized with Laboratory-Confirmed Coronavirus Disease 2019—COVID-19-NET, 14 States, March 1–30, 2020. *MMWR Morb. Mortal. Wkly. Rep.* **2020**, *69*, 458–464. [CrossRef]
21. Wu, Z.; McGoogan, J.M. Characteristics of and Important Lessons from the Coronavirus Disease 2019 (COVID-19) Outbreak in China: Summary of a Report of 72 314 Cases from the Chinese Center for Disease Control and Prevention. *JAMA* **2020**, *323*, 1239–1242. [CrossRef]
22. Nandy, K.; Salunke, A.; Pathak, S.K.; Pandey, A.; Doctor, C.; Puj, K.; Sharma, M.; Jain, A.; Warikoo, V. Coronavirus disease (COVID-19): A systematic review and meta-analysis to evaluate the impact of various comorbidities on serious events. *Diabetes Metab. Syndr.* **2020**, *14*, 1017–1025. [CrossRef]

23. Álvarez-Esteban, P.C.; Del Barrio, E.; Rueda, O.M.; Rueda, C. Predicting COVID-19 progression from diagnosis to recovery or death linking primary care and hospital records in Castilla y León (Spain). *PLoS ONE* **2021**, *16*, e0257613. [CrossRef]
24. Demeterco-Berggren, C.; Ebekozien, O.; Rompicherla, S.; Jacobsen, L.; Accacha, S.; Gallagher, M.P.; Alonso, G.T.; Seyoum, B.; Vendrame, F.; Haw, J.S.; et al. Age and Hospitalization Risk in People with Type 1 Diabetes and COVID-19: Data from the T1D Exchange Surveillance Study. *J. Clin. Endocrinol. Metab.* **2021**, *107*, 410–418. [CrossRef] [PubMed]
25. Williamson, E.J.; Walker, A.J.; Bhaskaran, K.; Bacon, S.; Bates, C.; Morton, C.E.; Curtis, H.J.; Mehrkar, A.; Evans, D.; Inglesby, P.; et al. Factors associated with COVID-19-related death using OpenSAFELY. *Nature* **2020**, *584*, 430–436. [CrossRef] [PubMed]
26. Westreich, D.; Edwards, J.K.; van Smeden, M. Comment on Williamson et al. (OpenSAFELY): The Table 2 Fallacy in a Study of COVID-19 Mortality Risk Factors. *Epidemiology* **2021**, *32*, e1–e2. [CrossRef] [PubMed]
27. Holman, N.; Knighton, P.; Kar, P.; O'Keefe, J.; Curley, M.; Weaver, A.; Barron, E.; Bakhai, C.; Khunti, K.; Wareham, N.J.; et al. Risk factors for COVID-19-related mortality in people with type 1 and type 2 diabetes in England: A population-based cohort study. *Lancet Diabetes Endocrinol.* **2020**, *8*, 823–833. [CrossRef]
28. Aggarwal, G.; Lippi, G.; Lavie, C.J.; Henry, B.M.; Sanchis-Gomar, F. Diabetes mellitus association with coronavirus disease 2019 (COVID-19) severity and mortality: A pooled analysis. *J. Diabetes* **2020**, *12*, 851–855. [CrossRef] [PubMed]
29. Yang, Y.; Cai, Z.; Zhang, J. Hyperglycemia at admission is a strong predictor of mortality and severe/critical complications in COVID-19 patients: A meta-analysis. *Biosci. Rep.* **2021**, *41*, BSR20203584. [CrossRef]
30. Kan, C.; Zhang, Y.; Han, F.; Xu, Q.; Ye, T.; Hou, N.; Sun, X. Mortality Risk of Antidiabetic Agents for Type 2 Diabetes With COVID-19: A Systematic Review and Meta-Analysis. *Front. Endocrinol.* **2021**, *12*, 708494. [CrossRef]
31. Giri, M.; Puri, A.; Wang, T.; Guo, S. Clinical features, comorbidities, complications and treatment options in severe and non-severe COVID-19 patients: A systemic review and meta-analysis. *Nurs. Open* **2021**, *8*, 1077–1088. [CrossRef]
32. Xie, J.; Wang, Q.; Xu, Y.; Zhang, T.; Chen, L.; Zuo, X.; Liu, J.; Huang, L.; Zhan, P.; Lv, T.; et al. Clinical characteristics, laboratory abnormalities and CT findings of COVID-19 patients and risk factors of severe disease: A systematic review and meta-analysis. *Ann. Palliat. Med.* **2021**, *10*, 1928–1949. [CrossRef]
33. Mehra, M.R.; Desai, S.S.; Kuy, S.; Henry, T.D.; Patel, A.N. Cardiovascular Disease, Drug Therapy, and Mortality in COVID-19. *N. Engl. J. Med.* **2020**, *382*, e102, Retraction in *N. Engl. J. Med.* **2020**, *382*, 2582. [CrossRef]

MDPI
St. Alban-Anlage 66
4052 Basel
Switzerland
www.mdpi.com

Journal of Clinical Medicine Editorial Office
E-mail: jcm@mdpi.com
www.mdpi.com/journal/jcm

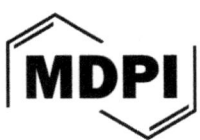

Disclaimer/Publisher's Note: The statements, opinions and data contained in all publications are solely those of the individual author(s) and contributor(s) and not of MDPI and/or the editor(s). MDPI and/or the editor(s) disclaim responsibility for any injury to people or property resulting from any ideas, methods, instructions or products referred to in the content.